REHABILITATION RESEARCH

Principles and Applications

FIFTH EDITION

REHABILITATION RESEARCH

Principles and Applications

Russell E. Carter, PT, EdD
Professor Emeritus
Department of Physical Therapy
College of Health and Human Services
Governors State University
University Park, Illinois

Jay Lubinsky, PhD, CCC-A/SLP, ASHA Fellow
Professor Emeritus
Department of Communication Disorders
College of Health and Human Services
Governors State University
University Park, Illinois

ELSEVIER

ELSEVIER

3251 Riverport Lane
St. Louis, Missouri 63043

REHABILITATION RESEARCH: PRINCIPLES AND APPLICATIONS, FIFTH EDITION   ISBN: 9781455759798

Notices

Knowledge and best practice in this field are constantly changing. As new research and experience broaden our understanding, changes in research methods, professional practices, or medical treatment may become necessary.

Practitioners and researchers must always rely on their own experience and knowledge in evaluating and using any information, methods, compounds, or experiments described herein. In using such information or methods they should be mindful of their own safety and the safety of others, including parties for whom they have a professional responsibility.

With respect to any drug or pharmaceutical products identified, readers are advised to check the most current information provided (i) on procedures featured or (ii) by the manufacturer of each product to be administered, to verify the recommended dose or formula, the method and duration of administration, and contraindications. It is the responsibility of practitioners, relying on their own experience and knowledge of their patients, to make diagnoses, to determine dosages and the best treatment for each individual patient, and to take all appropriate safety precautions.

To the fullest extent of the law, neither the Publisher nor the authors, contributors, or editors, assume any liability for any injury and/or damage to persons or property as a matter of products liability, negligence or otherwise, or from any use or operation of any methods, products, instructions, or ideas contained in the material herein.

Library of Congress Cataloging-in-Publication Data

Carter, Russell E.
 [Physical therapy research]
 Rehabilitation research : principles and applications. – Fifth edition / Russell E. Carter, PT, EdD, professor emeritus, Department of Physical Therapy, College of Health and Human Services, Governors State University, University Park, Illinois, Jay Lubinsky, PhD, CCC-A/SLP, ASHA Fellow, professor emeritus, Department of Communication Disorders, College of Health and Human Services, Governors State University, University Park, Illinois, author emerita, Elizabeth Domholdt, PT, EdD, Vice President for Academic Affairs, Professor of Physical Therapy, The College of St. Scholastica, Duluth, Minnesota.
   pages cm
 Revision of: Physical therapy research / Elizabeth Domholdt. c2000. 4th ed.
 Includes index.
 ISBN 978-1-4557-5979-8 (pbk.)
 1. Medical rehabilitation–Research. I. Lubinsky, Jay. II. Domholdt, Elizabeth, 1958- III. Title.
 RM930.D66 2016
 615.8'2072–dc23   2015006994

Executive Content Strategist: Kathy Falk
Content Development Manager: Jolynn Gower
Associate Content Development Specialist: Laurel Berkel
Publishing Services Manager: Hemamalini Rajendrababu
Project Manager: Umarani Natarajan
Design Direction: Renee Duenow

Printed in the United States of America
Last digit is the print number: 9 8 7 6 5 4 3 2 1

As in any work of this magnitude, authors need the support and patience of those whose time was intruded upon. In this case, our wives, Diane Carter and Arlene Lubinsky, provided both qualities and in generous quantity. We dedicate this book to them.

R. C.

J. L.

Preface

In this fifth edition of **Rehabilitation Research**, the intents and purposes of earlier editions, particularly the fourth edition, continue. We have especially kept and, we hope, enhanced, our emphases on providing a text to clearly address the needs of students in addition to those of practicing clinicians. Therefore, we have maintained and, where possible, increased the emphasis on the scientist-practitioner model and significantly enhanced information on single-subject research, feeling that rehabilitation clinicians will often rely on those designs in their everyday practice. We have maintained and, when possible, updated relevant information on evidence-based practice and have consistently encouraged readers to utilize its principles and methods. This book acknowledges that all rehabilitation professionals have several common needs as consumers and producers of research. The same holds true for students in the rehabilitation professions. Specifically, all need to understand the bases of research, methodologies, and uses. Perhaps most important, they need to understand not only how to apply the research findings of others in daily practice but also how to employ the rigorous methods of science to their daily practice. This is *sine qua non* of the scientist-practitioner. For these reasons, we have attempted to make this book *useful* to students and practicing professionals as well as to those whose primary function is research.

Rehabilitation professionals share a belief that the exercise of our professional expertise, in partnership with the patients or clients with whom we work, makes a difference in their lives. This deeply held belief is a positive force when it leads to the high levels of professionalism and commitment that are demonstrated daily by rehabilitation professionals around the globe. This belief, however, can also serve as a negative force when it leads practitioners to the uncritical acceptance of all of rehabilitation practice.

The purpose of research is not to give validity to what we do as rehabilitation professionals; it should determine purposes. This is an important distinction. The former leads to a search for weak evidence that supports our current practices; the latter leads to strong evidence that can help us improve our future practices.

Evidence-based practice in rehabilitation can be realized only by a joint effort of the producers and consumers of research. This is a textbook that will serve many needs of research consumers and can serve foundational needs of research producers. It does so by using straightforward language and relevant examples to capture the diversity and complexity of research that is of interest to rehabilitation professionals. Readers will note a great deal of updated literature relevant to the topics at hand. We have included updated studies for two reasons. First, having recent literature signifies the ongoing relevance of the type of research being discussed. Second, updated literature provides the reader with examples of the complexities and variations of research designs that might not otherwise be discussed in the text. At the same time that we have updated a great deal of examples from published literature, we have maintained some older references—even to "classic" studies—when we felt those studies best exemplified or clarified the discussion in the text.

The text is divided into nine sections. Although divided into sections, we have taken the view that information in all sections forms a unified whole for the location, understanding, consumption, production, and dissemination of research as relevant to clinical practice.

From the very first edition, this text has provided a solid grounding in traditional research design and analysis as well as an introduction to emerging research topics such as qualitative and single-system (now called single-subject) designs. Subsequent editions introduced even more emergent research paradigms, such as outcomes research and epidemiology (among others). More recently, and continuing into the present edition, the text has increasingly incorporated research from a broader array of rehabilitation professions in order to demonstrate the commonalities of their research methodologies. We think this is critical as we see increased incorporation of team and co-treatment approaches to rehabilitation.

In this fifth edition, we have endeavoured to impart enthusiasm for a few ways of thinking about rehabilitation research and a textbook on that topic. Those ways of thinking include usefulness, incorporation of a scientist-practitioner model, and use of evidence-based practice. We sincerely hope that readers find these appealing and helpful.

Russell E. Carter, PT, EdD
Jay Lubinsky, PhD, CCC-A/SLP, ASHA Fellow

Acknowledgment

Elizabeth Domholdt was the sole author of the first three editions of **Rehabilitation Research** and author emerita of the fourth edition. We wish to express our gratitude to her as this edition could not have been completed without her pioneering authorship. Her vision in previous editions, her knowledge coupled with outstanding writing and organization, and her commitment to bringing research principles and applications into the clinical milieu were invaluable stepping stones as we fashioned the new edition. We sincerely hope that we have enhanced her vision and labors.

Russell E. Carter, PT, EdD
Jay Lubinsky, PhD, CCC-A/SLP, ASHA Fellow

Contents

SECTION ONE
Research Fundamentals

1   Rehabilitation Research, *1*
2   Theory in Rehabilitation Research, *11*
3   Evidence-Based Practice, *23*
4   Finding Research Literature, *33*
5   Research Ethics, *42*

SECTION TWO
Research Design

6   Research Paradigms, *55*
7   Variables, *68*
8   Research Validity, *76*
9   Selection and Assignment of Participants, *92*

SECTION THREE
Experimental Designs

10   Group Designs, *107*
11   Single-Subject Designs, *120*

SECTION FOUR
Nonexperimental Research for Rehabilitation

12   Overview of Nonexperimental Research, *143*
13   Clinical Case Reports, *153*

SECTION FIVE
Research Beyond the Everyday

14   Qualitative Research, *159*
15   Epidemiology, *176*
16   Outcomes Research, *194*
17   Survey Research, *215*

SECTION SIX
Measurement

18   Measurement Theory, *231*
19   Methodological Research, *249*

SECTION SEVEN
Data Analysis

20   Statistical Reasoning, *259*
21   Statistical Analysis of Differences: The Basics, *281*
22   Statistical Analysis of Differences: Advanced, *298*
23   Statistical Analysis of Relationships: The Basics, *318*
24   Statistical Analysis of Relationships: Advanced, *329*

SECTION EIGHT
Being a Consumer of Research

25   Evaluating Evidence One Article at a Time, *345*
26   Synthesizing Bodies of Evidence, *363*

SECTION NINE
Implementing Research

27   Implementing a Research Project, *377*
28   Publishing and Presenting Research, *399*

Appendices

Appendix A: Random Numbers Table, *409*
Appendix B: Areas in One Tail of the Standard Normal Curve, *414*
Appendix C: Questions for Narrative Evaluation of a Research Article, *415*

Appendix D: Basic Guidelines for Preparing a Journal
Article Manuscript, *418*

Appendix E: American Medical Association Style:
Sample Manuscript for a Hypothetical
Study, *423*

Appendix F: American Psychological Association
Style: Sample Manuscript for a
Hypothetical Study, *443*

Appendix G: Sample Platform Presentation Script
with Slides, *463*

Index, 471

REHABILITATION RESEARCH

Principles and Applications

CHAPTER 1

Rehabilitation Research

CHAPTER OUTLINE

Definitions of Research
Research Challenges the Status Quo
Research Is Creative
Research Is Systematic
**Reasons for Developing
Rehabilitation Research**
Develop Body of Knowledge
Determine Whether Interventions
Work
Improve Patient and Client Care

Barriers to Rehabilitation Research
Lack of Funds
Lack of Research Mentors
Lack of Time
Lack of Familiarity with the Research
Process
Lack of Statistical Support
Ethical Concerns About Use of
Human Participants and
Animal Subjects

The Clinician-Researcher Dichotomy
Overcoming Barriers
The Scientist-Practitioner
Status of Rehabilitation Research
Professional Association Goals
Research Publication Vehicles
Educational Standards
Research Funding
Summary

Rehabilitation professionals believe that the work we do makes a difference in the lives of the people we serve. Rehabilitation research is the means by which we test that belief. In the rapidly changing and increasingly accountable world of health care, it is no longer enough to say that we do good work or to note that patients or clients feel better after we've intervened. Rather, we must be willing to search for, or even create, evidence about the value of our practices and then modify those practices in response to the evidence. Rehabilitation professionals who embrace evidence-based practice also embrace the challenge of learning about rehabilitation research.

Learning about rehabilitation research involves developing a diverse set of knowledge and skills in research methodologies, research design, statistical and qualitative analysis, presentation, and writing. At the same time a practitioner or student is acquiring these new skills, he or she is forced to reexamine the status quo, the conventional wisdom of the rehabilitation professions. This combination of trying to learn new

material while challenging previously held beliefs can engender frustration with the new material and doubt about previous learning. Some clinicians, unable to cope with such uncertainty, retreat to anecdotes and intuition as the basis for their work in rehabilitation. Others delight in the intellectual stimulation of research and commit themselves to developing an evidence-based practice. Such clinicians balance the use of existing but unsubstantiated practices with critical evaluation of those same practices through regular review of the professional literature and thoughtful discussion with colleagues. Furthermore, these professionals may participate in clinical research to test the assumptions under which they practice.

This introductory chapter defines research, examines reasons for and barriers to implementing rehabilitation research, and considers the current status of rehabilitation research. Based on this foundation, the rest of the book presents the principles needed to understand research and suggests guidelines for the application of those principles to rehabilitation research.

DEFINITIONS OF RESEARCH

Research has been defined by almost every person who has written about it. Kettering, an engineer and philanthropist, had this to say:

> "Research" is a high-hat word that scares a lot of people. It needn't; … it is nothing but a state of mind—a friendly, welcoming attitude toward change…. It is the problem-solving mind as contrasted with the let-well-enough-alone mind. It is the composer mind instead of the fiddler mind. It is the "tomorrow" mind instead of the "yesterday" mind.[1(p. 91)]

We think his words, published in 1961, still ring true.

Payton, a physical therapist who has written widely about research, indicates that "research should begin with an intellectual itch that needs scratching."[2(p. 8)] Kazdin, a psychologist, speaks about various research methods, noting that "they have in common careful observation and systematic evaluation of the subject matter."[3(p. 2)] Portney and Watkins,[4] Polit and Beck,[5] Stein and colleagues,[6] and Nelson,[7] who have written texts on clinical, nursing, occupational therapy, and communication disorders research, respectively, all emphasize the organized, systematic nature of research. Three important characteristics about research emerge from these different authors: (1) research challenges the status quo, (2) it is creative, and (3) it is systematic.

Research Challenges the Status Quo

Definers of research all indicate it as a way of answering questions. Thus, the first characteristic is that research challenges the status quo. Sometimes the results of research may support current clinical practices; other times the results point to treatment techniques that are not effective. But whether research does or does not lead to a revision of currently accepted principles, the guiding philosophy of research is one of challenge. Does this treatment work? Is it more effective than another treatment? Would this person recover as quickly without intervention? The status quo can be challenged in several ways, as illustrated in the three examples that follow.

One way of challenging the status quo is to identify gaps in our knowledge—for example, to identify common practices about which we know very little. Because much of our practice as clinicians is based on the collective wisdom of past professionals, we forget that much of this practice has not been verified in a systematic way. However, we are increasingly in the process of validating our clinical practices. Many clinicians, professional associations, and scientists are engaged in

outcomes research (see Chapter 16). Emphasis and literature on evidence-based practice (see Chapter 3) continue to grow. The increasing number of meta-analyses and critical reviews validates some of our clinical practices and challenges others (see Chapter 4). These recent developments suggest a powerful research agenda for rehabilitation providers.

Despite recent efforts, we continue many rehabilitation practices about which few, if any, data exist. A second approach to challenging the status quo, therefore, is to systematically test the effects of these practices.

A third way of challenging the status quo is to test novel or traditionally avoided treatments. Some examples of such treatments are (1) use of human magnetic fields to manage pain[8] and (2) application of sensory integration training to a very wide variety of clinical conditions.[9-11]

These examples of challenges to the status quo identified gaps in knowledge about rehabilitation practice, may provide support for one set of clinical practices, and suggest a need for review of another set of clinical beliefs. Research is about embracing these kinds of challenges. It is about the willingness to test our assumptions, to use what works, and to change our practices in light of new evidence.

Research Is Creative

The second characteristic of research is that it is creative. Rothstein, in an editorial, chastised physical therapists for their willingness to accept authoritarian views of their profession: "Our teachers and our texts tell us how it should be, and we accept this in our eagerness to proceed with patient care."[12(p. 895)] Researchers are creative individuals who move past the authoritarian teachings of others and look at rehabilitation in a different way. And, in at least a partial answer to Rothstein, we note the increasing emphasis on evidence-based practice and the emergence of the scientist-practitioner. Virtually every piece of research is the product of a creative question.[13] In any science, "the dualism between science and creativity is unfounded."[14] "Why?" and "Why not?" are core questions, as is, "What if …?"

Creative aspects of rehabilitation research are emphasized in Chapter 2, which presents information about the use of theory in practice and research, and Chapter 4, which provides a framework for the development of research problems.

Research Is Systematic

The third characteristic of research is that it is systematic. In contrast, much of our clinical knowledge is anecdotal, or is passed on by prominent practitioners who teach a particular treatment to eager colleagues or students. As Hicks noted,... "after all, many of the therapeutic techniques currently in practice have been developed over the years and consequently are tried and tested."[15(p. 3)] Anecdotal claims for the effectiveness of treatments are colored by the relationship between the clinician and patient and typically do not control for factors, other than the treatment, that may account for changes in the condition of the patient or client. The systematic nature of some research methodologies attempts to isolate treatment effects from other influences not ordinarily controlled in the clinic setting. Other methodologies focus on systematic description of the phenomenon of interest, rather than control of the research setting. Much of this text presents the systematic principles that underlie research methods: Sections 2 through 5 (Chapters 6 through 17) cover research design, Section 6 (Chapters 18 and 19) discusses measurement tools, and Section 7 (Chapters 20 through 24) introduces data analysis.

REASONS FOR DEVELOPING REHABILITATION RESEARCH

There are at least three reasons for conducting rehabilitation research: (1) to develop a body of knowledge for the rehabilitation professions, (2) to determine whether interventions work, and (3) to improve patient and client care. Each of these reasons is examined in the sections that follow.

Develop Body of Knowledge

The "body of knowledge" rationale for rehabilitation research is related to the concept of a profession. The characteristics of a profession have been described by many authors but include several common elements. Houle[16] divided the characteristics of a profession into three broad groups: conceptual, performance, and collective identity characteristics (Box 1-1). One of the critical performance characteristics is mastery of the theoretical knowledge that forms the basis for the profession.

The theoretical foundations of the rehabilitation professions, discussed further in Chapter 2, include concepts such as occupation, disablement, and movement science.

Although the knowledge base for our professions has grown and continues to grow, rehabilitation professionals and students still work to develop ways of identifying important theoretical constructs as well as ways of understanding them. Kinsella and Whiteford[17] offer, as an example, a way of structuring the concept of

---

Box 1-1

Characteristics of a Profession

Conceptual Characteristic
Establishment of a central mission

Performance Characteristics
Mastery of theoretical knowledge
Capacity to solve problems
Use of practical knowledge
Self-enhancement

Collective Identity Characteristics
Formal training
Credentialing
Creation of a subculture
Legal reinforcement
Public acceptance
Ethical practice
Penalties
Relations to other vocations
Relations to users of service

List developed from Houle CO. *Continuing Learning in the Professions.* San Francisco, Calif: Jossey-Bass; 1981.

"evidence-based practice," a concept that has achieved widespread recognition. Kenyon and Blackinton applied aspects of motor-control theory to a clinical case, further integrating theory and the development of the knowledge base for physical therapy.[18] The search for definition and understanding of what may seem like basic concepts is far from complete.

Determine Whether Interventions Work

The second major rationale we offer for performing rehabilitation research relates to determining whether interventions work.

The need for research on the effectiveness of rehabilitation interventions was highlighted by Brummel-Smith[19] when he summarized the research recommendations of a National Institutes of Health Task Force on Medical Rehabilitation Research and applied them to rehabilitation of older adults. He noted four major areas in need of study: the natural history of disability, functional assessment and performance evaluation, intervention issues, and rehabilitation service delivery. In discussing intervention issues, he identified a need both to "evaluate effectiveness of existing interventions and to develop novel approaches to care,"[19(p. 895)] noting that "current interventions have not received the type of careful scrutiny that is now expected of medical interventions."[19](p. 895) More recently, the sentiment is summarized by Hicks, who notes, "healthcare professionals have an imperative to ensure that their clinical decisions can be justified on empirical grounds ..." and further laments, "good quality research studies that address fundamental issues in care provision have not been as plentiful as is either desirable or necessary."[15](p. vii)

Improve Patient and Client Care

The third reason for rehabilitation research is perhaps the most important one: improving patient and client care. This, of course, is not completely separate from the reason of finding out whether our treatments work. However, once we find out what works and what does not, and under what circumstances, research can improve care by helping clinicians make good decisions about the use of existing practices or by providing systematic evaluation of the effectiveness of new practices.

When we know what has or has not been supported by research, we can make intelligent, evidence-based decisions about which clinical procedures to use with our clients. Clinical research about these procedures could provide additional evidence that would help practitioners make informed decisions about recommending the procedures.

Although there are many areas of rehabilitation practice for which evidence is thin, there are other areas in which clinicians who are committed to evidence-based practice can find a rich body of evidence on which to base their work. Chapter 4 gives a hint about the large and growing amount of literature available (and how to find it) to rehabilitation scientist-practitioners. The increase in meta-analyses and critical reviews (see Chapters 4 and 26) points to not only how much is available but also how useful it is. A search for meta-analyses and critical reviews in the period 2009 through 2012 for all journals related to physical therapy or occupational therapy indexed in the CINAHL search engine (see Chapter 4) yielded more than 16,000 results. Results of the same search for speech-language pathology in the same period yielded more than 11,000 results.

In addition to helping clinicians make judgments about the use of existing treatments, research can be used to test new procedures so that clinicians can make evidence-based decisions about whether to add them to their clinical repertoire. For example, body-weight–supported treadmill ambulation, although established, continues to undergo modifications in need of such testing. In theory, body-weight–supported treadmill ambulation should enable patients to improve their ambulation function by training in a way that ensures safety, does not require handheld assistive devices, uses relatively normal gait patterns, and has reduced energy demands when compared with unsupported walking. A recent innovation included the use of robots to assist with body-weight support.[20] Clinicians with a good knowledge base in research will be able to critically evaluate this article to determine whether they can apply the results to the clinical situations in which they work. Chapters 25 and 26 present guidelines for evaluating research literature.

BARRIERS TO REHABILITATION RESEARCH

In 1975, Hislop, a physical therapist, articulated one major philosophical barrier to research in the profession:

> A great difficulty in developing the clinical science of physical therapy is that we treat individual persons, each of whom is made up of situations which are unique and, therefore, appear incompatible with the generalizations demanded by science.[21](p. 1076)

Although this conceptual barrier may still loom large for some practitioners, many more concrete obstacles to rehabilitation research have been documented.[22–24] These obstacles include lack of familiarity with research methodology, lack of statistical support, lack of funding, lack of a mentor, and lack of time. An additional obstacle is concern for ethical use of humans or animals in research activities. Although the cited authors' comments go back several years, we think they are still valid; given the economy and demand for productivity at the writing of this book, they may be even more problematic than previously thought. However, this book should help to overcome several of the obstacles, particularly those pertaining to research methodology.

Lack of Funds

The scope of this text will not directly help in overcoming lack of funding, although information in Chapter 27 will help you gain access to funds that are available. Funding, especially from public sources, is largely a political process; we urge readers to take part in that arena to advocate for research budgets.

Lack of Research Mentors

Another example is lack of research mentors. Contemporary research is often done in teams. Ideally, novice researchers would be invited by experienced researchers to become members of working research teams with ongoing projects, external funding, and access to a network of colleagues engaged in similar work. The importance of research mentors—and the difficulty in finding them in the rehabilitation professions—has been discussed for several rehabilitation professions.[25-27] The picture is possibly made bleaker by the documented shortage of research-prepared doctoral faculty in academic programs,[28-30] and, at least at this writing, it is difficult to predict how the advent of required entry-level professional (i.e., clinical) doctorates will affect the situation. There may be at least one bright light in the situation, however. Although the traditional model of mentoring is that the mentor and protégé are in the same institution, professional associations have recently developed research-mentoring programs in which the mentor and protégé are not necessarily in the same institution, giving more flexibility to establishing possible mentor-protégé relationships.[31-33]

Lack of Time

A third barrier difficult to overcome is lack of time. Testa[34] outlined six major factors that influence the completion of research. Two of the six factors referred to "time" directly, and two more (complexity and funding) are indirectly related to the time that a researcher has available to devote to the task. Hegde noted, "Clinicians do not have the needed extra time for research."[35(p. 10)]

Indeed, it is difficult to separate the "time" issue from the "funding" issue because a lack of external funding generally limits the time available for research. In the absence of external funding, tasks with firm deadlines are given higher priority than research, and the immediate time pressures of the clinic and classroom may lead clinicians and academicians alike to postpone or abandon research ideas. One solution is to design studies that are relatively easy to integrate into the daily routine of a practice. Chapters 11, 13, and 16 present a variety of research designs particularly suitable for implementation in a clinical setting.

Despite these difficulties, there are barriers to research that can be overcome, which are addressed in this text. They include lack of familiarity with the research process, lack of statistical support, ethical concerns, and the clinician-researcher dichotomy.

Lack of Familiarity with the Research Process

Clinicians sometimes view rehabilitation research as a mysterious process that occupies the time of an elite group of professionals, far removed from patient or client care, who develop projects of little relevance to everyday practice. Although this characterization is a caricature, and evidence exists of ways to implement a research culture in a clinical environment,[36] even the most clinically grounded research uses the specialized language of research design and data analysis, and those who have not acquired the vocabulary are understandably intimidated when it is spoken. One goal of this text is to demystify the research process by clearly articulating the knowledge base needed to understand it.

Lack of Statistical Support

Another barrier we think can be overcome is lack of statistical support. Section 7 (Chapters 20 through 24) of this book provides the conceptual background needed to understand most of the statistics reported in the rehabilitation research literature.[37,38] A conceptual background does not, however, provide an adequate theoretical and mathematical basis for selection and computation of a given statistic on a particular occasion, particularly for complex research designs. Thus, many researchers will require the services of a statistician at some point in the research process. Guidelines for working with statisticians are provided in Chapter 27.

Ethical Concerns About Use of Human Participants and Animal Subjects

Often, rehabilitation research is halted by ethical concerns related to the use of either human participants or animal subjects. Those who choose to study animal models should follow appropriate guidelines for the use, care, and humane destruction of animal subjects. Clinicians who use human participants in their research must pay close attention to balancing the risks of the research with potential benefits from the results. Chapter 5 examines ethical considerations in detail; Chapter 27 provides guidelines for working with the committees that oversee researchers to ensure that they protect the rights of research participants.

The Clinician-Researcher Dichotomy

Yet another barrier to research implementation is the apparent and widely held belief that clinicians and researchers have little in common. We refer to this as the "clinician-researcher" dichotomy. The history of this situation is a long one, especially in clinical psychology, and accounts of its development are offered by Hayes and associates[39] and Merlo and colleagues.[40] Hayes and associates offer two primary reasons for the dichotomy: "(a) the almost universally acknowledged inadequacies of traditional research methodology to address issues important to practice and (b) the lack of a clear link between empiricism and professional success in the practice context."[39](p. 15) By "traditional research methodologies," the authors are referring to large-scale group-data experiments, especially clinical trials. Hegde also offers the doubt "regarding the extent to which research affects day-to-day practice."[35](p. 10) Fago confirms a "widening division between psychology's clinical investigators and clinical practitioners."[41](p. 15) Bishop notes the "general consensus ... that the translation of sport-science research to practice is poor."[42](p. 253) Clearly, if clinicians do not think that they have much in common with researchers (including time available, research training, etc.) and that the research that is completed has little applicability to their practice, the production and even consumption of research is going to be significantly curtailed.

Overcoming Barriers

Overcoming these barriers depends on leaders who are willing to commit time and money to research efforts, individuals who are willing to devote time and effort to improving their research knowledge and skills, and improved systems for training researchers and funding research. Cusick's qualitative study of clinician-researchers underscores the importance of making an individual commitment to becoming a researcher, accepting responsibility for driving the research process, and learning to negotiate the administrative and social systems that make clinical research possible.[43] Research is, however, rarely an individual effort. Therefore, one key to overcoming barriers to research is to develop productive research teams composed of individuals who, together, have all the diverse skills needed to plan, implement, analyze, and report research. The different rehabilitation professions are working to develop such teams in different ways: the Foundation for Physical Therapy in 2002 funded its first Clinical Research Network, designed to increase research capacity in physical therapy through collaborative arrangements between academic and clinical sites[44]; and building research capacity in the allied health professions has been of interest to policy-making bodies in the United States[45] and the United Kingdom.[46]

The Scientist-Practitioner

We wish to make special note of the possible solution to the barrier of the clinician-researcher dichotomy. That is the development of the scientist-practitioner model of education first developed in clinical psychology and later applied to other rehabilitative professions.

Thorough histories of the effort are offered by Hayes and associates[39] and Merlo and colleagues.[40] Essentially, the model seeks to provide education so that clinicians have good research training and researchers have good clinical training at least to the extent of good understanding of both roles.

The history of attempts at developing scientist-practitioners is far from over, but we see hopeful trends. In an abridged meta-analysis of 10 articles, Chang and colleagues[47] concluded that current education of scientist-practitioners is based on a flawed version of the model and needs to be more flexible and versatile. That is, with changed attitudes, attainment of the scientist-practitioner is a reasonable goal. Proposing an educational model based on dialectics, Fago[41] offers several suggestions for overcoming the clinician-researcher dichotomy and fostering development of the scientist-practitioner. In a survey of students from 163 Council of University Directors of Clinical Psychology (CUDCP) programs, the returns from 611 students, representing 55 programs, showed that students overwhelmingly "indicated that science training was very important to them. Overall, students reported experiencing a fairly balanced emphasis on science and clinical work, and endorsed receiving a good amount of high-quality training in science."[40](p. 58) Pettigrew[48] and Brobeck and Lubinsky[49] offer examples of how students in training are actually immersed in the scientist-practitioner model during the clinical rotations of their graduate programs in occupational therapy and/or speech-language pathology.

Although the past certainly has supported the notion of a clinician-researcher dichotomy, we are encouraged by the growth of and attention to "evidence-based practice" in academic programs and in the rehabilitation professions. Examination of academic curricula by one of the authors, an accreditation site visitor in communication sciences and disorders, reveals universal attention to ways in which students can incorporate an evidence base into their clinical practice. The Web site of the American Speech-Language-Hearing Association devotes considerable space to the subject,[50] as do the Web sites of the American Physical Therapy Association[51] and American Occupational Therapy Association.[52] Only time will tell if, and to what extent, the emphasis on evidence-based practice has influenced the everyday lives of rehabilitation clinicians.

We do not expect that all clinicians will be prolific (or even occasional) researchers, but we do ascribe in this text to the notion that the clinician who is a scientist-practitioner will be able to fulfill at least two of the three roles suggested by Hayes and associates[39]: (1) a knowledgeable consumer of new research, using scientifically based clinical procedures; (2) an evaluator of his or her own clinical practices; and (3) a producer of new data.

STATUS OF REHABILITATION RESEARCH

The rehabilitation professions are relative newcomers to the health care arena, as the "conflagrations of World War I and II provided the impetus for the development and growth of the field of rehabilitation."[53](p. 1) Mindful of the way in which new professions grow, in 1952 Du Vall, an occupational therapist, wrote about the development of the health care professions into research:

> A study of the growth and development of any well established profession will show that, as it emerged from the swaddling clothes of infancy and approached maturity, research appeared.[54](p. 97)

Research has indeed appeared across the rehabilitation professions. A great deal can be learned about the current status of rehabilitation research by examining the role of research in the professional associations of the various rehabilitation disciplines, by reviewing the development of research publication vehicles, by examining the educational standards for the different rehabilitation professions, and by reviewing research funding opportunities for rehabilitation and related research.

Professional Association Goals

All of the major professional associations that promote the rehabilitation professions take a leading role in advancing rehabilitation research. The American Occupational Therapy Association works "through standard-setting, advocacy, education, and research on behalf of its members and the public."[55] As part of its mission statement, the International Society for Prosthetics and Orthotics includes, "Promoting research and evidence based practice."[56] The American Physical Therapy Association developed a clinical research agenda in 2000 designed to "support, explain, and enhance physical therapy clinical practice by facilitating research that is useful primarily to clinicians."[57](p. 499) That association has recently revised and broadened the agenda to include all research, eliminating the limiting word "clinical."[58] Common Program Requirements of the Accreditation Council for Graduate Medical Education require that "the curriculum must advance residents' knowledge of the basic principles of research, including how research is conducted, evaluated, explained to patients, and applied to patient care" and also that "residents should

participate in scholarly activity."[59] Their recently introduced "core requirements" include the ability to "appraise and assimilate scientific evidence."[60] Furthermore, these associations do not simply make empty statements about their roles in research—they follow through with actions to promote research in their respective professions. For example, the American Speech-Language-Hearing Association's commitment to research is shown by its development of a national outcomes measurement system.[61]

Research Publication Vehicles

Dissemination of rehabilitation research findings in peer-reviewed journals is an important indicator of the status of rehabilitation research. Over the past several decades, the number of journals with a primary mission to publish research related to rehabilitation has increased dramatically, as a journey through any relevant database (see Chapter 4) will attest. As of February 2015, searching the CINAHL database (see Chapter 4) for journal titles added just since 2000 reveals that 40 new titles have been added relevant to physical therapy, 16 for occupational therapy and 32 for speech-language pathology and audiology. The increased importance of rehabilitation research across time is apparent both in the ability of the professions to sustain these new journals and in the emergence of new types of publications: specialty journals (e.g., *Journal of Pediatric Physical Therapy*), interdisciplinary journals (e.g., *Journal of Occupational Rehabilitation*), and international journals (e.g., *International Journal of Language and Communication Disorders*).

Educational Standards

As research becomes more important to a profession, the standards against which education programs that prepare new practitioners are evaluated can be expected to reflect this emphasis. A review of educational program requirements for the various rehabilitation professions shows that this is indeed the case, with requirements for research content, research activities, or both. The American Speech-Language-Hearing Association,[62] in its standards for educational program accreditation, requires that "the scientific and research foundations of the profession are evident in the curriculum" to prepare speech-language pathologists and audiologists. The Commission on Accreditation in Physical Therapy Education notes that "physical therapy upholds and draws on a tradition of scientific inquiry while contributing to the profession's body of knowledge," requires a "scholarly agenda," and requires "activities that systematically advance the teaching, research, and practice of physical therapy through rigorous inquiry."[63] The American Council on Occupational Therapy Education lists "researcher" among the roles to be mastered by occupational therapists in training and requires that graduates be prepared as an effective consumer of the latest research.[64] Finally, the Accreditation Council for Graduate Medical Education has enhanced its physical medicine and rehabilitation residency requirements to include formal curricular elements related to research design and methodology as well as opportunities to participate in research projects and conferences.[59,60]

Research Funding

The creation of a vast government-funded medical research enterprise began in earnest in the United States in the 1940s after World War II. One symbol of this expansion of the research enterprise was the transformation in 1948 of the National Institute for Health, formerly a "tiny public health laboratory,"[65(p. 141)] into the plural National Institutes for Health (NIH) that conduct and support research through many specialized institutes focusing on particular branches of medicine and health care. It was not until the 1980s, however, that NIH, as well as the Centers for Disease Control (in 1992 becoming the Centers for Disease Control and Prevention), became important sources of funding for rehabilitation research.[66] Today, the NIH's National Institute of Child Health and Human Development, National Institute on Aging, National Institute of Arthritis and Musculoskeletal and Skin Diseases, National Cancer Institute, National Institute of Mental Health, National Institute of Neurological Disorders and Stroke, and National Institute of Deafness and Other Communication Disorders are important sources of funding for rehabilitation researchers.[67,68] The National Institute for Disability and Rehabilitation Research, an arm of the U.S. Department of Education, is another important source of funding for rehabilitation research.[66] In addition, private foundations associated with the various rehabilitation professions, such as the American Occupational Therapy Foundation, the Foundation for Physical Therapy, and the American-Speech-Language-Hearing Foundation, provide nonfederal sources of research funding.[69–71] Thus, even though a lack of funding for rehabilitation research has been identified as a serious problem for rehabilitation and the rehabilitation professions, a broad set of government and private sources of funding are available to rehabilitation researchers who choose to compete for external funding of their research efforts. You can read more about funding sources and resources in Chapter 27.

Although the refrains to increase and improve rehabilitation research do not seem to change from one generation of providers to the next, this review of the status of rehabilitation research shows that, in the second decade of this century, professional associations for the rehabilitation disciplines include the development of research among their stated goals, that there is a wide variety of established and emerging journals in which to publish rehabilitation research, that educational standards for rehabilitation providers include criteria related to research, and that external funds for rehabilitation research are available from several sources. These signs of the recent strength of rehabilitation research must be tempered by the often chaotic economic and political influences that can limit research funding for government granting agencies and philanthropic donations to private ones. Yes, the barriers to research are significant. Yes, identifying and using available resources takes initiative and energy. Yes, making research a priority in a cost-containment environment is difficult. However, the incentives to overcome these barriers are substantial in that the future of rehabilitation within the health care system and society requires that we establish a firm base of evidence on which to build our practice.

SUMMARY

Research is the creative process by which professionals systematically challenge their everyday practices. Developing a body of rehabilitation knowledge, determining whether rehabilitation interventions work, and improving patient and client care are reasons for conducting rehabilitation research. Barriers to research are lack of familiarity with the research process, lack of statistical support, lack of funds, lack of mentors, lack of time, and concern for the ethics of using humans and animals in research. The importance of research to the rehabilitation professions is illustrated by professional association goals, publication vehicles for rehabilitation research, educational standards, and funding for rehabilitation research.

REFERENCES

1. Kettering CF: In Boyd TA, editor: *Prophet of progress*, New York, NY, 1961.
2. Payton OD: *Research: The Validation of Clinical Practice*, 3rd ed, Philadelphia, Pa, 1994, FA Davis.
3. Kazdin AE: *Research Design in Clinical Psychology*, 4th ed, Boston, Mass, 2003, Allyn & Bacon.
4. Portney LG, Watkins MP: *Foundations of Clinical Research: Applications to Practice*, 3rd ed, 2009, Upper Saddle River, NJ, Prentice Hall.

5. Polit DF, Beck CT: *Nursing Research: Principles and Methods*, 9th ed, Philadelphia, Pa, 2012, Lippincott Williams & Wilkins.

6. Stein F, Rice MS, Cutler SK: *Clinical Research in Occupational Therapy*, 5th ed, New York, NY, 2013, Delmar, Cengage Learning.

7. Nelson LK: *Research in Communication Sciences and Disorders*, 2nd ed, San Diego, Calif, 2013, Plural.

8. Westerlund S, Medina MEG, González OP: Effect of human electromagnetic fields in relief of minor pain by using a Native American method, *Integr Med Clin J* 11(1):39–44, 2012.

9. Cermak SA, Mitchell TW: Sensory integration. In McCauley RJ, Fey RE, editors: *Treatment of Language Disorders in Children*, Baltimore, Md, 2006, Paul H Brookes.

10. Devlin S, Healy O, Leader G, Hughes B: Comparison of behavioral intervention and sensory-integration therapy in the treatment of challenging behavior, *J Autism Dev Disord* 41:1303–1320, 2011.

11. Schaaf RC, Hunt J, Benevides T: Occupational therapy using sensory integration to improve participation in a child with autism: A case report, *Am J Occup Ther* 66:547–555, 2012.

12. Rothstein JM: Clinical literature [Editor's Note], *Phys Ther* 69:895, 1989.

13. Simonton DK: *Creativity in Science: Chance, Logic, Genius, and Zeitgeist*, Cambridge, UK, 2004, Cambridge University Press.

14. Bailey C, White C, Pain R: Evaluating qualitative research: Dealing with the tension between "science" and "creativity," *J Royal Geogr Soc* 31(2):169–183, 1999.

15. Hicks CM: *Research Methods for Clinical Therapists*, 5th ed, Edinburgh, UK, 2009, Elsevier.

16. Houle CO: *Continuing Learning in the Professions*, San Francisco, Calif, 1981, Jossey-Bass.

17. Kinsella EA, Whiteford GE: Knowledge generation and utilization in occupational therapy: Towards epistemic reflexivity, *Aust Occup Ther J* 56:249–258, 2009.

18. Kenyon LK, Blackinton MT: Applying motor-control theory to physical therapy practice: A case report, *Physiother Can* 63:345–354, 2011.

19. Brummel-Smith K: Research in rehabilitation, *Clin Geriatr Med* 9:895–904, 1993.

20. Lam T, Pauhl K, Krassioukov A, Eng JJ: Using robot-applied resistance to augment body-weight—supported treadmill training in an individual with incomplete spinal cord injury, *Phys Ther* 91:143–151, 2011.

21. Hislop HJ: Tenth Mary McMillan lecture: the not-so-impossible dream, *Phys Ther* 55:1069–1080, 1975.

22. Ballin AJ, Breslin WH, Wierenga KAS, Shepard KF: Research in physical therapy: Philosophy, barriers to involvement, and use among California physical therapists, *Phys Ther* 60:888–895, 1980.

23. Taylor E, Mitchell M: Research attitudes and activities of occupational therapy clinicians, *Am J Occup Ther* 44:350–355, 1990.

24. MacDermid JC, Fess EE, Bell-Krotoski J, et al: A research agenda for hand therapy, *J Hand Ther* 15:3–15, 2002.

25. Paul S, Stein F, Ottenbacher KJ, Yuanlong L: The role of mentoring on research productivity among occupational therapy faculty, *Occup Ther Int* 9:24–40, 2002.

26. Minichiello V, Kottler JA: *Qualitative Journeys: Student and Mentor Experiences with Research*, Thousand Oaks, Calif, 2010, Sage.

27. Jones ML, Cifu DX, Sisto SA: Instilling a research culture in an applied clinical setting, *Arch Phys Med Rehabil* 94(1):S49–S54, 2013.

28. Wetmore SW: The association between program characteristics and enrollment in postprofessional doctorate programs in physical therapy [Dissertation], Ann Arbor, Mich, 2010, ProQuest LLC.

29. Myotte T, Hutchins TL, Cannizzaro MS, Belin G: Understanding why speech-language pathologists rarely pursue a Ph.D. in communication sciences and disorders, *Comm Dis Q* 33:42–54, 2011.

30. Johnson CE, Danjhauer JL, Page AS, et al: AuD degree holders in tenure-track positions: Survey of program chairpersons and AuD degree holders, *J Am Acad Audiol* 24:425–446, 2013.

31. American Speech-Language-Hearing Foundation: Grants and awards. Available at: http://ashfoundation.org/grants/default.htm. Accessed November 11, 2014.

32. American Speech-Language-Hearing Association: Mentoring academic research careers. Available at: http://ashfoundation.org/grants/default.htm. Accessed November 11, 2014.

33. American Physical Therapy Association: Mentoring in academia. Available at: https://www.apta.org/APTALogin.aspx?RedirectTo=http://www.apta.org/PTinMotion/2007/12/MentoringinAcademia/. Accessed November 11, 2014.

34. Testa MH: The nature of outcomes assessment in speech-language pathology, *J Allied Health* 24:41–55, 1995.

35. Hegde MN: *Clinical Research in Communicative Disorders*, Austin, Tex, 2003, Pro-Ed.

36. Jones ML, Cifu DX, Sisto SA: Instilling a research culture in an applied clinical setting, *Arch Phys Med Rehabil* 94(1):S49–S54, 2013.

37. Zito M, Bohannon RW: Inferential statistics in physical therapy research: A recommended core, *J Phys Ther Educ* 4:13–16, 1990.

38. Schwartz S, Sturr M, Goldberg G: Statistical methods in rehabilitation literature: A survey of recent publications, *Arch Phys Med Rehabil* 77:497–500, 1996.

39. Hayes SC, Barlow DH, Nelson-Grey RO: *The Scientist Practitioner*, Boston, Mass, 1999, Allyn & Bacon.

40. Merlo LJ, Collins A, Bernstein J: CUDCP-affiliated clinical psychology student views of their science training, *Training and Education in Professional Psychology* Vol 2(1):58–65, 2008.

41. Fago DP: The evidence-based treatment debate: Toward a dialectical rapprochement [Comment], *Psychotherapy Theory, Research, Practice, Training* Vol 46(1):15–18, 2009.

42. Bishop D: An applied research model for the sport sciences, *Sports Med* 38(3):253–263, 2008.

43. Cusick A: The experience of clinician-researchers in occupational therapy, *Am J Occup Ther* 55:9–18, 2001.

44. Foundation news: CRN to explore effects of muscle strengthening exercises, *PT Magazine* 10(11):12, 2002.

45. Selker LG: Clinical research in allied health, *J Allied Health* 23:201–228, 1994.

46. Ilott I, Bury T: Research capacity: A challenge for the therapy professions, *Physiotherapy* 88:194–200, 2002.

47. Chang K, Lee I, Hargreaves TA: Scientist versus practitioner: An abridged meta-analysis of the changing role of psychologists, *Couns Psychol Q* 21(3):267–291, 2008.

48. Pettigrew CM: Bridging the gap: How therapists-in-training can facilitate research for clinicians, *Phys Ther Rev* 11(3):205–228, 2006.

49. Brobeck T, Lubinsky J: Using single-subject designs in speech-language pathology practicum, *Clin Issues Commun Sci Disord* 30:101–106, 2003.

50. American Speech-Language-Hearing Association. Available at: http://www.asha.org/members/ebp/. Accessed November 11, 2014.

51. American Physical Therapy Association. Available at: http://www.apta.org/EvidenceResearch/. Accessed November 11, 2014.

52. American Occupational Therapy Association. Available at: http://www.aota.org/Practice/Researchers.aspx. Accessed February 6, 2015.

53. Dillingham TR: Physiatry, physical medicine, and rehabilitation: Historical development and military roles, *Milit Trauma Rehabil* 13:1–16, 2002.

54. Du Vall EN: Research, *Am J Occup Ther* 6:97–99, 132, 1952.

55. American Occupational Therapy Association: AOTA Mission Statement. Available at: http://www.aota.org/AboutAOTA.aspx. Accessed February 6, 2015.

56. International Society for Prosthetics and Orthotics: *ISPO aims and objectives*. Available at: www.ispoint.org. Accessed November 11, 2014.

57. Clinical research agenda for physical therapy, *Phys Ther* 80:499–513, 2000.

58. Goldstein MS, Scalzitti DA, Craik RL, et al: The revised research agenda for physical therapy, *Phys Ther* 91:165–174, 2011.

59. American Council on Graduate Medical Education: Common program requirements. Available at: http://www.acgme.org/acgmeweb/Portals/0/PFAssets/ProgramRequirements/CPRs2013.pdf. Accessed November 11, 2014.

60. American Council on Graduate Medical Education: Core competencies. Available at: http://www.acgme.org/acgmeweb/Portals/0/PFAssets/ProgramRequirements/CPRs2013.pdf. Accessed February 6, 2015.

61. American Speech-Language-Hearing Association: National Outcomes Measurement System (NOMS). Available at: www.asha.org/members/research/NOMS/. Accessed November 11, 2014.

62. American Speech-Language-Hearing Association: Standards for accreditation of graduate education programs in audiology and speech-language pathology. Available at: www.asha.org/academic/accreditation/accredmanual/section3.htm. Accessed November 11, 2014.

63. American Physical Therapy Association: Evaluative criteria PT programs. Available at: http://www.capteonline.org/uploadedFiles/CAPTEorg/About_CAPTE/Resources/Accreditation_Handbook/EvaluativeCriteria_PT.pdf. Accessed November 11, 2014.

64. American Council for Occupational Therapy Education: 2011 ACOTE Accreditation Standards. Available at: http://www.aota.org/Education-Careers/Accreditation/StandardsReview.aspx. Accessed February 6, 2015.

65. Ludmerer KM: *Time to Heal: American Medical Education from the Turn of the Century to the Era of Managed Care*, New York, NY, 1999, Oxford University Press.

66. Cole TM: The 25th Walter J. Zeiter lecture: The greening of physiatry in a gold era of rehabilitation, *Arch Phys Med Rehabil* 74:231–237, 1993.

67. National Institutes of Health: Grants and funding. Available at: http://grants.nih.gov/grants/oer.htm. Accessed November 11, 2014.

68. Penner LA, Albrecht TL, Dovidio JF: Obtaining and evaluating research resources. In Cooper H, Camic PM, Long DL, et al, editors: *APA Handbook of Research Methods in Psychology, Vol. 1: Foundations, Planning, Measures, and Psychometrics*, Washington, DC, 2012:145–162, American Psychological Association.

69. American Occupational Therapy Foundation: Available at: http://aotf.org/. Accessed November 11, 2014.

70. Foundation for Physical Therapy: Research grants. Available at: http://foundation4pt.org/apply-for-funding/research-grants/. Accessed November 11, 2014.

71. American Speech-Language-Hearing Foundation: Grants and awards. Available at: http://www.ashfoundation.org/grants/default.htm. Accessed November 11, 2014.

2

Theory in Rehabilitation Research

CHAPTER OUTLINE

Relationships Among
   Theory, Research, and Practice
Definitions of Theory
   Level of Restrictiveness
      Least Restrictive Definition
      Moderately Restrictive Definition
      Most Restrictive Definition
   Tentativeness of Theory
   Testability of Theory
Scope of Theory
   Metatheory
   Grand Theory
   General, or Middle-Range, Theory

Specific, or Practice, Theory
Evaluating Theory
Putting Theory into Practice:
   Research, Questions,
   Hypotheses, and Problems
   Developing Answerable Research
      Questions
   Topic Identification and Selection
   Problem Identification and
      Selection
   Theoretical Framework
      Identification and Selection

Question Identification and
   Selection
Research Methods Identification
   and Selection
Criteria for Evaluating Research
   Problems
   Study Is Feasible
   Problem Is Interesting
   Problem Is Novel
   Problem Can Be Studied Ethically
   Question Is Relevant
Summary

All of us have ideas about how the world operates. We may even dub some of our ideas "theories." Think of the kind of banter that goes back and forth among a group of friends sharing a meal. "I have this theory that my car is designed to break down the week before payday." "The theory was that my mom and her sisters would rotate who cooks Christmas dinner." "Here's my theory—the electronics manufacturers wait until I buy a new gadget and then they come out with a new, improved model."

When do ideas about the nature of the world become theories? What distinguishes theory from other modes of thought? Is theory important to the applied disciplines of rehabilitation practitioners? Does theory drive practice, or does practice drive theory? The purpose of this chapter is to answer these questions by examining the relationships among theory, practice, and research; by defining theory and some closely related terms; by presenting examples of theories categorized by scope extent; and by suggesting a general approach to evaluating theory.

RELATIONSHIPS AMONG THEORY, RESEARCH, AND PRACTICE

Theory is important because it holds the promise of guiding both practice and research. Figure 2-1 presents a schematic drawing, showing the expected relationships among theory, research, and clinical practice. Theory is generally developed through reflection on experience (e.g., "It seems to me that patients who pay for their own therapy follow home exercise instructions better than those whose insurance companies cover the cost") or from logical speculation (e.g., "If pain is related to the accumulation of metabolic by-products in the tissues, then modalities that increase local blood flow should help reduce pain").[1] Theories developed by reflections on experience may draw on the careful observations of clinicians in practice or may flow from qualitative research studies that develop theories grounded in qualitative data (see Chapters 6 and 14 for more information). Theory, however it is generated, is then formally tested through research. Based on research results, the theory is confirmed or modified, as are clinical practices based on the theory. Unfortunately, theory and practice are often disconnected from one another, leading Kielhofner to "underscore the need for better ways to connect theoretical explanation and practice."[2(p. 14)] Further, he suggests that "when knowledge is developed and organized as a part of practical problem solving, the gap between theory and practice can be eliminated."[2(p. 14)]

If research is conducted with animals, with normal human participants, or with techniques that differ from typical clinical practice, then the results are not directly applicable to the clinical setting. However, such

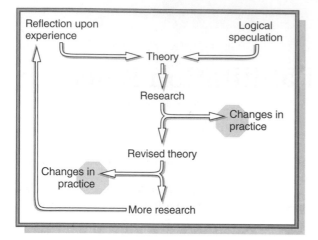

Figure 2-1 Relationships among theory, research, and practice.

research results may lead to modification of theory, and modification of theory may in turn lead clinicians to rethink the ways in which they treat their patients or clients. (The application of the general case—changes in theory—to the specific case—changes in the treatment of a client—is an illustration of deductive reasoning.) In contrast, if research is conducted with a clinical population and types of interventions that can be easily implemented in actual practice, then clinicians may be able to change their practices based on the research results. The accumulated results of clinical implementation can lead to modification of theory, which is an example of inductive reasoning. It is incumbent on the authors of research reports to help readers connect theory and practice through thoughtful discussion of the practical implications—both applicability and limitations—of their work.

DEFINITIONS OF THEORY

Theories are, by nature, abstractions. Thus, the language of theory is abstract, and there are divergent definitions of theory and its components. Instead of presenting a single definition of theory, this section of the chapter examines three elements of various definitions of theory: level of restrictiveness, tentativeness, and testability.

Level of Restrictiveness

Definitions of theory differ in their level of restrictiveness, and the level of restrictiveness of the definition then has an impact on the purposes for which a theory can be used. Table 2-1 summarizes the distinctions between the definitions and purposes of theories with different levels of restrictiveness. Restrictiveness addresses how inclusive or wide ranging are specific instances covered by a definition. As a theory becomes more restrictive, the requirements for inclusion are more specific. Different types of theory may be appropriate to different points in the development of a profession and its body of knowledge, with descriptive theory emerging first, predictive theory next, and finally explanatory theory.

To illustrate the differences among various levels of restrictiveness and their corresponding purposes, a simple example about hemiplegia is developed throughout this section of the chapter. This example is not meant to be a well-developed theory; it is merely an illustration based on a clinical entity that many rehabilitation professionals should have encountered at some point in their professional education or practice.

Least Restrictive Definition

The least restrictive form of theory, *descriptive theory*, requires only that a phenomenon be described—and

Table **2-1**

Level of Restrictiveness in Theory Definitions

| | LEVEL OF RESTRICTIVENESS | | |
	Least	**Moderate**	**Most**
Definition	Account for or characterize phenomena	Specify relationships between constructs	Specify relationships and form a deductive system
Purpose	Description	Prediction	Explanation
Comments	Subdivided into ad hoc and categorical theories	Sometimes referred to as conceptual frameworks or models	Can take the form of if-then statements

not predicted or explained—in some way, as in Fawcett's permissive definition: "A theory is a set of relatively concrete and specific concepts and the propositions that describe or link those concepts."[3(p. 4)] Thus, using this least restrictive definition, the statement "Individuals with hemiplegia have difficulty ambulating, eating, and speaking" is a simple form of theory because it describes (difficulty ambulating, eating, and speaking) a phenomenon (individuals with hemiplegia).

Moderately Restrictive Definition

Kerlinger and Lee have advanced a more restrictive definition of theory: "A theory is a set of interrelated constructs (concepts), definitions, and propositions that present a systematic view of phenomena by specifying relations among variables, with the purpose of explaining and predicting the phenomena."[4(p. 9)]

Although Kerlinger and Lee and others[3,4] draw distinctions between concepts and constructs—the former considered observable, the latter as abstract—we will consider them equivalent and use the terms interchangeably in this text. In addition, Kerlinger and Lee use *proposition* and *hypothesis* nearly interchangeably, as in Kerlinger and Lee's definition that a hypothesis is "a conjectural statement of the relation between two or more variables."[4] The hallmark of Kerlinger and Lee's definition of theory, then, is that it must specify relationships between or among concepts.

The earlier statement about individuals with hemiplegia would need to be developed considerably before Kerlinger and Lee would consider it to be theory. Such a developed (predictive) theory might read like this: "The extent to which individuals with hemiplegia will have difficulty ambulating is directly related to the presence of flaccid paralysis, cognitive deficits, and balance deficits and inversely related to prior ambulation status." This is no longer a simple description of several characteristics of hemiplegia; it is a statement of relationships between concepts and predicts an outcome.

Researchers who prefer the most restrictive definition of theory may consider descriptions at this moderately restrictive level to be conceptual frameworks or models. For example, Burns and Grove[5] consider theories as interrelated concepts that afford prediction, explanation, and control of a phenomenon that can be tested. By contrast, they consider concept models as more general, less well articulated than theories, and not testable.

Theory that meets Kerlinger and Lee's definition is known as *predictive theory* because it can be used to make predictions based on the relationships between variables. If the four factors in this hypothetical theory about hemiplegic gait were found to be good predictors of eventual ambulation outcome, rehabilitation professionals might be able to use information gathered at admission to predict long-term ambulation status.

Most Restrictive Definition

The most restrictive view of theory is that "theories involve a series of propositions regarding the interrelationships among concepts, from which a large number of empirical observations can be deduced."[6(p. 96)] This is the most restrictive definition because it requires both relationships between variables and a deductive system.

Deductive reasoning goes from the general to the specific and can take the form of if-then statements. To make the hypothetical theory of hemiplegic gait meet this definition, we would need to add a general gait component to the theory. This general statement might read, "Human gait characteristics are dependent on muscle power, skeletal stability, proprioceptive feedback, balance, motor planning, and learned patterns." The specific deduction from this general theory of gait is the statement, "In individuals with hemiplegia, the critical components that lead to difficulty ambulating independently are presence of flaccidity (muscle power), impaired sensation (proprioceptive feedback), impaired perception of verticality (balance), and processing difficulties (motor planning)." In an if-then format, this theory might read as follows:

1. *If* normal gait depends on intact muscle power, skeletal stability, proprioceptive feedback, balance, motor planning, and learned patterns, and
2. *If* hemiplegic gait is not normal,
3. *Then* individuals with hemiplegia must have deficits in one or more of the following areas: muscle power, skeletal stability, proprioceptive feedback, balance, motor planning, and learned patterns.

This theory, then, forms a deductive system by advancing a general theory for the performance of normal gait activities and then examining the elements that are affected in individuals with hemiplegia. Figure 2-2 presents this theory schematically. The six elements in the theory are central to the figure. In the absence of pathology, normal gait occurs, as shown above the central elements; in the presence of pathology, the elements are altered, and an abnormal gait results, as shown below the gait elements.

With a deductive system in place, theory can begin to be used to explain natural phenomena. *Explanatory theory* looks at the why and how questions that undergird a problem, generally in more explicit terms than illustrated in Figure 2-3. The hypothetical explanatory theory about gait begins to explain ambulation difficulty in terms of six elements needed for normal gait.

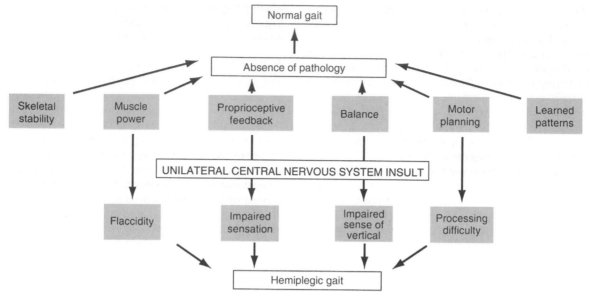

Figure 2-2 Diagram of the theory of gait in individuals with hemiplegia.

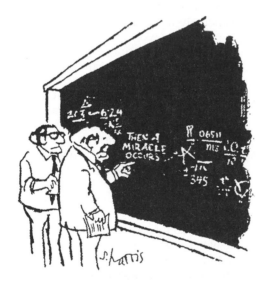

"I THINK YOU SHOULD BE MORE EXPLICIT HERE IN STEP TWO."

Figure 2-3 Then a miracle occurs ... (From Sidney Harris, with permission. ScienceCartoonsPlus.com.)

Tentativeness of Theory

The second element of the definition of theory is its tentativeness. The tentative nature of theory is emphasized by Portney and Watkins:

Therefore, our acceptance of a particular theory will reflect the present state of knowledge and must adapt to changes in that knowledge as technology and scientific evidence improve. Therefore, a theory is only a tentative explanation of phenomena.... Many theories that are accepted today will be discarded tomorrow.[7(p. 40)]

Thus, theory is not absolute; rather, it is a view that is acceptable, at the time, to the scientists studying the phenomenon. For example, the idea that the sun revolved around the earth (geocentric theory) suited its time. It was also a useful theory:

It described the heavens precisely as they looked and fitted the observations and calculations made with the naked eye; ... it fitted the available facts, was a reasonably satisfactory device for prediction, and harmonized with the accepted view of the rest of nature.... Even for the adventurous sailor and the navigator it served well enough.[8(p. 295)]

However, the small discrepancies between the geocentric theory and the yearly calendar were troublesome to Renaissance astronomers and led to the development of the heliocentric theory—the one we still believe—that the earth revolves around the sun. Perhaps a later generation of scientists will develop different models of the universe that better explain the natural phenomena of the changing of days and seasons. Natural scientists do not assume an unchangeable objective reality that will ultimately be explained by the perfect theory; there is no reason for rehabilitation researchers to assume that their world is any more certain or ultimately explainable than the natural world.

Testability of Theory

Testability has been described as a sine qua non (an indispensable condition) of theory.[9] If so, then every theory needs to be formulated in ways that allow the theory to be tested. However, theories cannot be proved true because one can never test them under all the conditions under which they might be applied. Even if testing shows that the world behaves in the manner predicted by a theory, this testing does not prove that the theory is true; other rival theories might provide equally accurate predictions. Theories can, however, be proved false by instances in which the predictions of the theory are not borne out.

For example, if one can accurately predict the discharge ambulation status of individuals with hemiplegia based on tone, sensation, vertical sense, and processing difficulty, then the theory is consistent with the data. However, rival theories might predict discharge ambulation status just as well. A cognitive or emotionally oriented practitioner might develop a theory that predicts discharge ambulation status as a function of the level of motivation of the patient, and a behaviorally oriented one might cite the extent to which the staff provide immediate rewards for gait activities. If the behavioral or cognitive theory accurately predicts discharge ambulation status of individuals with hemiplegia as well as the other theory does, it will also be consistent with the data. None of the theories can be proved in the sense that it is true and all others are false; all theories can, however, be shown to be consistent with available information.

SCOPE OF THEORY

Theories have been classified by different researchers in terms of their scope, often with four levels: metatheory, grand theory, general (or middle-range) theory, and specific, or practice, theory.[10,11]

Metatheory

Metatheory literally means "theorizing about theory." Therefore, metatheory is highly abstract, focusing on how knowledge is created and organized. The development of occupational science as a broad, organizing framework for occupational therapy has been described as metatheory.[10] In addition, the intellectual process of linking various theories to one another is a form of metatheory. For example, work that examines intersections, commonalities, and differences among the three grand theories described in the following paragraphs would be metatheoretical.

Grand Theory

Grand theories provide broad conceptualizations of phenomena. The World Health Organization's International Classification of Functioning, Disability, and Health (ICF) is a grand theory of importance to all rehabilitation practitioners (Fig. 2-4). A form of descriptive theory, it "provides a description of situations with regard to human functioning and its restrictions and serves as a framework to organize this information."[12(p. 7)] The ICF is divided into two parts: (1) functioning and disability, and (2) contextual factors.

Functioning and disability are further divided into body functions (physiology), body structures (anatomy), activities (individual functioning), and participation (societal functioning). The activities and participation classifications are further divided into capacity (what someone can do) and performance (what they actually

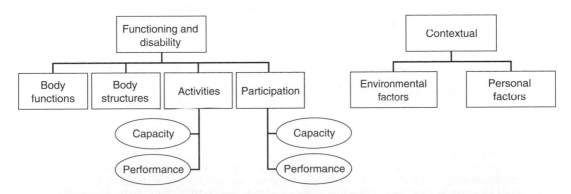

Figure 2-4 Schematic diagram of the International Classification of Functioning, Disability, and Health.

do) constructs. The contextual factors are divided into environmental and personal factors. Stephens and colleagues[13] used the ICF as a framework for studying the problems experienced by hearing-impaired older adults. They designed a new clinical questionnaire, built around the ICF framework, for use by older adults to identify problems associated with their hearing impairments. When older adults completed the new clinical questionnaire, they identified more participation limitations than they did with previous questionnaires. In this case, then, the link between theory and practice is that using the theoretical model of the ICF facilitated the development of more complete problem lists for use in treatment planning.

Hislop's[14] conceptual model of pathokinesiology and movement dysfunction is a grand theory related to physical therapy. This model looks at physical therapy using the overarching phenomena of movement disorders (others have modified the term from *disorders* to *dysfunction*) and pathokinesiology (the application of anatomy and physiology to the study of abnormal human movement). Figure 2-5 is an interpretation of Hislop's formulation of the pathokinesiological basis for physical therapy. Physical therapy is viewed as a triangle with a base of service values supplemented

by science, focusing on treatment of motion disorders through therapeutic exercise based on the principles of pathokinesiology. In this theory, physical therapy is viewed as affecting motion disorders related to four of six components of a hierarchy of systems ranging from the family to the cellular level of the body. The goal of physical therapy is either to restore motion homeostasis or to enhance adaptation to permanent impairment. This theory, presented in 1975, was groundbreaking in that no one before Hislop had advanced a coherent, comprehensive view of the work of physical therapists. This theory challenged physical therapists to think of themselves not as technicians who applied external physical agents to their patients, but as movement specialists who used a variety of tools to effect changes in troublesome movement patterns.

The model of human occupation (MOHO) is an example of grand theory that comes from the profession of occupational therapy. In the MOHO, people are viewed as having three subsystems (volitional, habituation, and mind-brain-body performance) that interact with the environment to produce occupational behavior.[15] The MOHO has been used in clinical practice to organize assessment and treatment activities, as in Pizzi's[16] case report of his work with an individual

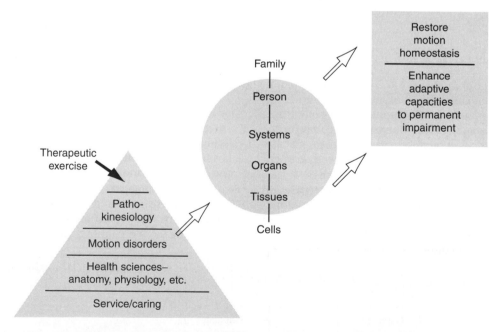

Figure 2-5 Interpretation of Hislop's pathokinesiological framework for physical therapy. The triangle represents the structure of physical therapy, the circle a hierarchy of systems affected by physical therapy, and the square the goals of physical therapy. (Modified from Hislop HJ, Tenth Mary McMillan lecture: The not-so-impossible dream, *Phys Ther* 55:1073, 1075, 1975. Reprinted from *Physical Therapy* with the permission of the American Physical Therapy Association.)

with acquired immunodeficiency syndrome. In addition, it has been used to structure research activities, as in Chen and colleagues'[17] work on factors influencing adherence to home exercise programs.

General, or Middle-Range, Theory

General, or middle-range, theories provide general frameworks for action, but do not purport to address large ideas (e.g., human functioning) or entire disciplines (e.g., physical therapy or occupational therapy) with a single theoretical context. Three examples of general theories illustrate the wide range of phenomena that can be viewed through a middle-range scope.

The gate control theory of pain, first presented in 1965 by Melzack and Wall, is an important general theory about the way that pain works. Before this theory was advanced, it was assumed that pain was largely a peripheral phenomenon, and treatments aimed at reducing or eliminating pain focused on peripheral solutions. In the words of Melzack himself, "The gate control theory's most important contribution to the biological and medical sciences ... was the emphasis on [central nervous system] CNS mechanisms. Never again, after 1965, could anyone try to explain pain exclusively in terms of peripheral factors. The theory forced the medical and biological sciences to accept the brain as an active system that filters, selects, and modulates inputs."[18(p. S123)] This theory led to the development of new physical modalities such as transcutaneous electrical nerve stimulation (TENS) and to a new emphasis on stress management and multidisciplinary approaches to modulating pain and pain behaviors.

The sensory integration model advanced by Ayres in the 1970s is a middle-range theory that hypothesizes a relationship between motor and learning difficulties and sensory processing problems. Concerned with how people integrate more than one source of sensory information, the sensory integration model focuses on tactile, vestibular, and proprioceptive information.[19] This theory is linked to practice by the development of assessment procedures designed to diagnose and classify sensory integration disorders[20] and by the development of treatment programs designed to have an impact on sensory processing.[21] The effectiveness of sensory integration programs has been studied in different groups of patients, including those with autism,[22] cerebral palsy,[23] and dementia.[24]

Mueller and Maluf[25] proposed the physical stress theory (PST) as a general theory with broad application to physical therapist practice, education, and research. In this theory, there is one basic premise: Changes in the relative level of physical stress cause a predictable adaptive response in all biological tissues. There are 12 fundamental principles, such as "physical stress levels that exceed the maintenance range (i.e., overload) result in increased tolerance of tissues to subsequent stresses (e.g., hypertrophy)" and "individual stresses combine in complex ways to contribute to the overall level of stress exposure."[25(p. 385)] There are also four categories of factors that affect the level of tissue stress or the adaptive response to stress: movement and alignment, extrinsic, psychosocial, and physiological factors. This theory will link to practice if therapists use it as a framework for determining factors contributing to excessive stress, for modifying stresses to permit tissue healing, and for studying the effectiveness of interventions.

Specific, or Practice, Theory

Specific, or practice, theories can be described as particular applications of grand or general theories. For example, current practice theory supports the early use of powered mobility for some children with disabilities.[26] This contemporary view is consistent with some key ideas put forward in the ICF: that disability exists within an environmental context and that social participation—not just individual activity—are important goals for most people. Using this framework, powered mobility becomes a tool that enables a child to explore his or her environment independently and to participate more fully in family and school activities. In this framework, children with disabilities may work on traditional motor development tasks during portions of their days, but they use powered mobility when they want to go long distances or keep up with a group. The grand theory advanced by the ICF is linked to practice through specific theory that conceptualizes powered mobility as a way of modifying the environment to promote participation.

The general gate control theory of pain is linked to practice through the specific theoretical propositions that led to the development of TENS as a treatment for pain.[27] The body of research that tests the effectiveness of TENS for different patient populations provides an indirect way of evaluating the gate control theory of pain.[27,28]

EVALUATING THEORY

Much of research is for the purpose of determining the validity of certain theoretical constructs. Theoretical constructs should be presented first in the literature review of a research manuscript and then reflected in the study question and hypothesis. In the Methods section of the manuscript, the participant features should be consistent with the theoretical concepts. That is, the participant features should be consistent with those features that the theoretical constructs include. In the description of the intervention or independent variable (IV), the intervention should reflect the theoretical constructs on which the IV was developed or implemented. Similarly, study outcomes are those proposed to be affected by the IV and thus should be a reflection of the theory's constructs. Clearly, theory, through its constructs, strongly guides a research study. It is imperative that the researcher present the theoretical constructs of interest in multiple places in a research manuscript.

When researchers and practitioners use theory to guide their work, they should critically evaluate those theories. In doing so, there may be a temptation to determine which of several competing theories is "correct." The answer is that none needs to be correct but each must be useful. The purpose of any theory is to organize constructs in ways that help us describe, predict, or explain phenomena of interest. Each theory—regardless of whether it meets restrictive or permissive definitions of theory and regardless of the scope of the theory—should be critically evaluated in terms of the extent to which it accurately describes the phenomenon, provides a framework for the study of the phenomenon, and influences practice. Different researchers will find that one or another theory provides a better framework for the questions they wish to ask, and different readers will simply find that some theories are more appealing to them than others. Stevens articulates her view of the folly of looking for one true theory in any discipline:

> Imagine what we would think of the field of psychology were it to dictate that each of its practitioners be Freudian. Indeed, it is the conflict and diversity among theories that account for much of the progress in any discipline. A search for conformity is an attempt to stultify the growth of a profession.[29(pp. xii–xiii)]

Rehabilitation practitioners need not choose a single framework to guide their actions. What they must do is develop, analyze, and use a rich set of different theories to enhance their understanding of the rehabilitation process they undertake with their patients and clients.

PUTTING THEORY INTO PRACTICE: RESEARCH, QUESTIONS, HYPOTHESES, AND PROBLEMS

We noted earlier that a hallmark of theory is its testability. Thus, regardless of the level of theoretical restriction or scope, a task of the scientist-practitioner is to verify, modify, or clarify theories via research. To do

so, however, requires consideration of crucial factors of generating research questions and hypotheses.

Developing Answerable Research Questions

Novice researchers usually have little difficulty identifying a general topic of interest: "I want to do something with the knee" or "My interest is in children with cerebral palsy." From these general statements, novice researchers often take a giant leap directly into asking research questions: "What is the relationship between hamstring strength and knee stability in patients with anterior cruciate ligament tears?" "Which individuals with spinal cord injury respond best to intrathecal baclofen for management of spasticity?"

Moving directly from topic to question, however, does not establish that the questions are relevant to problems within the field. This leap also fails to place the research question in a theoretical context. At the inception of a research project, researchers need to focus on broad problems within the profession, rather than on narrow questions. By focusing on problems, researchers are more likely to develop relevant questions.

The process of moving from a general topic to a specific research question involves four sets of ideas: (1) topic identification and selection, (2) problem identification and selection, (3) theoretical framework identification and selection, and (4) question identification and selection. A fifth step, determining the research methods, flows from the development of the ideas in the previous four steps. For each step, researchers must first be creative enough to generate many ideas and then must be selective enough to focus on a limited number of ideas for further study.

Topic Identification and Selection

Selecting a general topic is usually not a problem. However, if it is, direction can come from reading a wide range of literature and discussing problems with colleagues. From all the possible topics considered, one is selected for further study. At this point, all of the topics are often relatively broad because the practitioner or student may not yet know what is and is not known about each topic. Finding out more about each will allow the scientist-practitioner/student to determine which topics seem most likely to yield interesting and feasible research possibilities. Thus, the scientist-practitioner completes the first of the four cycles of expansion (identification of many possible topics) and contraction (selection of a single topic from the many) of ideas that takes place during the development of a research question.

Problem Identification and Selection

After a topic is selected, it is the job of the researcher to articulate important problems related to that topic area. One way of articulating research problems is to develop a series of logical statements that can be thought of as "givens," "howevers," and "therefores." The "given" is a statement of information that is generally accepted as true or at least what is known, based on research literature and common clinical practice. The "however" contradicts or casts doubt on the "given," pointing out gaps and conflicts in existing information. The conflict between the "givens" and the "howevers" creates the perplexing situation that is the research problem. The perplexing situation leads, "therefore," to the development of a research question. The conflicts that lead to research questions may be between actions, policies, or knowledge.

Conflicts of action and knowledge arise when scientist-practitioners act in ways that are not consistent with the formal knowledge of the profession: New therapies in all rehabilitation professions are constantly being introduced and, if involving saleable material or equipment, marketed. However, existing research may not support either the theoretical bases or claims of results of a particular therapy. A task of the scientist-practitioner is to engage in research to further justify (or not) the use of the therapy.

Knowledge-knowledge conflict is between different types of knowledge, often between general knowledge and scientifically based knowledge. Here, the scientist-practitioner must view commonly accepted descriptions or commonly used therapies with a skeptical eye. Good research serves to corroborate (or not) differences in types of knowledge.

Policy-action conflict examines the relationship between professional actions and internal or external rules. For example, professional associations often place limitations on the types of activities permitted to paraprofessional personnel. The scientist-practitioner may validly wonder if the limitations are overly restrictive or not restrictive enough, given the education and training of the paraprofessionals.

Knowledge void (self-explanatory) is probably the most common generator of problems. In fact, the mere lack of knowledge may well lead to the types of conflicts described previously. Scientist-practitioners may wish to engage in research to fill gaps in knowledge, help resolve conflicts, and help solve clinical problems.

Identifying and then selecting from among these potential problems is the second of the series of expansion and contraction of ideas that must occur before a research study is designed. Any given topic will yield many potentially researchable conflicts. The conflicts and voids that form the basis for research problems can be identified through a review of the professional literature. Table 2-2, based on the work of Kazdin,[30] shows how to develop ideas for rehabilitation research by adding novel "twists" to existing work found during the review of the literature. Details about finding relevant literature and synthesizing the results are presented in Chapters 4 and 26.

Theoretical Framework Identification and Selection

Defining and selecting a theoretical framework for the study is the third cycle of expansion (identification of possible frameworks) and contraction (selection of a framework) of ideas within the problem development process. After a problem is selected, it needs to be placed into a theoretical framework that will allow it to be viewed in relation to other research. Theoretical grounding provides a broad perspective from which to view the problem. Sometimes, a researcher will be drawn to a particular framework based on previous interests or education; other times, the researcher will need to read widely in several areas to settle on a framework that seems most promising for further study. Review information earlier in this chapter about theory to find a match between that information and the chosen problem.

Adopting a theoretical framework, then, is a way of choosing a lens through which one views the problem of interest. The framework helps the researcher define what will and will not be studied and helps the researcher select appropriate variables for study.

Question Identification and Selection

After the problem is identified and placed in a theoretical perspective, the researcher must develop the specific questions that will be studied. This is done through the fourth cycle of expansion (identification of many possible questions) and contraction (selection of a limited number of questions for study) of ideas within the problem development process.

A researcher may prefer to state the purpose of his or her study as a question; another may prefer to state his or her purpose as an objective, which takes the form of a declarative sentence. Either is acceptable, but researchers in rehabilitation should strive to develop research questions or statements of purpose for which results are measurable.

Table 2-2

Using Existing Research to Develop New Research Problems

General Form of Problem	Specific Hypothetical Question
Studying a well-known clinical phenomenon in the context of a new population	How does clinical depression present itself in individuals with acquired spinal cord injury?
Studying subgroups of clinical populations	What distinguishes adolescents with myelomeningocele who remain community ambulators from those who do not?
Developing research problems that apply basic research findings to clinical populations	Can the findings from animal research on tissue responses to overload stimuli from electrical stimulation be replicated in humans?
Extending previous work by modifying aspects of the independent variable	Would the same results have been achieved if speech therapy sessions were conducted more frequently?
Extending previous work by adding new dependent variables	Does aquatic therapy for individuals with knee osteoarthritis improve participation levels and health-related quality of life, in addition to its established impact on impairment measures such as strength and range of motion?
Extending previous work by studying new clinical populations or new health care settings	Can preschool-aged children with disabilities benefit from powered mobility to the same extent as the school-aged children who have been the subject of previous studies?
Studying the impact of covariates on the clinical phenomena	Do individuals from different cultures and from different socioeconomic strata perform differently on tests of aphasia?

After stating their purpose as either a question or an objective, many researchers advance a research hypothesis. The research hypothesis is the researcher's educated guess about the outcome of the study. This educated guess is generally based on the theoretical grounding for the study, previous research results, or the clinical experiences of the researchers. Having such a hypothesis enables a researcher to place his or her results into the context of the theory or experience that led them to conduct the study. Research hypotheses should not be confused with the statistical hypotheses within a study. The statistical hypotheses, subdivided into null and alternate hypotheses, are essentially given once a particular type of statistical analysis is selected. Statistical hypotheses are discussed in greater detail in Chapters 20 and 21.

Research Methods Identification and Selection

Only after the research question is determined can the investigator begin to consider which research methods are appropriate to answer the question. Research methods are discussed in detail in Chapters 5 to 16 and 19.

Criteria for Evaluating Research Problems

While proceeding through the steps of research problem development, the researcher is faced with several selection decisions. Which topic, problem, or question should be studied? Which research approach to the question should be adopted? Cummings and colleagues[31(p. 19)] believe that a good research problem is feasible, interesting, novel, ethical, and relevant; the acronym FINER can be used to remember these five characteristics.

Study Is Feasible

Feasibility should be assessed in terms of subjects, equipment and technical expertise, time, and money. Researchers need to be realistic about the technical resources available to them. If the proper equipment is not available, then another problem should be selected for study.

The time needed to complete a research study is often underestimated. As noted in Chapter 1, lack of time is a significant impediment for clinical researchers. Therefore, scientist-practitioners need to develop research questions that can be answered within the time constraints of their practices and students within the constraints of their classes or registrations for thesis or dissertation. Chapters on case reports (Chapter 13), single-subject designs (Chapter 11), and outcomes research (Chapter 16) introduce research methods that may fit well within the context of a busy clinical practice or academic calendar.

Financial resources needed to conduct research must also be considered. Direct costs such as equipment, postage, and printing must be met. Personnel costs may include salaries and benefits for the primary investigator, data collectors, secretaries, statisticians, engineers, and photographers. If there are no funds for statisticians and engineering consultants, then complex experimental designs with highly technical measures should not be attempted.

Problem Is Interesting

The research question must be of interest to the investigator. Because rehabilitation is practiced by a broad set of professionals and their research base is rapidly growing, a wide range of interesting unanswered questions exists. All rehabilitation practitioners should therefore be able to identify several questions that whet their intellectual appetites. Thus, interest in the topic must be high to motivate the researcher to move through the sometimes tedious steps necessary to reach the discovery.

Problem Is Novel

Good research is novel in that it adds to knowledge. However, novice researchers are often unrealistic in their desire to be totally original in what they do. Novelty can be found in projects that confirm or refute previous findings, extend previous findings, or provide new findings. Because many aspects of rehabilitation are not well documented, novel research ideas abound.

Problem Can Be Studied Ethically

An ethical study is one in which the elements of informed consent can be met and the risks of the research are in proportion to the potential benefits of the research, as described in Chapter 5. Readers should become familiar with ethical limitations to research.

Question Is Relevant

When developing research questions, rehabilitation practitioners need to answer an important relevancy question: "Who cares?" If the first phase of the problem development process was taken seriously, the researcher should be able to provide a ready answer to that question. If the researcher skipped that phase and generated

a research question without knowing how it related to a problem within rehabilitation, then the question may not be relevant to the field. Relevant rehabilitation research questions are grounded in day-to-day problems faced by scientist-practitioners.

SUMMARY

Theory, research, and practice are related through theories that are developed through reflection on experience or logical speculation, through research that tests theories, and through revisions of theory and clinical practice based on research results. Theory can be defined according to levels of restrictiveness, tentativeness, and testability. The different levels of theory are used for description, prediction, and explanation. Theories are also differentiated based on scope. Metatheory focuses on how knowledge is created and organized, as in the development of occupational science. Grand theories provide broad conceptualizations of phenomena, as in the World Health Organization's ICF,[12] Hislop's pathokinesiological framework for physical therapy,[14] and Kielhofner's MOHO.[15] General, or middle-range, theories provide general frameworks for action, as in the gate control theory of pain,[18] the sensory integration model,[19] and the PST.[25] Specific, or practice, theories are particular applications of grand or general theories, as in the application of ICF concepts to support the use of powered mobility for children with disabilities[26] and the role of the gate control theory of pain in the development of TENS.[27]

A hallmark of theory, especially for the scientist-practitioner, is its testability. Development of research questions begins with a general topic of interest but soon focuses on problems, often of a clinical nature. Problems arise from conflicts among and between knowledge, action, and policy. The resulting question needs to be viewed within a theoretical framework and should lead to research that is feasible, interesting, novel, ethical, and relevant and must take into account various potential barriers to its completion.

REFERENCES

1. Tammivaara J, Shepard KF: Theory: The guide to clinical practice and research, *Phys Ther* 70:578–582, 1990.
2. Kielhofner G: The organization and use of knowledge. In Kielhofner G, editor: *Conceptual Foundations of Occupational Therapy Practice*, 3rd ed, Philadelphia, Pa, 2003, FA Davis.
3. Fawcett J: *The Relationship of Theory and Research*, 3rd ed, Philadelphia, Pa, 1999, FA Davis.
4. Kerlinger FN, Lee HB: *Foundations of Behavioral Research*, 4th ed, Fort Worth, Tex, 2000, Harcourt College.

5. Burns N, Grove SK: *Understanding Nursing Research*, 5th ed, St Louis, Mo, 2011, Saunders.

6. Polit DF, Tatano Beck C: *Nursing Research: Generating and Assessing Evidence for Nursing Practice*, 9th ed, Philadelphia, Pa, 2012, Lippincott Williams & Wilkins.

7. Portney LG, Watkins MP: *Foundations of Clinical Research: Applications to Practice*, 3rd ed, Upper Saddle River, NJ, 2008, Prentice Hall.

8. Boorstin DJ: *The Discoverers: A History of Man's Search to Know His World and Himself*, New York, NY, 1985, Vintage.

9. Krebs DE, Harris SR: Elements of theory presentations in physical therapy, *Phys Ther* 68:690–693, 1988.

10. Reed KL: Theory and frame of reference. In Neistadt ME, Crepeau EB, editors: *Willard and Spackman's Occupational Therapy*, Philadelphia, Pa, 1998, JB Lippincott, pp 521–524.

11. Hagstrom F: Using and building theory in clinical action, *J Commun Disord* 34:371–384, 2001.

12. World Health Organization. International Classification of Functioning, Disability, and Health. Available at: http://www.who.int/classifications/icf/training/icfbeginnersguide.pdf. Accessed November 17, 2014.

13. Stephens D, Gianopoulos I, Kerr P: Determination and classification of the problems experienced by hearing-impaired elderly people, *Audiology* 40:294–300, 2001.

14. Hislop HJ: Tenth Mary McMillan lecture: The not-so-impossible dream, *Phys Ther* 55:1069–1080, 1975.

15. Kielhofner G: The model of human occupation. In Kielhofner G, editor: *Conceptual Foundations of Occupational Therapy*, 3rd ed, Philadelphia, Pa, 2004, FA Davis.

16. Pizzi M: The Model of Human Occupation and adults with HIV infection and AIDS, *Am J Occup Ther* 44:257–264, 1990.

17. Chen CY, Neufeld PS, Feely CA, Skinner CS: Factors influencing compliance with home exercise programs among patients with upper-extremity impairment, *Am J Occup Ther* 53:171–180, 1999.

18. Melzack R: From the gate to the neuromatrix, *Pain* 6:S121–S126, 1999.

19. Kielhofner G: The sensory integration model. In: Kielhofner G, editor: *Conceptual Foundations of Occupational Therapy*, 3rd ed, Philadelphia, Pa, 2004, FA Davis.

20. Ayres AJ, Marr DB: Sensory integration and praxis tests. In Bundy AC, Lane SJ, Murray EA, editors: *Sensory Integration: Theory and Practice*, 2nd ed, Philadelphia, Pa, 2002, FA Davis.

21. Bundy AC: The process of planning and implementing intervention. In Bundy AC, Lane SJ, Murray EA, editors: *Sensory Integration: Theory and Practice*, 2nd ed, Philadelphia, Pa, 2002, FA Davis.

22. Dawson G, Watling R: Interventions to facilitate auditory, visual, and motor integration in autism: A review of the evidence, *J Autism Dev Disord* 30:415–421, 2000.

23. Bumin G, Kayihan H: Effectiveness of two different sensory-integration programmes for children with spastic diplegic cerebral palsy, *Disabil Rehabil* 23:394–399, 2001.

24. Robichaud L, Hebert R, Desrosiers J: Efficacy of a sensory integration program on behaviors of inpatients with dementia, *Am J Occup Ther* 48:355–360, 1994.

25. Mueller MJ, Maluf KS: Tissue adaptation to physical stress: A proposed "physical stress theory" to guide physical therapist practice, education, and research, *Phys Ther* 82:383–403, 2002.

26. Wiart L, Darrah J: Changing philosophical perspectives on the management of children with physical disabilities—their effect on the use of powered mobility. *Disabil Rehabil* 24:492–498, 2002.

27. Rutjes AWS, Nuesch E, Sterchi R, et al: Transcutaneous electrostimulation for osteoarthritis of the knee (Review), *Cochrane Database Syst Rev* (1), 2010.

28. Osiri M, Welch V, Brosseau L, et al: Transcutaneous electrical nerve stimulation for knee osteoarthritis, *Cochrane Database Syst Rev*, 4: CD002823, 2000. Update in *Cochrane Database Syst Rev*, 4:CD002823, 2000.

29. Stevens B: *Nursing Theory: Analysis, Application, Evaluation*, 2nd ed, Boston, Mass, 1984, Little, Brown.

30. Kazdin AE: Selection of the research problem and design. In Kazdin AE, editor: *Research Design in Clinical Psychology*, 4th ed, Boston, Mass, 2003, Allyn & Bacon.

31. Cummings SR, Browner WS, Hulley SB: Conceiving the research question. In Hulley SB, Cummings SR, Browner WS, et al, editors: *Designing Clinical Research: An Epidemiological Approach*, 3rd ed, Philadelphia, Pa, 2001, Lippincott Williams & Wilkins, p 2007.

CHAPTER 3

Evidence-Based Practice

CHAPTER OUTLINE

The Need or Demand
What is Evidence-Based
   Practice?
Evidence-Based Practice Process
Evaluating Research Studies

Evaluating the Four Areas of
   Research Validity
Written Evaluations of Research
Instituting Evidence-Based Practice
Databases of Evaluated Studies

Limitations of Evidence-Based
   Practice
Summary

THE NEED OR DEMAND

The use of research results, or evidence, in health care practice is an important attribute of the health professions. Since the early 1990s, there has been an increased emphasis on use of evidence, prompted in part by health professionals but also by patients and third-party payers. The ethical principles of beneficence and nonmaleficence demand that health professionals use the best practices available, presumably those practices based on research, without inflicting harm on the patient. Although these principles have been at the heart of health care professions, the emphasis on using evidence to guide practice is relatively recent. Additionally, patients as consumers have been increasingly given the responsibility for determining their own health. As a result, patients are increasingly demanding that practitioners use the most effective interventions for a faster and/or most cost-effective recovery. Similarly, third-party payers are demanding that health care providers use the most cost-effective interventions with their insured patients in order to contain costs.

WHAT IS EVIDENCE-BASED PRACTICE?

In the early 1990s the evidence-based medicine (EBM) model was developed to increase physicians' use of published, peer-reviewed evidence in their patient care decision making.[1,2] Defined as "… the integration of the best research evidence with clinical expertise and patient values,"[3] EBM considers these three major aspects equally in clinical decision making. Although patients' reports, including their health and medical

history, and clinicians' observations are considered important evidence in health care practitioners' decision making, published research is considered the "evidence" in evidence-based practice.

Acknowledging that evidence can vary in its validity, the EBM model of practice developed a hierarchy of evidence to assist the physician in determining the validity of published research. The gold standard of the EBM evidence hierarchy is the randomized control trial (RCT). (Acknowledging that different research designs have different purposes, the American Academy of Cerebral Palsy and Developmental Medicine [AACPDM] has developed a separate hierarchy of evidence for single-subject studies that is comparable to the hierarchy of evidence for group studies.[4] The limitations of RCTs are discussed in Chapter 10 on group designs.) Further, the hierarchy considers quantitative studies to be stronger evidence than qualitative studies and multiple studies to be stronger than a single study, assuming equality of the studies.

The EBM practice model has five domains of medical practice and research. These are therapy/prevention/harm/etiology, prognosis, diagnosis, differential diagnosis/symptom prevalence, and economic and decision analysis. For each of the domains, there are five major levels of evidence (Table 3-1).[5] In four of the five domains of medical practice and research, the first three levels are further divided into sublevels of evidence. Specifically, in the first or highest level of evidence, there are three sublevels for the practice domains of therapy/prevention and etiology/harm. At the first sublevel (1a) are systematic reviews and meta-analyses of RCTs. In order for a systematic or meta-analytic review to be considered at this level, the review must meet

Table **3-1**

Levels of Evidence for Different Domains of Medical Practice and Medical Research

Level	Therapy/ Prevention, Etiology/Harm	Prognosis	Diagnosis	Differential Diagnosis/ Symptom Prevalence Study	Economic and Decision Analysis
1a	Systematic review (SR) (with homogeneity) of randomized controlled trials (RCTs)	SR (with homogeneity) of inception cohort studies; Clinical decision rule (CDR) validated in a single population	SR (with homogeneity) of level 1 diagnostic studies' CDR with 1b studies from different centers	SR of prospective cohort studies	SR of level 1 economic studies
1b	Individual RCT with narrow confidence interval (CI)	Individual inception cohort studies with >80% follow-up; CDR validated in a single population	Validating cohort study with good reference standards; CDR tested within one clinical center	Prospective cohort study with good follow-up	Analysis based on clinically sensible costs or alternatives; SR of the evidence and including multi-way sensitivity analyses
1c	All-or-none studies	All-or-none case studies	Absolute SpPins and SnNouts	All-or-none case series	Absolute better-value or worse-value analyses
2a	SR (with homogeneity) of cohort studies	SR (with homogeneity) of retrospective cohort studies or untreated control groups in RCTs	SR (with homogeneity) of level >2 diagnostic studies	SR of 2b and better studies	SR of level >2 economic studies
2b	Individual cohort study or low-quality RCT (e.g., <80% follow-up)	Retrospective cohort study or follow-up of untreated control patients in an RCT	Exploratory cohort study with good reference standards; CDR after derivation or validated only on split-sample databases	Retrospective cohort study, or poor follow-up	Analysis based on clinically sensible costs of alternatives; limited reviews of the evidence or single studies; and including multi-way sensitivity analyses
2c	Outcomes research; ecological studies	Outcomes research		Ecological studies	Audit or outcomes research
3a	SR (with homogeneity) of case-controlled studies		SR (with homogeneity) of 3b and better studies	SR of 3b and better studies	SR of 3b and better studies

Table 3-1—cont'd

Levels of Evidence for Different Domains of Medical Practice and Medical Research

Level	Therapy/ Prevention, Etiology/Harm	Prognosis	Diagnosis	Differential Diagnosis/ Symptom Prevalence Study	Economic and Decision Analysis
3b	Individual case-control study		Nonconsecutive study; or without consistently applied reference standards	Nonconsecutive cohort study or very limited population	Analysis based on limited alternatives or costs, poor-quality estimates of date but including sensitivity analyses incorporating clinically sensible variations
4	Case series and poor-quality cohort and case-control studies	Case series and poor-quality prognostic cohort studies	Case-control study, poor or non-independent reference standard	Case series or superseded reference standards	Analysis with no sensitivity analysis
5	Expert opinion without explicit critical appraisal or "bench" research studies	Expert opinion without explicit critical appraisal or "bench" research studies	Expert opinion without explicit critical appraisal or "bench" research studies	Expert opinion without explicit critical appraisal or "bench" research studies	Expert opinion without explicit critical appraisal or based on economic theory

Adapted from Oxford Centre for Evidence-Based Medicine: Levels of medicine (March 2009). Available at: www.cebm.net/index.aspx?o=1025. Accessed November 18, 2014.

specific criteria, including a criterion that the review provide sufficient information for replication of the review process. At the next sublevel (1b) are single RCT studies. The third sublevel (1c) is an all-or-none study, in which all subjects prior to the study die when they have the studied disease, but all subjects survive after the treatment is introduced.

At the next or second level in the hierarchy of evidence for the therapy/prevention/harm/etiology domain is cohort studies. In these, the experimenter identifies naturally occurring cohorts, each having different known risk factors for developing a particular adverse health condition. The groups are then followed to see which are more likely to develop the condition. Again, within this level, there are three sublevels of evidence, of which systematic reviews of cohort studies (2a) are considered the top of this level, followed by the individual cohort study or a low-quality RCT (2b). At the third level (2c) are outcomes research studies and ecological studies. The remainder of the hierarchy for the practice domains of therapy/prevention and harm/etiology, as well as for the other two domains of practice (i.e., prognosis and diagnosis) and of medical research, is presented in Table 3-1.

Further, Table 3-1 presents the EBM levels of evidence for each of the various domains of medical practice (e.g., prognosis, diagnosis, therapy/prevention, harm/etiology) based on the different methodological elements used in the research studies for each domain. From this table, it is clear that RCTs are a necessary methodological requirement for an intervention or therapy study to be at level 1 evidence, whereas for diagnostic and prognostic studies, cohort designs are considered necessary to achieve level 1 evidence.[6]

EVIDENCE-BASED PRACTICE PROCESS

As the EBM model was embraced by the medical community, the model was adopted by other health care professionals, including speech-language pathologists, audiologists, occupational therapists, and physical therapists. Termed *evidence-based practice* (EBP) by the wider health care community, Jewell[7] has used the term *evidence-based physical therapy* (EBPT) for the use of the paradigm by physical therapists. In this text, we will use the term EBP. Like EBM, EBP is a method of integrating the best available evidence (including the clinician's expertise) and patients' values into the scientist-practitioner's clinical decision making. In addition, EBP uses the same hierarchy of evidence as EBM. To implement the EBP, a five-step process is followed (Box 3-1).[3]

The EBP process begins with the scientist-practitioner formulating the patient care issue into an answerable question that will be, in part, answered by the best evidence. Remember, "best available evidence" is only one of three parts to the EBP clinical decision making. To assist the scientist-practitioner in formulating the patient care question, four considerations (i.e., patient characteristics, the intervention, the comparative intervention, and the outcomes), as represented by the acronym PICO, must be addressed.

- *P:* Represents the specific relevant patient characteristics and interests, such as the patient's health characteristics or condition, sex, age, lifestyle, avocations, and other interests, that may affect the patient's participation in the rehabilitation process.
- *I:* Represents the intervention, which the scientist-practitioner is considering for use in the patient's rehabilitation program. Often, when the scientist-practitioner

engages in the EBP process, he or she is seeking to determine whether one intervention is better than another intervention.

- *C:* Represents the comparison intervention. When a study compares the effect of an intervention to a control group that receives no intervention, the *C* represents the control group. Where the scientist-practitioner is considering what assessment instruments to use with a patient, the *I* stands for the assessment instrument under consideration, and the *C* represents the comparison assessment tool.
- *O:* Represents the outcome measures the scientist-practitioner will use to determine whether an intervention is likely to be effective or whether one intervention is more effective than another. Sometimes the outcome measures to be used will cover several different aspects of the patient's health. We suggest that the scientist-practitioner use the International Classification of Functioning, Disability, and Health (ICF) in determining which aspects of outcomes should be measured.[8] The ICF is further described in Chapter 16 on outcomes research.

Following these steps, the scientist-practitioner has now (1) identified the keywords that will be used to guide the literature search, and (2) developed a specific question to determine whether the found literature will help the scientist-practitioner in decision making.

After the keywords for the literature search have been identified, the literature search proceeds as described in Chapter 4. The found literature is then screened for relevance to the question. Typically, the found articles are screened or perused by title and abstract for relevance to the patient question. After the articles have been screened for relevance and accepted, the scientist-practitioner must evaluate the articles "... for (research) validity, for impact, and for clinical applicability."[3]

EVALUATING RESEARCH STUDIES

In the scientific arena, research results have been typically evaluated for validity or truthfulness by determining how rigorously the researchers restricted the influence of extraneous causes on the results. Even in studies in which the research is conducted in a clinical environment, as opposed to a laboratory setting, the emphasis is on the ability to state with confidence that study outcomes are due to the intervention and not some extraneous cause. Shadish and colleagues[9] proposed that a research study's validity be evaluated in four areas: (1) construct validity, (2) internal validity, (3) statistical validity, and (4) external validity. Table 3-2

Box 3-1

Five-Step Process for Implementing Evidence-Based Practice

Step 1	Formulating the question using the PICO steps*
Step 2	Identifying the evidence
Step 3	Critically appraising the evidence
Step 4	Applying the evidence
Step 5	Re-evaluating the application of the evidence

*See text for definition of the PICO steps.

Table 3-2

Manuscript Element×General Research Validity Types

Manuscript Element	Statistical Validity	Internal Validity	Construct Validity	External Validity
Introduction				
Literature Review			X	
Hypothesis, purpose			X	
Subjects				
Are the subjects representative of the population?				X
How were the subjects selected from a larger group of similar subjects?				X
Are the subjects similar to your patient?				X
What are the inclusion/exclusion criteria?			X	X
Were inclusion/exclusion criteria to increase likelihood of effect?	X	X		
Sample size ($N =$)				
Is the size large enough for the type of statistic used?	X			
Is the sample large enough for the desired effect size?	X			
How were the subjects assigned to groups?		X		
Were the subjects blind to their assignment?		X		
How many subjects completed the study?	X			X
If all did not complete the study, did they report why?		X		
Did subjects participate in activities that may have affected group outcomes?		X		X
Settings				
Was the setting sufficiently described to replicate the study?				X
How controlled was the setting?		X		X
Was the setting similar enough to your setting that you can apply the study to your setting?				X
Dependent Variable				
Are the outcome measures reflective of the purpose or hypothesis of the study?			X	
Was reliability reported? Are the measures reliable?	X			
What level of reliability was reported?*	X			
Was validity reported? Are the measures valid?	X			
Were reliability assessors independent?	X			
Design				
What threats to internal validity were controlled or not?		X		
What threats to external validity were controlled or not?				X
Was the study long enough to obtain reasonable outcomes?			X	X

Continued

Table 3-2—cont'd

Manuscript Element×General Research Validity Types

Manuscript Element	Statistical Validity	Internal Validity	Construct Validity	External Validity
	RESEARCH VALIDITY			
Was there follow-up to the outcomes after the study was completed?				X
Statistics				
Were the statistics used appropriate for the levels of measurements?	X			
Were the statistics used appropriate for the sample size?	X			
Were the statistics used appropriate for the number of groups?	X			
Were statistics used to control for confounding variables?	X			
Independent Variable (Intervention Procedures)				
Were the procedures described thoroughly enough for you to replicate the study?				X
Was the intervention consistent with the theory, hypothesis?			X	
Was there a "check" to see if the interventions were implemented as described?		X	X	
Were the therapists aware of the "check"?		X		
Were the observers blind to subject assignment?		X		
Were the therapists blind to the subject or intervention assignment?		X		
Results				
Did the results match what was stated in the purpose or hypothesis?			X	
Were the statistics appropriately used?	X			
Were all subjects analyzed?	X			
Was minimal clinically important difference presented?	X			
Discussion				
Did the authors interpret data correctly?	X	X	X	X

*Reliability (addressed by an *appropriate measure*):

Best reliability reported when the researchers have taken reliability measures *before* and *during* study, or if more than one phase, reliability measures taken during each phase.

Next best reliability reporting when the researchers have taken reliability measures *during* the study, or *during each phase* of the study, or *prior to* the start of a study.

Acceptable reliability reporting when researchers report reliability measures on same behaviors from other studies of *similar* subjects.

Less acceptable reliability reporting when researchers report reliability measures from other studies but of *disparate* subjects.

Least acceptable reliability reporting when researchers carefully describe dependent variable measurements.

Not acceptable reliability reporting when researchers have no report of reliability measures or acknowledgment of dependent variable reliability *or* present the wrong form of reliability for the use of the instrument.

presents which aspects of the different elements of a research manuscript address the four areas or subtypes of a research study's validity.

Evaluating the Four Areas of Research Validity

In the more traditional model of evaluating the construct validity of the research study, the scientist-practitioner is concerned with how well the theoretical constructs of the study are represented in the independent variable (IV) (i.e., the intervention) and the dependent variable (DV) in order to afford application to similar groups. That is, are these two variables sufficiently and specifically defined to ensure there is clarity and no confusion on (1) implementation of the intervention with the subjects of the study and (2) measurement of the dependent variables?

Construct validity is determined by how well the study controls for experimental bias and expectations (see Chapter 8) as well as by evaluating the rigor of the operational definitions of both the IV and DV. One way to reduce experimental bias is to conduct "procedural integrity checks" in order to ensure the IV was implemented as described in the procedures section of the study. In a single-subject investigation of the effectiveness of neurodevelopmental treatment (NDT) and a knee orthotic on knee flexion during gait, Embrey and colleagues[10] conducted a procedural integrity check by having an independent therapist record the delivery of the IV, any 1 of 10 specific NDT activities, in the intervention sessions. While watching the intervention sessions through a one-way mirror, the observing therapist recorded if the treating therapist was implementing any of the 10 activities correctly or incorrectly, or if no activity was being delivered, using a 10-second momentary time-sampling technique.

Although a carefully detailed, scripted procedures subsection, affording easy replication of the IV, will not ensure the IV has been implemented as described (i.e., has procedural integrity), the clarity and detail of the procedures suggest that the researchers were careful in implementing the procedures as described. A carefully detailed description of the IV or procedures will serve as an operational definition of the IV, if it meets the three criteria of a behavioral objective: measurable, clear, and complete.

The internal validity of a study is concerned with how well a study design controls factors or variables other than the intervention or IV for its influence on the study's results. Gliner and associates[11] have indicated that internal validity has two dimensions—the equivalence of groups and the control of extraneous

variables—that need to be considered when evaluating internal validity. Of course, in single-subject designs, in which there is no comparison group, internal validity is concerned only with the control of extraneous variables' influence on the DV. See Chapter 8 for a more extensive discussion of internal validity.

The third subtype of research validity to be evaluated, external validity, is concerned with how well the study results can be generalized to other populations similar to those in the study, or to a setting similar to the study setting. The factors affecting the external validity of a study, and how to control their influence, are presented in Chapter 8. Generally, the more a study has controlled for extraneous factors influencing the results (i.e., there is strong internal validity of the study), the less ability there is to generalize the results to other populations, settings, or treatments.[11]

A study's statistical validity addresses the statistical relationship of the IVs and DVs. Statistical validity is most frequently evaluated by examining the study's effect size, statistical power, appropriate use of statistical tests (sample size, scale of measurement), and measurement reliability (intraobserver or interobserver agreement/reliability) and variance.

By comparison, the EBP model of evaluating the research literature generally emphasizes three aspects of a study: (1) a study's validity, often emphasizing internal validity of the study; (2) a study's impact (e.g., treatment effect size); and (3) a study's clinical applicability (e.g., similarity of the study's intervention to the intervention being considered for use by the scientist-practitioner, the similarity of the study subjects to the scientist-practitioner's patient, the similarity of the study setting to the clinic).

When using the EBP model of evaluating a study's validity, impact, and clinical applicability, consideration of several criteria has been suggested. Two criteria sources are presented in Box 3-2. Jewell's criteria are a close adaptation of the Oxford Centre for Evidence-Based Medicine criteria for critically appraising RCTs.

Written Evaluations of Research

The Critically Appraised Topics (CAT),[12,13] intended as a one-page summary of a research study to be shared with colleagues, is a format for uniformly evaluating research studies using the EBP criteria presented in Box 3-2. The study's validity, impact, and clinical applicability are presumed to be evaluated when using these criteria. Typically, the CAT begins with the clinical question, followed by a "clinical bottom line,"

Box 3-2

Two Sources of Criteria for Determining an Intervention Study's Validity, Impact, and Clinical Applicability

Jewell*	Oxford Centre for Evidence-Based Medicine†
1. Did the investigators randomly assign (or allocate) subjects to groups?	1. Was the assignment of patients to treatments randomized?
2. Was each subject's group assignment concealed from people enrolling individuals in the study?	2. Were the groups similar at the start of the trial?
3. Did the groups have similar sociodemographic, clinical, and prognostic characteristics at the start of the study?	3. Aside from the allocated treatment, were groups treated equally?
4. Were subjects, clinicians, and outcome assessors masked (blinded) to the subjects' group assignment?	4. Were all patients who entered the trial accounted for? And were they analyzed in the groups to which they were randomized?
5. Did the investigators manage all of the groups in the same way except for the experimental intervention(s)?	5. Were the measures objective or were the patients and the clinicians "blind" to which treatment was being received?
6. Did subject attrition (e.g., withdrawal, loss to follow-up) occur over the course of the study?	6. How large was the treatment effect?
7. Did the investigators collect follow-up data on all subjects over a time frame long enough for the outcomes of interest to occur?	7. How precise was the estimate of the treatment effect?
8. Were subjects analyzed in the groups to which they were assigned?	

*Jewell DV: *Guide to Evidence-Based Physical Therapy Practice,* Sudbury, Mass, 2008, Jones and Bartlett, p 283.
†Oxford Centre for Evidence-Based Medicine: Critical appraisal tools. Available at: www.cebm.net/index.aspx?o=1157. Accessed November 18, 2014.

which is the evaluator's summary of the study's clinical applicability. Following the bottom line summary is the evaluator's summary of "key evidence" supporting the clinical bottom line. Finally, the evaluator presents an analysis of the study's strengths and weaknesses, particularly as the study meets the criteria, but also addressing other issues, such as factors other than the intervention that might have influenced the study's outcomes.

By contrast, the more traditional method of evaluating a study's research validity follows the same format in which the research manuscript is written. Each manuscript section (i.e., Methods, Results) and subsection (e.g., subjects and setting, DV, procedures/intervention) is evaluated for how well that section contributes to the four subtypes of research validity (see Table 3-2). However, each section or subsection does not have to address controls for all four subtypes of research validity. For example, in the Methods section of a manuscript, a traditional evaluation of statistical validity will note in the subject subsection if

the sample size was sufficient for the statistical tests used, and in the DV subsection what were the measurement reliability and validity of the DV measures; however, statistical validity will not be addressed within in the settings subsection. Furthermore, internal validity might be addressed, in part, in the subject subsection by the manner in which the subjects were recruited for the study and subsequently assigned to different groups and in the procedures subsection by how well each group received separate and distinct interventions.

INSTITUTING EVIDENCE-BASED PRACTICE

After the identified literature has been evaluated, the scientist-practitioner must determine whether the evidence from the literature evaluation supports or negates the specified intervention (or assessment instrument) or the comparative intervention (or assessment instrument) or whether there is insufficient evidence on which to base a decision. Regardless of the strength of evidence, the scientist-practitioner must consider the evidence in relationship to the other two aspects of the EBP model (i.e., clinical expertise and the patient's values and goals) when making a clinical decision. Examples of how scientist-practitioners have employed the EBP model are presented in *EBP Briefs*, a journal providing practicing speech-language pathologists with evidence-based reviews applicable to common clinical questions. Another source of examples on how to implement EBP was occasionally published in the journal *Physical Therapy*, under the feature *Evidence in Practice*, from 2004 through 2006. For example, in *EBP Briefs*, Murza and Nye[14] provided an evidence-based answer to the question, "Does explicit instruction in story grammar positively impact elementary school students' comprehension abilities in reading narrative text?" Keane-Miller and colleagues[15] described their use of EBP beginning with the PICO process to identify the keywords for the search process, a detailed description of the literature search, summaries of the selected studies, and the final decision of recommending patient placement on discharge from an acute care environment. Of note in the Keane-Miller and colleagues example was the authors' decision to ultimately base the patient's placement on the patient's values and goals because there was no definitive evidence on which to base a decision.

DATABASES OF EVALUATED STUDIES

As the use of EBP has grown, electronic collections or databases of reviewed articles on specific topics have emerged. These several databases are described in more detail in Chapter 4. Generally, these databases have specific criteria on which published research studies are evaluated. Some of these collections have professional staff conduct the evaluations (e.g., Cochrane Collection), whereas other databases have the evaluations conducted by volunteers (e.g., National Center for Evidence-Based Practice in Communication Disorders [N-CEP], Hooked on Evidence). Both the N-CEP and the Cochrane Collection conduct systematic reviews of topics using specified procedures and evaluative criteria for determining the strength of evidence for different interventions. These databases are meant as avenues for the busy scientist-practitioner to obtain reviews of research without actually having to read and evaluate the studies. The scientist-practitioner must decide whether the criteria by which the "evidence" is evaluated by these services are sufficiently rigorous to use the reviews without reading the original studies.

LIMITATIONS OF EVIDENCE-BASED PRACTICE

Despite the increased emphasis on the use of EBP, the process is not without its limitations. Several authors have suggested that the EBP emphasis on RCT studies as the gold standard is misleading,[16] in that not all RCTs can be considered better than alternative designs. Grossman and Mackenzie[16] and Bithell[17] argue that random assignment of studies with small sample sizes is likely to have an unbalanced distribution of variables among groups. Indeed, they suggest that matching on variables in small sample size studies may be a better design than an RCT. They also argue that an RCT may not be the best design for methodological reasons, such as the ethical basis of having a control group of no treatment. Others suggest that other methodological omissions in an RCT may make it a lesser design than other designs.[16–18] For example, a review of the EBP model for evaluating studies appears to emphasize the random assignment of subjects to groups, the blinding of assignment, the blinding of testing, and the blinding of treating, while de-emphasizing, or even disregarding, the importance of using measurement instruments that are reliable and valid and that have been developed for use with the specific population in the study.[16,18] Without reliable and valid measurements, a study's results are subject to strong suspicion, if not outright rejection.

Bluhm[19] argues that because RCTs are group designs, differences between groups are based on group averages, and the individual patient may not resemble the "average" patient. Others have suggested the apparent EBP model's emphasis on group studies, including RCTs, may lead the clinician to overlook the contributions of other designs, including qualitative and single-subject designs.[20] As noted earlier, the AACPDM's development of a separate "hierarchy of evidence" for single-subject design studies is a clear indication that designs other than RCTs may be of greater value in EBP than RCTs.[4,21]

SUMMARY

The EBP model has been embraced by the rehabilitation professions. One of the more significant issues facing EBP is how to implement EBP in the practice setting. The Internet has afforded the scientist-practitioner increased access to the research literature. The volume of research literature available to the health care professional reportedly doubles every 5 years.[22] This is a two-edged sword. Although the increased volume of published literature indicates that more information is available, it also means more literature for the scientist-practitioner to read and evaluate. Practitioners have argued that clinical productivity demands leave little or no time for the practitioner to remain abreast of the literature.[23] Relatedly, one of the largest barriers to the use of evidence in practice has been the practitioner's ability to understand and apply the literature.[23] Despite the multiple demands on the scientist-practitioner to remain current with research and to use evidence in practice, as well as the increased access to the literature, there is little evidence that the health care professional is routinely using evidence in practice. Yet the demands will continue for the practitioner to base practice on evidence. It is imperative that scientist-practitioners learn how to evaluate the evidence and import that evidence into their practice. Ultimately, perhaps the EBP model for the scientist-practitioner is supported by DiFabio's suggestion that "... the 'evidence' in evidence based practice is for each of us to decide."[24]

REFERENCES

1. Guyatt GH, Sackett DL, Cook DJ, for the Evidence-Based Medicine Working Group: Users' guides to the medical literature. II: How to use an article about therapy or prevention. A: What were the results and will they help me in caring for my patients? *JAMA* 270:2598–2601, 1993.
2. Guyatt GH, Sackett DL, Cook DJ, for the Evidence-Based Medicine Working Group: Users' guides to the medical literature. II: How to use an article about therapy or prevention. B: Were the results of the study valid? *JAMA* 271:59–63, 1994.
3. Sackett DL, Straus SE, Richardson WS, et al: *Evidence-Based Medicine: How to Practice and Teach EBM*, 2nd ed, Edinburgh, UK, 2000, Churchill Livingstone.
4. American Academy of Cerebral Palsy and Developmental Medicine. Methodology to develop systematic reviews of treatment interventions (revision 1.2), 2008 version. Available at: http://www.aacpdm.org/UserFiles/file/systematic-review-methodology.pdf. Accessed February 19, 2015.
5. Oxford Centre for Evidence-Based Medicine. Levels of medicine (March 2009). Available at: www.cebm.net/index.aspx?o=1025. Accessed November 18, 2014.
6. Toronto Centre for Evidence-Based Medicine. Is this a systematic review of evidence-based trials? Available at: www.cebm.utoronto.ca/practise/ca/therapysr/q1.htm. Accessed November 18, 2014.
7. Jewell DV: *Guide to Evidence-Based Physical Therapy Practice*, Sudbury, Mass, 2008, Jones and Bartlett.
8. World Health Organization. Family of international classifications: Definition, scope and purpose. Available at: www.who.int/classifications/en/FamilyDocument2007.pdf. Accessed November 18, 2014.
9. Shadish WR, Cook TD, Campbell DT: *Experimental and Quasi-Experimental Designs for Causal Inference*, Boston, Mass, 2002, Houghton Mifflin.
10. Embrey DG, Yates L, Mott DH: Effects of neurodevelopmental treatment and orthoses on knee flexion during gait: A single-subject design, *Phys Ther* 70:626–637, 1990.
11. Gliner JA, Morgan GA, Leech NL: *Research Methods in Applied Settings: An Integrated Approach to Design and Analysis*, 2nd ed, New York, NY, 2009, Taylor and Francis.
12. Oxford Centre for Evidence-Based Medicine. Critical appraisal tools. Available at: www.cebm.net/index.aspx?o=1157. Accessed November 18, 2014.
13. Fetter L, Figueiredo EM, Keane-Miller D, et al: Critically appraised topics, *Pediatr Phys Ther* 16:19–21, 2004.
14. Murza K, Nye C: A clinical language/literacy decision: Evidence-based story grammar instruction, *EBP Briefs* 3(4):1–14, 2008. Available at: www.speechandlanguage.com/ebp/pdfs/3-4-december-2008.pdf. Accessed November 18, 2014.
15. Keane-Miller D, Ellis T, Fetters L: Evidence in practice. Does the literature indicate that patients with a stroke have better outcomes after receiving rehabilitation from an acute rehabilitation facility than from a skilled nursing facility? *Phys Ther* 85:67–76, 2005.
16. Grossman J, Mackenzie FJ: The randomized controlled trial. Gold standard, or merely standard? *Perspect Biol Med* 48:516–534, 2005.
17. Bithell C: Evidence-based physiotherapy: Some thoughts on "best evidence," *Physiotherapy* 86:58–59, 2000.
18. Upshur RG: Looking for rules in a world of exceptions, *Perspect Biol Med* 48:477–489, 2005.
19. Bluhm R: From hierarchy to network: A richer view of evidence for evidence-based medicine, *Perspect Biol Med* 48:535–547, 2005.
20. Ritchie JE: Case series research: A case for qualitative method in assembling evidence, *Physiother Theory Pract* 17:127–135, 2001.
21. Romeiser Logan L, Hickman RR, Harris SR, Heriza CB: Single-subject research design: Recommendations for levels of evidence and quality rating, *Dev Med Child Neurol* 50:99–103, 2008.
22. Hook O: Scientific communications: History, electronic journals and impact factors, *Scand J Rehabil Med* 31:3–7, 1999.
23. Jette DU, Bacon K, Batty C, et al: Evidence-based practice: Beliefs, attitudes, knowledge, and behaviors of physical therapists, *Phys Ther* 83:786–805, 2003.
24. DiFabio RP: What is evidence? *JOSPT* 30:52–55, 2000.

CHAPTER 4

Finding Research Literature

CHAPTER OUTLINE

Reasons for Searching the Literature
Types of Information
Types of Professional Literature
Finding Literature
  Electronic Databases Not Site Specific
  Search Fields
  Boolean Operations
  Search Limits
Some Common Rehabilitation Databases

PubMed (MEDLINE)
EMBASE
Cumulative Index of Nursing and Allied Health Literature (CINAHL)
PsycINFO
Educational Resource Information Center (ERIC)
SPORTDiscus
Google Scholar
HighWire Press
Web of Science

Dissertation Abstracts International
Evidence-Based Review Databases
Library Catalogs
Reference Lists and Bibliographies
Single-Journal Indexes or Databases
Organizing Your Search
Summary

In this day of massive amounts of information, much of the available knowledge relevant to rehabilitation professions is in "the literature": that collection of journal articles, books, book chapters, conference papers, dissertations, essays, and opinion papers published to assist clinicians, researchers, scientist-practitioners, and aspiring professionals in developing and answering important questions. Although regular reading of the rehabilitation literature is an essential activity, just finding relevant literature has become a necessary skill in itself. Equally important, rehabilitation professionals and students must also learn how to sift through the information to identify and use manageable amounts of high-quality information. This chapter will help scientist-practitioners and students learn to use a wide array of contemporary tools to locate literature relevant to their practice or education. First, we identify reasons to search for literature and explain types of information and types of literature. We next present some basic information about the "nuts and bolts" of finding relevant literature, with particular emphasis on using electronic databases, and we provide a description of several relevant databases. We also give suggestions for using sources that are not database bound, both electronic and hard copy. We conclude the chapter with a strategy for using the information provided for an organized

search. Readers should recognize that they might need to modify the strategies and information in this chapter in response to the rapid pace of technological change in library and information services. In that regard, we will say it now, and again later: Do not hesitate to find and use the services of a professional medical librarian.

REASONS FOR SEARCHING THE LITERATURE

Chapter 3 developed the principles of evidence-based practice (EBP), and we have espoused these principles for effective clinical practice. Take note that the first word of EBP is "evidence," and that evidence resides in "the literature." Clinicians, researchers, and students all must incorporate evidence when deciding on courses of clinical application. To do so, they must find and analyze information about effectiveness and efficacy of particular treatment regimens, perhaps modified by application to specific populations and outcomes. They may wish to compare outcomes of more than one treatment. EBP simply cannot take place without some exploration of published information.

Locating literature is essential to developing a research question because research questions arise most often from those that have been explored before. Those

33

whose careers primarily involve research quite often continue a "research agenda," building one research question on others they have asked previously. But students, from undergraduate to doctoral, typically do not have that "line" (although doctoral students may be influenced by the agenda of their mentors). Thus, students typically start "cold," often without even an area of interest. It becomes critical to be able to find, then, even basic information about a topic, gradually collecting and analyzing the most recent and specialized literature so that a research question can be developed.

TYPES OF INFORMATION

The basic goal of any literature review is to discover what is known about a certain topic. Accomplishing this goal depends on at least four types of information about the topic: theory, facts, opinions, and methods. Some references provide primarily one type of information; others contain many different types of information. For example, a physical therapist who is interested in treating patients by means of continuous passive motion (CPM) therapy, or students learning about CPM, will likely want to know (1) theories about how CPM works, (2) factual information about protocols and results from other clinics, (3) opinions of therapists and surgeons about future directions for the clinical use of CPM, and (4) methods that others have used to measure the results of CPM use. A researcher planning a study in the area of CPM use after total knee arthroplasty needs to (1) place the topic of CPM into a conceptual, theoretical context, (2) know the facts (i.e., results) of previous investigations of CPM, (3) understand the opinions of other researchers about important areas still in need of study, and (4) be familiar with the methods others have used to measure and analyze data in previous studies.

TYPES OF PROFESSIONAL LITERATURE

The literature can be divided broadly into primary and secondary sources. We offer a third category, that of meta-analyses and critical reviews, which we consider a hybrid of primary and secondary literature.

Primary sources are those in which authors provide the original report of research they have conducted. Commonly encountered primary sources include journal articles describing original research, theses and dissertations, and conference abstracts and proceedings. Clinicians will probably seek out just a few primary articles from a literature review, selecting those that appear to have the most relevance to the particular types of patients they see or the settings in which they work. This

practice is consistent with our focus on EBP. Researchers tend to seek out many primary articles, selecting those that have the most potential to influence the work they plan to undertake. Students also need to learn to seek out primary articles for assigned papers, theses, and dissertations, and to become acculturated in the melding of clinical practice and consumption of professional literature.

Secondary sources of information are those in which the authors summarize their own work or the work of others. Books, book chapters, and journal articles that review the literature are considered secondary sources. We also consider editorials and opinion papers to be secondary sources. Secondary sources are useful because they organize the literature for the reader and provide a ready list of primary sources on the topic of interest.

In the past, secondary sources of information were often viewed as less important than primary sources, and researchers and clinicians alike were encouraged to always go to the primary source for their information. In today's world, with the explosion of information in all areas, including rehabilitation research, review articles and tutorials have gained new respect as a practical way for clinicians to update their knowledge regularly. For researchers, review articles can serve the important function of concisely summarizing gaps in the literature of interest and suggesting areas for further research. Although both clinicians and researchers can profitably use the secondary literature, both groups will likely wish to follow up with readings in the primary literature.

Critical reviews and meta-analyses review available literature on a topic but also go beyond simple description. In a sense, they—and especially meta-analyses—are "research about the research." In critical reviews, authors develop conclusions about a body of literature, often in response to a clinical question or treatment method. The review is based on rigorous criteria for examining research. In a meta-analysis, authors aggregate results from available studies and apply statistical procedures to draw conclusions. For example, in a combination critical review and meta-analysis, Smits-engelsman and colleagues[1] examined methods for improving motor performance in children with developmental disabilities. They reviewed 26 studies that met their inclusion criteria, finding strong effects for task-oriented intervention and physical and occupational therapies. In the field of speech-language pathology, Baker and McLeod[2] provided a review of studies on intervention methods used for children with speech-sound disorders. They reviewed 134 intervention studies, finding that nearly three fourths of the studies were quasi-experimental or nonexperimental. Finding seven different therapeutic approaches used, they concluded that the strength of evidence varied with therapeutic approach and research design.

FINDING LITERATURE

Electronic Databases Not Site Specific

Currently, anyone looking for literature may well start by searching electronic sources, particularly Web-based databases that do not represent only the holdings of a particular library or consortium of libraries. The essential function of databases is to provide a searchable aggregation of sources of information such as journal articles, books, book chapters, or dissertations. Some are very general (e.g., the familiar Google), but many are dedicated to providing access to information about specialized topics, including health-related topics.

Despite the presence of many databases—and their growing number—they have several common features, and learning these features will facilitate using any of them. We describe some we feel are the most commonly used, but the reader should not forget about using others when appropriate.

Search Fields

One common feature is that of search fields. These are categories that help limit your search to relevant items. An excellent start to the search process is to allow the database to do the searching and not choose a search field. However, if the topic is a common one, the search may yield several hundred or even several thousand results. In that case, an excellent next step is to use *keywords,* words that relate to the topic of interest and sometimes to the method of study (e.g., randomized clinical trial) or methods used to produce data. Keywords use familiar vocabulary. The Web site of the University of Illinois Library describes them as, "Natural language words describing your topic. A good way to start your search." In other words, using keywords is akin to a Google search. Though that seems simple—and often gives the results you want—because the terms you enter may not be recognized, it is possible to retrieve irrelevant results or to miss relevant results.[3]

Differing from the open language of keywords, using subject headings for searches is known as "controlled vocabulary searching" because only specific words or phrases are recognized as subject headings. Subject headings are provided by the Library of Congress or the National Library of Medicine (medical subject headings, or MeSH). Although catalogs have cross-referencing systems to help users who search under nonstandard subject headings, users who do not find the correct subject headings for their topic may miss valuable information. This is often the case when searching with outdated subject headings. A thesaurus of these subject headings should be available in the library, typically online, to help the practitioner determine the terms under which the desired information is likely to be found.

Taking a rather random example to explore subject terms, we found the article titled, "An exercise-based physical therapy program for patients with patellar tendinopathy after platelet-rich plasma injection"[4] in the CINAHL database (see later). Using "patellar tendinopathy" and "platelet-rich plasma" as subject terms, each yielded the article, meaning each one was a subject term to find this source.

Many journals now include keywords or subject terms in the articles themselves. For example, in the article cited above, in addition to "patellar tendinopathy" and "platelet-rich plasma," both of which appear in the title, the article also includes "growth substances" and "therapeutic exercise" as subject terms. Using those two as subject terms yielded the cited article (in fact, only that article).

One final note about subject headings as a field: Finding the exactly desired subject or subjects can become complex. To help, the CINAHL database has a very good online tutorial on using search terms.[5] PsycINFO and ERIC each has a thesaurus.[6,7] The National Library of Medicine's Web site contains an important section instructing viewers about MeSH and how to use it.[8] Using subject headings from MeSH only will facilitate searches.

One other useful search field is that of title. That is, entering "Title" as a search field will yield sources with your search terms in the title. Entering the entire title is not necessary. This is useful when looking for research that used a specific therapy regimen (e.g., "sensory integration"), published test (e.g., Peabody Picture Vocabulary Test), or published scale used as a dependent variable (e.g., "SF-36") or when looking for information about those procedures.

There are many other search fields, some more commonly used than others. One can search by author if the name of a particularly productive author is known or by publication name if results from one particular journal are needed. The list of fields is too long to review each one here, but we recommend getting to know the properties of at least several of them.

Boolean Operations

A very useful way of modifying searches is by Boolean operations. These operations form a set of ways to either limit or expand searches, and all databases use them. The operation AND will limit a search because the search engine needs to find two terms that appear together. For instance, searching for "spinal cord injury" AND "continuous passive motion" (with no other limits) yielded just seven results on CINAHL. The operation OR will expand a search because the search engine can produce either of two (or any of three) terms. Searching for "spinal cord injury" OR "continuous passive motion" yielded 8715 citations, a result of questionable utility. The NOT operator may also limit a search. This becomes useful if a search term that has similar terms is considered.

Search Limits

Another common feature of Web-based databases is that of limits. That is, searches can be limited using one or more parameters. These limits are most often found in the "advanced" search section of the database. One of the most common limits is that of publication date or a time span of publication, which is useful because often only the most recent sources are sought. Using the example of "spinal cord injury," a search on that term in CINAHL with no limits yielded 8424 sources—a distinctly unwieldy result. Limiting the search to the publication years 2010 to 2013 cut the result to 2380; this is better but still a lot of sources to filter.

Language can be limited to English or one of several other languages, although so much is written in English we find this limit not overly helpful. Limiting the spinal cord injury search to English language articles cut the result to 2309.

Limiting results by age of study participants can be helpful because researchers are often interested in a particular age group, especially if asking an EBP question. Limiting the spinal cord injury search to 65+ years resulted in 368 hits, a manageable number in our opinion.

Several other types of limits exist, but we will not review all of them. Different databases may have different types of limits, so researchers should become familiar with the most popular and useful ones and remember to use them. Using a combination of keywords, subject terms, Boolean operators, search fields, and limits, researchers should be well on the way to finding the literature needed. However, it is difficult to become an expert, and researchers should not hesitate to use the services of a trained medical librarian.

SOME COMMON REHABILITATION DATABASES

We are about to describe some of the more commonly used databases to find literature on rehabilitation. Because there are many databases, and because they are both complex and evolving, our review is necessarily cursory.

All of these databases are widely available in medical school libraries and the libraries of institutions with rehabilitation programs. The databases are supplied to libraries through various vendors or "platforms," so the looks and features of the database vary from library to library, but the contents remain the same. Individual access to each of these databases may also be available. Some databases (e.g., CINAHL and PsycINFO) have a link to the complete list of indexed journals; others (e.g., ERIC) do not. However, it is very easy to determine whether a database indexes a particular journal. All that is necessary is to enter the journal name as a limiting field and hit "Search." If there are no results, the database does not use that journal. The databases provide complete indexing of some of the journals and selective indexing of other journals. This means that, even though two databases include a particular journal, different articles from the journal may be selected for inclusion in each of the databases. Because of the irregular overlapping of coverage among databases, users who wish to be as comprehensive as possible should search several databases. Even though many of the same articles are identified by different databases, each database typically identifies unique resources not identified by others.

PubMed (MEDLINE)

The U.S. National Library of Medicine maintains a database of medically related information called MEDLINE and makes it available electronically as the database PubMed. The entries in the database are indexed according to the medical subject headings (MeSH) of the National Library of Medicine. It is available to anyone at www.ncbi.nlm.nih.gov/pubmed/. PubMed is probably the first database researchers will want for a medically related subject, even those subjects outside of the rehabilitation professions, such as the effects of various drugs. Although exceptionally complete, PubMed can be daunting to use. However, the site itself has various tutorials[8] as well as FAQs to help.

EMBASE

EMBASE is a proprietary database that combines MEDLINE with additional resources, particularly in biomedical research and pharmacology.[9] Available by subscription, most users gain access to this database through an academic library or an employer subscription.

Cumulative Index of Nursing and Allied Health Literature (CINAHL)

CINAHL Plus with Full Text (CINAHL) was developed in 1956 to meet the needs of nonphysician health care practitioners because some journals of interest to nurses and other health professionals may not be indexed in MEDLINE. CINAHL may provide a means to gain access to these journals. Recently, CINAHL has added a growing number of full-text articles to its database. We find it an extremely useful database for rehabilitation professionals. In addition to journals, CINAHL indexes books of interest to nurses and other health professionals and nursing dissertations. The CINAHL indexing terms are based on MeSH but provide for greater specificity in the terms related to each profession represented in the index. Wong and associates[10] found that, by combining indexing terms and search words, they were able to achieve high sensitivity and specificity in retrieving sound treatment studies and review articles in CINAHL. We provided some examples of the efficacy of CINAHL searches earlier. Libraries that serve health professionals generally subscribe to CINAHL. It is also available online by subscription to individual users.

PsycINFO

The PsycINFO database, produced by the American Psychological Association, provides extensive coverage of journals in psychology and related disciplines, as well as some book chapters, dissertations, and various university and government reports. Information is available at www.apa.org/psycinfo/. Most academic libraries and large employers with psychology services purchase an institutional subscription to PsycINFO, and searches are available through their Web pages. Individual subscriptions are available as well.

Among rehabilitation professions, we find PsycINFO particularly useful for speech-language pathology and audiology because speech, language, and audition are considered topics in or related to psychology. It is quite useful for rehabilitation when searching for generalized topics such as quality of life or cognitive changes with aging. It may be less useful in finding rehabilitation literature that is medically oriented or in finding information about treatments that have no psychological correlates. For example, a search on "patellar tendinopathy" (without any modifications) yielded only five results, whereas the same search on CINAHL yielded 190.

Educational Resource Information Center (ERIC)

The Educational Resource Information Center (ERIC) is a large database of education-related documents and articles. Funded by the U.S. Department of Education, it offers free database access at www.eric.ed.gov. Like PubMed, it can also be accessed through different interfaces available in academic libraries. Rehabilitation professionals who interface with the educational system through school-based services, physical education, and sports may find ERIC to be a good source of information on relevant topics. Note that, in addition to journal articles and other typical research literature, ERIC contains grant reports and other documents written by researchers, but without peer review. Sometimes there is review within a federal agency. Users of ERIC need to be rigorous in examining literature obtained on ERIC.

SPORTDiscus

SPORTDiscus is a large sport, fitness, and sports medicine bibliographic database (http://www.ebscohost.com/academic/sportdiscus-with-full-text). Based in Canada, it includes journal citations and book references, as well as access to relevant theses and dissertations. Many academic libraries and sports-related employers purchase institutional subscriptions to the database.

Google Scholar

Managed by the same company as the very familiar Google, Google Scholar indexes literature from a very broad array of professional literature, both within and outside of rehabilitation. According to its Web site (www.scholar.google.com/intl/en/scholar/about.html), researchers can "search across many disciplines and sources: articles, theses, books, abstracts and court opinions, from academic publishers, professional societies, online repositories, universities and other web sites."[11] A helpful feature is that articles are ranked by relevance. Another relevant feature is its citation search capability. That is, it will find sources that cite an article (or other source) you enter as a search term.

HighWire Press

HighWire is a service of Stanford University. Its Web site indicates that it disseminates electronically information from "1783 journals, reference works, books, and proceedings" with more than 5 million full-text articles from publishers, societies, associations, and university presses.[12] HighWire is limited to searching online journals, perhaps both an advantage and a limitation. One advantage is that online journals continue to increase in number. For example, all the professional journals of the American Speech-Language-Hearing Association (ASHA) and the American Physical Therapy Association are now available in online format. Thus, the user of HighWire is poised to easily take advantage of future electronic journal additions.

Web of Science

An often-effective search strategy is to find a useful article, and then search for other, more recent, articles and book chapters that have cited the older source. In the past, this was most often accomplished with the Science Citation Index and Social Science Citation Index (and, to a lesser extent, with the Arts and Humanities Citation Index). These sources have been incorporated into the newer Web of Science. Its Web site indicates that it provides "quick, powerful access to the world's leading citation databases. Authoritative, multidisciplinary content covers more than 12,000 of the highest impact journals worldwide, including Open Access journals and more than 150,000 conference proceedings."[13]

Dissertation Abstracts International

Master's theses and, more often, doctoral dissertations should be considered a fruitful source of information for searches. Dissertation Abstracts International now indexes virtually every dissertation written in the ProQuest Dissertation Abstracts International, and you will likely find what you are looking for in its ProQuest Dissertations and Theses (PQDT) database.[14] Both its sections (Section A, Humanities and Social Sciences; and Section B, Sciences and Engineering) may yield relevant information for rehabilitation professionals.

Evidence-Based Review Databases

Several reference products not only inform the user of relevant sources but also provide commentary or rate the quality of articles to assist in assessing the potential value of the literature.

The Cochrane Library is probably the best known of these.[15] It is an electronic collection of evidence-based reviews of health care research, each review culminating in a qualitative evaluation. Each review uses a systematic search of literature on the topic, with expert synthesis across sources of information. Subscribers, including many medical and academic libraries, have access to a searchable database of reviews and links to the full text of reviews. In addition, relevant Cochrane reviews are indexed in the major bibliographic databases, such as PubMed.

The Physiotherapy Evidence Database (PEDro) is a product of the Centre for Evidence-Based Physiotherapy at The George Institute for Global Health in Australia.[16] Full, free access to PEDro is available on the Internet (www.pedro.org.au). This database includes clinical trials, systematic reviews, and practice guidelines in physical therapy. The trials are rated with a 10-item checklist (the PEDro scale) to help readers assess the quality of the trial. OTseeker is a parallel project developed at the University of Queensland in Australia. It is "a database that contains abstracts of systematic reviews and randomised controlled trials relevant to occupational therapy."[17] Like PEDro, full, free access to OTseeker is available on the Internet (www.otseeker.com).

Hooked on Evidence is a relatively new initiative of the American Physical Therapy Association.[18] Volunteers, usually members of the association, extract and verify information from articles about physical therapy interventions. The abstracted variables include a variety of indicators of quality, such as research design, allocation methods, and the level of researcher and participant masking. However, the site cautions, "The database does not include practice guidelines, systematic reviews, articles on diagnostic and prognostic tests, or outcome measures"; thus, those seeking information about those categories need to search elsewhere. Members of the American Physical Therapy Association have full access to the database, including its search features.

A similar project, sponsored by the ASHA, is the National Center for Evidence-Based Practice (ASHA/N-CEP).[19] Part of the Center's activities include providing evidence-based systematic reviews of literature relevant to speech-language pathology and audiology. Each of these reviews is limited to a specific clinical question or clinical procedure.

LIBRARY CATALOGS

Although just about every library (or shared) catalog these days is an electronic database, catalogs differ from the databases described previously in that they index only the holdings of a particular library or consortium of libraries (such as all the colleges and universities in a particular state). One advantage is that researchers know materials will be readily available. Another is that material in all media will be represented, including film and sound recordings. Online library catalogs tend to differ from one institution to another, so most of them include search instructions. Essentially, the searching tools are not very different from those described for the databases that are not site specific.

REFERENCE LISTS AND BIBLIOGRAPHIES

Whether on paper or on the Internet, book chapters and articles will have a list of references (i.e., works cited in the text) and may have a bibliography (list of relevant related sources). Using these can provide valuable information sources, although researchers will probably not use them until they begin reading in their area. The obvious limitation, especially for book chapters, is that no sources listed can be more recent than the list currently being perused (although you may occasionally see a reference to a work "in press"). Despite the limitation, if the work seems valuable, it is likely the researcher will find other valuable sources in the reference list or bibliography. The advantages are that all the cited works will be relevant to the article or chapter just read, and the process of locating those related sources is a fast and easy one.

SINGLE-JOURNAL INDEXES OR DATABASES

Many professionals receive one or more journals regularly either as a benefit of belonging to a professional association or by subscribing to a journal of particular interest. One's own journals are a convenient starting point for a literature search, particularly if the journal is not indexed in one of the non-site-specific databases. Many journals publish an annual subject and author index in the last issue of each volume. Thus, readers with an interest in a particular topic can easily identify any pertinent citations from the journals in their own collection. Even if a professional decides not to retain all the journals he or she receives, this ready source of citations can be maintained by keeping the annual indexes from each journal. Alternatively, many journals maintain Web sites with searchable databases of contents. For example, ASHA's Web site (www.asha.org) has a searchable database for each of its four scholarly journals. Likewise, the journal *Physical Therapy* has a searchable database at http://ptjournal.apta.org/.[20] Several specialty sections of the American Physical Therapy Association publish journals with online databases.

ORGANIZING YOUR SEARCH

It is time to put together what we have discussed about the characteristics and locations of various sources of information for a literature search. This can be integrated into a series of logical steps so that the search is an organized and coherent one. We recommend beginning the search with Internet-based databases.

First, define the information needed. For example, in the case of a question of evidence-based practice, a researcher may wish to know about a treatment method, a particular population (e.g., an age group), an outcome, and how that treatment method compares with others.

Second, break the information needed into components. Components should flow from the question. It is common, however, to start a search without a well-defined question. This is often the case for students who need to develop a topic for a class paper or even dissertation. Do not be dismayed, but begin with whatever components are available, even if they are few and quite general.

Third, identify synonyms for each concept or component. This enables the researcher to start with a keyword search and use the information provided to refine the search by using standardized subject headings.

Fourth, construct logical relationships among the concepts, using the terms "AND," "OR," and "NOT." Figure 4-1 shows the relationships that are defined by the use of these terms. Recall that "AND" narrows a search, as does "NOT." This command lops off a portion of the search that is not of interest to the researcher. In

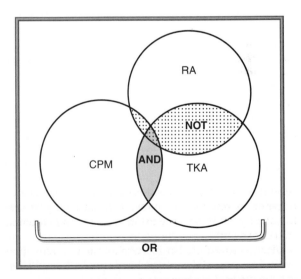

Figure 4-1 Illustration of Boolean relationships. Specifying "continuous passive motion (CPM) OR total knee arthroplasty (TKA)" would result in retrieval of articles in both circles, including the shaded intersection of both circles. Adding the command "NOT rheumatoid arthritis (RA)" would result in the elimination of all the stippled areas in the figure. Specifying "CPM and TKA NOT RA" would result in retrieval of articles in the shaded intersection, excluding the stippled, shaded region.

contrast, the use of "OR" broadens a search to include articles that include at least one of the specified terms.

Fifth, limit the search according to certain variables offered by the database. Common limits relate to "language" and "years of publication." See above for other common limits.

Do not limit a search to one database or other source. The literature of the different rehabilitation professions may be found in different databases. Even within one profession, different databases will return different search results because of the particular sources indexed in that database. For example, a mapping of the literature of selected health professions found that for physical therapy, CINAHL was the most productive database for finding journal articles, but other databases were helpful.[21] In contrast, a combined search of MEDLINE and PsycINFO would be more comprehensive for speech-language pathology.[22]

As the researcher proceeds in finding research literature, an extremely important step is to keep scrupulous records of searches, including databases used, keywords, Boolean operators, and results. This step is particularly important when preparing a systematic critical review of literature. Chapter 26 provides much detail on how to proceed.

We have recommended beginning with non-site-specific databases such as PubMed or CINAHL. However, do not neglect the other source types mentioned previously, particularly if they are convenient. Early on in the search, consult a recent textbook or recent journals in a personal collection or the collection of a nearby library.

We will conclude by noting that, much to many searchers' chagrin, the search process is not a linear one; there is not one path. Rather, literature searches contain loops, retracings, and refining of questions, necessitating repeated searches. Researchers may find just one or two articles of interest and, after reading them, look for other work by the same author or other relevant works in the same journal. Researchers may refine the research question by noting gaps and flaws in articles or chapters read, followed by looking for literature with a different set of keywords and synonyms, subject headings, and Boolean operations. No matter how it proceeds, it is critical to remain flexible and curious. And do not forget the medical librarian.

SUMMARY

The ability to locate published sources of information—"the literature"—has become an invaluable skill for today's rehabilitation scientist-practitioner or student, particularly with the ascendance of evidence-based practice. Rehabilitation professionals need to be aware of the types of and differences among sources of information. Secondary sources, such as textbooks, can serve an explanatory role as well as provide sources for further exploration. Systematic reviews and meta-analyses, also secondary sources, will be more current, will provide analyses of reviewed literature, and will also provide leads to more sources. Primary sources, especially journal articles, will provide the most current information and will allow readers to evaluate each source.

The ability to use electronic databases is at the heart of finding information. Scientist practitioners need to become familiar with at least the most common non-site-specific databases and learn to search through them using their various features such as search fields, Boolean operations, and search limits. Although seemingly daunting at times, we have provided several suggestions for organizing literature searches. And, we remind readers, do not forget the medical librarian.

REFERENCES

1. Smits-engelsman BCM, Blank R, van der Kaay AC, et al: Efficacy of interventions to improve motor performance in children with developmental coordination disorder: A combined systematic review and meta-analysis, *Dev Med Child Neurol* 55(3):229–237, 2013.
2. Baker E, McLeod S: Evidence-based practice for children with speech-sound disorders: Part 1 narrative review, *Lang Speech Hear Serv Schools* 42(2):102–139, 2011.
3. University of Illinois: Keyword searching vs. subject searching. Available at: http://www.library.illinois.edu/learn/research/keywordvssubject.html. Accessed February 7, 2015.
4. Van Ark M, Van den Akker-Scheek I, Meijer LTB, Zwerver J: An exercise-based physical therapy program for patients with patellar tendinopathy after platelet-rich plasma injection, *Phys Ther Sport* 14(2):124–130, 2013.
5. EBSCO. Using CINAHL/MeSH headings. Available at: http://support.ebsco.com/training/flash_videos/cinahl_mesh/cinahl_mesh.html. November 18, 2014.
6. EBSCO. PsycINFO thesaurus. Available at: http://gsuproxy.govst.edu:3962/ehost/thesaurus?sid=30265d62-ecd0-438a-9a5e-5080af1dead8%40sessionmgr4002&vid=2&hid=4212. Accessed February 7, 2015.
7. EBSCO. ERIC thesaurus. Available at: http://gsuproxy.govst.edu:3962/ehost/thesaurus?sid=856a8e59-aec2-46de-93c7-32a673f24a0a%40sessionmgr4005&vid=2&hid=4212. Accessed February 7, 2015.
8. National Library of Medicine. PubMed tutorial. Available at: www.nlm.nih.gov/bsd/disted/pubmedtutorial/015_010.html. Accessed November 18, 2014.
9. Elsevier. Embase biomedical database. Available at: http://www.elsevier.com/online-tools/embase. Accessed November 19, 2014.
10. Wong SSL, Wilczynski NL, Haynes RB: Optimal CINAHL search strategies for identifying therapy studies and review articles, *J Nurs Scholarsh* 38(2):194–199, 2006.

11. Google. Google scholar. Available at: scholar.google.com/intl/en/scholar/about.html. Accessed November 18, 2014.

12. Stanford University. HighWire Press. Available at: http://highwire.stanford.edu/about/. Accessed November 18, 2014.

13. Thomson Reuters. The web of science. Available at: http://thomsonreuters.com/web-of-science/. Accessed November 18, 2014.

14. ProQuest. Dissertation Abstracts International (DAI). Available at: http://www.proquest.com/products-services/proquest-dissertations-theses-full-text.html. Accessed February 7, 2015.

15. Cochrane Collaboration. The Cochrane Collaboration. Available at: www.cochrane.org/reviews/clibaccess.htm. Accessed November 18, 2013.

16. George Institute for Global Health. PEDro: Physiotherapy evidence database. Available at: www.pedro.org.au/. Accessed November 18, 2013.

17. OTseeker. Welcome to OTseeker. Available at: www.otseeker.com/. Accessed November 18, 2014.

18. American Physical Therapy Association. Hooked on Evidence. Available at: www.hookedonevidence.org/. Accessed November 18, 2014.

19. American Speech-Language-Hearing Association. ASHA/N-CEP evidence-based systematic reviews. Available at: http://www.asha.org/Members/ebp/EBSRs.htm. Accessed November 18, 2014.

20. American Physical Therapy Association. *Physical therapy*. Available at: http://ptjournal.apta.org/. Accessed November 18, 2014.

21. Fell DW, Burnham JF, Buchanan MJ, et al: Mapping the core journals of the physical therapy literature, *J Med Library Assoc* 99(3):202–207, 2011.

22. Slater LG: Mapping the literature of speech-language pathology, *Bull Med Libr Assoc* 85:297–302, 1997.

CHAPTER OUTLINE

Boundaries Between Practice and Research
Moral Principles of Action
 The Principle of Beneficence
 The Principle of Nonmaleficence
 The Principle of Utility
 The Principle of Autonomy
 Health Information Portability and Accountability Act
 Other Moral Principles

Informed Consent
Research Codes of Ethics
 Informed Consent
 Design Justifies Study
 Avoidance of Suffering and Injury
 Risk Is Commensurate with Potential Benefit
 Independent Review
 Publication Integrity
 Explicit Attention to Ethics

 Ethics in Professional Codes
Research Risks
 Physical Risks
 Psychological Risks
 Social Risks
 Economic Risks
Summary

The public expects, rightfully so, that researchers, perhaps most critically those engaged in research with human subjects, will conduct their research in an ethical manner. And it is probable that everybody has some notion of what that means—being honest, not being biased, and so on. And yet, unethical research behavior is common enough so that the U.S. Department of Health and Human Services has established the Office of Human Research Protection (OHRP).[1] The OHRP does investigate allegations of ethical misconduct, but it also provides a large amount of material on ethics policy and guidance and sponsors a substantial amount of educational activity. We emphasize from this that (1) ethics is likely more complex than most people's conception, (2) ethical misconduct is avoidable, and (3) learning about ethics is an ongoing process.

Complex ethical issues should be raised every time researchers ask others to assume the risks of their research—even seemingly low-risk research. The purpose of this chapter is to articulate ethical principles of importance to the conduct of research. First, attention is given to determining the boundaries between practice and research. Second, basic moral principles of action are presented. Examples of these moral principles in action are given for occurrences in everyday life, for treatment situations, and for research settings. Third, a special case of the moral principle of autonomy—informed consent—is examined in detail. Fourth, the application of the moral principles to research is illustrated through analysis of several widely used research

codes of ethics. Finally, a categorization of research risks is presented.

A note on terminology is required before moving into the content of the chapter. Contemporary usage favors the term research "participant" rather than "subject," emphasizing the active role played by individuals who consent to participate in research studies. However, this usage is sometimes confusing when writing about researchers and subjects because both are participants in the research process. In addition, in a chapter like this in which practice and research are contrasted, it is useful to sharpen the differences between patients or clients seeking services for their own benefit and subjects or research participants who should not expect benefits from their participation. Therefore, the term "subject" is used when "participant" would be confusing or would not set up the desired contrast.

BOUNDARIES BETWEEN PRACTICE AND RESEARCH

Every provider–patient relationship is predicated on the principle that the provider can render services that are likely to benefit the patient or client. The roles, relationships, and goals found in the treatment milieu can be, however, vastly different from those in the research setting. In the research setting, the health care professional becomes an investigator rather than a practitioner; the patient becomes a participant or subject. The patient seeks out a practitioner who may or may not decide to accept the patient for treatment;

the investigator seeks out potential subjects who may or may not agree to participate in the proposed research. The patient's goal is improvement; the investigator's goal is development of knowledge.

When standard health care is delivered in the context of provider–patient interaction, it is clear that the intent of the episode is therapeutic. When an innovative treatment technique is tested on a group of normal volunteers, it is clear that the intent of the episode is knowledge development. However, when a new technique is administered to a clinical population, the distinction between treatment and research becomes blurred. If the health care professional views each participant as a patient, then individualized treatment modifications based on each patient's response would be expected. Alternatively, if the clinician views each participant as a subject, then standardization of treatment protocols is often desirable. Protecting subjects from the risks of participating in research requires that one be able to distinguish research from practice. The National Commission for the Protection of Human Subjects of Biomedical and Behavioral Research, in its historic *Belmont Report*, developed a definition of research that makes such a distinction:

> Research (involving humans) is any manipulation, observation, or other study of a human being ... done with the intent of developing new knowledge and which differs in any way from customary medical (or other professional) practice.... Research may usually be identified by virtue of the fact that [it] is conducted according to a plan.[2(pp. 6,7)]

Three main elements of this definition warrant careful consideration: intent, innovation, and plan.

The Belmont definition recognizes that a fundamental difference between practice and research is that the two entities have different intents. Practice goals relate to individual patients; research goals relate to the development of new knowledge. Because of these disparate goals, different levels of protection from risk are needed for patients and subjects.

Health care rendered to an individual is always presumed to have some probability of benefit. When deciding whether to undergo a particular treatment, a patient will evaluate its risks against its potential benefits. In contrast, research on human participants is often of no benefit to the individual who assumes the risk of participation; rather, subsequent patients benefit from the application of the new knowledge. Some projects fall in a gray zone between research and practice. In this zone, innovative therapies with potential benefits are tested, providing both potential individual benefits and new knowledge.[2]

The second element of the Belmont definition is that the procedure differs in some way from customary practice. Simply reporting the treatment results of a series of patients who have undergone standard shoulder reconstruction rehabilitation would not be considered research. Because the treatment given is not innovative, the patients do not need special protection; the risk of being a patient whose results happen to be reported is no different than the risk associated with the treatment. Note, however, that if standard treatment calls for formal strength testing every 4 weeks, but the group in the series is tested every week, this should now be considered research. The risks of repeated formal strength testing, however minimal, are different than the risks of standard treatment alone. An implication of this component of the Belmont definition is that innovative therapies should be considered research and be conducted with appropriate research safeguards, until they can be shown to be effective and are adopted as accepted or customary practice.

The third element of the Belmont definition distinguishing research from practice is that research generally is conducted according to a plan. This implies a level of control and uniformity that is usually absent from clinical practice. However, you should note that single-subject research (see Chapter 11) is often very similar to clinical practice. And although the plan of single-subject research can be more flexible than that of group experiments, it is still planned research.[3] As such, single-subject experiments require the same attention to ethical treatment of participants as do group-design experiments.

MORAL PRINCIPLES OF ACTION

All professionals deal with complex, specialized issues for which the correct course of action may not be clear. Thus, professionals tend to be guided not by a rigid set of rules, but by general principles that demand that each practitioner assess a given situation in light of those principles and make decisions accordingly.

Although the content of the decisions one makes as a professional differs from one's personal decisions, the underlying principles that should guide these decisions are the same. This is also the case whether one is acting as a practitioner seeing a patient or as an investigator studying a research participant: The content of practice and research decisions may differ, but the underlying principles remain the same. Before presenting ethical principles for the conduct of research, it is therefore appropriate to lay a common groundwork of moral principles of action. Four major principles are discussed: beneficence, nonmaleficence, utility, and autonomy.

Examples from daily life, practice, and research are used to illustrate these principles.

The Principle of Beneficence

The principle of beneficence, particularly when considering research, requires that "there will be some benefit not only to those people participating in the study but also to the wider population."[4(p. 87)] Not only should we not harm them, but we should also attempt to help them. A daily example of the principle of beneficence is the person who goes grocery shopping for a homebound neighbor.

The professional–client relationship is based on the principle of beneficence. Patients would not come to health care professionals unless the patients believed that the professionals could help them. The extent of beneficence required is not always clear, however. Occasionally holding a family conference outside of usual clinic or office hours to accommodate family members who cannot attend during usual hours is a reasonable expectation of a professional. Never taking a vacation out of a sense of duty to one's patients is an unreasonable expectation.

The principle of beneficence presents conflicts for researchers. As noted previously, the individual participants who assume the risks of the research may not receive any benefits from the research project. Individuals who agree to be in a clinical trial to assess the effectiveness of a new drug to manage spasticity accept the risk that the drug may produce serious, unanticipated side effects. They may or may not experience any improvement in their spasticity as a result of participating in the trial. The researcher–subject relationship puts immediate beneficence aside for the sake of new knowledge that may eventually translate into benefits for future patients.

The Principle of Nonmaleficence

The principle of nonmaleficence "aims to protect participants from physical or mental danger."[4(p. 87)] In addition, the principle implies that we should not expose others to unnecessary risk. In daily life this means that one should not rob people at knifepoint in the subway, nor should one drive while intoxicated. People with backyard pools need to have them fenced properly to protect curious children from accidental drowning. Society levels civil and criminal penalties against members who violate the principle of nonmaleficence.

For health care providers, nonmaleficence means that one should neither intentionally harm one's patients nor cause unintentional harm through carelessness.

Suppose that a therapist is seeing a frustrating patient—one who demands much but does not appear to follow through with a suggested home program of exercise. The therapist decides to "teach the patient a lesson," being deliberately vigorous in mobilization techniques to make the patient "pay" for not following directions. This action would violate the principle of nonmaleficence because the regimen was intentionally sadistic, not therapeutic.

The practice of any of the rehabilitation professions does, however, require that we expose patients to various risks in order to achieve treatment goals. We cannot guarantee that no harm will come to patients in the course of treatment: They may fall, they may become frustrated, they may become sore, their skin may become irritated, they may experience adverse effects of medications. However, fulfilling the principle of nonmaleficence means exercising due care in the practice of one's profession. Due care requires the availability of adequate personnel during transfers and functional activities, planned progression of exercise intensity, monitoring of skin condition during procedures, screening for drug allergies and interactions, and considering the patient's or client's readiness to change.

In the conduct of research, we must also avoid exposing participants to unnecessary risk. Detailed delineation of the risks of research is presented later in this chapter. In general, however, the principle of nonmaleficence requires that we refrain from research that uses techniques we know to be harmful and that research be terminated if harm becomes evident. Although the risks of harm as a consequence of research can be great, there is also harm associated with not conducting research. If research is not performed to assess the effects of rehabilitation procedures, patients may be exposed to time-consuming, expensive, or painful treatments that may be ineffective or harmful. If researchers are to systematically assess the effects of treatments of unknown effectiveness, doing so will necessarily place someone at risk. The researcher must work carefully to minimize these risks.

The Principle of Utility

Classically, the principle of utility states that "actions or behaviors are right in so far as they promote *happiness* or *pleasure*, wrong as they tend to produce *unhappiness* or *pain*."[5] A family with limited financial resources needs to make utilitarian decisions. Should funds be spent on health insurance or life insurance? Which is potentially more devastating financially—an enormous hospital bill or loss of the primary earner's income? The answer that would bring about the most potential benefit and the least risk for harm would vary from family to family. If a practice cannot accommodate all the patients who desire appointments on a given day, decisions about who receives an appointment should focus on who will benefit most from immediate treatment and who will be harmed least by delayed treatment. Health services researchers may frame health care funding debates in terms of utility. For example, what will bring about the greatest benefit and the least harm: funding for prenatal care or funding for neonatal intensive care treatment for premature infants?

In the conduct of research, the principle of utility can guide the development of research agendas. Which projects will contribute most to the advancement of patient care in rehabilitation? Which projects involve risks that are disproportional to the amount of beneficial information that can be gained? Should a funding agency support a project that would assess the effects of different stretching techniques on prevention of injury in recreational athletes or a project that would provide augmented communication equipment for individuals with amyotrophic lateral sclerosis? The former project has the potential to reduce lost workdays for large numbers of full-time employees; the latter has the potential to improve quality of life and employability of small numbers of patients with the disease. Knowing about the principle of utility does not make allocation decisions easy!

The Principle of Autonomy

The principle of autonomy, particularly as applied to research, states that participants in the research must be allowed to make a free, independent, and informed choice without coercion."[6(p. 54)] Suppose that your elderly mother owns and lives alone in a house that badly needs a new roof. She indicates that it doesn't rain often, that it only leaks in the formal dining room, and that she won't live long enough to get her money's worth out of a new roof. The principle of autonomy indicates that you should respect her decision to determine whether her roof will be repaired. However, you may believe that because the house is your mother's primary financial asset and may be used to pay for her long-term care in the future, she will benefit from the preservation of that asset, even if you must violate her autonomy by hiring a roofer yourself. This violation of the principle of autonomy "for someone's own good" is known as *paternalism*.

Autonomy issues in patient treatment and research revolve around the concept of informed consent. Informed consent is an essential component of the research process and is therefore discussed in detail in the following section.

Health Information Portability and Accountability Act

The need for confidentiality took on a legal aspect with the passage of the Health Information Portability and Accountability Act (HIPAA, PL 104-191) of 1996. Following the passage of the act itself, the U.S. Department of Health and Human Services issued its "Privacy Rule" to assist health care providers in meeting the requirements of the law.[7]

The essence of HIPAA revolves around the concept of "protected health information." Essentially, that category includes all "forms of individuals' protected health information, whether electronic, written, or oral." It includes (1) current or previous health status, (2) health care services received, and (3) information regarding past, current, or future payments for health care. Thus, rehabilitation care providers cannot transmit any such information without express consent from the recipient.

HIPAA is intended to be flexible so that necessary transactions can take place. For example, a person receiving treatment can waive her or his right to protected health information (e.g., when protected information needs to be transmitted to a referral source). Also, providers may disclose protected information under certain circumstances. "Covered entities [providers] may rely on professional ethics and best judgments in deciding which of these permissive uses and disclosures to make."[8(p. 5)]

Other Moral Principles

Besides those mentioned previously, ethical behavior is also guided by several other principles. Below are a few common ones, although others exist.

Ethical behavior requires abstaining from conflict of interest, defined as "a situation in which personal and/ or financial considerations have the potential to influence or compromise professional judgment in clinical service, research, consultation, instruction, administration, or any other professional activity."[9] Note the inclusion of research in this definition. The avoidance of conflict of interest (and many say even the *appearance* of conflict of interest) has an aspirational quality in that a scientist-practitioner is expected to always strive for higher moral ground, even when personal gain must be sacrificed.

Another moral principle, particularly germane in our multicultural society, is nondiscrimination. The essence of nondiscrimination is an attitude of holding every individual as worthy. Although the federal government has defined categories in which discrimination is actually illegal (e.g., differential and usually derogatory treatment on the basis of age, ethnicity, sexual orientation, socioeconomic status), the practitioner should not focus solely on those but continually ask whether he or she is treating a research participant (or clinical case) differently for any unjustifiable reason.

As we said, there are other moral principles. The scientist-practitioner should continually try to hone his or her ethical sense. One good source is the book by Houser and Thoma.[10]

INFORMED CONSENT

Informed consent requires that patients or subjects give permission for treatment or testing and that they be given adequate information in order to make educated decisions about undergoing the treatment or test. Hicks notes that informed consent "demands that the participants knowingly, willingly, rationally, and freely agree to take part [in research]."[4(p. 87)] Four components are required for true autonomy in making either health care or research participation decisions: disclosure, comprehension, voluntariness, and competence.[11] In addition, as recommended by the 2002 Institute of Medicine's Committee on Assessing the System for Protecting Human Research Participants, informed consent should be viewed as an ongoing process within a research system, not as the isolated event of signing a consent form:

> The informed consent process should be an ongoing, interactive dialogue between research staff and research participants involving the disclosure and exchange of relevant information, discussion of that information, and assessment of the individual's understanding of the discussion.[12(p. 120)]

Information about treatment or research is needed before a patient or subject can make an informed decision from among several treatment options. Disclosure of treatment details should include the nature of the condition, the long-term effects of the condition, the effects of not treating the condition, the nature of available treatment procedures, anticipated benefits of any procedures, the probability of actually achieving these benefits, and potential risks of undergoing the procedure. Time commitments related to the treatment should be detailed, as should cost of the treatment. For patients undergoing routine, low-risk procedures, providing this information may be verbal or written. The practitioner explains the evaluative procedures to the patient, proceeds with an evaluation if the patient agrees, and then outlines the planned course of treatment to the patient. The patient then determines

whether the time, risks, and expense associated with the treatment is worth the anticipated benefit.

Disclosure of research details involves many of the same information items, depending on the nature of the research. Because research is usually not for the immediate benefit of the participant, more formal protection of the research subject is required than is needed for the patient. Thus, information about research risks and potential benefits must be written. If the research involves deception (e.g., disguising the true purpose of the study when full knowledge would likely alter participant responses), it is generally accepted that a "debriefing" procedure after completion of the study is important to fully inform participants about the true nature of the experiment.[13] Other instances in which debriefing may be appropriate are to "unmask" the assignment of participants to different placebo or treatment groups, to communicate research findings to interested subjects, or to bring closure to a research process that has required extended interactions of researchers and subjects (as in some qualitative research studies).

However, disclosing information is not enough. The practitioner or researcher must ensure that the patient or subject comprehends the information given. Practitioners who are sensitive to the comprehension issue describe procedures in lay language, prepare written materials that are visually appealing, provide ample time for explanation of procedures and for answering questions, and allow ample time before requiring a participation decision. Unfortunately, informed consent documents are often written at a level that may exceed the reading skills of the intended sample,[14] although in more recent years the readability of informed consent documents seems to have improved.[15]

The clinician or researcher also needs to ensure the voluntariness, or freedom from coercion, of consent. If free health care is offered in exchange for participation in a research study, will a poor family's decision to participate be truly voluntary? When a clinician requests that a man who is a patient participate in a study, and ensures him that his care will not suffer if he chooses not to participate, is it unreasonable for the patient to feel coerced based on the presumption that there might be subtle consequences of not participating? Practitioners and researchers need to be sensitive to real or perceived coercive influences faced by their patients or subjects.

Competence is the final component of informed consent. One must determine whether potential patients or research participants are legally empowered to make decisions for themselves. Consent from a legal guardian must be sought for minor children. If a legal guardian has been appointed for individuals who have a mental illness, have developmental disabilities, or are incompetent then consent must be sought from this party. When conducting research with populations in whom "proxy" consent is required, the researcher should also consider whether the subjects themselves "assent" or "dissent" to participation.[16] Suppose that an occupational therapist wishes to study the differences between in-class and out-of-class therapy for public school children with cerebral palsy. If out-of-class therapy has been the norm, a boy who voices a preference for out-of-class treatment should not be required to be a member of the in-class group even though his parents have given permission for him to be assigned to either group. A related problem occurs when a group is legally empowered to make decisions, but the characteristics of the group make informed consent difficult or impossible. For example, at state institutions for developmentally disabled adults, many of the residents may be their own legal guardians, with the legal ability to make their own decisions about participation in many activities. They might be unable, however, to comprehend the risks and potential benefits of participation in a research project, and therefore any consent they gave would not be informed. Swaine and colleagues offer some suggestions on ethically obtaining informed consent when incorporating compromised participants in research.[17]

It is clear that informed consent is required when experimental research that exposes participants to harm is undertaken, but what about research in which existing health care records are used to examine the outcomes of care that has already been delivered? In the recent past, individual consent to use personal health information in such studies was rarely sought, as long as researchers had reasonable procedures in place to maintain the anonymity of the records. In the United States, the implemented HIPAA requires dramatic change in this practice. In general, HIPAA requires specific authorization whenever protected health information (PHI) is disclosed. However, *institutional review boards* (IRBs) may authorize the research use of PHI under some circumstances even without individual consent. Six provisions of HIPAA have been described as "transformative" with respect to the conduct of research using medical records and insurance databases: (1) the need to track disclosures of PHI, (2) the need to ensure that research collaborators comply with the privacy rules, (3) the relationship between HIPAA and regulations for IRBs, (4) the principle that researchers should have access to only the minimum data necessary to carry out their work, (5) the requirement to de-identify data, and (6) the imposition of civil and criminal penalties for unlawful disclosure of PHI.[18] Similar issues have been raised in the United Kingdom with the implementation of the Data Protection Act.[19]

RESEARCH CODES OF ETHICS

The general moral principles of action discussed earlier become formalized when they are developed into codes of ethics to guide the practice of various professionals. There are three general codes of ethics that can provide rehabilitation researchers with guidance on ethical issues. The first of these is the Nuremberg Code developed in 1949 as a reaction to Nazi atrocities in the name of research.[20] The second is the World Medical Association (WMA) Declaration of Helsinki developed in 1964, most recently modified in 2008; as of 2013, the WMA is undertaking another revision with stronger emphasis on protecting compromised participants.[21,22] The third is the U.S. Department of Health and Human Services (DHHS) regulations that govern research conducted or funded by the department.[23] All are available online, either at the Internet addresses noted in the reference list or by doing an Internet search. Furthermore, readers wishing to solidify their knowledge of research ethics are encouraged to complete an online education program, prepared by the DHHS, through its National Institutes of Health, which reviews the history of human participant protections and the principles promulgated for the protection of human research subjects.[24]

Seven distinct ethical themes can be gleaned from these resources; most are present in more than one of the documents. The themes are informed consent, whether the research design justifies the study, avoidance of suffering and injury, risks commensurate with potential benefit, independent review of research protocols, integrity in publication, and explicit attention to ethics.

Informed Consent

One common principle is that of voluntary consent of the individual participating in the research. The responsibility for ensuring the quality of consent is with each individual who "initiates, directs, or engages in the experiment."[20(p. 1)] This means that the very important issues of consent should be handled by an involved researcher. Using clerical staff to distribute and collect informed consent forms does not meet this requirement. In addition to securing the consent of their human research participants, researchers should treat animal subjects humanely and respect the environment[21] in the course of their research. Box 5-1 highlights the Tuskegee Syphilis Study, an important historical example documented in a book,[25] a play,[26] and a film based on the play,[27] in which the principles of informed consent were violated in particularly egregious ways by the U.S. Public Health Service in its study of syphilis in African American men.

Box 5-1

Tuskegee Syphilis Study

The Tuskegee Syphilis Study, spanning 40 years from 1932 to 1972, is one of the most infamous cases of ethical abuses in health care research within the United States. The study was conducted by the U.S. Public Health Service in cooperation with a variety of other agencies, including the Alabama State Department of Health, the Macon County Health Department, and the Tuskegee Institute. The basic fact of the case is that approximately 400 black men with syphilis were left untreated for 40 years to study the "natural history" of the disease. Participants did not realize that they were being studied, did not know that they were being tested for syphilis, were not informed of the results of testing, and were not aware that treatment was being withheld.

Miss Eunice Rivers, a young black nurse, coordinated data collection within the study. She played a critical role by establishing credibility with participants and providing continuity throughout the extended study. The study itself involved physical examination of the men, radiographs, lumbar punctures, minimal treatment for the syphilis, and a variety of "perks" for participants, including free aspirin and tonics, burial funds, and some health care for their families. Therefore, Nurse Rivers both coordinated the nontreatment study and played an important public health role within the rural black community in Macon County.

There were several points at which it might have been "natural" to discontinue the study. The first was in the early 1940s when penicillin became available. If the researchers could justify the early years of the study because of the equivocal effectiveness of the then-available treatments for syphilis, they could no longer use this justification once penicillin became a known treatment. A second natural opportunity to stop the study and provide treatment to participants also occurred during the early 1940s when many participants received draft notices for World War II. If a man who was drafted was found to have syphilis, protocol indicated that he should receive treatment for the disease. However, special exceptions to this protocol were made for members of the Tuskegee study, who were neither inducted into service nor treated for their syphilis.

The problems with the study were exposed in 1972, nearly 40 years after its initiation. Hearings about the study resulted in the development of revised procedures for federally sponsored human experimentation. Contemporary guidelines under which most institutional review boards operate today are based on these post-Tuskegee regulations. Ultimately, surviving participants were provided with comprehensive medical care and cash settlements, and the heirs of deceased participants received cash settlements.

The Tuskegee experiment inspired the play *Miss Evers' Boys*,[25] which reminds us that responsible scientific inquiry rests on the moral choices of individual researchers:

> *Miss Evers [representing Nurse Rivers]:* There was no treatment. Nothing to my mind that would have helped more than it hurt.

> *Caleb [representing a participant]:* Maybe not in '33. But what about '46 and that penicillin? That leaves every year, every month, every day, every second right up to today to make a choice. It only takes a second to make a choice.

From Harvard Law School: Revisions to the Declaration of Helsinki. Available at: http://blogs.law.harvard.edu/billofhealth/2013/04/18/revisions-to-the-declaration-of-helsinki/. Accessed November 19, 2014.

Design Justifies Study

A link exists between research methodology and research ethics: "The experiment should be so designed ... that the anticipated results will justify the performance of the experiment."[20(p. 1)] The implication is that it is not appropriate to expose humans to risks for a study that is so poorly designed that the stated purposes of the research cannot be achieved. This, then, is essentially a utility issue: Why expose people to risk if the probability of benefit is low? Recent recommendations in the United States call for the development of separate scientific and ethical reviews of research proposals to ensure that the appropriate level of expertise is brought to bear on each review process.[12(pp. 72–82)]

Although this principle would seem to call for methodological rigor in the design of research studies, finding a balance between methodological and ethical rigor is complex. For example, consider the question of whether to use a placebo-controlled design versus an active-controlled design. In a placebo-controlled design, the control group receives a sham treatment, the experimental group receives the new treatment, and an effective treatment should show markedly different results than the placebo group. In an active-controlled design, the control group receives currently accepted treatment, the experimental group receives the new treatment, and an effective new treatment should be at least marginally better than the accepted current treatment. Researchers considering which design to use need to balance factors such as the number of participants needed to demonstrate a statistically significant effect (placebo-controlled studies typically require fewer participants than active-controlled studies because differences between groups are expected to be larger in the placebo-controlled studies), the impact of withholding currently accepted treatments, and the risks of both the current and new treatments.[28]

Avoidance of Suffering and Injury

Avoidance of suffering and injury is a nonmaleficence concern. Risks can be avoided through careful consideration during the design of a study and by careful protection of physical safety and avoidance of mental duress during the implementation of the study. A safety concern in the design phase of a study might occur for researchers deciding how to quantify the effects of exercise on the biceps brachii muscle. They might consider using various histological, strength, radiological, or girth measures to document change. The final decision about which measures to use would depend both on the specific research questions and on which measures are likely to cause the least amount of suffering or injury.

Safety issues during research implementation should be addressed as needed. For example, a speech-language pathologist implementing a study of techniques to improve swallowing for individuals with dysphagia would need to select appropriate food and drink for treatment sessions and attend to positioning to minimize the risk for aspiration during treatment or testing.

Privacy during evaluation and treatment, as well as confidentiality of results, can also be considered here as an issue of prevention of mental suffering. Seemingly innocuous portions of the research protocol may be stressful to the participant. For example, a protocol that requires documentation of body weight may be acceptable to a participant if the measure is taken and recorded by only one researcher. The same participant may be extremely uncomfortable with a protocol in which the body weight is recorded on a data sheet that accompanies the participant to five different measurement stations for viewing by five separate researchers.

In some qualitative research studies, participants may recall and explore upsetting events within their lives. For example, consider an occupational therapist using qualitative methods to explore the experiences of young adults with substance abuse problems. In the course of such a study, a research participant may share information about past sexual abuse or current suicidal ideation. Minimizing suffering requires that researchers implementing such studies plan for referral to appropriate mental health professionals. Even questionnaire-based research may be worrisome to participants or lead to expectations that cannot be met by the researchers. Researchers may, for example, ask respondents about such sensitive topics as sexual behavior, illegal activities, or questionable social attitudes, leading to possible dishonesty in responding owing to their desire to appear more acceptable.[29]

A final component of the safety issue relates to the issue of how a researcher should decide when to terminate a study prematurely. One end point is when injury or harm becomes apparent. A drug trial in the 1990s was halted after five patients died from liver failure and two patients survived only after receiving liver transplantation after taking long-term doses of the drug fialuridine to treat hepatitis B.[30] Although the injury or harm that may occur in much of rehabilitation research is less dramatic than liver failure and death, researchers must still conduct their trials in ways that allow them to identify safety concerns in a timely fashion. Another end point is when a new procedure is found to be superior to the comparison procedure. In opposing viewpoints about the ethical issues involved in premature termination of clinical trials, one set of authors reviewed a study they believed should have been stopped earlier than it was in order to permit new patients to take advantage of a treatment that proved to be superior to the control in reducing in-hospital deaths in patients being treated for acute myocardial infarction.[31] Another set of authors came to the very different conclusion that the statistical trends were not strong enough to justify a premature termination of the study and that 6-month survival data gave a different picture of the relative effectiveness of the techniques, justifying the continuation of the study to its original end point.[32] This point-counterpoint illustrates the complexity of putting research ethics into action.

Risk Is Commensurate with Potential Benefit

High-risk activities can only be justified if the potential for benefit is also great. Levine[2] noted that researchers are usually quick to identify potential benefits of their research, without always carefully considering all the potential risks to participants. Because of the subtle nature of many risks, and the duty of researchers to minimize and consider all risks, the last section of this chapter presents an analysis of risks associated with research.

Independent Review

Adequate protection of human participants requires that a body independent of the researcher review the protocol and assess the level of protection afforded to the human participants. The generic name for such an independent body in the United States is an *institutional review board* (IRB); in other countries it may be referred to as a research ethics committee, a research ethics board, or an independent ethics committee. In the United Kingdom, for example, qualifying research must be approved by a National Health Service Research and Ethics Commmittee.[4] By whatever name, the research ethics committee's charge is to examine research proposals to ensure that there is adequate protection of human participants in terms of safety and confidentiality, that the elements of informed consent are present, and that the risks of the study are commensurate with the potential benefits. Specific information about the nature of these committees and the procedures for putting the principles of informed consent into action are discussed in Chapter 27.

Publication Integrity

Researchers need to ensure the accuracy of reports of their work, should not present another's work as their own, and should acknowledge any financial support or other assistance received during the conduct of a research study. Chapter 28 provides specific guidelines for determining who should be listed as a study author and how to acknowledge the participation of those who are not authors.

Explicit Attention to Ethics

Researchers need to give explicit attention to ethical principles when they design, implement, and report their research. Researchers should change research projects for which they are responsible if ethical problems arise or should dissociate themselves from projects if they have no control over unethical acts. For example, assume that a prosthetist is collecting data in a study that is being conducted by a different primary investigator. If the prosthetist believes that patient consent is being coerced, he or she should seek to change the consent procedure with the primary investigator, discuss his or her concerns with the research ethics committee that approved the study, or refuse to participate further if no change occurs.

Ethics in Professional Codes

Rehabilitation professions, such as physical therapy, occupational therapy, speech-language pathology, and audiology, have professional associations that have developed codes of ethics. All of these contain references to research, indicating that the ethical conduct of research holds a high professional place alongside ethical clinical practice. The American Physical Therapy Association (APTA) Bylaws section III.B indicates that one of the functions of the association is to "maintain and promote ethical principles and standards of conduct for its members."[33] The APTA's Code of Ethics refers to research eight times, including in its Preamble, Principle 1 (nondiscrimination), Principle 2 (providing compassionate service), Principle 4 (demonstrating integrity), and Principle 5 (accountability).[34]

The Code of Ethics of the American Speech-Language-Hearing Association (ASHA) provides ethical guidance for speech-language pathologists and audiologists.[35] The code was revised in 2010 and now contains 18 specific references to research. Essentially, ASHA's Code holds researchers to the same ethical standards as practitioners. Besides its Code, ASHA also publishes "Issues in Ethics Statements," or IES, one of which is "Ethics in Research and Scholarly Activity." This IES notes that infused in ASHA's code are the ethical themes of (1) ethical treatment of research subjects, (2) competence, and (3) honesty.[36] In ethical treatment of participants, for example, Principle I, Rule C requires that ASHA members avoid discrimination in the conduct of research. Principle I, Rule F requires informing research participants of possible effects of research. The theme of competence is prominent, and ASHA's Code requires that adherents "provide all services (including research) competently" and are required to "achieve and maintain the highest level of professional competence." Regarding honesty, the ASHA Code requires truthful representation of research, truthful representation of credentials of research assistants, and accurate notation of the contributions of various people to research projects.

The whole structure of the Code of Ethics of the American Occupational Therapy Association (AOTA) is built on principles of moral action, with the Code's seven principles, respectively, based on (1) beneficence, (2) nonmaleficence, (3) autonomy and confidentiality, (4) social justice, (5) procedural justice, (6) veracity, and (7) fidelity. The AOTA Code is highly aspirational and notes that "commitment extends beyond service recipients to include professional colleagues, students, educators, businesses, and the community."[37] Some examples of germane rules in the AOTA Code are Principle 1.L., which requires that "occupational therapy research is conducted in accordance with currently accepted ethical guidelines"; Principle 1.N., which requires practice of "occupational therapy on the basis of current knowledge and research"; and Principle 5.D., which enjoins occupational therapists to make others—specifically employers—aware of their ethical obligations, including the ethical conduct of research.

In examining professional codes of ethics for the rehabilitation professions it becomes clear that, to a great extent, research is not parceled out for separate ethical consideration. Rather, research is seen as a professional activity requiring application of the same ethical principles as are used for other areas of practice. We trust the reader thus sees how this book's theme of the scientist-practitioner extends to ethical behavior.

RESEARCH RISKS

Much of the discussion in this chapter is related in some way to risk–benefit analysis. The risks of research can be categorized as physical, psychological, social, and economic.[2] Each category is described, and examples from the rehabilitation literature are presented.

Physical Risks

The physical risk associated with some research is well known. When a particular risk is known, participants should be informed of its likelihood, severity, duration, and reversibility. Methods for treating the physical harm should also be discussed if appropriate. If a strengthening study provides an eccentric overload stimulus to hamstring musculature, participants need to know that almost all will develop delayed muscle soreness, that it appears within 2 days after exercise, and typically lasts up to 8 days.[38] Higher-risk procedures, such as an invasive muscle biopsy or fine-wire electromyography, might include the risk for infection. Participants in such studies would need to receive information about signs and symptoms of infection and procedures to follow if infection occurs.

A different form of physical risk is the impact of *not* receiving treatment. A controversial aspect of the most recent revision of the Declaration of Helsinki is its Clause 32, which states the following:

> The benefits, risks, burdens and effectiveness of a new intervention must be tested against those of the best current proven intervention, except in the following circumstances:
>
> • The use of placebo, or no treatment, is acceptable in studies where no current proven intervention exists; or

> • Where for compelling and scientifically sound methodological reasons the use of placebo is necessary to determine the efficacy or safety of an intervention and the patients who receive placebo or no treatment will not be subject to any risk of serious or irreversible harm. Extreme care must be taken to avoid abuse of this option.[21(p. 5)]

This principle is ethically controversial because placebo conditions deny research participants access to a possibly beneficial treatment; at the same time, the actual treatment, because its effects are as yet unknown in an experiment, carries a degree of risk for harm. The WMA reaffirmed that "extreme care" must be taken in making use of a placebo-controlled trial but clarified that placebo-controlled trials may be acceptable even if proven therapies are available when there are "compelling and scientifically sound methodological reasons" for using them "and the patients who receive placebo will not be subject to an additional risk of serious or irreversible harm."[21(p. 5)] The related Clause 33 states the following:

> At the conclusion of the study, patients entered into the study are entitled to be informed about the outcome of the study and to share any benefits that result from it, for example, access to interventions identified as beneficial in the study or to other appropriate care or benefits.

Some critics believe that strict adherence to principles of the Helsinki Declaration, although appropriate for research in advantaged populations, may need to be revised, or at least carefully considered, in disadvantaged populations, for example, in developing nations.[39,40] The international research community needs to strike a balance between research that may exploit individuals in developing nations or other disadvantaged conditions by exposing them to all of the risks of research and few of the benefits of contemporary best health care practices and research that provides at least some care to communities that would not otherwise receive it.

Because rehabilitation research is often concerned with matters of long-term quality of life rather than immediate matters of life and death, it is often possible to delay treatments to some groups without additional risk for serious harm. However, even research on seemingly minor conditions requires careful consideration of the risks for both receiving and not receiving treatment. For example, Schaefer and Sandrey[41] performed a randomized controlled trial on three groups of participants with chronic ankle instability (CAI). They were interested to find out the effects of dynamic balance training (DBT) when supplemented by the Graston instrument-assisted soft tissue mobilization

(GISTM) technique. Always using DBT, they established three groups: DBT plus GISTM, DBT plus a sham (i.e., placebo) GISTM, and DBT alone. Interestingly, all participants improved on all direct measures of ankle function. More to the present point, their study provides an example of consideration of providing or not providing treatment for even a condition generally considered innocuous.

Risks of research may be population specific. For example, treatments such as the use of ultrasound over epiphyseal plates are relatively low risk in adults but may have high risks for children.[42] When delineating the risks of participation in a given study, researchers must consider whether the procedures they are using pose special risks to the population they are studying. In addition, physical risks of an intervention are not always known or may not become apparent for long periods. Researchers must always consider whether the potential benefit of a study is proportional to its long-term or hidden risks.

Psychological Risks

Although rehabilitation researchers may focus on the physical risks of their research, they must also consider psychological risks. Participant selection that requires normality can cause psychological harm to those identified as abnormal. Those receiving an experimental treatment may lie awake nights wondering what untoward effects they may experience. Or participants in a placebo-controlled study may be anxious about whether their condition is being undertreated with a placebo. Qualitative researchers must guard against psychological risks that arise from the interactions among researchers and participants that occur across time.[43] Participants in studies that investigate sensitive topics may have emotional reactions to data collection efforts.[29] Regardless of the type or topic of a study, researchers must carefully consider ways to minimize the psychological risks to participants in their studies.

Social Risks

The major social risk to individual research participants is the breach of confidentiality. As discussed earlier, legislation in both the United States and the United Kingdom provides protections to individuals relative to the privacy of their health information. These laws require that researchers be more vigilant than ever in protecting the privacy of research participants, including both those who are active participants receiving experimental measures or interventions and those who are more passive participants whose medical records or health insurance data are used to evaluate care that has already been delivered.

Economic Risks

When research has a combined knowledge and treatment effect, at least some portion of the payment for the research will generally be the responsibility of participants or the participants' health care insurers. Even if the treatment in question is not experimental, the participant may incur additional costs through lost work hours, baby-sitting fees while undergoing treatment, and transportation costs to and from the research facility.

Although it appears that many researchers build participant compensation into the costs of their research proposals, the result is not clear. In a survey of 353 IRB chairpersons reviewing six hypothetical studies, Ripley and colleagues found no evidence that investigators and IRB chairs actually compute participant costs.[44]

SUMMARY

The differences between practice and research demand that the participants in research receive special protection from the risks associated with research. The general moral principles of beneficence, nonmaleficence, utility, and autonomy form the base on which codes of ethics are built. Codes of ethics for the rehabilitation professions link ethics in research with other areas of practice. Informed consent requires that participation be a voluntary action taken by a competent individual who comprehends the risks and benefits of research participation as disclosed by the researcher. In addition to securing the informed consent of their participants, researchers must ensure that the design of a study justifies its conduct, that procedures are designed to minimize risk, that risk is commensurate with potential benefits, that an independent review body has approved the conduct of the research, that integrity is maintained in publication of the research, and that careful consideration is given to all ethical concerns related to the study. The risks associated with research may be physical, psychological, social, and economic.

REFERENCES

1. U.S. Department of Health and Human Services. Office for Human Research Protection (OHRP). Available at: http://www.hhs.gov/ohrp/. Accessed November 19, 2014.

2. Levine RJ: The boundaries between biomedical or behavioral research and the accepted and routine practice of

medicine. In National Commission for the Protection of Human Subjects of Biomedical and Behavioral Research, editors: *The Belmont Report: Ethical Principles and Guidelines for the Protection of Human Subjects of Research, Appendix, Volume I*, DHEW Publication OS 78–0013, Washington, DC, 1975, U.S. Government Printing Office.

3. Hayes SC, Barlow DH, Nelson-Gray R: *The Scientist Practitioner*, Boston, Mass, 1999, Allyn & Bacon.
4. Hicks CM: *Research Methods for Clinical Therapists*, 5th ed, Edinburgh, UK, 2009, Churchill Livingstone Elsevier.
5. White RF. The principle of utility. Available at: http://faculty.msj.edu/whiter/UTILITY.htm. Accessed August 1, 2013.
6. Holloway I, Wheeler S: *Qualitative Research in Nursing and Healthcare*, 3rd ed, West Sussex, UK, 2010, Wiley-Blackwell.
7. U.S. Dept. of Health and Human Services. Privacy rule. Available at: www.hhs.gov/ocr/privacy/hipaa/administrative/privacyrule/index.html. Accessed November 19, 2014.
8. U.S. Department of Health and Human Services. Summary of the HIPAA privacy rule. 2003. Available at: http://www.hhs.gov/ocr/privacy/hipaa/understanding/summary/privacysummary.pdf. Accessed July 26, 2013.
9. American Speech-Language-Hearing Association: Conflicts of professional interest (issues in ethics). 2011. Available at: http://www.asha.org/Practice/ethics/Conflicts-of-Professional-Interest/. Accessed February 9, 2015.
10. Houser RA, Thoma S: *Ethics in Counseling and Therapy: Developing an Ethical Identity*, Thousand Oaks, Calif, 2013, Sage.
11. Sim J: Informed consent: Ethical implications for physiotherapy, *Physiotherapy* 72:584–587, 1986.
12. Federman DD, Hanna KE, Rodriguez LL, and the Institute of Medicine (U.S.) Committee on Assessing the System for Protecting Human Research Participants: *Responsible Research: A Systems Approach to Protecting Research Participants*, Washington, DC, 2003, National Academies Press.
13. Kazdin AE: Ethical issues and guidelines for research. In Kazdin AE, editor: *Research Design in Clinical Psychology*, 4th ed, Boston, Mass, 2003, Allyn & Bacon, pp 497–544.
14. Paasche-Orlow MK, Taylor HA, Brancati FL: Readability standards for informed-consent forms as compared with actual readability, *N Engl J Med* 348:721–726, 2003.
15. Sand K, Eik-Nes NL, Loge JH: Readability of informed consent documents (1987-2007) for clinical trials: A linguistic analysis, *J Empir Res Human Res Ethics* 7(4):67–78, 2012.
16. Allmark P: The ethics of research with children, *Nurs Res* 10:7–19, 2002.
17. Swaine J, Parish SL, Luken K, Atkins L: Recruitment and consent of women with intellectual disabilities in a randomised control trial of a health promotion intervention, *J Intellect Disabil Res* 55:474–483, 2011.
18. Durham ML: How research will adapt to HIPAA: A view from within the healthcare delivery system, *Am J Law Med* 28:491–502, 2002.
19. Cassell J, Young A: Why we should not seek individual informed consent for participation in health services research, *J Med Ethics* 28:313–317, 2002.
20. Nuremberg Code. Available at: http://history.nih.gov/research/downloads/nuremberg.pdf. Accessed November 19, 2014.
21. World Medical Association. WMA Declaration of Helsinki: Ethical principles for medical research involving human subjects. Available at: http://www.wma.net/en/30publications/10policies/b3/. Accessed November 19, 2014.
22. Harvard Law School. Revisions to the Declaration of Helsinki. Available at: http://blogs.law.harvard.edu/billofhealth/2013/04/18/revisions-to-the-declaration-of-helsinki/. Accessed November 19, 2014.
23. U.S. Department of Health and Human Services. Office for human research protections. Available at: http://www.hhs.gov/ohrp/. Accessed November 19, 2014.
24. U.S. Department of Health and Human Services National Institutes of Health. Protecting human research participants. Available at: http://phrp.nihtraining.com/users/login.php. Accessed November 19, 2014.
25. Jones JH: *Bad Blood: The Tuskegee Syphilis Experiment*, new and expanded ed, New York, NY, 1993 Maxwell McMillan International.
26. Feldshuh D: *Miss Evers' Boys*, acting ed, New York, NY, 1995, Dramatists Play Service.
27. *Miss Evers' Boys*. Videotape. Distributed by: Home Box Office, 1997.
28. Miller FG, Shorr AF: Unnecessary use of placebo controls: The case of asthma clinical trials (commentary), *Arch Intern Med* 162:1673–1677, 2002.
29. Krumpal I: Determinants of social desirability bias in sensitive surveys: A literature review, *Quality Quantity Int J Methodol* 47(4):2025–2047, 2013.
30. Thompson L: The cure that killed, *Discover* 15:56, 58, 60–62, 1994.
31. Verdú-Pascual F, Castelló-Ponce A: Randomised clinical trials: A source of ethical dilemmas, *J Med Ethics* 27:177–178, 2001.
32. Hilden J, Gammelgaard A: Premature stopping and informed consent in AMI trials, *J Med Ethics* 28:188–189, 2002.
33. American Physical Therapy Association. Bylaws of the American Physical Therapy Association. 2011. Available at: http://www.apta.org/uploadedFiles/APTAorg/About_Us/Policies/General/Bylaws.pdf. Accessed November 19, 2014.
34. American Physical Therapy Association. Code of ethics for the physical therapist. Available at: http://www.apta.org/uploadedFiles/APTAorg/About_Us/Policies/Ethics/CodeofEthics.pdf#search=%22code of ethics%22. Accessed November 19, 2014.
35. American Speech-Language-Hearing Association. *Code of Ethics*. 2010. Available at: http://www.asha.org/docs/html/ET2010-00309.html. Accessed July 30, 2013.
36. American Speech-Language-Hearing Association. *Ethics in research and scholarly activity [Issues in Ethics]*. Available online at http://www.asha.org/policy/ET2008-00299/. Accessed November 19, 2014.
37. American Occupational Therapy Association. *Occupational Therapy Code of Ethics and Ethics Standards*. 2010. Available at: http://www.aota.org/~/media/Corporate/Files/AboutOT/Ethics/Code%20and%20Ethics%20Standards%202010.ashx. Accessed July 31, 2013.

38. Kellis E, Baltzopoulos V: Isokinetic eccentric exercise, *Sports Med* 19:202–222, 1995.

39. Tollman SM: Fair partnerships support ethical research, *BMJ* 323:1417–1423, 2001.

40. Giordano S: The 2008 Declaration of Helsinki: Some reflections, *J Med Ethics* 3(10):598–603, 2010.

41. Schaefer JL, Sandrey MA: Effects of a 4-week dynamic-balance-training program supplemented with Graston Instrument-Assisted Soft-Tissue Mobilization for chronic ankle instability, *J Sport Rehabil* 21(4):313–326, 2012.

42. McDiarmid T, Ziskin MC, Michlovitz SL: Therapeutic U.S. In Michlovitz SL, editor: *Thermal Agents in Rehabilitation*, Philadelphia, Pa, 1996, FA Davis, pp 168–212.

43. Glesne C: *Becoming Qualitative Researchers: An Introduction*, 2nd ed, New York, NY, 1999, Addison Wesley Longman, pp 113–129.

44. Ripley E, Macrina F, Markowitz M, Gennings C: Who's doing the math? Are we really compensating research participants? *J Empir Res Human Res Ethics* 5:57–65, 2010.

CHAPTER 6

Research Paradigms

CHAPTER OUTLINE

Quantitative Paradigm
Assumptions of the Quantitative
  Paradigm
  Assumption 1
  Assumption 2
  Assumption 3
  Assumption 4
  Assumption 5
Quantitative Methods
  Theory
  Selection
  Measurement
  Manipulation
  Control

Qualitative Paradigm
Assumptions of the Qualitative
  Paradigm
  Assumption 1
  Assumption 2
  Assumption 3
  Assumption 4
  Assumption 5
Qualitative Methods
  Theory
  Selection
  Measurement
  Manipulation and Control

Single-Subject Paradigm
Assumptions of the Single-Subject
  Paradigm
Single-Subject Methods
  Theory
  Selection
  Measurement
  Manipulation and Control
**Relationships Among the Research
  Paradigms**
Summary

Knowledge is continually evolving. What was believed to be true yesterday may be doubted today, scorned tomorrow, and resurrected in the future. Just as knowledge itself evolves, beliefs about how to create knowledge also evolve. Our beliefs about the methods of obtaining knowledge constitute *research paradigms*.[1(p. 15)] The beliefs that constitute a paradigm are often so entrenched that researchers themselves do not question the assumptions that undergird the research methodology they use. Although the details of various research methods are presented in later chapters, this chapter provides readers with a broad framework for thinking about the research paradigms that support those methods.

Although differences in the research approaches of the different rehabilitation professions can be seen, the dominant research paradigm across the rehabilitation disciplines is the quantitative paradigm. Two other common paradigms of importance are the qualitative and single-subject paradigms. The study of alternative research paradigms in rehabilitation is important for two reasons. First, research based on the various paradigms is reported in the rehabilitation literature, so consumers of the literature need to be familiar with the assumptions that undergird these paradigms. Second, differing research paradigms in any discipline emerge because of the inability of the dominant paradigm to answer all the important questions of the discipline. Researchers therefore need to consider research from differing paradigms not only in terms of the specific research questions addressed but also in terms of what the research implies about the limitations of the dominant paradigm.

The purpose of this chapter is to develop these three research paradigms for consideration. This is done by first emphasizing differences between the paradigms (some might say by presenting caricatures of each paradigm) and later examining relationships among the paradigms. The quantitative paradigm is discussed first.

This paradigm focuses on the study of groups whose treatment is often manipulated by the investigator. The qualitative paradigm is then discussed. This paradigm focuses on broad description and understanding of phenomena without direct manipulation. The final paradigm to be analyzed is the single-subject paradigm, which focuses on data from individual responses to manipulation.

Deciding on the terminology to use for the different research paradigms is difficult. The paradigms are sometimes described in philosophical terms, sometimes in terms of components of the paradigm, and sometimes in terms of the methods that usually follow from the philosophical underpinnings of the paradigm. Box 6-1 presents various names that have been used to identify what are being labeled in this chapter as quantitative, qualitative, and single-subject paradigms. Accurate use of the different philosophical labels requires a strong background in the history and philosophy of science, backgrounds that most scientist-practitioners do not have. To avoid imprecise use of the language of philosophy, the more "methodological" terms are used in this text rather than the more "philosophical" terms. This choice, however, may lead to the misconception that paradigms and methods are interchangeable. They

are not. A paradigm is defined by the assumptions and beliefs that guide researchers. A method is defined by the actions taken by investigators as they implement research. Adoption of a paradigm implies the use of certain methods but does not necessarily limit the researcher to those methods. The presentation of the assumptions of each paradigm is followed by general methodological implications of the paradigm. Later chapters present specific designs associated with these paradigms.

QUANTITATIVE PARADIGM

The quantitative paradigm is what has become known as the traditional method of science, including applied behavioral sciences such as rehabilitation. The term *quantitative* comes from the emphasis on measurement that characterizes this paradigm. The paradigm has its roots in the 1600s with the development of Newtonian physics.[2,3] In the early 1900s, the French philosopher Auguste Comte and a group of scientists in Vienna became proponents of related philosophical positions often labeled *positivism* or *logical positivism*.[4] This positivist philosophy is so labeled because of the central idea that one can only be certain, or positive, of knowledge that is verifiable through measurement and observation.

Assumptions of the Quantitative Paradigm

Just as there are multiple terms for each paradigm, there are also multiple views about the critical components of each paradigm. Lincoln and Guba[1(p. 37)] use five basic axioms to differentiate what they refer to as positivist and naturalistic paradigms. Their five axioms are presented here as the basis of the quantitative paradigm. The qualitative and single-subject paradigms are developed by retaining or replacing these with alternate axioms. Table 6-1 summarizes the assumptions of the three paradigms.

Assumption 1: Single Objective Reality

The first assumption of the quantitative paradigm is that there is a single objective reality. One goal of quantitative research is to determine the nature of this reality through measurement and observation of the phenomena of interest. This reliance on observation is sometimes termed *empiricism*. A second goal of quantitative research is to predict or control reality. After all, if researchers can empirically determine laws that regulate reality in some predictable way, they should be able to

---

Box 6-1

Alternate Names for the Three Research Paradigms

Quantitative Paradigm
Positivist
Received view
Logical positivist
Nomothetic
Empiricist

Qualitative Paradigm
Naturalistic
Phenomenological
Ethnographic
Idiographic
Postpositivist
New paradigm

Single-Subject Paradigm
Idiographic
$N=1$
Single system

Table **6-1**

Assumptions of the Three Research Paradigms

Assumption	PARADIGM		
	Quantitative	**Qualitative**	**Single-Subject**
Reality	Single, objective	Multiple, constructed	Single, objective
Relationship between investigator and subject	Independent	Dependent	Independent
Generalizability of findings	Desirable and possible	Situation specific	System specific
Cause-and-effect relationships	Causal	Noncausal	Causal
Values	Value free	Value bound	Value free

use this knowledge to attempt to influence that reality in equally predictable ways.

Assumption 2: Independence of Investigator and Subjects

The second basic assumption of the quantitative paradigm is that the investigator and subject, or object of inquiry, can be independent of one another. In other words, it is assumed that the investigator can be an unobtrusive observer of a reality that does not change by virtue of the fact that it is being studied. Researchers who adopt the quantitative paradigm do, however, recognize that it is sometimes difficult to achieve this independence. Rosenthal,[5] in his text on experimenter effects in behavioral research, related a classic story about "Clever Hans," a horse who could purportedly tap out the correct response to mathematical problems by tapping his hoof. Hans's skills intrigued a researcher, Pfungst, who tested Hans's abilities under different controlled conditions. Pfungst found that Hans could tap out the correct answer only when his questioner was a literate individual who knew the answer to the question. He found that knowledgeable questioners unconsciously raised their eyebrows, flared their nostrils, or raised their heads as Hans was coming up to the correct number of taps. Rosenthal notes:

> Hans' amazing talents ... serve to illustrate further the power of self-fulfilling prophecy. Hans' questioners, even skeptical ones, expected Hans to give the correct answers to their queries. Their expectation was reflected in their unwitting signal to Hans that the time had come for him to stop his tapping. The signal cued Hans to stop, and the questioner's expectation became the reason for Hans' being, once again, correct.[5(p. 138)]

Despite the recognition of the difficulty of achieving the independence of the investigator and subject, the assumption of the quantitative paradigm is that it is possible and desirable to do so through a variety of procedures that isolate subjects and researchers from information that might influence their behavior.

Assumption 3: Generalizability of Results

The third basic assumption of the quantitative paradigm is that the goal of research is to develop generalizable characterizations of reality. The generalizability of a piece of research refers to its applicability to other subjects, times, and settings. The concept of generalizability leads to the classification of quantitative research as *nomothetic*, or relating to general or universal principles. Quantitative researchers recognize the limits of generalizability as threats to the validity (discussed in greater detail in Chapter 8) of a study; however, they believe generalizability is an achievable aim, and research that fails to be reasonably generalizable is flawed.

Assumption 4: Determining Causation

The fourth basic assumption of the quantitative paradigm is that causes and effects can be determined and differentiated from one another. Quantitative researchers are careful to differentiate experimental research from nonexperimental research on the basis that causal inferences can only be drawn if the researcher is able to manipulate an independent variable (the "presumed cause") in a controlled fashion while observing the effect of the manipulation on a dependent variable (the "presumed effect"). Quantitative researchers attempt to eliminate or control extraneous factors that might interfere with the relationship between the independent and dependent variables (see Chapters 10, 11, and 12 for more information on experimental and nonexperimental research).

Assumption 5: Value Free

The final assumption of the quantitative paradigm is that research is value free. The controlled, objective nature of quantitative research is assumed to eliminate the influence of investigator opinions and societal norms on the facts that are discovered. Inquiry is seen as the objective discovery of truths and the investigator as the impartial discoverer of these truths.

Quantitative Methods

The adoption of these quantitative assumptions has major implications for the methods of quantitative research. Five methodological issues are discussed in relation to the assumptions that underlie the quantitative paradigm: theory, selection, measurement, manipulation, and control. These five issues, as well as the issues of data types, are summarized in Table 6-2. Quotes from a single quantitative piece of research are used to illustrate the way in which each of these methodological issues is handled within the quantitative paradigm.

Theory

The first methodological issue relates to the role of theory within a study. Quantitative researchers are expected to articulate *a priori* theory, that is, theory developed in advance of the conduct of the research. The purpose of the research is then to determine whether the components of the theory can be confirmed. This top-down notion of theory development was presented in Chapter 2 on theory. Klein and colleagues[6] used a quantitative research approach when they compared the effects of exercise and lifestyle modification on the overuse symptoms in polio survivors. As such, an *a priori* theoretical perspective guided the study:

Symptoms of upper-extremity overuse are also common among people with mobility impairments. In such cases shoulder disorders result when the arms are used repetitively to compensate for weak leg muscles during weight-bearing tasks such as getting up from a chair or using an assistive device while walking.... If lower-extremity weakness predisposes to upper-extremity overuse, then the relevant lower-extremity muscle groups must be strengthened and/or behavioral patterns leading to overuse must be altered.[6(pp. 708–709)]

The elements of this theory are (1) if shoulder disorders in polio survivors result from overuse as a result of lower-extremity weakness, (2) then treatment that improves lower-extremity muscle strength or alters the behavioral patterns leading to overuse should improve the overuse symptoms. The purpose of the study, then, was to test this "if-then" hypothesis. A further indication of the importance of theory to this study is seen in the prediction of outcomes based on the theory:

We predicted that the subjects who received both interventions [exercise and lifestyle modification instruction] would show the most improvement, and this improvement would be associated with an increase in leg strength.[6(p. 709)]

Selection

The second methodological issue relates to the generalizability of the research. Because quantitative researchers want to be able to generalize their findings to subjects similar to those studied, they often articulate an elaborate set of inclusion and exclusion criteria so that readers can determine the group to which the research can be generalized:

Table **6-2**

Methods of the Three Research Paradigms

Method	PARADIGM		
	Quantitative	Qualitative	Single-Subject
Theory	*A priori*	Grounded	*A priori*
Number and selection of subjects	Groups, random	Small number, purposive	One, purposive
Measurement tools	Instruments	Human	Instruments
Type of data	Numerical	Language	Numerical
Manipulation	Present	Absent	Present
Control	Maximized	Minimized	Flexible

Subjects were recruited from a pool of 194 polio survivors.... Other inclusion criteria for this study were bilateral knee-extensor and hip-extensor strength ≥ grade 3 but less than a grade 5 on manual muscle testing and shoulder pain with daily activity for at least 30 days. Exclusion criteria included any major disabilities or conditions unrelated to polio that could cause weakness or overuse problems (e.g., stroke, amputation, inflammatory arthritis...), serious illness such as heart or lung disease that could make exertion during a strength test unsafe (e.g., severe emphysema, poorly controlled asthma, recent heart attack), history of shoulder trauma, and recent fracture or surgery.... Subjects with significant upper-extremity weakness who could not use their arms to push out of a chair were also excluded.[6(p. 709)]

After individuals are selected for a quantitative study, the way they are placed into treatment groups is also viewed as an important control mechanism, with random assignment to groups being the preferred way to maximize the chances that the groups have similar characteristics at the start of the study.

Measurement

The third methodological issue relates to a desire for a high level of precision in measurements as an expression of the belief in an objective reality. Klein and colleagues[6] carefully document their measurement procedures and their own reliability in using the measurement tools used within their study:

The dynamometer was placed proximal to the malleoli on the anterior aspect of the tibia. For each muscle group, the maximum force generated in each of 3 trials was recorded. Subjects had a minimum of 30 seconds to rest between trials. The reliability of these measurements was established previously in a sample of 2 polio survivors and 4 adults with no history of polio.... All [intraclass correlation coefficients] were greater than .910, with the exception of hip extension on the dominant side, which was .787.[6(p. 709)]

Measurement theory, presented later in this text, is largely based on the concept that researchers use imperfect measurement tools to estimate the "true" characteristics of a phenomenon of interest and that the best measures are those that come closest to this "truth" on a consistent basis.

Manipulation

The fourth methodological issue is related to the role of manipulation within a study. Quantitative researchers believe that the best research for documenting the effect of interventions is that which allows one to determine causes and effects in response to controlled manipulations of the experimenter. Klein and colleagues[6] show this preference for experimental evidence when they identify one source of evidence—clinical observation—as insufficient to establish the causal link their study addresses:

Based on clinical observation, survivors who comply with the recommended changes [muscle strengthening and lifestyle changes] often experience a reduction in their pain and fatigue. To date, however, there have been no published studies that compare the effectiveness of lifestyle modification therapy with exercise in reducing pain and maintaining function in polio survivors. Therefore, this study sought to compare the effectiveness of 2 interventions (exercise and lifestyle modification instruction) alone and in combination in alleviating shoulder overuse symptoms in polio survivors with lower-extremity weakness.[6(p. 709)]

Quantitative researchers place a great deal of emphasis on this type of controlled manipulation as the only valid source of evidence for the effectiveness of interventions.

Control

The fifth and final methodological issue is related to the control of extraneous factors within the research design. Klein and colleagues[6] included many control elements in their study. Each subject received similar education and educational materials at the beginning of the study: a visit with a therapist, an educational videotape, and printed materials. Intensity, duration, and frequency of exercise were standardized across subjects. In addition, the total time spent with a therapist in follow-up visits across the study was the same across subjects, regardless of group assignment. Because of these controls, the treatments administered within this study likely differed from routine clinical practice, with more initial education and more regular follow-up than might be typical. Researchers who adopt the quantitative paradigm generally believe that control of extraneous variables is critical to establishment of cause-and-effect relationships, even when such control leads to the implementation of experimental procedures that may not be fully representative of typical clinical practices.

These, then, are examples of how five methodological issues—theory, selection, measurement, manipulation, and control—are handled by researchers who work within the framework of the quantitative paradigm.

QUALITATIVE PARADIGM

Just as the mechanistic view of Newtonian physics provided the roots for the development of the quantitative paradigm, the relativistic view of quantum mechanics provided the roots for the development of the qualitative paradigm. Zukav[2] contrasted the "old" Newtonian physics with the "new" quantum physics:

> The old physics assumes that there is an external world which exists apart from us. It further assumes that we can observe, measure, and speculate about the external world without changing it.... The new physics, quantum mechanics, tells us clearly that it is not possible to observe reality without changing it. If we observe a certain particle collision experiment, not only do we have no way of proving that the results would have been the same if we have not been watching it, all that we know indicates that it would not have been the same, because the results that we got were affected by the fact that we were looking for it.[2(pp. 30–31)]

Because the quantitative paradigm has proved inadequate even for the discipline of physics, a seemingly "hard" science, qualitative researchers argue that there is little justification for continuing to apply it to the "soft" sciences in which human behavior is studied.

Assumptions of the Qualitative Paradigm

The assumptions that form the basis for the qualitative paradigm are antithetical to the assumptions of the quantitative paradigm. Once again, Lincoln and Guba's[1] concepts, but not their terminology, form the basis for this section of the chapter. What Lincoln and Guba label the *naturalistic paradigm* is referred to in this text as the *qualitative paradigm*. Table 6-1 provides an overview of the assumptions of the qualitative paradigm.

Assumption 1: Multiple Constructed Realities

The first assumption of the qualitative paradigm is that the world consists of multiple constructed realities. "Multiple" means that there are always several versions of reality; "constructed" means that participants attach meaning to events that occur within their lives, and that this meaning is an inseparable component of the events themselves. Refer to Box 6-2 for a simple test of the phenomenon of multiple constructed realities. It is easy to demonstrate how multiple constructed realities may be present within clinician-patient interactions. For example, if one man states that his physician is cold and unfeeling, that is his reality. If a woman states that the same physician is professional and candid, that is

---

Box 6-2

Test of the Phenomenon of Multiple Constructed Realities

Instructions: Count the number of "F"s in the quote below:

"FABULOUS FITNESS FOLLOWS FROM YEARS OF FREQUENT WORKOUTS COMBINED WITH FOCUSED FOOD CHOICES."

Solution: If you are like most adults, you counted seven "F"s in the sample. Read it again:

"FABULOUS FITNESS FOLLOWS FROM YEARS OF FREQUENT WORKOUTS COMBINED WITH FOCUSED FOOD CHOICES."

There are 7 "F" sounds (fabulous, fitness, follows, from, frequent, focused, food), but 8 "F"s (of). People who understand the relationship between letters and sounds intuitively search for the "F" sound when doing this exercise. In doing so, the task that is completed is different than the task that was assigned. If it is possible to interpret even a simple letter-counting exercise in different ways, think of the difficulty in developing "objective" measures that are more complicated! Qualitative researchers believe that such attempts are futile and instead embrace the depth of understanding that accompanies different ways of seeing the world.

---

her reality. The notion of a single, objective reality is rejected. Researchers who adopt the qualitative paradigm believe that it is fruitless to try to determine the physician's "true" manner because the physician's demeanor does not exist apart from how it is perceived by different patients.

Assumption 2: Interdependence of Investigator and Subjects

The second assumption of the qualitative paradigm is that investigator and subject are interdependent; that is, the process of inquiry itself changes both the investigator and the subject. Whereas quantitative paradigm researchers seek to eliminate what is viewed as undesirable interdependence of investigator and subject, qualitative paradigm researchers accept this interdependence as inevitable and even desirable. For example, a qualitative researcher would recognize that a physician who agrees to participate in a study of clinician demeanor is likely to change, at least in subtle ways, his or her demeanor during the period that he or she is observed.

Assumption 3: Results Specific to Time and Context

The third assumption of the qualitative paradigm is that knowledge is time and context dependent. Qualitative paradigm researchers reject the nomothetic approach and its concept of generalizability. In this sense, then, qualitative research is *idiographic*, meaning that it pertains to a particular case in a particular time and context. The goal of qualitative research is a deep understanding of the particular. Researchers who adopt the qualitative paradigm hope that this particular understanding may lead to insights about similar situations. Although not generalizable in the quantitative tradition, themes or concepts found consistently in qualitative research with a small number of subjects may represent essential components of phenomena that, with further investigation, would also be found in larger samples.

Assumption 4: No Causation

The fourth assumption of the qualitative paradigm is that it is impossible to distinguish causes from effects. The whole notion of cause is tied to the idea of prediction, control, and an objective reality. Researchers who adopt the qualitative paradigm believe it is more useful to describe and interpret events than it is to attempt to control them to establish oversimplified causes and effects. In the physician demeanor example, qualitative researchers believe that it would be impossible to determine whether a certain physician demeanor caused better patient outcomes or whether certain patient outcomes caused different physician demeanors. Because of their belief in the inability to separate causes from effects, qualitative researchers would instead focus on describing the multiple forces that shape physician-patient interactions.

Assumption 5: Value Laden

The fifth assumption of the qualitative paradigm is that inquiry is value bound. This value-laden quality is exemplified in the type of questions that are asked, the way in which constructs are defined and measured, and the interpretation of the results of research. The traditional view of scientists is that they are capable of "dispassionate judgment and unbiased inquiry."[7(p. 109)] Qualitative researchers, however, believe that all research is influenced by the values of the scientists who conduct research and the sources that fund research. The status of research about the use of hormone replacement therapy during menopause provides one example of the value-laden quality of the research enterprise. In July 2002, the results of a randomized controlled trial of combined estrogen and progestin versus placebo on coronary heart disease and invasive breast cancer for postmenopausal women were published.[8] The study had been halted in May 2002, approximately 3 years earlier than planned, because increased risks for development of coronary heart disease and invasive breast cancer were found. The results of this trial received widespread publicity and comment in both the popular media and the health care literature. The following exchange, from a U.S. National Public Radio science program, illustrates some of the ways in which the health care and research environments may be influenced by cultural values and business interests:

Dr. GRADY [physician guest]: I object to the word "replacement" and try never to use it. And that's because a normal postmenopausal woman is not sick. This is a normal transition in life, just like puberty.

FLATOW [program host]: This whole idea of using hormone replacement to create this so-called fountain of youth for women, is this a male-dominated research item made by a man that …

Dr. RICHARDSON [physician guest]: Well, I don't think there's been enough research done on this in general anyway. I mean, we don't know what the physiology of hot flashes is. And one of my fond hopes with all of this publicity is that maybe someone will fund more research so we can figure out what causes hot flashes and fix them.

FLATOW: Well, I was thinking more as a marketing technique to make money on a replacement therapy more than, you know, if men had to do it for themselves, they wouldn't have been so fast to do it, as they used to talk about men and birth control pills.

Dr. BARRETT-CONNOR [physician guest]: Well, you know, it's very interesting that now that testosterone patches are being developed for men in their older years when their testosterone levels fall—this is a fairly popular treatment, but it's been hard to get trials of it because both the scientists and the people who sponsor studies are worried about prostate cancer.[9]

In this short exchange in the popular media, we hear many value-laden questions: whether male-dominated health care and research interests influenced the widespread adoption of hormone replacement therapy even in the absence of randomized controlled trials, why mechanisms behind menopausal symptoms have not been studied more fully, whether economic factors related to the profitability of hormone replacement therapy influenced the research agenda, and how safety concerns may be influencing trials for testosterone replacement therapy for men.

Researchers who adopt the qualitative paradigm recognize that they are unable to separate values from inquiry. They do not believe that it is productive to pretend that science is objective, particularly in light of questions such as those raised by the recent hormone replacement therapy controversy.

Qualitative Methods

These five assumptions have an enormous impact on the conduct of qualitative paradigm research. The roles of theory, selection, measurement, manipulation, and control are all vastly different in qualitative research than in quantitative research, as summarized in Table 6-2. Dudgeon and associates[10] used the qualitative paradigm to structure their study of physical disability and the experience of chronic pain. This study is used to provide examples of the methods that flow from adoption of the beliefs of the paradigm.

Theory

The first methodological issue relates to the role of theory. Because researchers who adopt the qualitative paradigm accept the concept of multiple constructed realities, they do not begin their inquiry with a researcher-developed theoretical framework. They begin the research with an idea of what concepts or constructs may be important to an understanding of a certain phenomenon, but they recognize that the participants in the inquiry will define other versions of what is important. A rigid theoretical framework of the researcher would constrain the direction of the inquiry and might provide a less-than-full description of the phenomenon of interest. Dudgeon and colleagues[10] express this in the broad, exploratory language of their purpose statement:

> The purpose of this study was to explore the nature of pain that accompanies physical disability, getting an insider's views about experiencing and dealing with pain as part of daily living and communicating.[10(p. 229)]

In addition, the authors do not advance a set of predictions about their findings, as was the case with the quantitative study example cited earlier in the chapter.

Selection

The second methodological issue relates to the way in which subjects are selected. Rather than selecting a randomized group of individuals, qualitative researchers purposely select individuals who they believe will be able to lend insight to the research problem. Dudgeon and colleagues[10] describe just such a method:

> We asked the health care liaisons to identify participants who they regarded as representative of

the specific clinical population [spinal cord injury, amputation, or cerebral palsy] and who were particularly fluent in describing their views.[10(p. 229)]

In this example, purposive sampling procedures led to the selection of only nine individuals, three from each of the diagnostic groups of interest. Most traditional quantitative researchers would find this sample to be insufficient because it would not likely be representative of a larger group and because small samples do not lend themselves to statistical analysis. Because neither representativeness nor statistical analysis is required for a qualitative study to be valid, these issues are not considered to be problematic.

Measurement

The third methodological issue relates to the primary measurement tool of qualitative research: the "human instrument." Because of the complexity of the multiple realities the qualitative researcher is seeking to describe, a reactive, thinking instrument is needed, as noted by Dudgeon and associates:[10]

> The interviews were open ended and relatively unstructured.... Because we wanted the participants to guide the interviews, the protocol was flexible and the order of discussion often shifted, depending on the direction taken by the individual.[10(p. 230)]

The data collected in qualitative studies are usually not numerical but, rather, are verbal and consist of feelings and perceptions rather than presumed facts. Researchers gather a great deal of descriptive data about the particular situation they are studying so that they can provide a "rich" or "thick" description of the situation.

Manipulation and Control

Fourth and fifth, the qualitative researcher does not manipulate or control the research setting. Rather, the setting is manipulated in unpredictable ways by the interaction between the investigator and the participants. The mere fact that the researcher is present or asks certain questions is bound to influence the participants and their perception of the situation.

The natural setting is used for qualitative research. Because everything is time and context dependent, researchers who adopt the qualitative paradigm believe there is little to be gained—and much to be lost—from creating an artificial study situation. Dudgeon and associates,[10] for example, interviewed participants in their homes or in the researchers' offices, whichever was preferred by the participant. Researchers guided by the quantitative paradigm would probably view this as an undesirable source of uncontrolled variation. Being guided by the qualitative paradigm, however, meant that researchers were unconcerned about the location of the interviews and presumably assumed that the location preferred by the participants would yield the richest conversation about their pain experiences.

It is clear from this example that these five methodological issues—theory, selection, measurement, manipulation, and control—are handled very differently within a qualitative framework compared with a quantitative one. Theory unfolds during the study instead of directing the study. Small numbers of participants are selected for their unique ability to contribute to the study. Measurement is done with a "human instrument" who can react and redirect the data-gathering process rather than being done with a standardized measurement protocol. The object of the study is observed rather than manipulated. And finally, the setting for data collection is natural and uncontrolled rather than artificial and tightly controlled.

SINGLE-SUBJECT PARADIGM

The single-subject paradigm developed out of a concern that the use of traditional group research methods focused away from the unit of clinical interest: the individual. Assume that a group study of the effectiveness of a particular gait-training technique on gait velocity is implemented with 30 patients who have undergone transtibial amputation. If gait velocity improves for 10 patients, remains the same for 10 patients, and declines for 10 patients, then the average velocity for the group does not change very much, and the group conclusion is likely to be that the treatment had no effect. This group conclusion ignores the fact that the treatment was effective for 10 patients but detrimental for 10 other patients. A clinically relevant conclusion might be that the treatment has the potential to improve velocity but that clinicians should also recognize that the opposite effect is also seen in some patients. An appropriate focus for future research would be the identification of those types of patients for whom this technique is effective.

Unfortunately, this type of subgroup analysis rarely occurs, and practitioners are left with the general group conclusion that the new technique is not effective. Single-subject research eliminates the group conclusion and focuses on treatment effects for individuals.

Box 6-1 lists several different names for single-subject research. Kazdin[11] uses the term *single-case experimental design* to emphasize the controlled manipulation that is characteristic of this paradigm. Ottenbacher[12(p. 45)] uses the term *single system* rather than the more common *single subject* because there are some instances in which the single unit of interest would itself be a group rather than an individual. For example, a rehabilitation administrator might wish to study departmental productivity before and after a reorganization. If the concern was not with changes in individual therapist productivity, but only with the productivity of the department as a whole, the effect of the reorganization could be studied as a single system. The use of "single system" here is correct because it is referring back to how Ottenbacher used the term. However, the defining feature of single-subject research is that data—even if the participants form a group—are not pooled but considered individually. If the departmental improvement data represent a group average, this is more properly a group study and not similar to the single-subject research we are discussing here.

Assumptions of the Single-Subject Paradigm

The single-subject paradigm has its roots in behavioral research, which focused much research on the influence of environmental stimuli (e.g., settings, verbal cues, physical cues) on subject behaviors. Thus, the basic assumption of the single-subject paradigm is that the effectiveness of treatment is subject and setting dependent. Single-subject researchers believe that research should reflect the idiographic nature of practice by focusing on the study of individuals. Except for this focus on individuals rather than groups, the rest of the assumptions of the single-subject paradigm are those of the quantitative paradigm, as shown in Table 6-1. In fact, the single-subject paradigm focuses exclusively on experimental problems in which there is active manipulation of the individual under study.

The single-subject paradigm is sometimes confused with the clinical case report or case study. The two are very different. The case report or case study is a description, very often a retrospective description, of a course of treatment of an individual (see Chapter 13). Single-subject research, on the other hand, uses a systematic process of introduction and withdrawal of treatments to allow for controlled assessment of the effects of a treatment (see Chapter 11).

Single-Subject Methods

Because many assumptions are shared between the quantitative and single-subject paradigms, many methods are shared as well, as shown in Table 6-2. Hannah and Hudak's[13] study of splinting for radial nerve palsy and Washington and associates'[14] study of adaptive seating on sitting posture and hand manipulation are used to illustrate these methods in practice. We have chosen to use two examples from the single-subject literature to illustrate how these methods may apply.

Hannah and Hudak compared the effects of three different types of splints for an individual with radial nerve palsy: static volar wrist cock-up splint, dynamic tenodesis suspension splint, and dorsal wrist cock-up splint with dynamic finger extension splint. Washington and associates examined the effects of different adaptive seatings (i.e., foam liner and a contoured foam seat in a highchair) on the sitting posture and hand manipulation of four infants with neuromotor impairments.

Theory

First, single-subject paradigm research generally operates from an *a priori* theoretical foundation. Hannah and Hudak established the rationale for intervening with splinting, stating:

> One of the challenges for hand therapists during this period of nerve regeneration is to fabricate a splint that prevents over-stretching of denervated extensor musculature while maximizing hand function.[13(p. 195)]

Thus, splints that are consistent with this theoretical framework should include elements that position and protect the hand to prevent over-stretching and elements that address functional use of the hand.

Similarly, Washington and associates indicated early in their introduction that two motor control theories, dynamical systems and neuromaturational, "... have been applied to adaptive seating...."[14(p. 1065)] Later, they further expanded on how these two theories may impact the sitting posture and hand manipulation of infants:

> According to neuromaturational theory, adaptive seating is aimed at decreasing the influence of primitive reflexes, normalizing the resistance of muscles to stretching, and providing proximal stability to promote distal mobility and function.[14(p. 1065)]

Selection

Second, selection of the individual for study is purposive. Single-subject researchers would not choose to study someone for whom they did not believe the interventions were uniquely appropriate. For example, Washington and associates developed six selection criteria (e.g., were able to reach and grasp toys from a midline position) that the four infants with neuromotor impairments had to meet in order to be included in their study.[14] This is in contrast to a group approach in which 30 infants with neuromotor impairments would be randomly assigned to different adaptive seating conditions or 30 participants who had radial nerve palsy

would be studied with a randomly assigned splint. How likely is it that the assigned adaptive seating would be designed specifically for each infant or that a provided splint would be uniquely appropriate for each of these 30 subjects? As noted by Hannah and Hudak:

> A randomized controlled trial is not the best way to determine the treatment of choice for a specific patient, since results are based on average improvement scores for all subjects and therefore do not provide information on the performance of individual subjects.[13(pp. 195–196)]

The single-subject paradigm requires that the individual studied have a specific need for the treatment implemented and enables the researcher to observe treatment effects in that individual.

Measurement

Third, precise measurement is an integral part of the single-subject paradigm. Repeated measures taken during baseline and treatment phases are compared. Thus, measurement accuracy and reliability are critical to the ability to draw conclusions about the effects of treatment. The importance of employing reliable measurements is evident in the Washington and associates study, in which the authors presented operational definitions for their behavioral outcomes and reported that they established interrater reliability between raters on the occurrence of these behaviors with each infant during both baseline and intervention phases.[14]

Furthermore, this measurement focus is apparent in Hannah and Hudak's study:

> Four established outcomes measures were chosen to assess the following variables—performance of the upper extremity during activities of daily living (Test Evaluant Les Members Supèriuurs des Personnes Agèes, TEMPA), self-reported level of disability (Disabilities of the Arm, Shoulder and Hand questionnaire, DASH), self-perceived performance in activities of daily living (Canadian Occupational Performance Measure, COPM), and strength of specific muscle groups (manual muscle testing).... High reliability as well as content, face, and preliminary construct validity in this population have been reported [for the TEMPA]. Preliminary results provide evidence of the reliability and convergent validity of the DASH.... Preliminary results provide evidence of test-retest reliability of the COPM as well as of content validity and responsiveness to clinical change.[13(pp. 197–198)]

This focus on the use of standardized tools with documented reliability and validity is important to single-subject designs.

Manipulation and Control

Experimental manipulation is an essential part of the definition of single-subject research. This is illustrated in Hannah and Hudak's[13] study by their manipulation of four phases of the study: baseline without any splint, with the static cock-up splint, with the dynamic tenodesis splint, and with the dynamic finger extension splint. Similarly, Washington and associates employed two phases in their study: baseline and intervention. The baseline phase consisted of each infant sitting in an unadapted highchair, whereas the intervention phase consisted of each infant sitting alternately in a highchair adapted with a foam liner or a contoured foam seat.[14]

Finally, control of extraneous factors is important in the conduct of single-subject research, as it is in any quantitative research. Hannah and Hudak[13] controlled the experimental setting by randomly determining the order in which the patient would test the splints, by having the same therapist fabricate each splint, and by standardizing the instructions for wear and care of each splint. In addition, the patient was asked to keep a log showing the time spent wearing each splint, in part to establish that each splint had received a fair trial during the 3-week period assigned for its use. Control of extraneous factors was similarly asserted by Washington and associates.[14] For one infant, they extended the baseline phase because the infant demonstrated great variability of the measured behaviors. For all infants, the order in which each experienced the experimental conditions was randomly determined, as was the presentation of the toys used to determine hand manipulation. Additionally, the study was conducted about the same time each day. Table 6-2 indicates, however, that the control in single-subject paradigm research may be more flexible than that of traditional group designs. In group designs, researchers usually attempt to control the nature of the treatment administered so that all individuals within the group receive approximately the same treatment. With the single-subject designs, the treatment can be administered as it would be in the clinic. Thus, the intervention can be tailored to accommodate scheduling changes, status changes, or varying patient moods. Chapter 11 presents several designs that use the general methods associated with the single-subject paradigm.

RELATIONSHIPS AMONG THE RESEARCH PARADIGMS

There are those who believe that the paradigms are mutually exclusive, that in adopting the assumptions of one paradigm, the assumptions of the others must be forsaken. Lincoln and Guba[1] make a case for the separateness of the quantitative and qualitative paradigms:

> Postpositivism is an entirely new paradigm, *not* reconcilable with the old.... We are dealing with an entirely new system of ideas based on fundamentally *different*—indeed sharply contrasting—assumptions.... What is needed is a transformation, not an add-on. That the world is round cannot be added to the idea that the world is flat [emphasis in original].[1(p. 33)]

A more moderate view is that the assumptions underlying the different paradigms are relative rather than absolute. Relative assumptions need not be applied to every situation; they can be applied when appropriate to a given research problem. This text adopts the moderate view that all forms of study have the potential to add to knowledge and understanding. The contrasting assumptions of the paradigms can be managed as we all manage many belief-action clashes on a daily basis. For example, many people believe that the world is round. However, in daily activities, they act as if the world is flat by using flat maps to get from place to place and by visualizing the part of the world they are most familiar with as flat. They hold one belief but find it useful to suspend that belief in their daily activities.

Likewise, a belief in multiple constructed realities need not prevent one from studying a certain problem from the perspective of a single objective reality. A belief that it is impossible to study any phenomenon without affecting it in some way need not prevent one from attempting to minimize these effects through the design control methods developed in Chapters 7 through 18. The potential contributions of the different research paradigms are best realized when investigators recognize the assumptions that undergird their methods and make explicit the limitations of their methods.

Furthermore, the development of a line of research on a particular topic may benefit from the use of different research paradigms at different points in time. Consider the example of research on constraint-induced movement therapy, a technique that restrains the unaffected upper extremity of a person with hemiplegia to force the use of the hemiparetic limb. Over the past 20 years or so, this technique has been studied through all three research paradigms. In 1981, an early report on the technique used a single-subject experimental design with an adult with hemiplegia.[15] In 1989, a group quantitative paradigm study of the technique was reported with adults with stroke and head injury.[16] By the early 2000s, the technique had been extended to new aspects of stroke rehabilitation (treating aphasia with constraint-induced principles applied to communication, studied through quantitative paradigm methods)[17] and to new patient populations (children with hemiplegia, studied with case report methods).[18] Basic science research in the quantitative tradition has also been conducted on this treatment technique, both with human participants assessed with magnetic resonance imaging[19] and with rats assessed with skill testing and measurement of tissue losses.[20] Finally, a qualitative study was published in 2003, looking at perceptions and experiences of patients who participated in constraint-induced therapy home programs.[21] This brief, incomplete history of research on constraint-induced therapy demonstrates the complex interplay between what is known and not known about a topic and the ways in which new knowledge about a topic can be developed.

The moderate view adopted in this text also implies that the paradigms can be mixed within a study to address different aspects of a research problem. For example, Bat-Chava and Martin's[22] study of the impact of child and family characteristics on sibling relationships of deaf children combined quantitative and qualitative methods. Parents of 37 children who were deaf were interviewed about the quality of sibling relationships. In addition to the identification of themes about sibling relationships from the interview data, as would be expected in a qualitative study, the authors also constructed a scale to measure the quality of sibling relationships. They then used this scale in a quantitative way to search for factors such as birth order, gender, family size, and so forth that could explain differences in sibling relationships in different families.

Patton,[23] in his text on qualitative research methods, offers a contemporary analogy about the mixing of research paradigms:

> Mixing parts of different approaches is a matter of philosophical and methodological controversy.... In practice, it is altogether possible, as we have seen, to combine approaches, and to so do creatively. Just as machines that were originally created for separate functions such as printing, faxing, scanning, and copying have now been combined into a single integrated technological unit, so too methods that were originally created as distinct, stand-alone approaches can now be combined into more sophisticated and multifunctional designs.[23(p. 252)]

SUMMARY

Research paradigms are the beliefs that underlie the conduct of inquiry. The dominant paradigm in rehabilitation research is currently the quantitative paradigm, which emphasizes generalizable measurement of a single objective reality with groups of subjects that are often manipulated by the investigator. The competing qualitative paradigm emphasizes the study of multiple constructed realities through in-depth study of particular settings, with an emphasis on determining underlying meanings within a particular context. The single-subject paradigm, on the other hand, includes many of the beliefs of the quantitative paradigm with the important exception of the concept of generalizability; single-subject studies look at changes in individuals because the individual is the unit of interest within a discipline such as rehabilitation. Some researchers believe that adoption of one paradigm precludes the use of other paradigms; others believe—as we do—that all three paradigms are useful when applied to appropriate questions.

REFERENCES

1. Lincoln YS, Guba EG: *Naturalistic Inquiry*, Beverley Hills, Calif, 1985, Sage.
2. Zukav G: *The Dancing Wu Li Masters: An Overview of the New Physics*, New York, NY, 1979, Bantam Books.
3. Irby DM: Shifting paradigms of research in medical education, *Acad Med* 65:622–623, 1990.
4. Phillips DC: After the wake: Postpositivistic educational thought, *Educ Res* 12:4–12, 1983.
5. Rosenthal R: *Experimenter Effects in Behavioral Research*, enlarged ed, New York, NY, 1976, Irvington.
6. Klein MG, Whyte J, Esquenazi A, et al: A comparison of the effects of exercise and lifestyle modification on the resolution of overuse symptoms of the shoulder in polio survivors: A preliminary study, *Arch Phys Med Rehabil* 83:708–713, 2002.
7. Mahoney MJ: *Scientist as Subject: The Psychological Imperative*, Cambridge, Mass, 1976, Ballinger.
8. Rossouw JE, Anderson GL, Prentice RL, et al: Risks and benefits of estrogen plus progestin in healthy postmenopausal women: Principal results from the Women's Health Initiative randomized controlled trial, *JAMA* 288:321–333, 2002.
9. Risks and benefits of hormone replacement therapy. Distributed by: National Public Radio, July 26, 2002.
10. Dudgeon BJ, Gerrard BC, Jensen MP, et al: Physical disability and the experience of chronic pain, *Arch Phys Med Rehabil* 83:229–235, 2002.
11. Kazdin AE: Observational research: Case-control and cohort designs. In Kazdin AE, editor: *Research Design in Clinical Psychology*, 4th ed, Boston, Mass, 2003, Allyn & Bacon.
12. Ottenbacher KJ: *Evaluating Clinical Change: Strategies for Occupational and Physical Therapists*, Baltimore, Md, 1986, Williams & Wilkins.
13. Hannah SD, Hudak PL: Splinting and radial nerve palsy: A single-subject experiment, *J Hand Ther* 14:195–201, 2001.
14. Washington K, Deitz JC, White OR, Schwartz IS: The effects of a contoured foam seat on postural alignment and upper-extremity function in infants with neuromotor impairments, *Phys Ther* 82:1064–1076, 2002.

15. Ostendorf CG, Wolf SL: Effect of forced use of the upper extremity of a hemiplegic patient on changes in function: A single-case design, *Phys Ther* 61:1022–1028, 1981.

16. Wolf SL, Lecraw DE, Barton L, Jann BB: Forced use of hemiplegic upper extremities to reverse the effect of learned nonuse among chronic stroke and head-injured patients, *Exp Neurol* 104:125–132, 1989.

17. Pulvermuller F, Neininger B, Elbert T, et al. Constraint-induced therapy of chronic aphasia after stroke, *Stroke* 32:1621–1626, 2001.

18. Glover JE, Mateer CA, Yoell C, Speed S: The effectiveness of constraint-induced movement therapy in two young children with hemiplegia, *Pediatr Rehabil* 5:125–131, 2002.

19. Schaechter JD, Kraft E, Hilliard TS, et al. Motor recovery and cortical reorganization after constraint-induced movement therapy in stroke patient: A preliminary study, *Neurorehabil Neural Repair* 16:326–338, 2002.

20. DeBow SB, Davies ML, Clarke HL, Colbourne F: Constraint-induced movement therapy and rehabilitation exercises lessen motor deficits and volume of brain injury after striatal hemorrhagic stroke in rats, *Stroke* 34:1021–1026, 2003.

21. Gillot AJ, Holder-Walls A, Kurtz JR, Varley NC: Perceptions and experiences of two survivors of stroke who participated in constraint-induced movement therapy home programs, *Am J Occup Ther* 57:168–176, 2003.

22. Bat-Chava Y, Martin D: Sibling relationships of deaf children: The impact of child and family characteristics, *Rehabil Psychol* 47:73–91, 2002.

23. Patton MQ: *Qualitative Research and Evaluation Methods*, 3rd ed, Thousand Oaks, Calif, 2002, Sage.

CHAPTER 7

Variables

CHAPTER OUTLINE

Independent Variables
Levels of Independent Variables
Active and Assigned Variables
  Dependent Variables
  Intervening Variables

Confounding and Extraneous
  Variables
Extraneous Variables in the Setting
Extraneous Variables Related to
  Participants

Functional Relationships
Graphs
Summary

Surely, one of the most important functions of clinical science—and science in general—is to determine cause and effect. A basic question is, "When there is a change in 'A,' does a change in 'B' result?" If the answer is yes, we can infer that the change in "A" was the cause of the change in "B." This is most true when the change in "A" is controlled by the researcher. Necessarily, in that condition, the change in "A" will not have happened before the research began (i.e., the study is *prospective*). When we engage in this type of study, the study is an *experiment*.

As both clinicians and scientists, we are constantly applying empirical methods. In looking for cause-and-effect relationships, we attempt to assess the effectiveness of our treatments, or we try to find cause-and-effect relationships. That is, we manipulate a treatment in some way. We introduce, withdraw, or modify it, to see if any of those changes has an effect on an outcome, usually some behavior we are attempting to help our clients change.

To understand cause and effect, the concept of *variables* must be understood. As the term implies, variables change within the course of an experiment, whether clinical treatment or not. If there is no change to an aspect, that aspect is a *constant*, not a variable. For example, assume a physical therapist tries two different treatments for low back pain on a series of 70-year-old patients. Because treatment varied (i.e., there were two), treatment is a variable. Because age did not vary (i.e., all patients were 70 years old), age was not a variable, but a constant.

INDEPENDENT VARIABLES

Independent variables are aspects of a study that a scientist-practitioner either controls or chooses. They are independent because they do not rely on other variables for their changes. They are causes of outcomes or at least presumed causes of outcomes. A typical independent variable for all rehabilitation professionals is treatment. When we vary the type of treatment, treatment becomes an independent variable. Even when we first implement a treatment, we are going from a condition of no treatment to one of implementation. Thus, again, treatment is a variable.

LEVELS OF INDEPENDENT VARIABLES

Any independent variable must have at least two values; if there is only one value, the aspect does not vary, and it is a constant, not a variable. Each value of an independent variable is called a *level* of the variable. For example, if a researcher is studying the effect of three different types of acoustic conditions—white noise, 12-speaker babble, and ambient room noise—on decision making in children with learning disability, the independent variable of *acoustic condition* would have three levels, that is, the three acoustic conditions. It is important to note that the independent variable is identified by the aspect that has changed, not by the three conditions that result from producing the change.

If a physical therapist wants to determine the effect of four treatment types for shoulder pain—(1) cryotherapy and transcutaneous electrical nerve stimulation (TENS), (2) hot packs and TENS, (3) TENS alone, and (4) sham treatment—the independent variable of *treatment type* has four levels. Again, the variable is identified by the aspect that has changed—in this case, treatment type. Each type of treatment is not a variable, but one level of the variable.

ACTIVE AND ASSIGNED VARIABLES

Some independent variables allow the researcher to have complete control. For example, if a scientist-practitioner is comparing the effects of two different treatments on a population of 12-year-old children with autism, the researcher can choose the treatments and, further, the children can be assigned randomly to either treatment. Likewise, in the noise study mentioned previously, the researcher has complete freedom to choose the acoustic conditions. Thus, not only are treatment or acoustic conditions independent variables, they also are *active* variables over which the researcher has complete control. Having at least one active independent variable is essential for an experiment and drawing a conclusion of cause and effect.

On the other hand, there are some conditions of interest in which participants cannot be randomly assigned or the researcher can choose, but not control. A common paradigm in rehabilitation research includes comparison of typically developing individuals with those who have some clinical condition. Say, for example, we are interested in finding out about some motor ability in children with cerebral palsy compared with children with typical motor ability. Children with cerebral palsy cannot be in the group of physically typical participants, and the physically typical participants cannot be in the group of individuals with cerebral palsy. In this case, motor ability might be an independent variable, but it is an *assigned* (also known as *attribute*) variable. The most common assigned independent variables are participant characteristics, such as age, health status, or intelligence.

In this example, the presence of an assigned independent variable might tempt a researcher to attribute any group differences in motor ability to the presence of cerebral palsy. However, this interpretation is limited because the researcher had no control over who went into each group and because the groups were formed before the research began; that is, it is not prospective. Thus, a case like this does not constitute a true experiment and we cannot truly assign cause and effect.

Dependent Variables

Dependent variables are the outcomes of a study, whether clinical intervention or not. In the case of clinical intervention, they are the behaviors we wish to help change. They are *dependent* because their values *depend* on changes in the independent variable. When a scientist-practitioner manipulates an active independent variable, and the result is a change in a dependent variable, we infer a cause-and-effect

relationship. In physical therapy, some common dependent variables are range of motion, pain rating, and performance on outcome measures, such as the Functional Independence Measure.[1] In communication sciences and disorders, some common dependent variables are speech fluency, articulatory precision, and speech recognition ability. In occupational therapy, some common dependent variables are self-dress ability, hand dexterity, and success in using adaptive equipment.

It is critical to recognize that, for purposes of an experiment, a dependent variable must be operationally defined. That is, the researcher must decide how to *measure* the outcome. It is not enough to say that range of motion is being measured; the metric used (degrees, in this case) must be specified. Likewise, it is not enough to measure "fluency"; the researcher must specify how the value will be determined (e.g., by counting the number of dysfluencies per 100 words).

There are a few very common parameters that are most often used to operationally define dependent variables. Often, they relate to physical parameters, such as distance or sound intensity. They may also be nonphysical, such as percent correct, some subjective rating, or the outcome on some standardized and validated test.

In an example of using a common physical parameter, John and colleagues[2] evaluated the ability of (1) elderly participants with sensorineural hearing loss, (2) elderly participants with essentially normal hearing, and (3) normally hearing young adults to detect silent gaps within 6-second segments of white noise. Gaps were simply measured in milliseconds (msec) of duration, in this case from 2 to 20 msec.

However, dependent variables are not always measurable in such a straightforward manner. For example, Fukuda and colleagues[3] examined the effect of pulsed shortwave (PSW) treatment for knee osteoarthritis in 121 women (mean age = 60 years). One of the outcome measures was change in pain. But how does a researcher truly measure "how much" pain someone experiences? We do not have a simple physical measure of it. In this case, and in many experiments of similar design, researchers need to rely on participants' report of a subjective measure such as pain intensity. In this case, the researchers used an 11-point pain rating scale and the Knee Injury Osteoarthritis Outcome Score (KOOS) to measure their dependent variable of pain (they also measured other outcomes). They were careful to note that both measures have been shown to be valid. We emphasize here that, when either evaluating research or conducting research/clinical practice, it is critical to determine the validity of measures of dependent variables, particularly when those measures involve subjective procedures such as rating scales.

Sometimes scientist-practitioners do not have either a physical measure or a validated subjective indicator to measure outcomes and must develop their own creative ways of measuring dependent variables. Koutsoftas and colleagues[4] examined the effect of a certain intervention, called "Tier 2," on phonemic awareness skills of preschool children from low-income families. Tier 2 intervention is used for children not progressing as well as their peers in achieving various curricular benchmarks. Koutsoftas and colleagues indicate it "typically consists of high-quality, short-term explicit instruction that is carried out in small groups by teachers, reading specialists, speech-language pathologists (SLPs), or other educators."[4(p. 117)] "Phonemic awareness" was the dependent variable, and it may seem like a rather abstract one. After all, how does a researcher know that somebody is "aware" of something?

Koutsoftas and colleagues[4] operationally defined dependent variables in several ways. First, they measured the pretreatment and posttreatment ability of participants to produce the first sound in words (consonant-vowel, consonant-vowel-consonant, or vowel-consonant, none of which had first sounds that were taught in class) when shown a picture representing a word. Second, they measured preintervention and postintervention outcomes on the Harcourt Trophies Pre-K curriculum for language and early literacy development curriculum benchmarks.[5] Third, they measured fall and spring performance on the Beginning Sound Awareness Subtest of the Phonological Awareness Literacy Screening for Preschool.[6]

Operationally defining a dependent variable can be challenging. However, the scientist-practitioner needs to be creative in developing ways of measuring seemingly difficult concepts. One of the authors was supervising a student in a speech-language pathology practicum. One of her assignments was to develop an outcome that would be beneficial to her. She chose "greater independence." How could she measure this internalized concept? The solution in this case was to count the number of times per week she went to her on-site supervising speech-language pathologist before finalizing her treatment plans for each of her clients.

Intervening Variables

Hegde[7] describes a type of variable he labels "intervening." These are largely mental processes that supposedly "intervene" between input and outcome. Examples are intelligence, motivation, and executive function. In this book, we do not deny the existence of these processes.

However, we note that they are extremely difficult to measure, if measurable at all. Thus, their experimental value is questionable at best.

Confounding and Extraneous Variables

One of the goals of experiments as we currently construct them is to be able to validly pinpoint the cause-and-effect relationship between independent and dependent variables. In our current conception of experiments, we try our hardest to make sure that changes in a dependent variable are due to only those independent variables the researcher manipulated or chose. That is, before the experiment, we try to account for possible causes of outcomes that are not related to the chosen independent variables and minimize them as best we can.

At times, there are circumstances outside our experiments/clinical interventions that have an effect on outcomes and that either we are not aware of or are beyond our control. We may consider extraneous variables in the research/clinical setting and those related to research participants/patients.

Extraneous Variables in the Setting

We need to control the clinical/research setting as best we can. Control of extraneous variables includes, for example, keeping the temperature, lighting, and time of day of testing constant to rule out differences in these factors as possible explanations for any changes in the dependent variable.

Extraneous Variables Related to Participants

Control of extraneous variables related to the participant is another means of control within research design. Researchers usually attempt to hold factors other than the independent variable constant for all participants or groups. In this way, extraneous variables are controlled because they will affect all participants or groups equally. When researchers do not, or cannot, control extraneous variables, the study is vulnerable to various threats to its internal validity. Chapter 8 provides detail on ways to prevent, or at least minimize, these threats to internal validity.

FUNCTIONAL RELATIONSHIPS

In an experiment or in a clinical intervention, we look for some causal relationships between inputs (independent variables) and outcomes (dependent variables). That is, we look for a *functional relationship* between or among variables. When we see what looks like a cause-and-effect relationship, we say that a change in outcome *is a function of* the change in input.

We note two important types of functional relationships. A *linear* relationship exists when the independent variable changes by a constant amount (if the variable is quantifiable); that is, the change between each level of the independent variable is the same from one to the next, and each change is accompanied by a constant amount of change in the dependent variable. Table 7-1 shows a data set of a hypothetical linear relationship. This example shows the presumed relationship between lower extremity muscle strength (an assigned independent variable) and distance in feet walked in 6 minutes (the dependent variable) among participants 80 years old and weighing between 160 and 170 lb. Muscle strength is defined as the number of squats performed in 1 minute. The data show that as number of squats increases by a given amount (e.g., 2 per minute), distance increases by a constant amount (175 feet). Figure 7-1 shows a graph of the results, and the results describe a straight line.

In a *nonlinear* functional relationship, constant changes in the independent variable (or any level of an independent variable) produce nonequal changes in a dependent variable. Table 7-2 shows a data set from the same type of relationship as described previously between muscle strength and distance walked. This time, however, the outcome changes in a nonlinear way. As number of squats increases by two, the distance walked increases less and less. Figure 7-2 shows a graph of these data, and the results describe a curving (i.e., nonlinear) line rather than a straight one.

A very important case of functional relationship occurs in experiments in which there are more than one indepen-

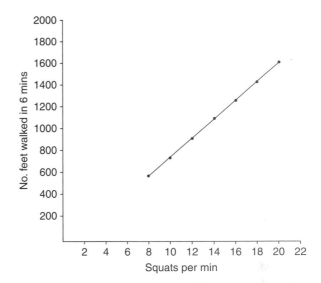

Figure 7-1 Graph of data in Table 7-1. Squats per minute is on the X-axis, and number of feet walked in 6 minutes is on the Y-axis.

dent variable, called a *factorial* experiment (see Chapter 10 for a complete description). Nelson notes, "An important advantage of factorial designs is that researchers can investigate not only the effect of each independent variable, but also how independent variables work together or influence one another.... Interaction effects occur in a factorial research design when the outcomes associated with one independent variable are different depending on the level of the other independent variable."[8(p. 118)]

Table **7-1**

Number of Feet Walked in 6 Minutes by 80-Year-Old Participants Varying in Lower Extremity Muscle Strength*

Squats/Minute	Distance Walked in 6 Minutes (ft)
8	600
10	775
12	950
14	1125
16	1300
18	1475
20	1650

*Defined as number of squats repeated in 1 minute. The data describe a linear functional relationship.

Table **7-2**

Number of Feet Walked in 6 Minutes by 80-Year-Old Participants Varying in Lower Extremity Muscle Strength*

Squats/Minute	Distance Walked in 6 Minutes (ft)
8	600
10	775
12	925
14	1050
16	1150
18	1225
20	1275

*Defined as number of squats repeated in 1 minute. The data describe a nonlinear functional relationship.

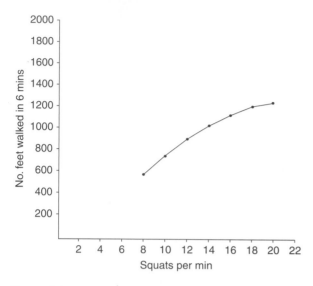

Figure 7-2 Graph of data in Table 7-2. Squats per minute is on the X-axis, and number of feet walked in 6 minutes is on the Y-axis.

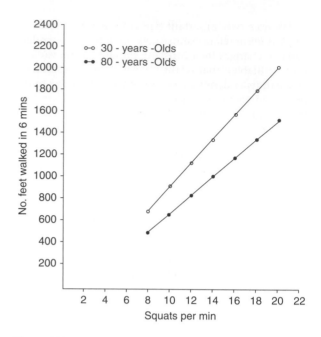

Figure 7-3 Graph of data from Table 7-3. Squats per minute is on the X-axis, and number of feet walked in 6 minutes is on the Y-axis. Data points from 30-year-olds are represented by *open circles*. Data points from 80-year-olds are represented by *filled circles*.

Table **7-3**

Number of Feet Walked in 6 Minutes by 80-Year-Old Participants and 30-Year-Old Participants Varying in Lower Extremity Muscle Strength*

Squats/Minute	Distance Walked in 6 Minutes— 30-Year-Old	Distance Walked in 6 Minutes— 80-Year-Old
8	800	600
10	1025	775
12	1250	950
14	1475	1125
16	1700	1300
18	1925	1475
20	2150	1650

*Defined as number of squats repeated in 1 minute. The data describe a linear functional relationship.

In Table 7-3, the data set shows a hypothetical example of the effect of muscle strength on distance walked per unit time. However, this time, the investigation was applied to two different groups: adults 80 years old and adults 30 years old (all the same weight). Thus, "client age" is the second (assigned) independent variable. The effect of increased muscle strength was that it was consistently accompanied by increased walking distance. However, even though this was true for both young and old participants, a constant increase in muscle strength produced greater improvement for the younger group than for the older participants. Thus, the outcome associated with increases in number of squats per minute varied depending on the level of the second independent variable (in this case, age). The graph in the case of an interaction has characteristic nonparallel lines (Fig. 7-3).

GRAPHS

Certainly one of the best ways to understand functional relationships among variables is by representing them on graphs. Most graphs that researchers see or use are two-dimensional, that is, have a horizontal axis (the "abscissa") and a vertical axis (the "ordinate") that intersect at some point, creating a right angle. Although it is not necessary, it is customary to label the abscissa with values of the independent variable and to label the ordinate with values of the dependent variable.

These simple graphs are almost always one of two kinds: a *line* graph or a *bar graph*. We use line graphs when the independent variable represents a continuum of some kind. For example, the data sets in Tables 7-1 and 7-2 describe increasing values of muscle strength in squats per minute, that is, a continuum. It is a continuum because, from left to right, each strength value must be followed by a larger one. The distances associated with each respective strength value are connected by a line. Refer again to Figures 7-1 and 7-2 showing simple line graphs depicting the data sets for the hypothetical cases described previously.

There are two special cases of line graphs to consider. One is when the experiment had a factorial design, that is, had more than one independent variable. In that case, the abscissa represents either one of the independent variables, and the other independent variable(s) is/are represented as a *parameter*. Figure 7-3 shows this example, representing the data set (see Table 7-3) in which varying degrees of muscle strength produce distance walked in 6 minutes in two age groups. In Figure 7-3, the abscissa represents one independent variable, muscle strength, and the ordinate represents distance walked in 6 minutes, the dependent variable. The parameter is the second independent variable, age, with two values, represented by open circles (young adult) and filled circles (older adults). In this case, there was an interaction of the independent variables, and the characteristic nonparallel lines are the result.

It is just as possible to have represented the data from Table 7-3 with age, rather than strength, on the abscissa and have strength as the parameter value. This is depicted in Figure 7-4. The X-axis now represents the two age groups. Because age is a continuum, the data from 30-year-olds are to the left and those of 80-year-olds are to the right. For the sake of demonstration, we will consider only the data from participants who produced 8 (open circles), 14 (filled circles), and 20 (open squares) squats per minute. Distance is still represented on the Y-axis. Once again, because age is a continuum, the data points are connected by lines. It is important to note that the results still have the same nonparallel lines as when the X-axis represented muscle strength.

There is one other special case for line graphs: the case of single-subject designs. In these designs, treatment is always the independent variable. One of the aspects that make these designs unique is that the treatment is always applied over time. It is customary, then, to have the abscissa represent elapsed time, rather than values of the independent variable. The ordinate still represents values of the dependent variable; it is understood that the independent variable (treatment) is always operating, and its values are incorporated into the line graph. Note that the graph is a line graph because elapsed time is always on a continuum.

Figure 7-5 shows the results of one participant in a study using a single-subject design. The study by Gutman, an occupational therapist, and colleagues[9] examined the effects of a motor-based social skills intervention in two participants with high-functioning

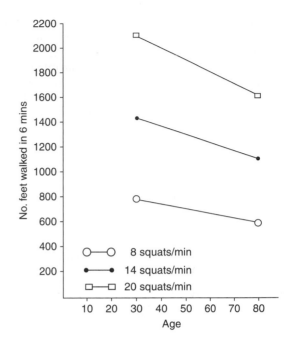

Figure 7-4 Graph of data from Table 7-3 with age on the X-axis. The parameter is muscle strength, showing 8 *(open circles)*, 14 *(filled circles)*, and 20 *(open squares)* squats per minute. Distance walked (ft) in 6 minutes is on the Y-axis.

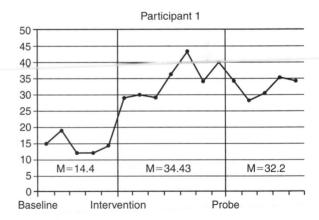

Figure 7-5 Results of a motor-based social skills intervention for one adolescent with high-functioning autism. (Modified from Gutman SA, Raphael EI, Ceder LM, et al: The effect of a motor-based, social skills intervention for adolescents with high-functioning autism: Two single-subject design cases, *Occup Ther Int* 17:188–197, 2010.)

autism. The outcome measure was the average frequency of aggregated social skills, collected in series of 20-minute observation periods. In this line graph, the abscissa shows data collection times (i.e., on a time continuum) divided into baseline (pretreatment),

treatment, and probe (postintervention) phases. The ordinate shows the frequency of outcome measures.

Up to now we have considered the appropriate use of line graphs. On the other hand, there are often cases in which the values of the independent variable are not in any hierarchical order. That is, any value of the independent variable could be represented in any position. In this case, the appropriate graph to use is a bar graph. Figure 7-6 shows the results from a data set (not shown) of three different therapy methods for increasing use of the upper extremity of persons who have had a cerebrovascular accident (CVA). For this hypothetical example, interventions are constraint-induced movement therapy, progressive resistance exercise, and neurodevelopmental treatment, each applied in separate but similar populations, for 1 month. The dependent variable is number of minutes of use per day of an upper extremity paralyzed by the CVA. After data are collected, the researcher may wish to represent the values of the independent variable according to the outcomes of the dependent variable (e.g., from lowest to highest), but it is not required, nor even conventional. The critical

point is that the three values of the independent variable (i.e., the three therapy methods) do not represent a hierarchical order of some kind. Thus, the values of the dependent variable generated by the three methods are not connected by a line, but rather are represented by the height of a vertical bar.

SUMMARY

Variables are aspects that change over the course of research, whether clinical or not, as well as clinical practice itself. Understanding their nature and function is critical, certainly for clinical practice, and, in research, particularly for experimentation. They are broadly designated as *independent* and *dependent* variables, with the former presumed to be causes and the latter presumed to be effects of those causes. If the independent variables are *active*, that is, controlled or chosen by the scientist-practitioner, then a true cause-and-effect relationship may be inferred. If the independent variables are *assigned*, that is, with categories not manipulable by the researcher, then the outcome must be considered correlational, rather than causal. However, both types are valuable and commonly used by scientist-practitioners. Every independent variable must have at least two *levels* or values; otherwise, the property is a constant, not a variable.

Dependent variables are the outcomes of a study. Although sometimes difficult, scientist-practitioners should make every effort to define dependent variables in some measurable way. Sometimes the definition can be with common physical measures, such as elapsed time, velocity, or sound intensity. Often researchers may use outcomes on a standardized and validated test or other clinical instrument. Sometimes, scientist-practitioners just need to be creative in operationalizing their outcomes.

Scientist-practitioners also need to be aware of intervening and extraneous variables, those they wish to exclude from affecting results. Although it is not always possible to exclude every possible extraneous effect, good science and clinical practice demand that we try, or at least acknowledge the possibility of those factors affecting results.

Independent and dependent variables will form a *functional relationship*, showing how (or whether) a change in an independent variable produced a change in a dependent variable. A *linear* relationship shows a constant change in a dependent variable as a value of an independent variable changes by a constant amount. In a *nonlinear* relationship, as the independent variable changes by a constant amount, the change in the dependent variable is something other than a constant one.

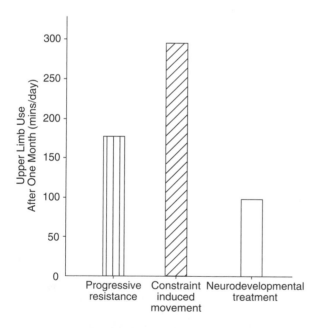

Figure 7-6 Bar graph showing results in minutes of use per day of cerebrovascular accident–affected upper limb for three therapy methods. The left-most bar shows results for progressive resistance (180 min). The middle bar shows results for constraint-induced movement (300 min). The right-most bar shows results for neurodevelopmental treatment (100 min).

Functional relationships are easily depicted by *graphs,* which often facilitate understanding of the relationship. Graphs in most rehabilitation research are two-dimensional, with a horizontal (X) axis (the abscissa) showing independent variables and a vertical (Y) axis (the ordinate) showing the dependent variable. Data points are connected by lines when the values of the independent variable form a continuum. If the values do not form a continuum, then data are represented by unconnected bars, each as high as the value of the dependent variable.

REFERENCES

1. Linacre JM, Heinemann AW, Wright BD, et al: The structure and stability of the Functional Independence Measure, *Arch Phys Med Rehabil* 75:127–132, 1994.
2. John AB, Hall JW, III. Kreisman BM: Effects of advancing age and hearing loss on gaps-in-noise test performance, *Am J Audiol* 21:242–250, 2012.
3. Fukuda TY, da Cunha RA, Fukuda VO, et al: Pulsed short-wave treatment in women with osteoarthritis: A multicenter, randomized, placebo-controlled clinical trial, *Phys Ther* 91:1009–1017, 2011.
4. Koutsoftas AD, Harmon MT, Gray S: The effect of Tier 2 intervention for phonemic awareness in a response-to-intervention model in low-income preschool classrooms, *Lang Speech Hear Serv Schools* 40:116–130, 2009.
5. Harcourt School Publishers: *Scientific Research Base, Harcourt Trophies*, Orlando, Fla, 2002, Author.
6. Invernizzi M, Sullivan A, Meier J: *Phonological Awareness Literacy Screening for Preschool*, Charlottesville, Va, 2001, University Press.
7. Hegde MN: *Clinical Research in Communicative Disorders*, 3rd ed, Austin, Tex, 2002, Pro-Ed.
8. Nelson LK: *Research in communication sciences and disorders*, 2nd ed, San Diego, Calif, 2013, Plural.
9. Gutman SA, Raphael EI, Ceder LM, et al: The effect of a motor-based, social skills intervention for adolescents with high-functioning autism: two single-subject design cases, *Occup Ther Int* 17:188–197, 2010.

CHAPTER 8

Research Validity

CHAPTER OUTLINE

Internal Validity
Threats to Internal Validity
History
Maturation
Testing
Instrumentation
Statistical Regression to the Mean
Assignment (Subject Selection)
Subject Attrition
Interactions Between Assignment
   and Maturation, History, or
   Instrumentation

Diffusion or Imitation of Treatments
Compensatory Equalization of
   Treatments
Compensatory Rivalry or Resentful
   Demoralization
Construct Validity
Construct Underrepresentation
Experimenter Expectancies
Interaction Between Different
   Treatments
Interaction Between Testing and
   Treatment

External Validity
Selection
Setting
Time
External Validity in Single-Subject
   Research
External Validity in Qualitative
   Research
**Relationships Among Types
   of Validity**
Summary

The validity of a piece of research is the extent to which the conclusions of that research are believable and useful. Cook and Campbell[1] have outlined four types of validity, and this chapter relies to a great extent on their now classic work. When determining the value of a piece of research, readers need to ask four basic questions:

1. In an experiment, is the research designed so that there are few alternative explanations for changes in the dependent variable other than the effect of the independent variable? Factors other than the independent variables that could be related to changes in the dependent variable are threats to *internal validity*.
2. Are the research constructs defined and used in such a way that the research can be placed in the framework of other research within the field of study? Poor definition of constructs or inconsistent use of constructs is a threat to *construct validity*.
3. To whom can the results of this research be applied? Sampling and design factors that lead to limited generalizability are threats to *external validity*.
4. Are statistical tools used correctly to analyze the data? Irregularities in the use of statistics are threats to *statistical conclusion validity*.

The purpose of this chapter is to provide a discussion of the first three types of validity. Because understanding statistical conclusion validity requires a background in statistical reasoning, its threats are discussed in Chapter 20 after statistical reasoning is introduced.

Each of the remaining three types of validity has several identifiable threats that can be illustrated either in examples from the rehabilitation literature or in examples of hypothetical rehabilitation research. For each of these threats, at least one example is presented, and mechanisms for controlling the threat are suggested. The chapter ends with an examination of the interrelationships among the types of validity.

INTERNAL VALIDITY

Internal validity is the extent to which the results of a study demonstrate that a causal relationship exists between the independent and dependent variables. In experimental research, the central question about internal validity is whether the treatments (or the various levels of the independent variable) caused the observed changes in the dependent variable. The classic randomized controlled trial, with random assignment to experimental and control groups, is considered by many to be the best way to control threats to internal validity when studying interventions.

We should not forget, however, that much of clinical practice is experimental in nature, in the sense that we attempt to draw a causal link between our treatment or intervention (independent variable) and desired changes in our clients' abilities (dependent variables). Thus, in clinical practice we also wish to show that those behavior changes are due to our interventions and not to extraneous variables.

In nonexperimental research designed to delineate differences between groups in the absence of controlled manipulation by the researcher, the question becomes less "causal" and instead focuses on whether the independent variable is a plausible explanation of group differences on the dependent variable. In nonexperimental research designed to describe a phenomenon or establish relationships among variables, internal validity is not an issue in that no comparisons between levels of the independent variable are being made.

However, some nonexperimental research looks experimental except that the independent variable is an attribute, rather than active variable. For example, Nippold and colleagues[2] measured various outcomes of syntactic ability (dependent variables) in adolescents with history of specific language impairment (SLI), nonspecific language impairment (NLI), and typical language development (TLD)—three levels of an independent variable (diagnostic category). Generally, TLD participants outperformed those in other categories on all measures, and on a standardized test, SLI participants outperformed those in the NLI group. In this case, although we cannot prove cause and effect, the case for a significant correlation is strengthened if the only plausible reason for the outcome is changes in the (assigned) independent variable. In fact, Nippold and colleagues[2] were cautious (and correct) in analyzing results as correlations. Because the researcher will at least choose, if not control, independent variables and their levels and will measure outcomes as these change, attention to internal validity in these quasi-experiments is certainly warranted.

The general strategy that researchers use to increase internal validity is to maximize their control over all aspects of the research project, as first described in Chapter 6. The researcher carefully monitors the control and experimental groups to ensure that experimental groups receive the intervention as designed and that control groups do not inadvertently receive components of the intervention. Randomized assignment of participants to treatment groups maximizes the probability that extraneous participant characteristics will be evenly distributed across groups. To check randomization, the researcher can collect information about participant characteristics that threaten internal validity to determine whether the characteristics in question were equally represented across groups. Eliminating extraneous variables through control of the experimental setting removes them as plausible causes of changes in the dependent variable. Research assistants are carefully trained to collect and record information accurately and reliably. Information about which participants are receiving which treatment is concealed, when possible, from both the participants as well as the researchers who collect data and interact with participants.

We also need to address internal validity in a certain class of experimental designs known as within-subjects or repeated measures designs. The designs are explained fully in Chapter 10, but, suffice to say that in the most typical of these, there is one group of subjects, each of whom receives each experimental condition, or, put another way, each level of each independent variable. For example, a physical therapist may wish to explore the effect of each of three treatment methods on range of motion after an intervention of different proprioceptive neuromuscular facilitation (PNF) strengthening exercises. In a group of, say, six participants, each would receive each treatment. Experimental control is largely gained by varying the order of the treatments among the participants in order to reduce or eliminate spurious outcomes that are the result of the order of treatments (see Chapter 10). However, it is critical to note that the varying of treatment order does not prevent the incursion of the threats to internal validity described subsequently.

Yet another type of experiment for which we need to consider internal validity is the single-subject experiment. Single-subject experiments (see Chapter 11) are those in which data for each participant are considered individually, rather than as part of a group. Because each participant's results are considered by themselves, each participant serves as his or her own control, rather than the research including a control group. However, single-subject experiments are susceptible to many of the threats to internal validity described later.

Threats to Internal Validity

When developing research proposals, investigators should carefully consider each threat to internal validity to determine whether their design is vulnerable to that threat. If it is, the researchers must decide whether to institute additional controls to minimize the threat, collect additional information to document whether the threat materialized, or accept the threat as an unavoidable design flaw. There is no perfect research design, and high levels of internal validity may compromise construct or external validity, as discussed at the end of the chapter. Eleven of Cook and Campbell's[1] threats to internal validity are important for rehabilitation researchers and are discussed later.

History

History is a threat to internal validity when events unrelated to the treatment of interest occur during the course of the study and may plausibly change the dependent variable.

Bhatt[3] led a study in which one group of participants with Parkinson's disease (PD) received training via audiovisual cues for stability control during sit-to-stand tasks. Other groups in the study were participants with PD who did not receive training and a group of non-PD older adults matched for body mass and height. At the end of 4 weeks of training, the trained group exhibited much greater stability and center-of-mass velocity compared with the untrained PD group.

Bhatt's study did not seem to have suffered from the historical threat to internal validity in that only the trained group improved. However, none of the participants was under the researchers' constant surveillance, and historical threats may well have appeared. The researchers did not report any efforts, for example, to limit external cue strategies in the participants' homes. They did not report any efforts to limit practice on the sit-to-stand task, such as from other sources of physical therapy. Had any of these occurred, results might have spuriously been different, such as not demonstrating a training effect. The lesson here is that, first, investigators must, to the best of their ability, try to predict sources of the threat of history. Second, after a study, researchers are well advised to investigate possible sources of historical threat that may have arisen.

Researchers can use three strategies to minimize the effects of history: planning, use of a randomly selected control group, and description of unavoidable historical events. In experimental studies, careful planning by the researcher can minimize the chances that historical events will influence the study. If a geographical region is usually snowed in during February, a study that requires participant attendance at treatment sessions 5 days per week should probably be scheduled at another time of year. If testing of participants requires a full day with half-hour rests between measurements, it might be wise to isolate participants and researchers from radios and televisions so that news that happens to occur on the day of testing does not influence participant or researcher performance.

Use of a control group provides the researcher with some ability to separate the effects of history from the effects of the treatment. Random assignment of participants to groups is the best way to minimize the effects of history because the different groups will likely be affected equally by the historical event.

In some instances, historical events that cannot be avoided may occur. In retrospective nonexperimental studies, control of history is impossible because the historical events have already occurred. If an uncontrolled historical event that may cause changes in the dependent variable does occur, it is important to collect and present information about the event.

Clark and colleagues[4] completed a retrospective study of the effects of early mobilization in a trauma and burns intensive care unit (ICU). They completed the study by examining medical records. Results indicated that the patients who had received early mobilization treatment had fewer airway, pulmonary, and vascular complications. However, Clark and colleagues pointed out—and rightly so—that their results were not conclusive because they could not account for changes in patient care other than early mobilization that may have affected patient outcomes. As illustrated in this study, when unable to control a threat, researchers have a responsibility to present information about the threat so that readers may form an opinion about its seriousness.

In single-subject designs, the threats from history are minimized in one or more of a few ways. One way is by establishing a stable pretreatment baseline, sometimes in more than one client or for more than one behavior (i.e., "multiple baselines"). If historical events were having an effect, they might happen in some period before treatment. If there is no change in client behavior once treatment begins, we can conclude that the history threat did not affect the experiment, at least during that period.

Another tactic in single-subject studies is withdrawing and reinstating treatment. Particularly in the early stages of treatment (experiment), if the treatment is effective, behavior should change toward desired values when it is applied and not change positively when it is not applied. By successively applying and withdrawing treatment (and this can be done several times during the course of treatment), the clinician can determine whether some extraneous variable—possibly from experimental history—is accounting for behavior change.

A variation on treatment withdrawal is *treatment reversal*. Although counterintuitive, in reversal, the treatment is actually applied to a behavior that is opposed to the desired behavior. The purpose is to show the effective behavior control of the treatment, rather than to sustain the reversed behavior. However, as Hayes and associates note, "The true reversal is seldom seen in applied situations, both for ethical reasons and because many interventions are not 'reversible.'"[5(p. 226)]

A third control mechanism is rapidly alternating between two treatments or between treatment and no treatment. As in treatment application and withdrawal, effects of the two treatment conditions should produce concomitant time-locked effects on the outcome. If the outcome does not change in a time-locked way with treatment alternation, the clinician must at least suspect the participation of the history threat.

A fourth control mechanism for the history threat is that of criterion-referenced change. In applying a criterion-referenced change, the clinician systematically "raises the bar" for reinforcement; if effective, behavior should change concomitantly. Hegde notes, "… if whenever the criterion is changed the dependent variable also changes in accordance with the new criterion in force, then the experimental control is demonstrated."[6(p. 111)]

A fifth control mechanism for history is replication, both within a study and in a series of studies. As Richards and colleagues note, "The more replications included within a study, the less changes in the dependent variable are attributable to extraneous or confounding variables."[7(p. 96)]

Maturation

Maturation—that is, changes within a participant caused by the passage of time—is a threat to internal validity when it occurs during the course of a study and may plausibly cause changes in the dependent variable. Participants get older, more experienced, or bored during the course of a study. Patients with neurological deficits may experience spontaneous improvement in their conditions; participants with orthopedic injuries may become less edematous, have less pain, and be able to bear more weight with time.

As was the case with historical threats to internal validity, single-group studies do not provide a basis from which the researcher may separate the effects of maturation from the effects of treatment. This becomes readily apparent in studies that take place over a relatively long period of time, such as a school year. Imagine a study being carried out by a school-based occupational therapist who has devised an intervention program for fine motor skill development. She identifies a group of first-graders who do not seem to have the fine motor skills typical of their age peers[8] and tests them in September. Then she implements her intervention and retests in April. Happily, she finds that 75% of the participants have improved and pats herself on the back. Of course, many factors other than the intervention may have contributed to or even caused the results. In studies of treatment effectiveness in single groups, readers must always consider the possibility that seemingly effective treatments may have been aided by extraneous factors.

Maturation effects can be controlled in several ways. The first is through use of a control group, preferably with random assignment of participants to either the control or the experimental group. Use of the control group allows the effects of maturation alone to be observed in the control group. The treatment effects are then evaluated in terms of how much the treatment group improved in comparison with the control group.

A second way to control for the effects of maturation is to take multiple baseline measures of participants before implementing the treatment. Suppose that you have a group of patients with ankle sprains who have persistent edema despite protected weight bearing, compression bandage wrap, elevation when possible, and use of ice packs three times daily. Documentation of baseline volume over a period of several days or weeks would provide appropriate comparison measures against which the effects of a compression and cryotherapy pump regimen could be evaluated. Figure 8-1 shows three patterns of baseline measurements: stable, irregular, and steadily progressing. Results after the intervention are interpreted in light of the baseline pattern documented before the intervention. Patients in Figure 8-1A had no change in the weeks before intervention but showed dramatic improvements after treatment. Patients in Figure 8-1B had weekly fluctuations in edema before treatment and marked improvement after treatment. Patients in Figure 8-1C showed consistent, but slow, improvement in the weeks before treatment and more rapid improvement after treatment.

Maturation effects may be seen in repeated treatment research designs. Any time participants receive more than one treatment, they may respond differently to later treatments than to earlier treatments. Performance on the dependent variable may improve for later treatments because of increased experience with the treatment, or performance may decline because of fatigue or boredom. For example, Tyrell and associates[9] investigated the effects of treadmill speed on gait kinematics in 20 patients who had had a stroke. They hypothesized that a fast treadmill speed would produce the best measures of walking. Their four treadmill speeds were (1) patient self-selected (slowest), (2) therapist-determined maximum, and (3,4) two intermediate speeds. Results indicated that, with the greatest speed, gait kinematics generally improved the most.

Perhaps a logical way for Tyrell to have proceeded would have been to start with slow speeds and work up to the fastest speed. But this would have masked the effects of the greatest speed, and results could have been attributed to practice or some other factor. Instead, the investigators chose to present the speeds randomly. Doing so isolated the effect of the fast speed and eliminated the maturation threat.

In single-subject research, the controls for the threat from maturation are the same as those for history: (1) stable baseline, (2) treatment withdrawal or reversal, (3) rapid treatment alternation, (4) criterion-referenced change, and (5) replication. As in controlling for history, if effects

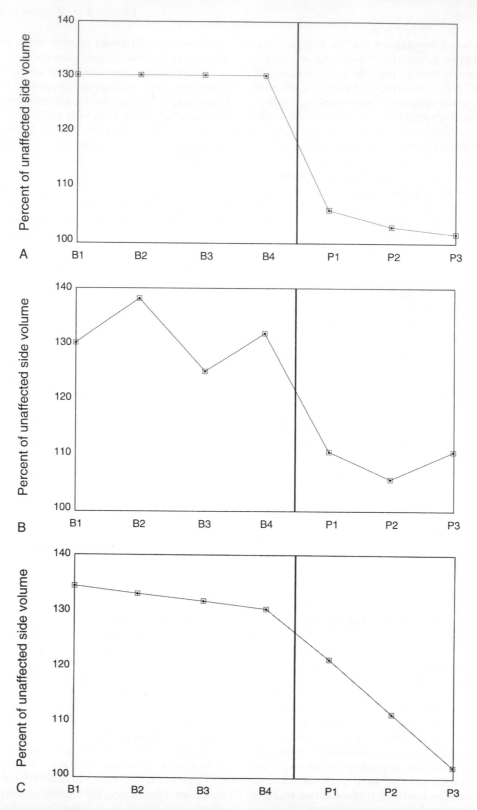

Figure 8-1 Patterns of baseline (*B*) measurements in relation to posttreatment (*P*) measurements. **A,** Stable baseline. **B,** Irregular baseline. **C,** Baseline with a downward trend.

of maturation are taking place, they will show up during periods of nontreatment or will show up in a carefully repeated study. In addition, if applicable, the researcher may design a study so that the total time span is not overly long; in this way, possible maturation effects may not have a chance to manifest themselves.

Testing

Testing is a threat to internal validity when repeated testing itself is likely to result in changes in the dependent variable. For example, on the first day of speech therapy, a child who has a speech delay may feel uncomfortable in the surroundings and intimidated by the speech-language pathologist, giving worse-than-normal responses to testing. Improved measurements on subsequent days may reflect familiarization with the testing procedure and the therapist rather than effectiveness of the treatment.

Three basic design strategies can be used to minimize testing effects. The first is to use randomly selected experimental and control groups so that the effects of testing in the control group can be removed by comparison with the effects of testing and treatment in the experimental group. This is analogous to the removal of the effects of history and maturation through use of a control group.

The second strategy is to eliminate multiple testing through use of a posttest-only design. However, in the absence of a pretest to establish that control and experimental groups were the same at the start of the experiment, posttest-only studies must have effective random assignment of participants to groups. In practice, posttest-only strategies, while theoretically minimizing the testing effect, make measurements of treatment effects difficult.

The third design strategy is to conduct familiarization sessions with the testing personnel or equipment so that the effects of learning are accounted for before the independent variable is manipulated. To determine the extent of familiarization needed, the researcher should conduct a pilot study to determine how much time or how many sessions are needed before performance is stable. One drawback of multiple testing is the possibility that the familiarization process will itself constitute a "treatment." For example, if participants familiarize themselves with a strength-testing protocol once a week for 4 weeks, they may have exercised enough during familiarization to show a training response.

Because of the clinical nature of single-subject research, measurement of the dependent variable both before and during (and after) treatment almost always takes place, giving some room for the testing threat. However, the behavioral nature of single-subject research often precludes effects of the testing threat. Specifically, single-subject research avoids the use of *reactive measures*, such as attitudes or opinions, which are known to change with repeated measures. Instead, the operationally defined dependent variables of single-subject research offer some measure of protection from the testing threat.

Instrumentation

Instrumentation is a threat to internal validity when changes in measuring tools themselves are responsible for observed changes in the dependent variable. Many tools that record physical measurements need to be calibrated with each testing session. Calibration is a process by which the measuring tool is compared with standard measures to determine its accuracy. If inaccurate, some tools can be adjusted until they are accurate. If a tool has limited adjustability, the researcher may need to apply a mathematical correction factor to convert inaccurate raw scores into accurate transformed scores. If temperature or humidity influences measurement, these factors must be controlled, preferably through testing under constant conditions or, alternatively, through mathematical adjustment for the differences in physical environment.

Researchers themselves are measuring tools ("human instruments"). An example of the variability in the human instrument has surely been felt by almost any student; it is almost impossible for an instructor to apply exactly the same criteria to each paper in a large stack. Maybe the instructor starts out grading leniently but "cracks down" as he or she proceeds through the stack of papers. Maybe the instructor who is a stickler at first adopts a more permissive attitude when the end of the stack is in sight. Maybe a middling paper is graded harshly if it follows an exemplary paper; the same paper might be graded favorably if it followed an abysmal example. A variety of observational clinical measures, such as perception of voice characteristics, identification of gait deviations, functional levels, or abnormal muscle tone, may suffer from similar problems. Measurement issues in rehabilitation research are addressed in detail in Section Six.

Control of the instrumentation threat is no different in single-subject and group designs. Scientist-practitioners must make sure their mechanical instruments are working properly and, if appropriate, calibrated. Human "instruments" must be trained and "calibrated" to make reliable and valid judgments of behavior.

Statistical Regression to the Mean

Statistical regression is a threat to internal validity when participants are selected based on extreme scores on a single administration of a test. A hypothetical example illustrates the mathematical principle behind statistical regression to the mean: We have three recreational runners, each of whom has completed ten 10-km runs in an average time of 50 minutes and a range of times from 40 to 60 minutes. The distribution in Figure 8-2A represents the race times of the three runners.

Suppose we wish to test a new training regimen designed to decrease race times to see whether the regimen is equally effective with runners at different skill

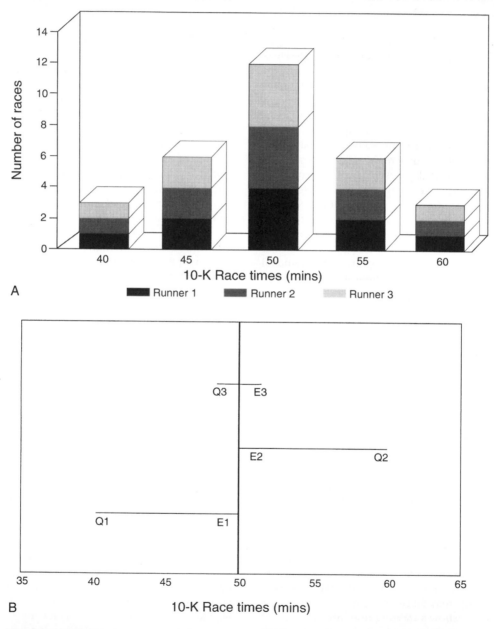

Figure 8-2 Statistical regression toward the mean. **A,** The distribution of race times for three runners, as shown by the different shading patterns on the bars. All three runners have an average race time of 50 minutes. **B,** The effect of statistical regression toward the mean if the runners are placed into different groups based on qualifying times at a single race. *Q* represents qualifying times for each runner; *E* represents the runners' evaluation times at a subsequent race. Runner 1 appears to have slowed from 40 to 50 minutes, Runner 2 appears to have speeded up from 60 to 50 minutes, and Runner 3 stayed approximately the same.

levels. We place runners into categories based on a single qualifying race time, have them try the training regimen for 1 month, and record their times at an evaluation race completed at the end of the 1-month training period. At the qualifying race, we place runners into one of three speed categories based on their time in that race: Participants in the fast group finished in less than 45 minutes, participants in the average group finished between and including 45 and 55 minutes, and participants in the slow group finished in greater than 55 minutes.

The times marked with a Q in Figure 8-2B show that Runner 1 performed much better than average on the day of the qualifying race (40 minutes), Runner 2 performed much worse than usual on the qualifying day (60 minutes), and Runner 3 gave an average performance (49 minutes). Runners 1 and 2 gave atypical performances on the qualifying day and in subsequent races would be expected to perform closer to their "true" running speed. Thus, even without intervention, Runner 1 would likely run the next race slower and Runner 2 would likely run the next race faster. Runner 3, who gave a typical performance, is likely to give another typical performance at the next race. In other words, the extreme scores tend to "regress toward the mean." This regression toward the mean for the evaluation race is represented by the times marked with an E in Figure 8-2B. If we do not consider the effects of statistical regression, we might conclude that the training program has no effect on average runners, speeds up the slow runners, and slows down the fast runners.

In general, the way to control for statistical regression toward the mean is to select participants for groups based on reliable, stable measures. If the measures used to form groups are inherently variable, participants are best assigned to groups based on a distribution of scores collected over time, rather than by a single score that might not reflect true ability. In single-subject designs, the effects of statistical regression to the mean can be controlled, or at least monitored, by the five control mechanisms noted for history and maturation.

Assignment (Subject Selection)

Assignment to groups is a threat to internal validity when groups of participants are different from one another on some variable that is related to the dependent variable of interest. Cook and Campbell labeled this particular threat "selection."[1] The term *assignment* is more precise and differentiates between this internal validity threat related to group assignment and the external validity threat, presented later, of participant selection.

Assignment threatens internal validity most often in designs in which participants are not randomly assigned to groups or in nonexperimental designs in which study group membership cannot be manipulated by the investigator. For example, Mäenpää and Lehto[10] used a retrospective nonexperimental design to determine the relative success of three different nonoperative ways to manage patellar dislocation. The three different groups were immobilized as follows: plaster cast, posterior splint, and bandage/brace. Because the treatment received was based on physician preference, there is no way to determine why individual participants were treated with a particular immobilization method and no randomization process to increase the likelihood that the groups would be similar on important extraneous variables. For example, the bandage/brace group consisted of proportionately more women than the other groups. Because women may have more predisposing anatomical factors for patellar dislocation than men, perhaps the higher re-dislocation rate for the bandage/brace group is related to the higher proportion of women, rather than to the type of immobilization.

Control of assignment threats is most effectively accomplished through random assignment to groups within a study (see Chapter 9). When random assignment to groups is not possible, researchers may use statistical methods to "equalize" groups (see Chapter 22).

Obviously, in single-subject research, group assignment is not a threat to validity because there are no assigned groups. Because data from single-subject research are treated individually rather than as group data, subject selection poses no threat to internal validity. Subject assignment or selection is also not a threat in within-subject designs because there is only one subject group.

Subject Attrition

Attrition is a threat to internal validity when participants are lost from the different study groups at different rates or for different reasons. Despite the best efforts of the researcher to begin the study with randomly assigned groups who are equivalent on all important factors, differential attrition can leave the researcher with very different groups by the end of the study. Assume that a researcher has designed a strengthening study in which one group of 50 participants begins a combined concentric and eccentric program of moderate intensity and another group of 50 participants begins a largely eccentric program of higher intensity. Forty-five of the participants in the moderate group complete the program, with an average increase in strength of 20%. Because of its strenuous nature, just 15 of the participants in the high-intensity group complete that program, with an average increase in strength of 40%. Concluding that the high-intensity program was superior to the moderate-intensity program would ignore the differential attrition of participants from the two groups. Investigators would need to explore the possibility that only the most physically fit of the high-intensity group were able or wanted to finish.

Researchers can control experimental attrition by planning to minimize possible attrition and collecting information about the lost participants and about reasons for the loss of participants.

Researchers need to make adherence to an experimental routine as easy as possible for participants while maintaining the intent of the experiment. Administering treatments at a place of work or at a clinic where participants are already being treated will likely lead to better attendance than if patients have to drive across town to participate in the study. Developing protocols that minimize discomfort is likely to lead to higher levels of retention within a study. Testing and treating on a single day avoids the loss of participants that inevitably accompanies a protocol that requires several days of participation.

When answering the research question requires longer term participation and its attendant loss of participants, researchers should document the characteristics of the participants who drop out of the study to determine whether they are similar to those who remain in the study. If the dropouts have characteristics similar to those of participants who remain in the study, and if the rate and character of dropouts are similar across study groups, then differential attrition has not occurred. Such a loss of participants is random and affects the study groups equally.

Because data from single-subject research are treated individually rather than as group data, subject attrition poses no threat to internal validity.

Interactions Between Assignment and Maturation, History, or Instrumentation

Assignment effects can interact with maturation, history, or instrumentation to either obscure or exaggerate treatment effects. These interactions occur when maturation, history, or instrumentation effects act differently on treatment and control groups.

A hypothetical example of an Assignment×History interaction would be seen in Bhatt's[3] study if all participants with PD—treated and untreated—also received cues for sit-to-stand and also practiced that task (historical threat). It is possible that those historical factors may have interacted with the treatment to produce what looked like solely a treatment effect. This problem might be described as follows in a journal article:

> A limitation to this study was that the investigators did not control or query the participants' home environment to ensure they did not receive any unintended practice or cues/instruction for the sit-to-stand task. If participants did receive unintended instruction, rather than comparing treatment to nontreatment, the study would have compared uncontrolled treatment (i.e., the historical factors) to uncontrolled plus controlled treatment.

In this scenario, the hypothetical threat of an Assignment×History interaction to internal validity was uncontrollable but explainable. Such threats can be explained only if researchers remain alert to possible threats and collect information about the extent to which participants were affected by the threat.

An interaction between assignment and maturation occurs when different groups are maturing at different rates. If a study of the effectiveness of a rehabilitation program for patients who have had a cerebral vascular accident (CVA) compared one group of patients 6 months after their CVA with another group 2 months after their CVA, the group with the more recent CVA would be expected to show greater spontaneous improvement.

An Assignment×Instrumentation interaction occurs when an instrument is more or less sensitive to change in the range at which one of the treatment groups is located. For example, assume that a researcher seeks to determine which of two methods of instruction, lecture or Web based, results in superior student achievement in pharmacology. The students in the different instructional groups take a pretest that has a maximum score of 100 points. The group being taught by the lecture method has an average pretest score of 60; the group being taught via the Web-based approach has an average pretest score of 20. The traditional group can improve only 40 points; the Web-based group can improve up to 80 points. Thus, the interaction between assignment and instrumentation exaggerates the differences in gain scores between the two groups by suppressing the gain of the group who started at 60 points. When scores "top out" and an instrument cannot register greater gains, this is termed a *ceiling effect;* when scores "bottom out" and an instrument cannot register greater declines, this is termed a *basement* or *floor effect.*

Control of interactions with assignment is accomplished through the same means that assignment, history, maturation, and instrumentation are controlled individually: random assignment to groups, careful planning, and collection of relevant information when uncontrolled threats occur. As is the case with assignment threats alone, mathematical equalization of groups can sometimes compensate for interactions between assignment and history, maturation, or instrumentation.

Diffusion or Imitation of Treatments

Diffusion of treatments is a threat to internal validity when participants in treatment and control groups share information about their respective treatments. Assume that an experiment evaluates the relative effectiveness of plyometrics versus traditional resistive exercise in restoring quadriceps torque in patients who have undergone anterior cruciate ligament reconstruction in a single clinic. Can you picture a member of the plyometrics group and a member of the traditional group discussing their respective programs while icing their knees down after treatment? Perhaps a man in the traditional group decides that low-intensity jumping is just the thing he needs to speed his rehabilitation program along and a man in the plyometrics group decides to buy a cuff weight and add some leg lifts to his program. If this treatment diffusion occurs, the difference between the intended treatments will be blurred.

Researchers can control treatment diffusion by minimizing contact between participants in the different groups, masking participants when possible, and orienting participants to the importance of adhering to the rehabilitation program to which they are assigned. Sometimes researchers offer participants the opportunity to participate in the alternate treatment after the study is completed if it proves to be the more effective treatment. This offer should make participants less tempted to try the alternate treatment during the study period.

Another way of viewing treatment diffusion is when positive behavior changes continue even in the absence of treatment. The behavioral view of this phenomenon is that some unintended and uncontrolled factor is now acting as the treatment, or independent variable. Treatment diffusion can be particularly insidious in single-subject research because of its natural inclusion of therapy methods. As in controlling several other threats to internal validity, the effects of a diffuse treatment can be detected and perhaps controlled by application of the five processes noted for the history threat. Aside from these, as in the example previously cited, researchers must take every precaution to limit treatment to the one they are providing. For example, a speech-language pathologist examining the effects of a new treatment for vocabulary acquisition in children might do well to notify the subjects' teachers of the experiment in an attempt to prevent the teacher from teaching the same vocabulary.

Compensatory Equalization of Treatments

Compensatory equalization of treatments is a threat to internal validity when a researcher with preconceived notions about which treatment is more desirable showers attention on participants who are receiving the treatment the researcher perceives to be less desirable. This extra attention may alter scores on the dependent variable if the attention leads to increased adherence to treatment instructions, increased effort during testing, or even increased self-esteem leading to a general sense of well-being.

Researchers should control compensatory equalization of treatments by avoiding topics about which they are biased or by designing studies in which their bias is controlled through researcher masking. In addition, if there is strong existing evidence that one treatment is more desirable than the other, researchers need to consider whether it is ethical to contrast the two treatments in another experimental setting.

Likewise, another control is an "integrity check" in implementing the independent variable(s). In this procedure, an independent researcher/clinician records delivery of treatment or other independent variable. See Chapter 3 for further detail.

Compensatory Rivalry or Resentful Demoralization

Rivalry and demoralization are threats to internal validity when members of one group react to the perception that they are receiving a less desirable treatment than other groups. This reaction can take two forms: compensatory rivalry (a "we'll show them" attitude) and resentful demoralization (a "why bother" attitude). Compensatory rivalry tends to mask differences between control and treatment groups; resentful demoralization tends to exaggerate differences between control and experimental groups. Researchers can control rivalry and resentment by controlling the information given to participants, masking themselves and participants to group membership, and having a positive attitude toward all groups.

CONSTRUCT VALIDITY

Construct validity is concerned with the meaning of variables within a study. Construct validity is an issue in all research studies. One of the central questions related to construct validity is whether the researcher is studying a "construct as labeled" or a "construct as implemented." An example of the difference between these two constructs is illustrated by a hypothetical example wherein a researcher uses active range of motion as a dependent measure of shoulder function. The construct as labeled is "function"; the construct as implemented is "active range of motion." Some readers might consider active range of motion to be a good indicator of function, but others might consider it an incomplete indicator of function. Those who are critical of the use of active range of motion as a functional indicator are questioning the construct validity of the dependent variable.

Cook and Campbell[1] described 10 separate threats to construct validity. Their list is collapsed into the four threats described in the following sections. The general strategy for controlling threats to construct validity is to develop research problems and designs through a thoughtful process that draws on the literature and theory of the discipline (see Chapter 2 for discussion of theory).

Construct Underrepresentation

Construct underrepresentation is a threat to construct validity when constructs are not fully developed within a study. One occurrence is the underrepresentation of constructs in independent variables.

A common—and often difficult—task in the real world is that of listening to speech in varying amounts of noise or other acoustic degradations (e.g., very rapid speech) and with varying amounts of language context (e.g., semantically relevant vs. irrelevant). Often, these interact, such that the ability to understand speech is greatly reduced if context is minimal and is also in a noisy background. Aydelott and Bates[11] conducted a study to examine the effects of semantic context and acoustic quality on participants' reaction times (RT) to indicating whether a word following a sentence (context) was either real or nonsense. However, Goy and colleagues[12] reasoned that the construct of distortion, including semantic and acoustic, was underrepresented. They note, "It is possible that the differential effects of the two types of distortion on facilitation observed by Aydelott and Bates (2004) could have resulted from the two distortion conditions differing in the *amount* of distortion as well as the *type* of distortion [their italics] ... selection of the distortion conditions [by Aydelott and Bates] (low-pass filtering at 1000 Hz and 50% time compression) likely confounded the amount of distortion with the intended comparison between types of distortion."[11(p. 8)] In response, Goy and colleagues devised two experiments using two amounts of distortion for each of three types of distortion. Thus, the construct of distortion of speech and its effects on RT were much more completely represented, and the authors posited that their results represented greater construct validity.

Construct underrepresentation may also be a concern related to the dependent variables within a study. Continuing the example of the ability to understand speech, it is instructive to note that, both in clinical practice and in more isolated research, that ability is measured by the accuracy of repetition of speech materials, usually single words or sentences. However, the two studies presented earlier[11,12] both note that an accuracy measure is often inadequate; it is common, for example, for people with hearing loss to be able to understand speech almost perfectly in favorable conditions, yet it takes more attention and processing time to do it. Thus, both Aydelott and Bates[11] and Goy and colleagues[12] used a time-sensitive measure (RT) to get a fuller picture of speech understanding.

Construct underrepresentation can also apply to the intensity of a construct. Kluzik and associates[13] studied the effect of a neurodevelopmental treatment (NDT) on reaching in children with spastic cerebral palsy. They analyzed reaching motions before and after a single NDT. In an invited commentary accompanying publication of Kluzik and associates'[13] article, Scholz noted the following:

> Something, albeit subtle, has resulted from the intervention. Expecting a more dramatic improvement in the reaching performance of this population following only one treatment is probably too much to ask in the first place. Future work should focus on the evaluation of long-term effects.[14(p. 77)]

Scholz thus recognized that the construct has been underrepresented because it was applied only once and recommended future work with a more intense representation of the construct. It should be noted that two of the original authors, Fetters and Kluzik,[15] shortly thereafter published follow-up work that addressed this concern by comparing the impact of 5 days of NDT with that of 5 days of practice of reaching tasks. Scholz's comments and the further work by Fetters and Kluzik[15] on more intensive NDT also gave impetus to additional investigation of intensive NDT.[16]

Experimenter Expectancies

Experimenter expectancy is a threat to construct validity when the participants are able to guess the ways in which the experimenter wishes them to respond, creating a mismatch between "construct as labeled" and "construct as implemented." In Chapter 6, "Clever Hans" was introduced during the discussion of whether it is possible to have independence of the investigator and participant. Recall that Clever Hans was a horse that could provide the correct response to mathematical problems by tapping his foot the correct number of times. His talents could be explained by the fact that questioners apparently unconsciously raised their eyebrows, flared their nostrils, or raised their heads as Hans was coming up to the correct number of taps. Rosenthal, who wrote about Hans, framed the issue in terms of the expectation of the examiner:

> Hans' questioners, even skeptical ones, expected Hans to give the correct answers to their queries. Their expectation was reflected in their unwitting signal to Hans that the time had come for him to stop his tapping. The signal cued Hans to stop, and the questioner's expectation became the reason for Hans' being, once again, correct.[17(p. 138)]

In the story of Clever Hans, the construct as labeled was "ability to do mathematics." The construct as implemented, however, was "ability to respond to experimenter cues."

There are several variations of this effect, most often involving one or more observers (not the investigator) and additional participants who perform some behavior recorded by the observers. In one variation, the Pygmalion effect (also known as the Rosenthal effect, named for the classic work by Rosenthal and Jacobson[18]), the experimenter induces expectations in an observer or observers. It then often turns out that participants in a task perform in accordance with the observers' expectations. In another variation, the investigator takes note of observers' expectations but does not purposely induce them. In a third variation, participants may behave in accordance with what they believe are the observers' expectations, whether that belief is valid or not; this often is manifest as the Hawthorne effect, in which participants' behavior is modified only because they know they are being observed.

Researchers can control experimenter expectancy effects by limiting information given to participants and themselves, by having different researchers who bring different expectations to the experimental setting replicate their study, and by selecting topics from which they can maintain an objective distance. Often, the threat is eliminated by a "double-blind" study. In this arrangement of a group research design (see Chapter 10), the investigators do not know to which group any participant has been assigned, and the participants do not know which group they are in (i.e., control or experimental).

Interaction Between Different Treatments

Interaction between different treatments is a threat to construct validity when treatments other than the one of interest are administered to participants. In

the population of rehabilitation patients, quite often the additional treatment is medication. For example, patients with PD often receive medical treatments while they might be participants in a study examining effects of rehabilitation therapy. Schenkman and colleagues[19] completed a study of the effects of three exercise programs on participants with early- to late-stage PD. They do not describe the medication schedules of their participants, but judging from their discussion, patients were off and on medication during the study. They did randomly assign participants to the treatment groups and note, "We did not collect data in the 'off-medication' state. However, we did control for levodopa [medication] equivalents, which should have adjusted for any bias due to medication effects."[19(p. 1407)] Here, the authors acknowledge the threat to construct validity that must be attended to by having more than one treatment at the same time. Had they not been cautious, they could not have known whether effects were due to physical therapy or an interaction of physical therapy and medication.

Control of interaction between different treatments is often difficult to achieve because of ethical considerations in clinical research. For example, if it would be unsafe for patients with Parkinson's disease to be off their medication temporarily, then Schenkman and colleagues[19] would have had no choice but to study the combined impact of stimulation and medication. However, researchers can document who receives additional treatment and can analyze data by subgroups if not all participants are exposed to the additional treatments. If all participants are exposed to multiple treatments, researchers need to carefully label the treatments to make this obvious.

Interaction Between Testing and Treatment

Interaction between testing and treatment is a threat to construct validity when a test itself can be considered an additional treatment. As discussed in the section on testing as a threat to internal validity, controlling for the threat to internal validity made by familiarization with the test may sometimes constitute an additional treatment. In the case of strength testing, for example, repeated familiarization sessions with the equipment may constitute a training stimulus. The treatment as labeled may be "nine strength training sessions"; the treatment as implemented may be "nine strength training sessions and three strength testing sessions."

One way to control for interaction between testing and treatment is to compare a treatment group that was pretested, a treatment group that was not pretested, a control group that was pretested, and a control group that was not pretested. This allows the researcher to compare the effects of the test and treatment combined with the effects of treatment alone, the test alone, and neither the test nor the treatment. Few examples of this design (known as a Solomon four-group design) can be found in the rehabilitation literature, presumably because of the large number of participants that would be required to form all four groups; a search in the CINAHL database (see Chapter 4) using "Solomon four-group design" as the keyword and searching from 2010 through September 2013 yielded only two examples. In addition, researchers can control for interaction between testing and treatment by limiting testing to the end of the study. However, as noted in the section on testing as threat to internal validity, not having pretreatment data makes measurement of treatment effects difficult.

EXTERNAL VALIDITY

External validity concerns to whom, in what settings, and at what times the results of research can be generalized. Cook and Campbell[1] distinguished between generalizing across groups, settings, or times and generalizing to particular persons, settings, or times. One can generalize to groups, settings, or times similar to the ones studied. One can generalize across groups, settings, or times if one has studied multiple subgroups of people, settings, or times. If researchers study the effect of a progressive resistive exercise technique on the biceps strength of elderly women, they can generalize their results only to elderly women. If they study the same question with a diverse group of men and women with an average age of 35 years, they can generalize their results to other diverse groups with an average age of 35 years. Even though the researchers have tested men and women of different age groups in the second example, they cannot generalize across age groups or sexes unless they analyze the diverse group according to subgroups. In this example, the overall group might show an increase in strength even if the elderly individuals in the group showed no change.

As was the case with construct validity, the question of generalizability of research results is equally applicable to descriptive research, relationship analysis, or difference analysis. Unlike internal validity and construct validity, both of which depend a great deal on the design of the study, external validity is influenced by not only the design of the study but also the research consumer who hopes to use the study findings as well. From a design perspective, controlling the threats to external validity requires thoughtful consideration of the population to whom the results of the study can be

applied, combined with practical considerations of the availability of participants for study and with attention to how closely the research resembles clinical practice. From a consumer perspective, external validity will relate to how closely the research participants and settings match the patients or clients to whom, and settings to which, the reader will apply the findings.

Selection

Selection is a threat to external validity when the selection process is biased in that it yields participants who are in some manner different from the population to which the researchers or readers hope to generalize the results. Individuals who are willing to serve as research participants may differ from the general population. As stated by Cook and Campbell, "Even when respondents belong to a target class of interest, systematic recruitment factors lead to findings that are only applicable to volunteers, exhibitionists, hypochondriacs, scientific do-gooders, those who have nothing else to do, and so forth."[1(p. 73)]

For example, consider a hypothetical experimental study in which a speech-language pathologist seeks volunteers to participate in a program to reduce foreign language accents among nonnative speakers of English. The program, which proves to be successful with the initial volunteer group, is considered for implementation by several corporations seeking to improve English language skills of their workers who are nonnative speakers. One consideration for these corporations must be how well the results from volunteers could be generalized to nonvolunteers. Volunteers who have a personal goal to reduce their accents would likely adhere to recommendations for practice outside the therapy environment. Contrast these volunteers with employees participating in a mandatory program imposed by their employers. If the employees in the imposed program do not practice recommended speech activities outside the therapy environment, their results may be substantially different from those found with the volunteers who do.

As an example of possible threats to external validity due to participant selection strategies, consider the study by Ebert and colleagues.[20] These investigators examined the effects of three interventions for language development in 59 school-aged (5:6 to 11:2 years), Spanish-English speaking, bilingual children with primary language impairment (PLI); that is, their communication difficulties were largely due to a language impairment per se rather than to their bilingual status. Fifty of the children were boys, and nine were girls. All were receiving special education language services at the time of the study.

The children in each of the treatment groups made language gains, although the gains were described as "modest." That speaks well for the intervention strategies, though perhaps the treatments need refining. Yet we need to consider the generalizability of results. These results cannot be generalized to populations much younger or older than the study participants. Results may well not be valid for bilingual children whose non-English language is something other than Spanish. They might not be generalizable to girls (9 out of 59), even Spanish-English speaking ones of school age.

Researchers can control selection as a threat to external validity by carefully considering the target population to whom they wish to generalize results, selecting participants accordingly, and carefully writing their research conclusions to avoid making inferences to groups or across subgroups who have not been studied. A selection issue receiving increased attention today is the need to ensure racial, ethnic, age, and gender representativeness of research participants to maximize generalizability across and to these groups. On the positive side, then, having these limitations from selection strategies invites a series of additional studies.

Setting

Setting is a threat to external validity when peculiarities of the setting in which the research was conducted make it difficult to generalize the results to other settings. We may easily continue our analysis of the study by Ebert and colleagues.[20] Their treatments were limited to being implemented in the children's schools, all in Minneapolis. Although schools are the single-most common locale for language therapy, they are not the only ones. We need to consider the generalizability of results to other therapy settings, for example, a private communication disorders clinic or hospital, or even at home. Again, these limitations invite further inquiry. Control of threats to external validity posed by setting requires that researchers simulate as closely as possible the setting to which they hope to generalize their results. Researchers who hope their studies will have clinical applicability must try to duplicate the complexities of the clinical, or even home, setting within their studies. Researchers who wish to describe participants or settings as they exist naturally must make the research process as unobtrusive as possible.

Time

Time is a threat to external validity when the results of a study are applicable to limited time frames. Many surveys investigating clinical or educational procedures are limited in their time generalizability because of ongoing developments in knowledge and trends in clinical practice. For example, Chan and associates[21] completed a survey of Australian speech-language pathologists, querying the degree to which they relied on evidence-based practice (EBP) to treat voice disorders. Because of an overall lack of higher levels of published evidence, the vast majority of respondents relied heavily on the "clinical expertise" part of EBP rather than on published research. Of course, as research progresses, new knowledge about voice disorders and their treatments will come to light, presumably influencing clinical practice. In addition, it is entirely possible that clinicians will increasingly rely on published evidence as the practice of EBP increases. Thus, results from Chan's study are not automatically generalizable to future times, and it would behoove researchers to replicate the study.

Time threats to external validity can be managed by authors through timely submission of research results for publication and by description of known changes that make the research results less applicable than when the data were collected. In addition, when articles are used some years after their publication date, readers have the responsibility to incorporate contemporary knowledge into their own review of the usefulness of the results to current practice.

External Validity in Single-Subject Research

Single-subject research poses some questions of external validity different from those posed by group designs. Because the very nature of single-subject research focuses on individuals, rather than group averages, generalizing to other participants/clients, settings, and times is challenged by the typically small number of participants. The question of generalizing to a population group is particularly daunting.

Without doubt, the most useful tactic for establishing generality from single-subject research is that of replication. Because no two individuals are assumed to be alike, replication of single-subject research can never be of *exactly* the same participant population. It could even be said that, because of the passage of time and prior exposure to the treatment, even replication on the same participant(s) is not of *exactly* the same people. However, the scientist-practitioner can at least begin to establish generality by replication on participants highly similar (e.g., on several important attributes) to those in the first study or by replication with the same participants after a period of some time. If the same results are obtained, some degree of generality of time and participant can be logically established. Once replication of highly similar, but not exact, circumstances shows similar effects, the researcher may replicate with some new variations, perhaps a change in degree of disability, age, a slightly different setting, or different clinician.

Barlow and Hersen[22] distinguished between "direct" and "systematic" replication. In the former, a study (whether of single-subject or group design) is replicated as closely as possible. Participants, settings, investigators, and all relevant conditions are repeated to the extent possible. In the latter, the investigator systematically introduces variations, such as those of client population characteristics, setting, or clinician. We take the view that the process is incremental rather than dichotomous. Replication for generality must be achieved in small steps, with each step another variation from the original research. Over time, with enough replication of results, generality becomes established.

External Validity in Qualitative Research

Qualitative research moves away from the types of controlled experimental studies we have been describing in order to investigate the unique characteristics of a population or phenomenon of interest (see Chapter 14 for more detail). As such, it is the very uniqueness of the various populations or phenomena studied that gives qualitative research its value. The concept of generalizability is not an issue. As Holloway and Wheeler note,

> Generalisability [sic] is difficult to achieve in qualitative research. Many qualitative researchers, however, do not aim to achieve generalisability as they focus on specific instances or cases not necessarily representative of other cases or populations... Indeed, the concept of generalisability is irrelevant if only a single case or a unique phenomenon is examined.[23(p. 300)]

RELATIONSHIPS AMONG TYPES OF VALIDITY

Numerous threats to validity have been presented. These threats are not, however, independent entities that can be controlled one by one until the perfect research design is created. The relationship between the validity threats can be either cumulative or reciprocal.

Cumulative relationships occur when a change that influences one of the threats influences other threats in the same way. For example, researchers may initially think to use a randomly assigned control group in a study because they want to control for the effects of maturation. By controlling for maturation in this way, they also control for history, assignment, testing, and so on.

Reciprocal threats occur when controlling a threat to one type of validity leads to realization of a different threat to validity. For instance, if a researcher wants to achieve the highest level of internal validity possible, he or she will standardize the experimental treatment so that there are few extraneous variables that could account for changes in the dependent measures. However, this standardization compromises external validity because the results can be applied only to settings in which the treatment would be equally well controlled. These reciprocal threats form the basis for the differentiation between research to test the efficacy of an intervention (testing effects under tightly controlled conditions with high internal validity) and effectiveness of an intervention (testing clinical usefulness under clinic-like conditions with high external validity). These concepts are explored further in Chapter 16 on outcomes research.

The reciprocal relationship between validity threats is illustrated in Mäenpää and Lehto's[10] study of conservative care of patients with patellar dislocation. As noted earlier, one of the groups of patients seemed to have a higher proportion of women patients than the other two groups. This represents an assignment threat to internal validity. To eliminate this threat from this retrospective study, the authors could have chosen to study only men or only women. In doing so, they would have reduced external validity by narrowing the group to whom the results of the study could be generalized. Mäenpää and Lehto couldn't win. If they studied men and women, they had to cope with a possible threat to internal validity. Conversely, if they studied only men, they would have limited external validity.

SUMMARY

Threats to the believability and utility of research can be classified as threats to internal, construct, or external validity. Internal validity concerns whether the treatment caused the effect; construct validity concerns the meaning attached to concepts used within the study; and external validity concerns the persons, settings, or times to which or across which the results can be generalized. Many of the threats to validity are reciprocal because controlling one leads to problems with another.

REFERENCES

1. Cook T, Campbell D: *Quasi-Experimentation: Design and Analysis Issues for Field Settings*, Chicago, Ill, 1979, Rand McNally.
2. Nippold MA, Mansfield TC, Billow JL, Tomblin JB: Syntactic development in adolescents with a history of language

impairments: A follow-up investigation, *Am J Speech Lang Pathol* 18(3):241–251, 2009.

3. Bhatt T, Feng Y, Mak MKY, et al: Effect of externally cued training on dynamic stability control during the sit-to-stand task in people with Parkinson disease, *Phys Ther* 93:492–503, 2013.

4. Clark DE, Lowman JD, Griffin RL, et al: Effectiveness of an early mobilization protocol in a trauma and burns intensive care unit: A retrospective cohort study, *Phys Ther* 93:186–196, 2013.

5. Hayes SC, Barlow DH, Nelson-Gray R: *The Scientist Practitioner*, Boston, Mass, 1999, Allyn & Bacon.

6. Hegde MN: *Clinical Research in Communicative Disorders*, 3rd ed, Austin, Tex, 2003, Pro-Ed.

7. Richards SB, Taylor RL, Ramasamy R: *Single Subject Research: Applications in Educational and Clinical Settings*, 2nd ed., Belmont, Calif, 2014, Wadsworth/Thompson Learning.

8. Kid Sense. Fine motor development chart. Available online at http://www.childdevelopment.com.au/home/183. Accessed February 10, 2015.

9. Tyrell CM, Roos MA, Rudolph KS, Reisman DS: Influence of systematic increases in treadmill walking speed on gait kinematics after stroke, *Phys Ther* 91:392–403, 2011.

10. Mäenpää H, Lehto M: Patellar dislocation: The long-term results of nonoperative management in 100 patients, *Am J Sports Med* 25:213–217, 1997.

11. Aydelott J, Bates E: Effects of acoustic distortion and semantic context on lexical access, *Lang Cogn Proc* 19:29–56, 2004.

12. Goy H, Pelletier M, Coletta M, Pichora-Fuller MK: The effects of semantic context and the type and amount of acoustical distortion on lexical decision by younger and older adults, *J Speech Lang Hear Res* 56(6):1715–1732, 2013.

13. Kluzik J, Fetters L, Coryell J: Quantification of control: A preliminary study of effects of neurodevelopmental treatment on reaching in children with spastic cerebral palsy, *Phys Ther* 70:65–76, 1990.

14. Scholz JP: Commentary, *Phys Ther* 70:76–78, 1990.

15. Fetters L, Kluzik J: The effects of neurodevelopmental treatment versus practice on the reaching of children with spastic cerebral palsy, *Phys Ther* 76:346–358, 1996.

16. Tsorlakis N, Evaggelinou C, Grouios G, Tsorbatzoudis C: Effect of intensive neurodevelopmental treatment in gross motor function of children with cerebral palsy, *Dev Med Child Neurol* 46(11):740–745, 2004.

17. Rosenthal R: *Experimenter Effects in Behavioral Research*, enlarged ed, New York, NY, 1976, Irvington.

18. Rosenthal R, Jacobson L: *Pygmalion in the Classroom*, New York, NY, 1968, Holt, Rinehart, Winston.

19. Schenkman M, Hall DA, Barón AE, et al: Exercise for people in early- or mid-stage Parkinson disease: A 16-month randomized controlled trial, *Phys Ther* 92(11):1395–1410, 2012.

20. Ebert KD, Kohnert K, Pham G, et al: Three treatments for bilingual children with primary language impairment: Examining cross-linguistic and cross-domain effects, *J Speech Lang Hear Res* 57(1):172–186, 2014.

21. Chan AK, McCabe P, Madill CJ: The implementation of evidence-based practice in the management of adults with functional voice disorders: A national survey of speech-language pathologists, *Int J Speech Lang Pathol* 15(3):334–344, 2013.

22. Barlow DH, Hersen M: *Single Case Experimental Design: Strategies for Studying Behavior Change*, 2nd ed, Elmsford, NY, 1984, Pergamon.

23. Holloway I, Wheeler S: *Qualitative Research in Nursing and Healthcare*, 3rd ed, West Sussex, UK, 2010, Wiley-Blackwell.

CHAPTER 9

Selection and Assignment
of Participants

CHAPTER OUTLINE

Significance of Sampling and Assignment
Population and Samples
Probability Sampling
  Simple Random Sampling
  Systematic Sampling
  Stratified Sampling
  Cluster Sampling
Nonprobability Sampling
  Samples of Convenience
  Snowball Sampling
  Purposive Sampling
Assignment to Groups
  Random Assignment by Individual
Random Assignment by Block
Systematic Assignment
Matched Assignment
Consecutive Assignment
Deciding on an Assignment Method
Sample Size
Summary

Researchers rarely have the opportunity to study all the individuals who possess the characteristics of interest within a study. Fiscal and time constraints often limit researchers' ability to study large groups of participants. In addition, the study of very large groups may be undesirable because it takes time and resources away from improving other components of the research design.[1(p. 3)] Sampling is the process by which a subgroup of participants is selected for study from a larger group of potential participants. Assignment is the process by which participants in the sample are assigned to groups within the study. This chapter acquaints readers with the major methods of selecting participants and assigning them to groups.

SIGNIFICANCE OF SAMPLING AND ASSIGNMENT

If a rehabilitation team is interested in studying, for example, rehabilitation outcomes in patients who have undergone total knee arthroplasty (TKA), they must somehow determine which of thousands of possible participants will be studied. The way in which participants are identified for study, and for groups within the study, profoundly affects the validity of the study.

Sampling methods influence the characteristics of the sample, which, in turn, influence the generalizability, or external validity, of a piece of research. If, for example, a sample of patients with TKA includes only participants older than 75 years, the research results cannot be generalized to younger patient groups.

The method by which participants are assigned to groups within the study influences the characteristics of participants within each group, which in turn influences the internal validity of the study. Assume that we design an experiment on the effect of postoperative femoral nerve block (FNB) on early knee range of motion after TKA. We use a design that includes one experimental group (routine rehabilitation plus FNB) and one control group (routine rehabilitation only). The threats to internal validity posed by history, maturation, testing, and assignment can all be controlled by assignment procedures that yield groups of patients with similar ages, medical problems, preoperative ambulation status, and the like.

POPULATION AND SAMPLES

The distinction between a population and a sample is an important one. A population is the total group of interest. A sample is a subgroup of the group of interest. Sampling is the procedure by which a sample of units or elements is selected from a population. In clinical research, the sampling unit may be the individual or a group of related individuals, such as graduating classes of practitioners or patients treated at particular clinics.

Defining the population of interest is not a simple matter. There are generally two types of populations that are considered in research: the target population and the accessible population. The target population is the group to whom researchers hope to generalize their findings. The accessible population is the group of potential research participants who are actually available for a given study.

Hulley and colleagues[2(p. 28)] listed four types of characteristics that define populations: clinical, demographic, geographical, and temporal. Clinical and demographic characteristics define the target population. The target population for our TKA study might be defined as individuals who have undergone a unilateral TKA and were at least 60 years of age at the time of the surgery. Geographical and temporal characteristics define the accessible population. The accessible population for our TKA study might consist of individuals with the aforementioned clinical and demographic characteristics who underwent surgery in any one of eight Indianapolis hospitals during the 5-year period from 2010 to 2014. Table 9-1 presents a hypothetical distribution of patients at the eight hospitals during this period. This accessible population of 3000 patients provides the basis for many of the examples in this chapter.

After the researcher has defined the accessible population in a general way, he or she needs to develop more specific inclusion and exclusion characteristics. We already know that patients aged 60 years or older who underwent unilateral TKA at one of eight hospitals from 2010 to 2014 are included in our accessible population. Some patients who fit this description should, nevertheless, be excluded from participation in the study. For

example, we need to decide whether to exclude patients who experienced postoperative infection, surgical revision, or rehospitalization soon after the TKA.

The decision to include or exclude participants with certain characteristics must be made in light of the purpose of the research. If the purpose of our study is to provide a description of functional outcomes after TKA, then excluding cases with complications would artificially improve group outcomes by eliminating those likely to have a poor outcome. In contrast, if the purpose of a study is to describe the functional outcomes that can be expected after completion of a particular rehabilitation regimen, then exclusion of patients who could not complete therapy seems reasonable.

After the researcher specifies inclusion and exclusion criteria, he or she needs a sampling frame from which to select participants. A sampling frame is a listing of the elements in the accessible population. In our TKA study, we would ask that someone in the medical records department in each of the eight hospitals create a sampling frame by developing a list of patients aged 60 years or older who underwent a TKA from 2010 through 2014.

Existing sampling frames are available for some populations. If we wish to study occupational and physical therapists' opinions on the use of assistants in delivering rehabilitation services, we could use either a professional association membership list or a professional licensing board list as our sampling frame. Use of an existing sampling frame necessarily defines the target population for the research. If we use the professional association membership list, we can generalize only to other professional association members; if we use the licensing board list, we can generalize to licensed occupational and physical therapists regardless of whether they belong to the professional association.

The most basic distinction between sampling methods is between probabilistic and nonprobabilistic methods. Generation of probability samples involves randomization at some point in the process; generation of nonprobability samples does not. Probability samples are preferable when the researcher hopes to generalize from an accessible population to a target population. This is because probability samples tend to have less sampling error than nonprobability samples. Sampling error "refers to the fact that the vagaries of chance will nearly always ensure that one sample will differ from another, even if the two samples are drawn from exactly the same target population in exactly the same random way."[3(pp. 45,46)] Probability samples tend to be less variable and better approximations of the population than nonprobability samples.

Table 9-1

Hypothetical Sample of Patients Who Underwent Total Knee Arthroplasty by Hospital and Year

Hospital	2010	2011	2012	2013	2014	Total
A	22	25	28	26	24	125
B	50	55	60	40	45	250
C	48	49	52	51	50	250
D	80	78	75	71	71	375
E	72	72	77	77	77	375
F	95	107	98	97	103	500
G	100	103	95	100	102	500
H	120	130	130	122	123	625
Total	587	619	615	584	595	3000

PROBABILITY SAMPLING

Four types of probability sampling are presented in this section. As required by definition, all involve randomization at some point in the sampling process. The extent of randomization, however, differs from technique to technique.

Simple Random Sampling

Simple random sampling is a procedure in which each member of the population has an equal chance of being selected for the sample, and selection of each subject is independent of selection of other participants. Assume that we wish to draw a random sample of 300 participants from the accessible population of 3000 patients in Table 9-1. To literally "draw" the sample, we would write each patient's name on a slip of paper, put the 3000 slips of paper in a rotating cage, mix the slips thoroughly, and draw out 300 of the slips. This is an example of *sampling without replacement* because each slip of paper is not replaced in the cage after it is drawn. It is also possible to *sample with replacement*, in which case the selected unit is placed back in the population so that it may be drawn again. In clinical research, it is not feasible to use the same person more than once for a sample, so sampling without replacement is the norm.

Drawing a sample from a cage, or even from a hat, may work fairly well when the accessible population is small. With larger populations, it becomes difficult to mix the units thoroughly. This apparently happened in the 1970 U.S. draft lottery, when troops were being deployed to Vietnam. Capsules representing days of the year were placed in a cage for selection to determine the order in which young men would be drafted into the armed forces. Days from the later months of the year were selected considerably earlier than days from months earlier in the year. Presumably, the capsules were not mixed well, leading to a higher rate of induction among men with birthdays later in the year.[3(pp. 5–7)]

The preferred method for generating a simple random sample is to use random numbers that are provided in a table or generated by a computer. Table 9-2 shows a portion of the random numbers table reproduced in Appendix A.[4] Internet sites for random number generation are also available;[5] however, we have kept the table for completeness and to show the basis of random selection. Before consulting the table, the researcher numbers the units in the sampling frame. In our TKA study, the patients would be numbered from 0001 to 3000. Starting in a random place on the table, and moving in either a horizontal or vertical direction, we would include in our sample any four-digit numbers from 0001 to 3000 that we encounter. Any four-digit numbers greater than 3000 are ignored, as are duplicate numbers. The process is continued until the required number of units is selected. From within the boldface portion of Table 9-2 in column 7, rows 76 through 80, the following numbers, which correspond to individual participants, would be selected for our TKA sample:

Table 9-2

Segment of a Random Numbers Table*

| Row | COLUMN | | | | | | | | | | | | | |
	1	2	3	4	5	6	7	8	9	10	11	12	13	14
71	91227	21199	31935	27022	84067	05462	35216	14486	29891	68607	41867	14951	91696	85065
72	50001	38140	66321	19924	72163	09538	12151	06878	91903	18749	34405	56087	82790	70925
73	65390	05224	72958	28609	81406	39147	25549	48542	42627	45233	57202	94617	23772	07896
74	27504	96131	83944	41575	10573	08619	64482	73923	36152	05184	94142	25299	84347	34925
75	37169	94851	39177	89632	00959	16487	65536	49071	39782	17095	02330	74301	00275	48280
76	11508	70225	51111	38351	19444	66499	7**1945**	05442	13442	78675	48081	66938	93654	59894
77	37449	30362	06694	54690	04052	53115	6**2757**	95348	78662	11163	81651	50245	34971	52924
78	46515	70331	85922	38379	57015	15765	9**7161**	17869	45349	61796	66345	81073	49106	79860
79	30986	81223	42416	58353	21532	30502	3**2305**	86482	05174	07901	54339	58861	78418	46942
80	63798	64995	46583	09765	44160	78128	8**3991**	42865	92520	83531	80377	35909	81250	54238

*Complete table appears in Appendix A.
From Beyer WH, ed: *Standard Mathematical Tables*, 27th ed, Boca Raton, Fla, 1984, CRC Press.

1945, 2757, and 2305. Alternatively, if we used an Internet random number generator, we would enter the upper and lower limits of the accessible population, 3000 and 1, respectively, and then select the option that did not give duplicate selections. Upon then activating the generator, all 3000 numbers would be listed in random order. To obtain our 300-number sample, we would simply select the first 300 numbers from the list of random ordered numbers. For example, on the referenced date that the random number generator was accessed, a listing of random numbers with a lower and upper limit of 1 and 3000 was selected. The first 10 numbers produced on that list were as follows: 250, 1890, 403, 1360, 2541, 1921, 1458, 45, 170, and 1024. The remaining 290 numbers for the sample would follow from that list. On a second effort of generating a random listing of numbers with the same parameters, the following first 10 numbers were produced: 1036, 848, 1734, 1898, 2533, 1708, 254, 1631, 2221, and 1281. Thus, a second effort of obtaining a random order of 3000 numbers produced an entirely different order than from the first effort.

Simple random sampling is easy to comprehend, but it is sometimes difficult to implement. If the population is large, the process of assigning a number to each population unit becomes extremely time consuming when using a random numbers table. Alternatively, employing a random numbers generator on the Internet makes the simple random sampling a more reasonable process. The other probability sampling techniques are easier to implement than simple random sampling and may control sampling error as well as simple random sampling. Therefore, the following three probability sampling procedures are used more frequently than simple random sampling.

Systematic Sampling

Systematic sampling is a process by which the researcher selects every nth person on a list. To generate a systematic sample of 300 participants from the TKA population of 3000, we would select every 10th person. The list of 3000 patients might be ordered by patient number, Social Security number, date of surgery, or birth date. To begin the systematic sampling procedure, a random start within the list of 3000 patients is necessary. To get a random start, we can, for example, point to a number on a random numbers table, observe four digits of the license plate number on a car in the parking lot, reverse the last four digits of the accession number of a library book, or ask four different people to select numbers between 0 and 9 and combine them to form a starting number. There are endless ways to select the random

starting number for a systematic sample. If the random starting number for a systematic sample of our TKA population is 1786, and the sampling interval is 10, then the first four participants selected would be the 1786th, 1796th, 1806th, and 1816th individuals on the list.

Systematic sampling is an efficient alternative to simple random sampling, and it often generates samples that are as representative of their populations as simple random sampling.[6] The exception to this is if the ordering system used somehow introduces a systematic error into the sample. Assume that we use dates of surgery to order our TKA sample and that for most weeks during the 5-year period 10 surgeries were performed. Because the sampling interval is 10, and there were usually 10 surgeries performed per week, systematic sampling would tend to overrepresent patients who had surgery on a certain day of the week. Table 9-3 shows an example of how patients with surgery on Monday might be overrepresented in the systematic sample; the boldface entries indicate the units chosen for the sample. If certain surgeons usually perform their TKAs on Tuesday, their patients would be underrepresented in the sample. If patients who are scheduled for surgery on Monday typically have fewer medical complications than those scheduled for surgery later in the week, this will also bias the sample. It is unlikely that the assumptions made to produce this hypothetical bias would operate so systematically in real life—the number of cases per week is likely more variable than presented here, and surgeons likely perform TKAs on more than one day of the week. However, possible systematic biases such as this should be considered when one is deciding how to order the population for systematic sampling.

Stratified Sampling

Stratified sampling is used when certain subgroups must be represented in adequate numbers within the sample or when it is important to preserve the proportions of subgroups in the population within the sample. In our TKA study, if we hope to make generalizations across the eight hospitals within the study, we need to be sure there are enough patients from each hospital in the sample to provide a reasonable basis for making statements about the outcomes of TKA at each hospital. On the other hand, if we want to generalize results to the "average" patient undergoing a TKA, then we need to have proportional representation of participants from the eight hospitals.

Table 9-4 contrasts proportional and nonproportional stratified sampling. In proportional sampling, the percentage of participants from each hospital is the same in the population and the sample (with minor

Table 9-3

Systematic Bias in a Systematic Sample*

Subject	Date of Surgery	Surgeon
1786	**1-6-2010 (Monday)**	**A**
1787	1-6-2010 (Monday)	A
1788	1-7-2010 (Tuesday)	B
1789	1-7-2010 (Tuesday)	B
1790	1-8-2010 (Wednesday)	C
1791	1-8-2010 (Wednesday)	C
1792	1-9-2010 (Thursday)	D
1793	1-9-2010 (Thursday)	D
1794	1-10-2010 (Friday)	E
1795	1-10-2010 (Friday)	E
1796	**1-11-2010 (Monday)**	**A**
1797	1-11-2010 (Monday)	A

*Boldface rows indicate the patients selected for the study. If the sampling interval is 10, and approximately 10 surgeries are performed per week, patients of Surgeon A, who usually performs total knee arthroplasties on Monday, will be overrepresented in the sample.

deviations because participants cannot be divided in half; compare columns 3 and 5). However, the actual number of participants from each hospital in the sample ranges from 12 to 62 (column 4). In nonproportional sampling, the percentage of participants from each hospital is different for the population and the sample (compare columns 3 and 7). However, the actual number of participants from each hospital is the same (column 6, with minor deviations because participants cannot be divided in half).

Stratified sampling from the accessible population is implemented in several steps. First, all units in the accessible population are identified according to the stratification criteria. Second, the appropriate number of participants is selected from each stratum. Participants may be selected from each stratum through simple random sampling or systematic sampling. More than one stratum may be identified. For instance, we might want to ensure that each of the eight hospitals and each of the 5 years of the study period are equally represented in the sample. In this case, we first stratify the accessible population into eight groups by hospital, then stratify each hospital into five groups by year, and finally draw a random sample from each of the 40 Hospital×Year subgroups.

Stratified sampling is easy to accomplish if the stratifying characteristic is known for each sampling unit. In our TKA study, both the hospital and year of surgery are known for all elements in the sampling frame. In fact, those characteristics were required for placement of participants into the accessible population. A much different situation exists, however, if we decide that it is important to ensure that certain knee replacement models are represented in the sample in adequate numbers. Stratifying according to this characteristic would

Table 9-4

Proportional and Nonproportional Stratified Sampling of Patients at Eight Hospitals

Hospital	POPULATION DISTRIBUTION		PROPORTIONAL SAMPLE		NONPROPORTIONAL SAMPLE	
	N	%	N	%	N	%
A	125	4.1	12	4.0	37	12.3
B	250	8.3	25	8.3	37	12.3
C	250	8.3	25	8.3	37	12.3
D	375	12.5	38	12.7	37	12.3
E	375	12.5	38	12.7	38	12.7
F	500	16.7	50	16.7	38	12.7
G	500	16.7	50	16.7	38	12.7
H	625	20.8	62	20.6	38	12.7
Total	3000	100.0	300	100.0	300	100.0

require that someone read all 3000 medical charts to determine which knee model was used for each subject. Because of the inordinate amount of time it would take to determine the knee model for each potential subject, we should consider whether simple random or systematic sampling would likely result in a good representation of each knee model.

Another difficulty with stratification is that some strata require that the researcher set classification boundaries. The strata discussed so far (hospital, year, and knee model) are discrete categories of items. Consider, however, the dilemma that would occur if we wanted to stratify on a variable such as "amount of inpatient rehabilitation." If we wanted to ensure that differing levels of rehabilitation are represented in the sample, we would need to decide what constitutes low, medium, and high amounts of inpatient rehabilitation. Not only would we have to determine the boundaries between groups, we would also have to obtain the information on all 3000 individuals in the accessible population. Once again, we should consider whether random or systematic sampling would likely result in an adequate distribution of the amount of rehabilitation received by patients in the sample.

In summary, stratified sampling is useful when a researcher believes it is imperative to ensure that certain characteristics are represented in a sample in specified numbers. Stratifying on some variables will prove to be too costly and must therefore be left to chance. In many cases, simple random or systematic sampling will result in an adequate distribution of the variable in question.

Cluster Sampling

Cluster sampling is the use of naturally occurring groups as the sampling units. It is used when an appropriate sampling frame does not exist or when logistical constraints limit the researcher's ability to travel widely. There are often several stages to a cluster sampling procedure. For example, if we wanted to conduct a nationwide study on outcomes after TKA, we could not use simple random sampling because the entire population of patients with TKA is not enumerated—that is, a nationwide sampling frame does not exist. In addition, we do not have the funds to travel to all the states and cities that would be represented if a nationwide random sample were selected. To generate a nationwide cluster sample of patients who have undergone a TKA, therefore, we could first sample states, then cities within each selected state, then hospitals within each selected city, and then patients within each selected hospital. Sampling frames for all of these clusters exist: The 50 states are known, various references list cities and populations within each state,[7] and other references list hospitals by city and size.[8]

Each step of the cluster sampling procedure can be implemented through simple random, systematic, or stratified sampling. Assume that we have the money and time to study patients in six states. To select these six states, we might stratify according to region and then randomly select one state from each region. From each of the six states selected, we might develop a list of all cities with populations greater than 50,000 and randomly select two cities from this list. The selection could be random or could be stratified according to city size so that one larger and one smaller city within each state are selected. From each city, we might select two hospitals for study. Within each hospital, patients who underwent TKA in the appropriate time frame would be selected randomly, systematically, or according to specified strata. Figure 9-1 shows the cluster sampling procedure with all steps illustrated for one state, city, and hospital. The same process would occur in the other selected states, cities, and hospitals.

Cluster sampling can save time and money compared with simple random sampling because participants are clustered in locations. A simple random sample of patients after TKA would likely take us into 50 states and hundreds of cities. The cluster sampling procedure just described would limit the study to 12 cities in six states.

Cluster sampling can occur on a smaller scale as well. Assume that some researchers wish to study the effectiveness of a speech therapy approach for children who stutter, and the accessible population consists of children who seek treatment for stuttering in a single city. This example is well suited to cluster sampling because a sampling frame of this population does not exist. In addition, it would be difficult to train all speech-language pathologists within the city to use the new approach with their clients. Cluster sampling of a few speech therapy departments or practices, and then a few therapists within each department or practice, would be an efficient use of the researcher's time for both identifying appropriate children and training therapists with the new modality.

Cluster sampling may also be necessitated by administrative constraints. Assume that researchers wish to determine the relative effectiveness of two educational approaches to third graders' developing awareness of individuals with physical disabilities: In one approach, children simulate disabilities themselves, and in the other approach, individuals with disabilities make presentations to the students. A superintendent is unlikely to allow the study to take place if it requires a random sampling of third graders across the school system with disruption of

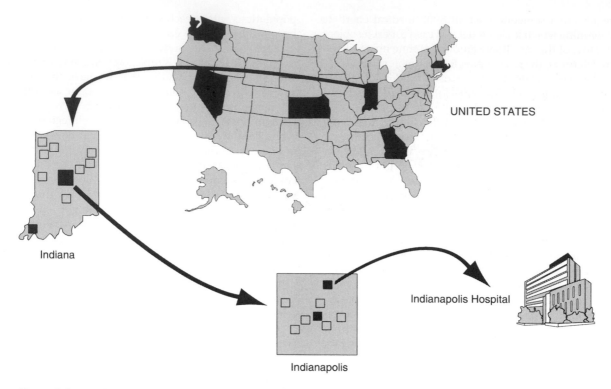

Figure 9-1 Partial example of cluster sampling. Six of 50 states are selected, two cities are selected in each state, and two hospitals are selected from each city. Selected units are shaded; only one state, city, and hospital are illustrated.

classrooms. Because third graders exist in clusters, it seems natural to use schools or classrooms as the sampling unit, rather than the individual pupil.

NONPROBABILITY SAMPLING

Nonprobability sampling is widely used in rehabilitation research and is distinguished from probability sampling by the absence of randomization. One reason for the predominance of nonprobability sampling in rehabilitation research is limited funding. Because many studies are self-funded, subject selection is confined to a single setting with a limited number of available patients, so the researcher often chooses to study the entire accessible population. Three forms of nonprobability sampling are discussed: convenience, snowball, and purposive sampling.

Samples of Convenience

Samples of convenience involve the use of readily available participants. Rehabilitation researchers commonly use samples of convenience of patients in certain diagnostic categories at a single clinic. If we conducted our

study of patients after TKA by using all patients who underwent the surgery from 2010 to 2014 at a given hospital, this would represent a sample of convenience. If patients who undergo TKA at this hospital are different in some way from the overall population of patients who have this surgery, our study would have little generalizability beyond that facility.

The term "sample of convenience" seems to give the negative implication that the researcher has not worked hard enough at the task of sampling. In addition, we already know that probability samples tend to have less sampling error than nonprobability samples. But before one totally discounts the validity of samples of convenience, it should be pointed out that the accessible populations discussed earlier in the chapter can also be viewed as large samples of convenience. An accessible population that consists of "patients post-TKA who are 60 years old or older and had the surgery at one of eight hospitals in Indianapolis from 2010 to 2014" is technically a large sample of convenience from the population of all the individuals in the world who have undergone TKA. Figure 9-2 shows the distinctions among a target population, an accessible population, a random sample, and a sample of convenience.

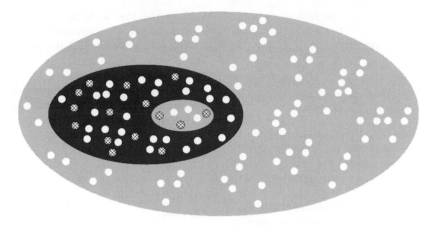

Figure 9-2 Distinctions among target populations, accessible populations, samples of convenience, and random samples. The *white dots* represent elements within the population. The *large gray ellipse* represents the target population. The *black ellipse* represents the accessible population. The *small gray ellipse* represents a sample of convenience. The *cross-hatched dots* represent a random sample from the accessible population.

Consecutive sampling is a form of convenience sampling. Consecutive samples are used in a prospective study in which the population does not exist at the beginning of the study; in other words, a sampling frame does not exist. If researchers plan a 2-year prospective study of the outcomes of TKA at a particular hospital beginning January 1, 2010, the population of interest does not begin to exist until the first patient has surgery in 2010. In a consecutive sample, all patients who meet the criteria are placed into the study as they are identified. This continues until a specified number of patients are collected, a specified time frame has passed, or certain statistical outcomes are seen.

Snowball Sampling

A snowball sample may be used when the potential members of the sample are difficult to identify. In a snowball sample, researchers identify a few participants who are then asked to identify other potential members of the sample. If a team of researchers wishes to study patients who return to sports activities earlier than recommended after ligament reconstruction surgery, snowball sampling is one way to generate a sufficient sample. The investigators will not be able to purchase a mailing list of such patients, nor will they be able to determine return-to-sport dates reliably from medical records because many patients will not disclose their early return to the health care providers who advised against it. However, if the researchers can use personal

contacts to identify a few participants who returned early, it is likely that those participants will be able to identify other potential participants from among their teammates or workout partners.

Purposive Sampling

Purposive sampling is a specialized form of nonprobability sampling that is typically used for qualitative research. Purposive sampling is used when a researcher has a specific reason for selecting particular participants for study. Whereas convenience sampling uses whatever units are readily available, purposive sampling uses handpicked units that meet the researcher's needs. Random, convenience, and purposive samples can be distinguished if we return to the hypothetical study of different educational modes for teaching children about physical disabilities. If there are 40 elementary schools in a district and the researchers randomly select two of them for study, this is clearly a random sample of schools from the accessible population of a single school district. For a sample of convenience, the researchers might select two schools in close proximity. For a purposive sample, the researchers might pick one school because it is large and students are from families with high median incomes and pick a second school because it is small and draws students from families with modest median incomes. Rather than selecting for a representative group of participants, the researchers deliberately pick participants who illustrate different levels of variables they believe may be important to the question at hand. Patton succinctly contrasts random sampling with purposive sampling:

> The logic and power of random sampling derive from statistical probability theory. A random and statistically representative sample permits confident generalization from a sample to a larger population.[9(p. 230)]

The logic and power of purposeful sampling lie in selecting information-rich cases for study in depth. Information-rich cases are those from which one can learn a great deal about issues of central importance to the purpose of the inquiry.

Purposive sampling was used by Pizzari and associates[10] in their study of adherence to anterior cruciate ligament rehabilitation. Because the purpose of their study was to "identify variables that influence adherence to rehabilitation after ACL reconstruction,"[10(p. 91)] they wanted to sample in a way that ensured that their participants reflected a full range of adherence to rehabilitation recommendations. To do so, they selected five participants whose self-report diaries indicated completion of more than 80% of recommended home exercises, one participant who reported completion of 60% to 70% of exercises, and five participants who reported completion of less than 60% of exercises. This purposive sampling strategy is known as a "maximum variability" or "heterogeneity" sampling, 1 of 16 purposive sampling strategies delineated by Patton.[9] Further information on qualitative research methods can be found in Chapter 14.

ASSIGNMENT TO GROUPS

When a study requires more than one group, the researchers need a method for assigning participants to groups. Random assignment to groups is preferred and is appropriate even when the original selection procedure was nonrandom. Thus, many studies in the rehabilitation literature use a sample of convenience combined with random assignment to groups. The goal of group assignment is to create groups that are equally representative of the entire sample. Because many statistical techniques require equal group sizes, a secondary goal of the assignment process is often to develop groups of equal size.

There are four basic ways to randomly assign participants to groups within a study. These methods can be illustrated by a hypothetical sample of 32 patients who have undergone TKA; age and sex are listed for each patient in Table 9-5. The sample has a mean age of 68 years and consists of 50% women and 50% men.

Each of the four assignment techniques was applied to this sample; the processes are described in the following four sections, and the results are presented in Tables 9-6 to 9-9.

Table 9-5

Existing Sample Characteristics: Case Number, Sex, and Age*

1. F, 70
2. M, 60
3. M, 71
4. F, 64
5. F, 65
6. F, 68
7. M, 68
8. M, 69
9. F, 62
10. F, 78
11. F, 68
12. M, 81
13. F, 69
14. F, 60
15. M, 66
16. M, 66
17. M, 70
18. F, 63
19. M, 71
20. F, 76
21. F, 61
22. M, 67
23. M, 65
24. M, 63
25. M, 76
26. F, 72
27. F, 77
28. F, 67
29. F, 69
30. M, 67
31. M, 65
32. M, 62

*Mean age is 68 years; 50% of sample is female.
F, Female; *M*, male.

Table 9-6

Random Assignment by Individual

Group 1:* CPM/FNB	Group 2:† CPM/No-FNB	Group 3:‡ No-CPM/FNB	Group 4:§ No-CPM/No-FNB
5. F, 65	4. F, 64	1. F, 70	6. F, 68
9. F, 62	14. F, 60	2. M, 60	7. M, 68
17. M, 70	15. M, 66	3. M, 71	8. M, 69
21. F, 61	20. F, 76	10. F, 78	11. F, 68
	24. M, 63	12. M, 81	18. F, 63
	28. F, 67	13. F, 69	19. M, 71
	30. M, 67	16. M, 66	22. M, 67
	31. M, 65		23. M, 65
	32. M, 62		25. M, 76
			26. F, 72
			27. F, 77
			29. F, 69

*$n=4$, mean age = 64.5 years, women = 75.0%.
†$n=9$, mean age = 65.5 years, women = 44.4%.
‡$n=7$, mean age = 70.7 years, women = 42.8%.
§$n=12$, mean age = 68.8 years, women = 50.0%.
CPM, continuous passive motion; *FNB*, femoral nerve block; *F*, female; *M*, male.

Table 9-7

Random Assignment by Block

Group 1:* CPM/FNB	Group 2:† CPM/No-FNB	Group 3:‡ No-CPM/FNB	Group 4:§ No-CPM/No-FNB
1. F, 70	2. M, 60	8. M, 69	10. F, 78
3. M, 71	4. F, 64	11. F, 68	12. M, 81
7. M, 68	5. F, 65	15. M, 66	13. F, 69
16. M, 66	6. F, 68	18. F, 63	14. F, 60
21. F, 61	9. F, 62	19. M, 71	20. F, 76
22. M, 67	17. M, 70	23. M, 65	26. F, 72
24. M, 63	25. M, 76	30. M, 67	28. F, 67
27. F, 77	31. M, 65	32. M, 62	29. F, 69

*Mean age = 67.9 years, women = 37.5%.
†Mean age = 66.3 years, women = 50.0%.
‡Mean age = 66.3 years, women = 25.0%.
§Mean age = 71.5 years, women = 87.5%.
CPM, continuous passive motion; *FNB*, femoral nerve block; *F*, female; *M*, male.

Table 9-8

Systematic Assignment

Group 1:* CPM/FNB	Group 2:† CPM/No-FNB	Group 3:‡ No-CPM/FNB	Group 4:§ No-CPM/No-FNB
1. F, 70	2. M, 60	3. M, 71	4. F, 64
5. F, 65	6. F, 68	7. M, 68	8. M, 69
9. F, 62	10. F, 78	11. F, 68	12. M, 81
13. F, 69	14. F, 60	15. M, 66	16. M, 66
17. M, 70	18. F, 63	19. M, 71	20. F, 76
21. F, 61	22. M, 67	23. M, 65	24. M, 63
25. M, 76	26. F, 72	27. F, 77	28. F, 67
29. F, 67	30. M, 67	31. M, 65	32. M, 62

∗Mean age = 67.5 years, women = 75.0%.
†Mean age = 66.9 years, women = 62.5%.
‡Mean age = 68.9 years, women = 25.0%.
§Mean age = 68.5 years, women = 37.5%.
CPM, continuous passive motion; *FNB*, femoral nerve block; *F*, female; *M*, male.

Table 9-9

Matched Assignment

Group 1:* CPM/FNB	Group 2:† CPM/No-FNB	Group 3:‡ No-CPM/FNB	Group 4:§ No-CPM/No-FNB
14. F, 60	21. F, 61	9. F, 62	18. F, 63
31. M, 65	24. M, 63	32. M, 62	2. M, 60
28. F, 67	4. F, 64	5. F, 65	6. F, 68
15. M, 66	22. M, 67	16. M, 66	23. M, 65
1. F, 70	29. F, 69	11. F, 68	13. F, 69
30. M, 67	7. M, 68	17. M, 70	8. M, 69
10. F, 78	27. F, 77	20. F, 76	26. F, 72
3. M, 71	19. M, 71	25. M, 76	12. M, 81

*Mean age = 68.0 years, women = 50.0%.
†Mean age = 67.5 years, women = 50.0%.
‡Mean age = 68.1 years, women = 50.0%.
§Mean age = 68.4 years, women = 50.0%.
CPM, continuous passive motion; *FNB*, femoral nerve block; *F*, female; *M*, male.

The design of our hypothetical study calls for four groups of patients, each undergoing a different post-TKA management. The four programs are variations based on whether or not the patient receives continuous passive motion (CPM or no-CPM) or a femoral nerve block (FNB or no-FNB) after surgery. CPM is one independent variable, and FNB is the second independent variable. One group receives CPM and FNB, one group receives CPM but no-FNB, one group receives FNB but no-CPM, and the final group receives no-CPM and no-FNB.

Random Assignment by Individual

The first method of random assignment is to randomly assign each individual in the sample to one of the four groups. This could be done with a roll of a die, ignoring rolls of 5 and 6. When this assignment technique was applied to the hypothetical sample in Table 9-5, the CPM/FNB condition was represented by a roll of 1, the CPM/no-FNB condition by a roll of 2, the no-CPM/FNB condition by a roll of 3, and the no-CPM/no-FNB condition by a roll of 4. The results of the procedure are shown in Table 9-6. Note that the group sizes range from 4 to 12 participants.

The advantage of assignment by individual is that it is easy to do. The main disadvantage is that with a small sample size, the resulting group sizes are not likely to be equal. With a larger sample size, the probability that group sizes will be nearly equal is greater.

Random Assignment by Block

The second assignment method uses blocks of participants to ensure equal group sizes. Say that in our sample of patients who underwent TKA, we wish to have four groups of eight participants. To assign by block, we can use a random numbers table to select eight numbers for the first group, eight for the second group, and so on. Looking at the last two digits in each column and proceeding from left to right beginning in column 1 of row 71 of the random numbers table (see Table 9-2), the numbers between 01 and 32 are bold and italic, skipping any duplicates. The first eight participants who correspond to the first eight numbers constitute the first group. The next eight numbers constitute the second group, and so on. The complete results of this assignment procedure are shown in Table 9-7. Random assignment to groups by block can become time consuming with large samples.

Systematic Assignment

The process of systematic assignment is familiar to anyone who has taken a physical education class in which teams were formed by "counting off." Researchers count off by using a list of the sample and systematically placing subsequent participants into subsequent groups. Table 9-8 shows the groups generated by systematic assignment for this example. The first person was assigned to the CPM/FNB group, the second person to the CPM/no-FNB group, the third person to the no-CPM/FNB group, the fourth person to the no-CPM/no-FNB group, the fifth person to the CPM/FNB group, and so on.

Matched Assignment

In matched assignment, participants are matched on important characteristics, and these subgroups are randomly assigned to study groups. In our sample of TKA patients, participants were matched on both age and sex. The four youngest women in the sample were placed in a subgroup and then were randomly assigned to study groups. To randomly assign the matched participants to groups, four different-colored poker chips, each representing a study group, were placed into a container. As shown in Table 9-9, the first chip drawn placed the youngest woman into the CPM/FNB group; the second chip drawn placed the next youngest woman into the CPM/no-FNB group; and so on. The four youngest men were then placed into a subgroup and were assigned randomly to study groups. This procedure continued for the next youngest subgroups until all participants were assigned to groups.

The matched assignment procedure is somewhat analogous to stratified sampling and has some of the same disadvantages as stratified sampling. First, it ensures relatively equal distributions only on the variables that are matched. The possibility that other characteristics may not be evenly distributed across the groups may be forgotten in light of the homogeneity on the matched variables. In addition, the information needed for matching on some variables is difficult and expensive to obtain. If we wanted to match groups according to range of motion and knee function before surgery, we would have had to collect these data ourselves or depend on potentially unreliable retrospective data.

Consecutive Assignment

The four assignment methods presented thus far are used when an existing sample is available for assignment to groups. This is not the case when consecutive sampling is being used, for example, to identify patients as they undergo surgery or enter a health care facility. When a consecutive sample is used, assignment to groups needs to be consecutive as well. The basic strategy used for consecutive assignment is the development of an ordered list with group assignments made in advance. As participants enter the study, they are given consecutive numbers and assigned to the group indicated for each number.

Deciding on an Assignment Method

The best assignment method ensures that group sizes are equal, group characteristics are similar, and group characteristics approximate the overall sample characteristics. Assignment by individuals leads to a situation in which group sizes are not necessarily equal; this is more of a problem with small group studies than with large group studies. Matched assignment obviously often leads to the least variability between groups on the matched variables, but it may not randomize other extraneous factors. In addition, it may be expensive and time consuming to collect the information on which participants will be matched. The difference in assignment outcomes between block assignment and systematic assignment is often minimal, unless the researcher suspects some regularly recurring pattern in participants that would suggest that block assignment would be more appropriate. However, because random allocation of participants to groups is seen as critical to the quality of many trials, block assignment is usually preferred to systematic assignment because it introduces random elements as each block is allocated.

SAMPLE SIZE

The preceding discussion of sampling and assignment was based on one major assumption—that the researcher knows how many participants should be in the sample and in each group. In the real world, researchers must make decisions about sample size, and these decisions have a great deal of impact on the validity of the statistical conclusions of a piece of research. A complete discussion of the determination of sample size is deferred until the statistical foundation of the text is laid, but one general principle of sample size determination is presented here.

This general principle is that larger samples tend to be more representative of their parent populations than smaller samples. To illustrate this principle, consider our hypothetical sample of 32 patients who underwent TKA as an accessible population from which we shall draw even smaller samples. From the population of 32 participants, four independent samples of two participants and four independent samples of eight participants are selected. An independent sample is drawn, recorded, and replaced into the population before the next sample is drawn.

Tables 9-10 and 9-11 show the results of the sampling, and Figure 9-3 plots the distribution of the mean age of participants in the different-sized samples. Note that mean ages for the samples of eight participants are clustered more closely around the actual population age than are the mean ages for the smaller samples. This, then, is a visual demonstration of the principle that large samples tend to be more representative of their parent populations. In addition, this clustering of sample characteristics close to the population characteristics means that there is less variability from sample to sample with the larger sample sizes.

For experimental research, group sizes of about 30 participants are often considered the minimum size needed to make valid generalizations to a larger population and to meet the assumptions of certain statistical tests.[1,11] For descriptive research, the precision of the description depends on the size of the sample. For

Table **9-10**

Characteristic with Sample Sizes of Two

Sample 1	Sample 2	Sample 3	Sample 4
7. M, 68	27. F, 77	21. F, 61	10. F, 78
17. M, 70	11. F, 68	4. F, 64	25. F, 76

Note: In samples 1 though 4, the mean ages are 69.0, 72.5, 62.5, and 77.0 years, respectively. The percentage of women in each sample ranges from 0.0% to 100.0%.
F, Female; *M*, male.

Table **9-11**

Characteristic with Sample Sizes of Eight

Sample 1	Sample 2	Sample 3	Sample 4
1. F, 70	1. F, 70	3. M, 71	3. M, 71
3. M, 71	6. F, 68	4. F, 64	5. F, 65
6. F, 68	7. M, 68	5. F, 65	6. F, 68
14. F, 60	17. M, 70	6. F, 68	9. F, 62
15. M, 66	22. M, 67	7. M, 68	16. M, 66
29. F, 69	25. M, 76	14. F, 60	17. M, 70
30. M, 67	27. F, 77	24. M, 63	26. F, 72
32. M, 62	30. M, 67	27. F, 77	32. M, 72

Note: In samples 1 though 4, the mean ages are 66.6, 70.4, 67.0, and 68.3 years, respectively. The percentage of women in each sample ranges from 37.5% to 68.3%.
F, Female; *M*, male.

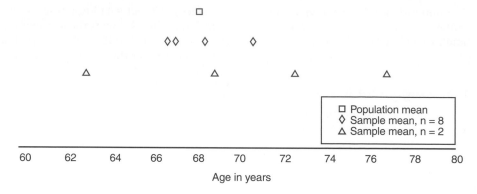

Figure 9-3 Effect of sample size on the stability of sample mean age.

example, a survey of 100 respondents shows that 60% prefer Brand X handheld dynamometer and 40% prefer Brand Y. Without going into any of the statistical theories underlying how researchers determine the precision of their results, with this result with 100 participants we could be 95% certain that the true preference for Brand X is between 50.2% and 69.8%. With 1000 participants, we could be 95% certain that the true preference for Brand X is between 56.9% and 63.1%. With 2000 participants, we could be 95% certain that the true preference for Brand X is between 57.8% and 62.2%. As a researcher, one has to determine whether the increase in precision from 100 to 1000 to 2000 participants is worth the additional time and money associated with the larger samples.

When deciding on sample size, researchers should always account for anticipated experimental attrition. If a subject's participation is required on only 1 day, retention of selected participants should be relatively high. If participation requires a commitment of a great deal of time, over a longer time period, researchers should expect that experimental mortality will be high.

Sometimes researchers are glibly advised to "get as many participants as you can." If only 20 participants are available, it is good advice—the researcher should try to use them all. However, if several hundred participants are available, such advice may be inappropriate. First, recommending that sample sizes be as large as possible is ethically questionable because this means large numbers of individuals are exposed to procedures with unknown benefits. Second, very large samples can create administrative problems that detract from other aspects of the research process. Third, sometimes the results of research on very large groups produce statistical distinctions that are trivial in practice, as is discussed in greater detail in Chapter 20.

SUMMARY

Selection and assignment of participants influence the internal, external, and statistical conclusion validity of research. Populations are total groups of interest; samples are subgroups of populations. Probability samples use some degree of randomization to select participants from the population. Common methods of probability sampling are simple random, systematic, stratified, and cluster sampling. Nonprobability samples do not rely on randomization. Common methods of nonprobability sampling are convenience, snowball, and purposive sampling. Assignment to groups within a study can be accomplished randomly regardless of whether or not the method used to select the sample was random. Common forms of assignment are individual, block, systematic, and matched assignment. A general principle in determining an appropriate sample size is that larger samples tend to be more representative of their parent populations than smaller samples.

REFERENCES

1. Fink A: *How to Sample in Surveys*, 2nd ed, Thousand Oaks, Calif, 2002, Sage.
2. Hulley SB, Newman TB, Cummings SR: Choosing the study subjects: Specification, sampling, and recruitment. In Hulley SB, Cummings SR, Browner WS, et al, editors: *Designing Clinical Research*, 2nd ed, Philadelphia, Pa, 2001, Lippincott, Williams & Wilkins.
3. Williams B: *A Sampler on Sampling*, New York, NY, 1978, John Wiley & Sons.
4. Beyer WH, editor: *Standard Mathematical Tables*, 27th ed, Boca Raton, Fla, 1984, CRC Press.
5. True Random Number Service. Available at: www.random.org. Accessed November 24, 2014.
6. Floyd JA: Systematic sampling: Theory and clinical methods, *Nurs Res* 42:290–293, 1993.

7. *2009 Commercial Atlas and Marketing Guide*, Chicago, Ill, 2010, Rand McNally.
8. *AHA Guide*, 2010 ed, Chicago, Il, 2010, American Hospital Association.
9. Patton MQ: *Qualitative Research and Evaluation Methods*, 3rd ed, Thousand Oaks, Calif, 2002, Sage.
10. Pizzari T, McBurney H, Taylor NF, Feller JA: Adherence to anterior cruciate ligament rehabilitation: A qualitative analysis, *J Sport Rehabil* 11:90–102, 2002.
11. Kraemer HC, Thiemann S: *How Many Subjects? Statistical Power Analysis in Research*, Newbury Park, Calif, 1987, Sage.

CHAPTER 10

Group Designs

CHAPTER OUTLINE

Assumptions of Group Designs
Randomized Controlled Trials
  Practical Considerations in RCTs
  Cautions About RCTs
Single-Factor Experimental Designs
  Pretest–Posttest Control Group
    Design
  Posttest-Only Control Group Design

Single-Group Pretest–Posttest
    Design
Nonequivalent Control Group
    Design
Time Series Design
Repeated Measures or Repeated
    Treatment Designs
**Multiple-Factor Experimental
    Designs**

Questions That Lead to a Multiple-
    Factor Design
Factorial Versus Nested Designs
Completely Randomized Versus
    Randomized-Block Designs
Between-Groups, Within-Group,
    and Mixed Designs
Summary

Experimental research, as defined in Chapter 6, is characterized by controlled manipulation of an active independent variable or variables by researchers. This controlled manipulation can be used with groups of participants or with individuals. In this chapter, experimental designs for groups of participants are described in detail. We should be clear that "group" refers to treatment of the data, rather than how the treatment is administered. That is, treatment (independent variable) may be administered to one participant at a time, but data from those individuals are "grouped" for analysis. In fact, although it is certainly possible to administer an independent variable to groups of participants simultaneously, in clinical research, administration to individuals, with subsequent grouping of their data, is much more the norm. First, the randomized controlled trial (RCT) is presented. Then, several of different single- and multiple-factor research designs are outlined.

We should also be clear that "experiment" requires at least one active independent variable, that is, one the

researcher can control. A very common research strategy is to examine the values of some dependent variable on nonmanipulable groups, such as clinical versus healthy populations, or young versus old populations, or comparison among various ethnic groups. Because the researcher cannot manipulate these categories (e.g., cannot put an aphasic participant in a nonaphasic group and vice versa), research like this is not experimental but, rather, correlational and will not show cause-and-effect relationships. Correlational research is discussed in Chapter 12.

The purpose of this chapter is to introduce readers to the terminology and information necessary to understand how group experimental designs are structured. There is, however, much more to designing valid experiments than just arranging for group allocation, measurement, and intervention, as noted in the many designs presented in this chapter. The control elements presented in Chapter 6 and the selection and assignment procedures presented in Chapter 9 must be implemented carefully to control the threats to validity outlined in Chapter 8. Chapter 27 presents implementation ideas for group experiments as well as other types of research. In addition, statistical tools, presented in Chapters 20 through 24, must be used correctly. Finally, the report of the experiment in the literature (Chapter 28) must present readers with the information needed to assess the quality of the trial.

ASSUMPTIONS OF GROUP DESIGNS

It is possible to learn about group designs, commit their details to memory, and implement them to good effect. Before doing so, however, it is very important to understand some of the assumptions that underlie their use.

One of the major concerns of experimentation, particularly with humans, is the variability that appears in data. Researchers will not find any reported experiment, in any body of literature, in which all human subjects produced the same results. What are the causes of this variability? One, as discussed in Chapter 8, is that it is difficult to control all the factors that might lead to experimental results coming from something other than manipulation of independent variables. That much is known. Apart from experimental error, however, we need to make assumptions about the sources of variability.

Group experimental designs assume that variability is intrinsic to human subjects, rather than coming from sources external to the people involved. The myriad factors could fill a page—age differences, intelligence, motivation, health status, and so on. The critical point is that these are all factors that experimenters cannot control very well, if at all. That leads to the notion that, if an experimenter uses a large enough sample and the sample is randomly drawn from the population and randomly assigned to the groups in the research, all those intrinsic factors will be balanced out between experimental and control groups, and the only effects left (aside from experimental errors) will be those of the independent variable or treatment.

Using this process, it becomes clear that, because emphasis is on the data of each of the groups in an experiment, rather than the individuals in the groups, experimenters must compare the averages of the groups, and differences between group averages are derived by application of inferential statistics. The underlying assumption is that the statistically significant differences will represent true differences between or among groups, at least to a satisfactory degree of probability. Writers in several rehabilitation disciplines[1-3] note the fallacy of this assumption, pointing out that statistical significance may be reached, even when the effect

of treatment is rather small. As Polit and Beck[3] state, "A careful analysis of study results involves evaluating whether, in addition to being statistically significant, the effects are large and clinically important."[(p. 477)]

To apply these assumptions, a further assumption must be that it is possible to create truly random samples of a population (to represent the population of interest) and to truly randomly assign participants to groups (to ensure the pre-experimental equivalence of groups on dependent variables of interest). We will have more to say about the reality of this assumption later.

A final assumption of group experimental designs, based on random selection and assignment, is that results of a valid experiment can be generalized to the population as a whole. We will also address this assumption later on. An interesting history of the development of group designs is presented by Hegde.[4]

RANDOMIZED CONTROLLED TRIALS

This textbook presents a broad view of research, acknowledging the value of different research paradigms (quantitative, qualitative, and single-system paradigms), different research purposes (description, relationship analysis, and difference analysis), and both experimental and nonexperimental designs. Notwithstanding the value of these diverse types of research, there is strong consensus that one particular type of research—the randomized controlled (or clinical) trial, or RCT—can provide strong evidence for one particular research purpose: determining whether clinical interventions work.

RCTs are prospective and experimental, meaning that (1) the independent (treatment) variable is subject to the controlled manipulation of the investigator and (2) the dependent (measurement or outcome) variables are collected under controlled conditions. The independent variable consists of at least two levels, including a treatment group and some form of comparison, or control, group. The "randomized" component of the RCT refers to random allocation of participants to treatment and control groups. RCTs may take many forms, but all contain the elements noted above. By definition, then, all RCTs are experimental designs. However, not all experimental designs are RCTs, in that there are many nonrandom ways of placing participants into groups.

Although the RCT is considered a strong form of evidence about the effect of an intervention, RCTs are not appropriate to answer all questions, nor is every topic of study ready for RCTs. For example, if one wanted the strongest possible evidence about whether cigarette smoking causes lung cancer, one would design and implement an RCT comparing a smoking group to a nonsmoking group. Given the strength of evidence from nonrandomized trials, would it be ethical to randomly assign a large group of nonsmoking adolescents to smoking and nonsmoking groups and follow them throughout their lives to determine the relative rates at which they develop lung cancer? Clearly not.

In the development of new pharmacological agents, researchers conduct a well-established sequence of trials on humans, termed phases 0 through 4.[5] A phase 0 trial involves very limited human drug exposure, with no therapeutic or diagnostic goals. Phase 1 studies are usually conducted with healthy volunteers and emphasize safety. The goal is to find out what the drug's most frequent and serious adverse events are. In phase 2, researchers gather preliminary data on whether the drug works in people who have a certain disease or condition. For example, participants receiving the drug may be compared with similar participants receiving a different treatment, usually an inactive substance (placebo) or a different drug. Safety continues to be evaluated, and short-term adverse events are studied. Phase 3 includes studies that gather more information about safety and effectiveness by studying different populations and different dosages and by using the drug in combination with other drugs. Last, phase 4 studies occur after the U.S. Food and Drug Administration has approved a drug for marketing. These include postmarket requirement and commitment studies that are required of or agreed to by the sponsor. These studies gather additional information about a drug's safety, efficacy, or optimal use.

Rehabilitation research does not have this tradition of a standardized, named progression of increasingly rigorous research about our interventions. However, the same type of progression is appropriate to the study of many rehabilitation interventions. For example, this progression can be seen in the literature related to the technique of body-weight-supported treadmill training for individuals with locomotor disabilities. Some of the earliest literature about this technique documented the responses in men without locomotor disabilities, similar in concept to a phase 0 or 1 drug study.[6] Next, researchers published the results of nonrandomized trials of small numbers of individuals with spastic paretic gait that determined the impact of treadmill training with or without body weight support on gait patterns, similar in concept to phase 3 trials.[7,8] Later, RCTs comparing body-weight-supported treadmill training to traditional gait training were published, similar to phase 4 trials[9,10] Finally, we see the emergence of the review article to help summarize the growing body of evidence about body-weight-supported treadmill training.[11]

Practical Considerations in RCTs

Sequences of studies like the above are not nearly as common in rehabilitation research as in medical research, and there are several practical reasons for this. Hegde[4] noted that treatments in medical research (e.g., drug administration) are much more consistent and straightforward than in rehabilitation. Imagine the difficulty in getting several rehabilitation therapists to administer treatment in exactly the same way, even with the development of a strict treatment protocol.

Another difficulty, and a very significant one, is simply getting the numbers of patients needed for a good RCT. Typical drug and other medical RCTs have patient populations in the hundreds or even thousands and often take place across multiple treatment centers in a variety of geographical regions. Many clinical populations for rehabilitation are just not that numerous. Small sample sizes limit the external validity of a study.

Medical RCTs ideally are "double-blinded," meaning that the participant does not know whether she or he is receiving the experimental treatment and that the health care provider does not know whether she or he is providing the experimental treatment (vs. a placebo or standard treatment). We think this would be very difficult to accomplish in rehabilitation research. Lack of double-blinding increases the likelihood of threats to validity from various forms of bias (see Chapter 8).

Yes, rehabilitation researchers should be working toward the implementation of high-quality RCTs to test the effectiveness of our interventions. Every study of treatment effectiveness that is not an RCT, however, should not be dismissed simply because it uses a less rigorous or different design. Instead, these studies should be examined in the light of related literature to determine whether they are important, either in their own right or as building blocks toward RCTs.

Cautions About RCTs

Although it is clear that RCTs offer a powerful way to examine cause-and-effect relationships, researchers should be aware of several factors to take into account in either designing an RCT or interpreting the results from one. Probably the most cogent factor is that it is practically impossible to obtain a true random sample of a population. Hegde notes that, in random selection, "all members of the defined population are available and willing to participate in the study."[4(p. 93)] Further, random sampling assumes that all members of a population have an equal chance of being selected for a study.

There are at least two roadblocks to the true random selection. First, it is very difficult, if not impossible, to identify all members of a clinical population. For example, in research on therapy for severe ankle sprain, many members will not be identified because they did not seek medical services and, thus, there is no record of their having sprained ankles. Not identifying all members of a population means that all members did not have an equal chance of being selected.

Second, because of present-day research ethics, researchers can only use participants who volunteer. Thus, all participants in clinical research are self-selected. Self-selected participants may not truly represent the population. For example, in occupational therapy for handwriting after hand surgery, only those with the most severe degrees of writing deficit might seek treatment. Once we see that the selected group might not represent the population, we must question the inferential generality of an experiment's results to the population at large.

In addition to difficulties with random selection, Hayes and colleagues[12] point out several other factors that limit the effectiveness of RCTs in answering clinical questions. Interestingly, they note that "as far back as 1949 the participants at the Boulder conference [a well-known conference to discuss the split between researchers and clinicians in psychology] also recognized that traditional experimental research approaches were probably not fully adequate for use by the majority of clinicians in studying clinical problems."[12(p. 17)] Among the reasons for their skepticism, Haynes and colleagues note that RCTs are fraught with "enormous practical difficulties,"[12(p. 17)] such as finding and matching large samples of relatively homogeneous participants. They also note, importantly in our opinion, that in RCTs, patients are (perhaps) randomly assigned to fixed treatment conditions. However, intervention in the real world is highly individualized. Hegde[4] also notes that there is no assumption that results of a group-design experiment are generalizable to any particular individual because results are based on averages and the "average" person probably does not exist.

Hayes and colleagues summarize cautions about RCTs and point to them as a primary cause for "the appalling lack of influence of traditional clinical research on practice."[12(p. 63)] They list some critical clinical questions not addressed by RCTs (e.g., How effective are clinical procedures? For whom will they work?) and note that RCTs do not generally address these questions. For example, an RCT cannot tell which participants in a sample improved because of treatment and which ones improved because of extraneous factors. "The very nature of the question, 'who improves due to treatment' requires that we distinguish the effect of treatment *at the level of the individual* [their italics], not merely the group."[12(p. 63)]

SINGLE-FACTOR EXPERIMENTAL DESIGNS

Single-factor experimental designs have one independent variable. Although multiple-factor experimental designs, which have more than one independent variable, are becoming increasingly common, single-factor designs remain an important part of the rehabilitation literature. In 1963, Campbell and Stanley[12] published what was to become a classic work on single-factor experimental design: *Experimental and Quasi-Experimental Designs for Research*. Their slim volume diagrammed 16 different experimental designs and outlined the strengths and weaknesses of each. Such a comprehensive catalog of single-factor designs cannot be repeated here, but several of the more commonly observed designs are illustrated by studies from the rehabilitation literature. It should be noted that some of the studies presented included secondary purposes that involved an additional independent variable. If readers go to the research reports themselves, they will find that some of the studies are more complex than would be assumed from reading this chapter.

Pretest–Posttest Control Group Design

The first design example is the pretest–posttest control group design, one of the classic RCT designs. The design calls for at least two groups randomly selected (as well as possible) from the population of interest and randomly assigned to one group or another. Pretreatment performance on the dependent variable(s) is measured and, often, group equivalence on the dependent variable(s) is determined statistically. Typically, when there are two groups, one group will then receive treatment (the independent variable), and the other group will not. At the end of the treatment period, performance on the dependent variable(s) is measured again. The pretest–posttest control group design is represented by the following notation from Campbell and Stanley[13(p13)]:

$$R \quad O \quad X \quad O$$
$$R \quad O \qquad\quad O$$

The R indicates that participants were assigned randomly to the two groups. The Os represent observation, or measurement. The X represents an intervention, or manipulation. The blank in the second row represents the control group. The intervention and the control, therefore, constitute the two levels of the independent variable. Another term for this type of design is a *between-subjects design* or a *between-groups design* because the differences of interest are those differences that occur between subject groups. This may also be referred to as a parallel-group design, wherein each group receives only one of the levels of the independent variable. The control group in this design may be referred to as a passive control group because it receives no treatment at all or else receives a sham or placebo treatment.

Siemonsma and colleagues[13] reported on a study designed to compare the effectiveness of cognitively treating illness perception versus no treatment in 156 adult patients with chronic low back pain. The study was a prospective RCT. Participants were randomly assigned to treatment or waiting-list (nontreatment) groups with an assessor blinded for group allocation. Intervention was through a previously developed protocol for cognitive treatment of illness perception (CTIP). The primary dependent variable was change in patient-relevant physical activities. The secondary outcome measures were changes in illness perceptions and generic physical activity level. All dependent variables were measured by changes in validated scales. Measurements were taken at baseline (before treatment) and after treatment (18 weeks). The authors concluded that results "showed statistically significant and clinically relevant improvements in patient-relevant physical activities and significant changes in illness perceptions for at least 18 weeks."[14(p. 444)]

Although the study was a well-designed RCT, some limitations to external validity should be noted. For one, participants spanned an age range from 18 to 70 years. For another, treatments were provided by four physical therapists and three occupational therapists, although they all received training in CTIP and a treatment protocol was developed. A third is that patients were limited to those invited to participate and only from the authors' clinic. The authors were wise to note, "Further studies are needed to estimate the effectiveness in comparison with active control groups and to determine for whom [e.g. what age] and under what circumstances CTIP can best be implemented in clinical practice. Longer-term results on the effectiveness of CTIP, as well as comparative intervention studies, also are needed."[14(p. 444)]

In clinical research, the pretest–posttest control group design is often altered slightly, as follows:

$$R \ O \ X_1 \qquad O$$
$$R \ O \ X_2 \qquad O$$

Here, X_1 and X_2 refer to two different treatments. This alteration is made when the researcher does not believe it is ethical to withhold treatment altogether and so provides the experimental treatment to one group and a treatment of known effectiveness (often called the "standard" treatment) to the "control" group. A control group receiving a standard treatment can be referred to as an active control group.

The design may also be used when two treatments are known to be effective and the researcher wishes to compare their effectiveness. In this version of the RCT, one group receives a typical treatment, and the other group receives the experimental treatment. Had Siemonsma and associates[14] provided a known treatment to their control group subjects rather than put them on a treatment waiting list, they would have satisfied the conditions for this design.

Additional variations on the classic pretest–posttest control group design include taking more than two measurements and using more than two treatment groups. Narciso Garcia and colleagues[15] employed the multiple-measures design in their comparison of the effectiveness of Back School versus McKenzie methods for treating chronic, nonspecific low back pain. Both methods were known to be "good active therapy options,"[15(p. 730)] although evidence on their effectiveness was conflicting. The pretest measure was an evaluation by a blinded (i.e., did not know to which group a patient was assigned) assessor of self-rated pain intensity and a measure of disability. Treatments were provided for 4 weeks per protocol, and the same measures used before treatment were assessed again at 1, 3, and 6 months after randomization. Results indicated that patients in the McKenzie group had greater improvements in disability at 1 month but not for pain. The Campbell and Stanley notation for their experiment is as follows:

$$R \ X_1 \quad O \ O \ O$$
$$R \ X_2 \quad O \ O \ O$$

As mentioned above, other variations are possible and are notable with the Campbell and Stanley system.

Posttest-Only Control Group Design

A second design is the posttest-only control group design. Researchers use this design when they are not able to take pretest measurements. Having a posttest-only study may also reduce the testing threat to internal validity, particularly if a pretest allows practice on or sensitization to an upcoming task or is a reactive measure (see Chapter 8). Therefore, the posttest is the only basis on which to make judgments about the effect of the independent variable on the dependent variable. Like the pretest–posttest control group design, this design is an RCT and a between-groups design. The basic Campbell and Stanley[13] notation for this design is as follows:

$$R \quad X \quad O$$
$$R \qquad\quad O$$

Baty and associates[16] used this design to compare the effects of a carbohydrate-protein supplement (CHO-PRO) versus a placebo on resistance exercise performance of young, healthy men. The study was double-blinded as well, meaning that neither the participants nor the judges knew which treatment was given to which participants. The 34 participants were randomly assigned to either the CHO-PRO (experimental) or placebo condition and asked to perform a set of eight resistance exercises. Performance of the exercises did not vary significantly between groups, although the researchers concluded that the CHO-PRO inhibited muscle damage to a greater degree than did the placebo based on posttreatment measures of myoglobin and creatine kinase.

It may be tempting to use posttest-only designs because of their noted reduction in the testing threat. We would caution, however, that without a pretest, it might be difficult to draw conclusions about treatment effectiveness because it would not be known that study groups are equivalent on the outcomes measures before treatment.

Single-Group Pretest–Posttest Design

The Campbell and Stanley[13] notation for the single-group pretest–posttest design is as follows:

$$O \quad X O$$

Unlike the pretest–posttest control group design and the posttest-only control group design, the single-group design is neither an RCT nor a between-groups design. Because there is only one group, there is no opportunity for random allocation of participants into groups, nor is there any between-groups comparison to be made. Instead, comparisons are made within the single experimental group, making this a within-group design. Meline[17] notes, though, that "single-group designs are weak because they lack scientific comparability, which is a basic requirement for scientific inquiry. In addition, without a comparison group, an important control for extraneous is missing."[(p. 103)]

Investigators may want to use the single-group, pretest–posttest design in pilot studies before committing to a large-scale RCT. Arya and Pandian[18] did just that in their study on the effect of mirror therapy on motor recovery in stroke patients. Using a convenience sample (see Chapter 9) of 13 stroke patients, their participants engaged in a task-based mirror therapy program for 4 weeks. Although some outcome measures did not show improvement, they did find improvement in hand function.

Nonequivalent Control Group Design

The nonequivalent control group design is used when a nonrandom control group is available for comparison. The Campbell and Stanley[13] notation for this design is as follows:

$$O \quad X \quad O$$
$$- - - - - - - - -$$
$$O \qquad\quad O$$

The dotted line between groups indicates that participants were not randomly assigned to groups (note the lack of the "R" notation). Thus, this design is not considered a randomized controlled design. It is, however, a between-groups design because the comparison of interest is between the nonrandom groups.

Zingmark and Bernspång[19] used a nonequivalent-groups design in their study of the effect of occupational therapy on participants who had bathing difficulties. Participants in the treatment group received occupational therapy, and those in the control group received home help for bathing. Activities of daily living, quality of life, and home help allocation were assessed at the baseline and after 15 weeks. Overall, participants in the treatment group needed much less home help and scored better in health-related quality of life and performance of activities for daily living. The authors concluded that occupational therapy could be beneficial for bathing difficulties but cautioned against overvaluing that conclusion. For example, the authors note, "A circumstance that must be considered is that clients in the control group reported significantly greater difficulties in bathing at baseline…. Based on these findings, it is logical that clients in the control group were allocated a home help to provide assistance with bathing more frequently."[(p. 169)]

Given the limitations of the study, we may ask why the investigators did not randomize their participants into treatment and control groups. Although they did not speak specifically to the issue, it is notable that, in order to get a reasonable sample for the study, the

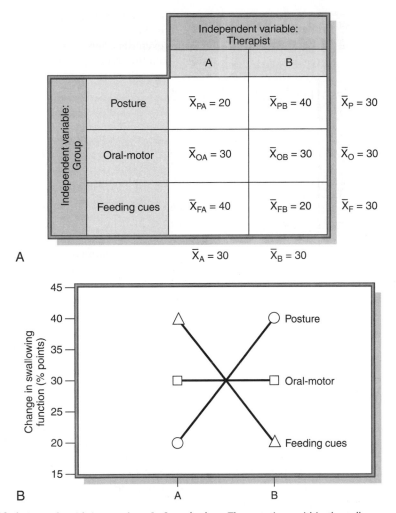

Figure 10-4 Example with interaction. **A,** Sample data. The notations within the cells represent the mean ($\bar{X}$) scores for participants for each combination. The means in the margins are the overall means for the column or row. **B,** Graph of sample data. Nonparallel lines indicate an interaction between therapist and treatment.

manipulable variables, and participants were assigned randomly to both treatment group and therapist.

Sometimes a *randomized-block design* is used, in which one of the factors of interest is not manipulable. That is, one of the independent variables is active (manipulable); the other is very often an attribute variable, such as age or clinical status. If, for example, we had wanted to look at the factors of patient sex and treatment, sex would have been a classification or attribute variable. Participants would be placed into blocks based on sex and then randomly assigned to treatments. This arrangement is also known as a *mixed design* and is quite common in rehabilitation research. Most often, the within-subjects factor is the manipulable,

active independent variable; all participants receive all the levels of treatment. The within-subjects factor is usually the groups in the research, very often based on an attribute variable (e.g., typically developing versus hearing-impaired children).

Between-Groups, Within-Group, and Mixed Designs

In summary, within the category of multiple-factor experimental designs, we can have between-subjects, within-subjects, and mixed designs. In the between-subjects arrangement, different groups get different levels of researcher-manipulable treatments. In the

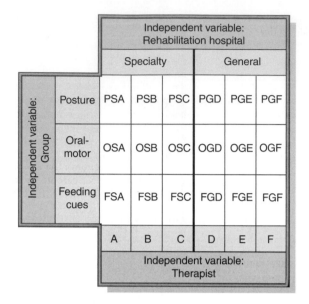

Figure 10-5 Schematic diagram of three-factor, nested design. Treatment (*P, O, F*) and rehabilitation hospital (*S, G*) are crossed factors. Therapist (*A–F*) is nested within hospital.

within-subjects arrangement, all participants receive all experimental conditions. In the mixed design, there is at least one between-subjects factor and one within-subjects factor. Very often, one of the independent variables is manipulable (active variable, commonly the within-subjects factor) and one is not (assigned or attribute variable, commonly the between-subjects factor).

The Treatment×Therapist example could also be termed a *between-groups design* for both factors. Different participants were placed into each of the six cells of the design (three groups×two therapists). The research questions relate to the interaction between treatment and therapist, to differences between groups that received different treatments, and to differences between groups that had different therapists.

An example of a two-factor between-groups design from the literature is Chin and colleagues'[26] work on the use of physical exercise and enriched foods for functional improvement in frail older adults. One factor (variable) was "exercise program" with two levels: exercise and no exercise. One factor was an "enriched food regimen" with two levels: enriched food and no enriched food. These two levels were crossed to yield four cells for the design, each with different participants: 39 participants exercised but did not eat enriched foods, 39 participants ate enriched foods but did not exercise, 42 participants exercised and ate enriched foods, and 37 participants served as controls who

neither exercised nor ate enriched foods. There was no interaction between exercise and eating enriched foods; the exercisers demonstrated significant improvements in functional performance compared with nonexercisers; and there were no significant differences between those who did and did not eat enriched foods.

In a within-group design, one group of participants receives all levels of the independent variable. The work of Jeyasura and colleagues[25] described above is a good example. As noted previously, a mixed, or split-plot, design contains a combination of between-subjects and within-subjects factors.

Blake[27] used a mixed design to study effects of context constraint on the ability to make inferences in adults with right-hemisphere damage (RHD). Participants were 14 adults with RHD and 14 with no cerebral damage. Thus, those groups constituted the between-subjects factor based on an assigned variable. Every participant read stories in which the outcome was highly predictable or not. Thus, "predictability" was the active independent variable with two levels (high and low) and, because every participant was exposed to both levels, constituted the within-subjects factor. As it turned out, adults with no brain damage made predictive inferences in both conditions of predictability; those with RHD made more inferences only when predictability was high. Thus, there was an interaction between groups and predictability.

SUMMARY

Experimental research is characterized by controlled manipulation of variables by the researcher. Although RCTs provide good evidence for determining whether a clinical intervention works, some questions related to interventions cannot be answered with RCTs, and some rehabilitation topics are not yet ready for rigorous testing with RCTs. In addition, RCTs face formidable practical problems because of the difficulty of achieving truly randomized samples, compromising their inferential generality or external validity. Single-factor experimental designs are those in which the researcher manipulates only one variable. Common single-factor designs include the pretest–posttest control group design, the posttest-only control group design, the single-group pretest–posttest design, the nonequivalent control group design, the time series design, and the repeated treatment design. Multiple-factor research designs are those in which the researcher studies more than one variable and is interested in the interactions among variables. Common forms of multiple-factor designs include factorial and nested designs; completely randomized and randomized-block designs; and between-groups, within-group, and mixed designs.

REFERENCES

1. Haynes WO, Johnson CE: *Understanding Research and Evidence-Based Practice in Communication Disorders*, Boston, Mass, 2009, Pearson Education.
2. Hicks CM: *Research Methods for Clinical Therapists*, 5th ed, Edinburgh, UK, 2009, Churchill Livingstone.
3. Polit DF, Beck CT: *Nursing Research*, 9th ed, Philadelphia, Pa, 2012, Wolters Kluwer/Lippincott Williams & Wilkins.
4. Hegde MN: *Clinical Research in Communicative Disorders*, 3rd ed, Austin, Tex, 2003, Pro-Ed.
5. U.S. National Institutes of Health: Clinicaltrials.gov. Glossary of Common Site Terms. Available at: https://clinicaltrials.gov/ct2/info/glossary. Accessed February 11, 2015.
6. Finch L, Barbeau H, Arsenault B: Influence of body weight support on normal human gait: Development of a gait retraining strategy, *Phys Ther* 71:842–855, 1991.
7. Waagfjord J, Levangie P, Certo CM: Effects of treadmill training on gait in a hemiparetic patient, *Phys Ther* 70:549–558, 1990.
8. Visintin M, Barbeau H: The effects of parallel bars, body weight support and speed on the modulation of the locomotor pattern of spastic paretic gait: A preliminary communication, *Paraplegia* 32:540–553, 1994.
9. Visintin M, Barbeau H, Korner-Bitensky N, Mayo N: A new approach to retrain gait in stroke patients through body weight support and treadmill stimulation, *Stroke* 29:1122–1128, 1998.
10. Nilsson L, Carlsson J, Danielsson A, et al: Walking training of patients with hemiparesis at an early stage after stroke: A comparison of walking training on a treadmill with body weight support and walking training on the ground, *Clin Rehabil* 15:515–527, 2001.
11. Hesse S, Werner C, von Frankenberg S, Bardeleben A: Treadmill training with partial body weight support after stroke, *Phys Med Rehabil Clin North Am* 14:S111–S123, 2003.
12. Hayes SC, Barlow DH, Nelson-Gray R: *The Scientist Practitioner*, Boston, MA, 1999, Allyn & Bacon.
13. Campbell DT, Stanley JC: *Experimental and Quasi-Experimental Designs for Research*, Chicago, Ill, 1963, Rand McNally College.
14. Siemonsma PC, Stuive I, Roorda LD, et al: Cognitive treatment of illness perceptions in patients with chronic low back pain: A randomized controlled trial, *Phys Ther* 93:435–448, 2012.
15. Narciso Garcia A, da Cunha Menezes Costa L, Mota da Silva T, et al: Effectiveness of back school versus McKenzie exercises in patients with chronic nonspecific low back pain: A randomized controlled trial, *Phys Ther* 93:729–747, 2013.
16. Baty JJ, Hwang H, Ding Z, et al: The effect of a carbohydrate and protein supplement on resistance exercise performance, hormonal response, and muscle damage, *J Strength Cond Res* 21(2):321–329, 2007.
17. Meline TA: *A Research Primer for Communication Sciences and Disorders*, Boston, Mass, 2010, Pearson.
18. Arya KN, Pandian S: Effect of task-based mirror therapy on motor recovery of the upper extremity in chronic stroke patients: A pilot study, *Top Stroke Rehabil* 20(3):210–217, 2013.
19. Zingmark M, Bernspång B: Meeting the needs of elderly with bathing disability, *Aust Occup Ther J* 58(3):164–171, 2011.
20. Chang F-Y, Huang H-C, Lin K-C, Lin L-C: The effect of a music programme during lunchtime on the problem behaviour of the older residents with dementia at an institution in Taiwan, *J Clin Nurs* 19(7–8):939–948, 2010.
21. Shaughnessy JJ, Zechmeister EB, Zechmeister JS: *Research Methods in Psychology*, 8th ed, New York, NY, 2009, McGraw-Hill.
22. Winer BJ: *Statistical Principles in Experimental Design*, 2nd ed, New York, NY, 1971, McGraw-Hill.
23. Kirk RE: *Experimental Design: Procedures for the Behavioral Sciences*, 3rd ed, Belmont, Calif, 1995, Thomson Brooks/Cole Publishing.
24. The Latin Square Design. Available at: www.tfrec.wsu.edu/ANOVA/Latin.html. Accessed November 24, 2014.
25. Jeyasura J, van der Loos HFM, Hodgson A, Croft AE: Comparison of seat, waist, and arm sit-to-stand assistance modalities in elderly population, *J Rehabil Res Dev* 50(6):835–844, 2013.
26. Chin A, Paw MJM, de Jong N, et al: Physical exercise and/or enriched foods for functional improvement in frail, independently living elderly: A randomized controlled trial, *Arch Phys Med Rehabil* 82:811–817, 2001.
27. Blake ML: Inferencing processes after right hemisphere brain damage: Effects of contextual bias, *J Speech Lang Hear Res* 52:373–384, 2009.

11

Single-Subject Designs

CHAPTER OUTLINE

When to Use Single-Subject
    Designs
Problems with Group Designs
Characteristics of Single-Subject
    Designs
Single-Subject Designs
    A-B Designs
    Withdrawal Designs

Multiple-Baseline Designs
Alternating-Treatments Designs
Interaction Designs
Changing-Criterion Designs
Graphing Single-Subject Data
    Graphing Data for Alternating-
        Treatments Designs

Considerations When Using Single-
    Subject Designs
Limitations of Single-Subject
    Designs
Summary

The scientist-practitioner's focus is on changing the performance of the individual client or patient. The need to document and examine the performance of individuals is central to the scientist-practitioner's practice. Hislop, in her McMillian lecture, so eloquently expressed the argument of studying individuals instead of groups:

> A great difficulty in developing … clinical science … is that we treat individual persons, each of whom is made up of situations which are unique and, therefore, appear incompatible with the generalizations demanded of science.[1(p. 1076)]

Single-subject designs were developed largely by behaviorists, influenced by scientists such as Skinner, Sidman, Bijou, and others to demonstrate the influence of setting and other intervention variables on the performance of research participants and to document the individual variability of participants' performance in response to these variables.[2,3] Group designs lose this sensitivity to setting influences and individual variability by applying the same treatment to all subjects, by virtue of their "averaging" the performance of all subjects in a study, and other limitations as noted in Chapter 6. In addition to this basic philosophical argument in favor of single-subject designs, advocates of this paradigm also cite many practical disadvantages of group designs in rehabilitation research.

In this chapter, we suggest that with only minimal effort and care on the part of the scientist-practitioner, the single-subject design has great clinical applicability, if not daily, then for special cases. Single-subject designs may be known by any of several different labels, including single-case designs, single-system designs, and $N=1$ designs (time series, within-subject).[4] Although single-subject designs may be used with groups of people, we have elected to use the more traditional term of *single-subject designs* because of its familiarity of use. It may be helpful to note that the term *single-subject* refers to the treatment of data (i.e., data from each research participant are analyzed separately) rather than to the number of participants in the study.

WHEN TO USE SINGLE-SUBJECT DESIGNS

The scientist-practitioner may use single-subject designs in any of several different situations. A single-subject design may be used when withholding treatment is considered unethical or when random assignment of subjects may not be possible. Also, single-subject designs may be used where it is too difficult to get enough participants for a group design study. The most frequent reason for using a single-subject design is to obtain detailed information about factors, such as participant features, setting descriptions, and specific intervention procedures, on the variability of a participant's performance.

PROBLEMS WITH GROUP DESIGNS

First, it is often difficult to structure powerful group designs in rehabilitation settings. Although a complete discussion of statistical power is deferred until Chapter 20, for now it is enough to know that powerful designs are those in which the data have the mathematical characteristics that make it likely that any true differences between groups will be detected by the statistical tools used to analyze the data. These mathematical characteristics include large sample sizes, participants who have similar values on the dependent variable at the beginning of the study, and large differences between groups at the conclusion of the study. Because of the difficulty in obtaining a sufficient sample size for a group study, and the time to conduct the study, many group studies have few participants in each group, and the participants are heterogeneous, varying greatly on the dependent variable at the beginning of the study. Often the studies are conducted for too short a period to adequately determine the effectiveness of the intervention. When a study lacks power and no difference between groups is identified, it is difficult to determine whether there is, in fact, no benefit to the experimental treatment or whether there is, in fact, a real benefit that was not detected because the design did not create the mathematical conditions needed to identify a difference. Advocates of single-subject research believe that carefully crafted single-subject designs provide clinicians with more useful information (e.g., detailed study participant characteristics, setting features, intervention procedures, and participant performance variability) than do group designs.

Second, group designs typically only call for measurement of participants a few times within the study. When participants are only measured at the beginning and end of a study, the researcher is unable to determine the typical pattern of fluctuation in the dependent variable in the absence of an experimental manipulation. A difference from pretest to posttest may be part of a pattern of natural fluctuation, rather than a difference related to the independent variable. As shown later in the chapter, single-subject designs are characterized by extended baselines that establish the extent of natural fluctuation on the variables of interest within the study, as well as frequent measurements during the intervention phase.

Third, group designs often have problems with external validity. Because of the need to standardize treatment across participants within the study, there may be a mismatch between some participants and the intervention that is planned. On average, the treatment may be appropriate for the participants within the group, but it may not be ideal for each participant. In addition, the standardization that is typical of group designs means that treatment is controlled in ways that may not be typical of clinical practice. Thus, the standardization of treatments restricts the scientist-practitioner from adjusting the intervention to the changing needs of the study participants. When a statistical advantage

is found in an experimental group compared with a control group, clinicians know that the treatment, when applied to groups similar to the one that was studied, is likely to be effective for the group as a whole. The group design, however, usually provides little information about which subgroups responded best—or did not respond at all. This means that the results of group designs often provide clinicians little guidance on whether a treatment is likely to be effective with a particular individual with particular characteristics. The generalizability of results from group studies can be described as "sample-to-population" generalizability.

In contrast, single-subject designs are characterized by experimental treatments that are tailored to the needs of the specific participant being studied. In addition, the participant is usually described in detail. This means that clinicians can determine the similarity of one of their patients to the single participant under study and make an educated clinical judgment about the applicability of the treatment to their patient. Sim[5] refers to this as "case-to-case generalizability" and believes that this kind of generalizability is important to clinicians trying to make evidence-based treatment decisions. Generalizability of single-subject designs can be enhanced by the replication of the design across several individuals. In a replicated single-subject design, the unit of analysis remains the single case. However, the researchers then discuss the case-to-case generalizability of the replicated results: Consistent results across cases provide generalized evidence about the intervention, whereas inconsistent results point to the need for further research to determine which subgroups of patients are most likely to benefit from a certain intervention.

CHARACTERISTICS OF SINGLE-SUBJECT DESIGNS

Single-subject designs are often confused with clinical case reports or case studies. The two are very different. The case report or case study is a description, very often a retrospective description, of a course of treatment of an individual. The case report is therefore a nonexperimental form of inquiry, which is covered in more detail in Chapter 13. Single-subject designs, in contrast, include *controlled manipulation* of an independent variable and are conducted prospectively. Kazdin[6] indicated that case reports and case studies could be greatly improved by simply adding single-subject design elements, such as when objective measures and frequent assessments are used.

Single-subject designs have several key characteristics: baseline assessment, stability of performance, continuous assessment, and use of different phases.[6]

An extended baseline assessment provides a picture of how the subject is currently performing or "behaving" before introduction of the intervention. In addition, we assume the baseline performance is how the subject performed before assessment and how the subject will continue to perform if the baseline assessments are continued. Typically, in single-subject designs, three data points are considered the minimum necessary to determine a subject's performance pattern, particularly the trend of performance (i.e., an increasing trend, a decreasing trend, or staying the same); however, three data points may be insufficient to determine a subject's pattern of performance variation. Thus, more than three baseline data points are often observed in single-subject studies.

As noted earlier, all subjects will have some variation in performance. Change in conditions (e.g., introduction of the intervention after a baseline assessment) is typically not introduced to a subject until a subject's performance has stabilized or a steady trend in pretreatment behavior change is observed. In a subject whose performance is highly variable, stability of performance may occur as a "pattern of variable performance."

Continuous assessment, when conducted at sufficient frequency, affords determination of normal changes in performance. All participants have some fluctuations or variations in performance even when conducted under the same conditions. If the assessment is too infrequent, normal patterns of performance variation may be missed. When an intervention is introduced to a participant, change in performance is expected. Continuous assessment allows us to determine what are normally occurring fluctuations in a patient's performance versus those changes in performance that are due to the introduction of the intervention.

The experimental nature of single-subject designs is shown by the controlled way in which the independent variable is implemented and the dependent variables are measured. Single-subject designs have at least two levels of the independent variable: typically a baseline phase and an intervention phase. The participant serves as his or her own control through the collection of an extended series of baseline measurements, which are contrasted to a series of measurements obtained during the intervention phase. Interpretation of single-subject design results is simplified if stable performance during the baseline phase is documented.

The importance of reliable dependent variable measurements is not unique to single-subject designs, but because of the frequency of assessment, and the emphasis on the detection of individual performance changes, it is imperative that reliable assessment measures are used in single-subject designs. When a measurement instrument with suspect reliability is used in a study, any changes in performance are similarly suspect because we cannot accurately determine whether performance changes actually occurred, if the performance changes are normal variations, or if the performance changes are due to the introduction of the intervention. Of course, the importance of having reliable measurements cannot be overly emphasized when an unreliable measure fails to accurately detect a deteriorating performance.

Single-subject designs are used when behaviors are expected to change as conditions are introduced or withdrawn. As noted earlier, when conditions are unchanged, as in baseline assessment, performance is expected to continue unchanged until a condition is introduced. Because of this assumption, by convention, assessment of subject performance occurs only in adjacent phases, when conditions change. That is, where more than two phases occur, comparison of performance in nonadjacent phases is prohibited. In addition, subject performance is usually evaluated by visual analysis of the subject's graphed data. Because single-subject designs emphasize the examination of a subject's unique fluctuations of performance, and because of the rules for using statistical analyses of subject data (e.g., sample size), visual analysis is the preferred method of evaluating subject performance in single-subject designs. Typically, subject data are analyzed for changes in levels, trends, slope, and stability. Visual analysis of single-subject studies is described in more detail in Chapter 22.

The prospective nature of single-subject designs is illustrated by the deliberate, planned intervention. Even though the researcher may deviate from the original treatment plan to accommodate the specific needs of the patient, these changes are carefully documented and recorded. Because of the planned nature of the study, researchers go through standard institutional review board processes to obtain approval to do the study, and they seek formal informed consent from the individuals who participate in the research.

SINGLE-SUBJECT DESIGNS

Several authors have categorized single-subject designs in different ways.[5,7–9] This chapter presents five basic variations (A-B designs, withdrawal designs, multiple-baseline designs, alternating-treatments designs, and changing-criterion designs) and adds a sixth (interaction designs) based largely on the classifications of Kazdin.[6] Each of these designs is described in this chapter. Readers needing a more complete enumeration of examples of the different designs should consult the previously referenced sources.[6–9]

When examining single-system designs, a basic nomenclature is used to describe the designs. By convention, a phase in which no intervention has been implemented is represented by the letter A. These typically include baseline (i.e., before any treatment) and any phases after implementation of treatment in which no treatment is present (e.g., treatment withdrawal). Phases in which an initial treatment is present are represented by the letter B. Thus, when initial assessment or baseline data are taken with a patient or research participant, that phase would be represented by the letter A. When the patient begins receiving the intervention, that phase would be represented by the letter B. If treatment is withdrawn in the next phase, that phase is represented by A, and if treatment is reintroduced following the phase at which it was withdrawn, the designation is a B. If a second (i.e., different) intervention is introduced, it would receive the designation C. Thus, we may have a design that examines two different interventions, such as ABACAB or BCB. Sometimes, when only a small variation in one of the interventions is made, rather than assign a new letter to the variation, a prime mark (′) is placed immediately after the letter representing the major intervention. Thus, when one intervention is represented by the letter B, the intervention with the small variation would be represented as B′. Thus, we might have a design as follows: BAB′. Sometimes, researchers will indicate the order of occurrence of similar phases with a numerical subscript. For example, in an ABAB withdrawal design, the first baseline phase may be indicated as A_1 and the second non-treatment phase labeled A_2. Similarly, the intervention phases, in which more than one of the same condition occurs, may be labeled with a numerical subscript indicating the order of occurrence. Thus, the ABAB study may be presented as $A_1B_1A_2B_2$.

A-B Designs

The most basic of single-subject designs, the A-B design, has been described as the foundation of single-subject research, even though it is considered a pre-experimental design.[6]

An A-B design consists of a baseline phase, A, followed by a treatment phase, B. The researcher collects multiple measures over time during the baseline phase to document the patient's status before implementation of the treatment. When the treatment is initiated, the measurements continue, and, following established convention of comparing only adjacent phases, the pattern of change during the treatment phase is compared with the pattern established during the baseline.

The A-B design most closely approximates the sequence of clinical practice of most rehabilitation professionals. The initial patient examination is analogous to the A phase in this design, whereas the intervention is, of course, comparable to the B phase of the A-B design. The single largest difference between this design and clinical practice is the presence of an extended baseline phase (e.g., continuous assessment). Generally, a single-subject design requires a minimum of three data points in any phase, including the baseline phase. A single data point informs us only how the subject/patient performed at that one instance. Having two data points increases our knowledge of the subject/patient's performance, but does not give us the information we need to determine whether the subject/patient's performance is increasing, decreasing, stabilized, or fluctuating. Adding a third data point in any phase provides the minimum information necessary to estimate the direction of a subject's performance, affording a comparison to the subject's performance in the preceding or following phase.

With recognition that few payers will permit payment for three occasions of assessment without providing some sort of intervention services, how may the scientist-practitioner implement this design? There are several options to adapting this design for clinical use. One option is to use a single data point. With only one data point, our assumptions concerning a patient's performance are very restricted, as noted earlier; however, this single data point gives us information on the patient's performance at that point in time. This is certainly no less than what is obtained in any clinical practice. Alternatively, the scientist-practitioner may obtain the first data point during the initial examination and obtain a second baseline data point at the beginning of the patient's second appointment, before the start of the intervention. The most acceptable adaptation is to obtain the first data point early in the initial examination, obtain the second data point later in the initial examination, and obtain the third data point at the beginning of the patient's second appointment, before initiating the patient's intervention phase. Now the scientist-practitioner has three data points, the minimum information necessary to estimate the patient's performance if the patient did not receive the intervention, and there has been no delay in the patient beginning the intervention phase.

Another alternative to having an extended baseline of no treatment is when an initial intervention already clinically in place (B) is considered as the control or baseline phase, and a new intervention (C) is implemented. Thus, the design would be represented as B-C. In this adaptation, there is no need to be concerned with an extended baseline of no treatment because the first phase is an intervention (B) that is in place, and the scientist-practitioner wants to see if a second intervention (C) changes the patient's performance. Because the patient is getting the B intervention, the concerns of an extended baseline are mitigated.[6]

One weakness of the A-B design is that it does not control for events or extraneous factors that might act simultaneously with the implementation of the treatment. If present, such factors, rather than the treatment, might be the cause of any changes seen in the dependent variables.

Marklund and Klässbo[10] used an A-B design to investigate the effects of a 2-week trial of intensive constraint-induced movement therapy (CIMT) for the lower extremity (LE) with five persons who had experienced a stroke. Both the baseline (A) and intervention (B) consisted of daily activities for 6 hours a day, 5 days a week, for 2 weeks each, with assessments occurring thrice weekly, and again at 3- and 6-months after the study. During the A phase, the participants engaged in nonorganized training. During the B phase, the participants had their uninvolved LE immobilized while they engaged in a variety of LE training activities, including sit to stand and return, stair training, and walking on uneven surfaces indoors and outdoors. Assessment measures included the 6-minute walk test, step test, Timed Up and Go, Fugl-Meyer subitems for the LE, weight distribution during standing, and walking ability.

If differences in any of the performance measures were seen during the B phase, a simple A-B design would not control for historical influences, such as a change in spasticity medications, that might influence LE performance during the study.

Withdrawal Designs

Withdrawal designs, sometimes referred to generically as A-B-A designs, are characterized by at least one implementation and withdrawal of treatment over the course of the study. In an A-B-A design, a baseline phase (A) is followed by a treatment phase (B) and then by another baseline (A). These designs were developed to answer the important clinical question, "Does this treatment work?" Other variants either reverse the order of treatments and baselines (B-A-B) or have multiple cycles of application and withdrawal of treatment (A-B-A-B).[2] When studying a phenomenon that is expected to change as the intervention is implemented and withdrawn (i.e., reverse trend from the previous phase), these designs provide good control of extraneous factors by enabling the researcher to determine whether the hypothesized change occurs each time the treatment is

applied or withdrawn. The strength of the intervention's effectiveness is borne out by the change in performance (e.g., trend, level, slope) over the multiple introductions and withdrawals of the interventions. Indeed, the more times the dependent variable changes with the repeated introductions and withdrawals of the intervention, the stronger is the evidence for control against the internal validity threats of history and maturation. Clearly, the threat of attrition is not an issue with single-subject designs unless the patient ceases to participate in the intervention, nor is the threat of selection an issue because the patient was specifically selected for the intervention. When the scientist-practitioner uses reliable measurements and conducts periodic interrater reliability assessments during the different phases, then instrumentation is controlled as a threat. It is obvious that this single-subject design controls many significant threats to internal validity.

One potential difficulty with withdrawal designs is that the researcher must consider the ethical implications of withdrawing a treatment that appears to be successful. Alternatively, because the effectiveness of many interventions is truly unknown, withdrawing a treatment, as in an ABAB design, in order to prove its effectiveness may be argued as acceptable. A second potential difficulty with withdrawal designs is that the expected pattern of change in the dependent variable with each new phase of the study will occur only if the changes are reversible. For example, Cross and Tyson,[11] using an A-B-A design, examined the effects of a slider shoe on the walking speed, walking efficiency, and Physiological Cost Index of four persons with a hemiplegic gait. In this instance, the authors expected the participants' performance to return to baseline levels when the intervention, use of the slider shoe, was withdrawn. They reported that although all four participants' performance returned toward baseline when the slider shoe was removed, only one participant's performance, subject 1, in the withdrawal phase actually returned to baseline levels (Fig. 11-1). Thus, only subject 1 presented good evidence that the treatment, and not some extraneous factor, was the cause of the changes in walking speed. Alternatively, there were "carry-over effects" (i.e., near or maintenance of performance at the intervention level) into the withdrawal phase for the other three participants, even though their performance fell off of the levels observed during the B phase.

If performance in the second nontreatment phase remains the same as in the treatment phase or fails to return to baseline levels, the more conservative and accepted interpretation is that some factor other than the treatment is considered as causing the sustained change. Others might argue that such a pattern

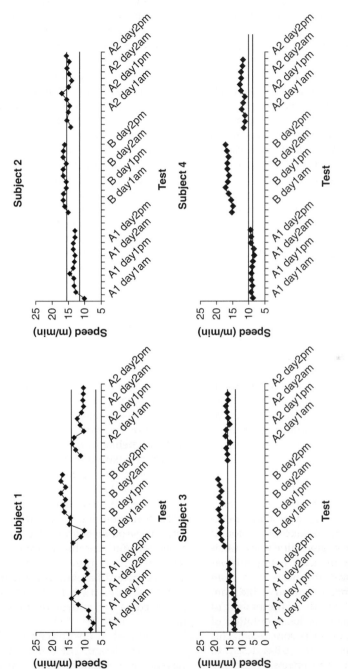

Figure 11-1 Graphs to show the effect of the slider shoe on walking speed (m/min) on each subject (subjects 1-4). The lines indicate the 2 standard deviations (2SD) from phase A1 (mean+2SD and mean−2SD) bands. (From Cross J, Tyson SF: The effect of a slider shoe on hemiplegic gait, *Clin Rehabil* 17:817–824, 2003. Reprinted by permission of SAGE.)

of evidence, rather than providing weak evidence of treatment effectiveness, provides strong support for the long-term impact of the treatment.[12] Thus, it is difficult to interpret the results of A-B-A designs with variables that are not expected to change when the intervention is removed. We argue that the more conservative interpretation of the data is likely the better interpretation.

Deitz and colleagues[13] conducted an A-B-A single-subject design to study the effect of powered mobility on child-initiated movement, contact with others, and affect for two children with complex developmental delays. First, performance on the dependent variables was collected during gym class or outdoor recess during the A_1 phase when the children did not have powered mobility. Then the children were trained in the use of a powered riding toy car. Data were collected during the B phase when the children used the car for mobility during gym class or outdoor recess activities. This B phase with the car was followed by an A_2 phase during which the car was not available. For both children, self-initiated movements increased markedly with the introduction of the car in the B phase and decreased markedly with the withdrawal of the car in the A_2 phase, thereby providing strong evidence that the car was the cause of the change in mobility (Fig. 11-2).

In contrast to this classic use of an A-B-A design with a variable that is expected to return to baseline on withdrawal of the treatment, Miller[12] used an A-B-A design to study the impact of body-weight-supported treatment and overground training in a woman 19 months after having a stroke. In this situation, an effective treatment would be reflected by improvements during the intervention phase and retention of those improvements after the treatment was completed. Measures of gait and balance were collected 10 times during the A_1 baseline phase. During the B intervention phase, gait training with the partial body-weight-support system was implemented three times per week for 8 weeks, with collection of gait and balance data twice a week. The gait and balance measures were then collected another 10 times during the A_2 withdrawal phase after treatment was complete. In general, improvements were seen from phase A_1 to B, and performance remained stable from B to A_2. For a study such as this, then, the benefit of an A-B-A design is that it allows for documentation of carryover effects after intervention is concluded. This is in contrast to the original use of the A-B-A design to control for history and maturation effects by looking for patterns of change at both the initiation and withdrawal of an intervention with a short-lived effect.

Although the three-phase A-B-A design is sufficient to demonstrate that the treatment's control over the behavior is exerted when the treatment is withdrawn in the second A phase, ethically it is difficult, if not impossible, to justify ceasing the study at this point. Reinstatement of the intervention (i.e., adding a second B phase), regardless of continuing to collect data, is the ethical action for the scientist-practitioner and also may demonstrate additional control. Obviously, if the behavior does not change after the intervention has been withdrawn, the ethical challenge of removing the intervention without reinstatement is moot; however, as noted earlier, the effectiveness of the intervention must be questioned if the participant's performance does not return toward baseline when the intervention has been withdrawn.

When removing the intervention in the second A phase, it is not necessary for the participant's performance to return completely to baseline, but a distinct trend toward the return to baseline levels is sufficient. Remember, at least three data points are needed to establish a trend. When the participant's performance is variable, determining that trend may be difficult. When a return to baseline is especially detrimental to the participant, it is better to err on the side of caution if there is doubt about the performance trend toward baseline levels. Thus, if a participant's initial behavior was highly detrimental to her health, such as impulsively standing up when standing balance was very poor, then a single data point in the withdrawal phase that indicated a participant's return to impulsive standing up on removal of the intervention may be sufficient to reinstate the intervention. In Chapter 22, we present various methods to analyze data in order to determine trends.

The phase length of withdrawal designs is generally dictated by the participant's performance. When a participant's behavior presents an immediate threat to her health, the baseline length will only be long enough to establish the pattern of behavior or the immediate threat to health. In either situation, the intervention is then implemented. Typically, the intervention will be implemented until the participant achieves some pre-established criterion level for the behavior, at which time the intervention is then removed. The reinstatement of the intervention does not occur until a trend toward baseline is evident or until the return of the participant's behavior toward baseline levels is perceived as an immediate threat to the participant's health.

Sometimes, the withdrawal design is referred to as a "reversal" design. The true reversal design is a special case of the withdrawal design in which the intervention is not removed but is actually reversed.[14] As Hayes and colleagues[14] note, the use of the reversal design in clinical practice is rarely observed because of the ethical prohibitions and because few interventions are subject to being reversed.

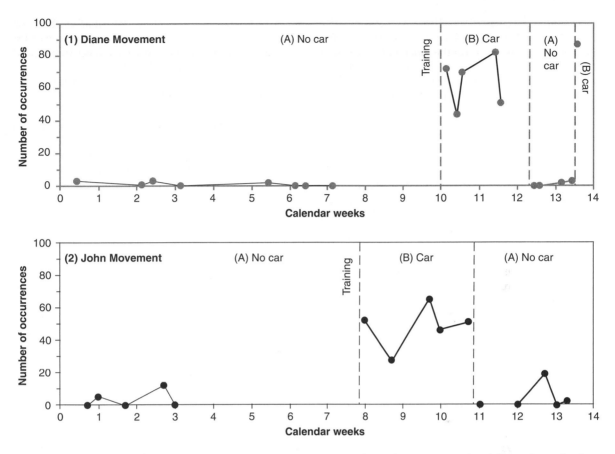

Figure 11-2 Child-initiated movement occurrences. (From Deitz J, Swinth Y, White O: Powered mobility and preschoolers with complex developmental delays, *Am J Occup Ther* 56:86–96, 2002.)

Multiple-Baseline Designs

Multiple-baseline designs, like withdrawal designs, answer the question of whether a treatment is effective. As we will see, they avoid the ethical dilemma of withholding an effective treatment.

Multiple-baseline design, and its variations (e.g., multiple-probe design), can be used to examine intervention effects with the different behaviors ("multiple baseline across behaviors" [e.g., heel-strike gait, straight swing through of the leg, and reciprocal arm swing]), across several different patients ("multiple baseline across participants" [e.g., the same treatment with three different patients]), with the patient's same behavior, but across different settings ("multiple baseline across settings" [e.g., heel-strike gait on a tile floor, carpeted floor, and grass lawn, or verbal interaction in a classroom, kitchen, and shopping mall]), or the same behavior but across different persons ("multiple baseline across therapists" [e.g., different therapists delivering the same treatment to the same patient or the patient verbally interacting with a school peer, a teacher, and a sales representative]). Traditionally, a

minimum of three different behaviors, settings, patients, or therapists is considered necessary for demonstration of intervention effectiveness when using this design.

There are several variations of the multiple-baseline designs. However, they all share the same purpose: to control for threats to internal validity without requiring that treatment be withdrawn.[8] The general format for the multiple-baseline study is to conduct several single-subject studies, with baselines at different times or for different durations. More specifically, after an intervention is introduced to the first patient (or first behavior, setting, or therapist), baseline data continue to be collected with the other patients until the first patient's intervention phase performance is stable. Subsequently, the intervention is provided to the second patient. Again, baseline data collection is continued with the remaining patients until the second patient's performance in the intervention phase is stabilized, and this pattern is followed until all patients have received the intervention. If, during baseline, any of the patients' data show changes in the desired direction of the intervention before receiving the intervention, conservative practice says baseline data should be collected until the baseline data stabilize. The strength of this design rests on the independence of each baseline to the introduction of the intervention with previous subjects (or behaviors or settings).

For example, Wambaugh[15] combined an alternating-treatments design with a multiple-baseline-across-behaviors design to investigate the relative effectiveness of phonological or semantic cueing on the word-retrieving abilities of a 44-year-old man with chronic anomic aphasia. In her study, the baseline for word sets 3 and 4 was extended until the upward trend ceased, even after the criterion was reached for word sets 1 and 2, because the baseline for sets 3 and 4 started to go up when the intervention phase began for word sets 1 and 2 (Fig. 11-3). Thus, Wambaugh was able to establish independence of behaviors by extending the baseline for the second behavior until it achieved a steady state.

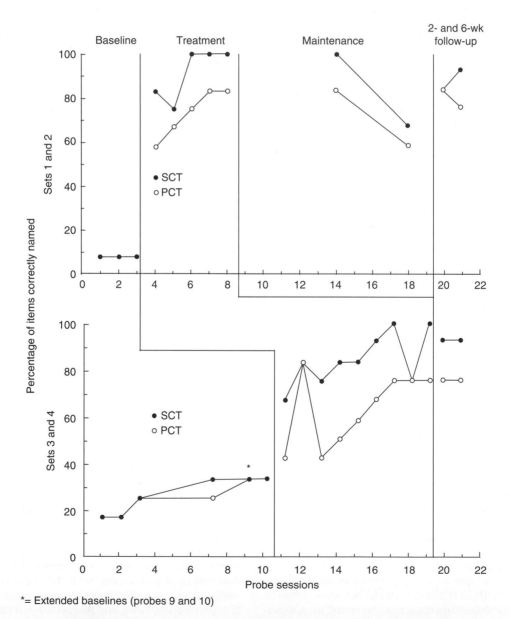

*= Extended baselines (probes 9 and 10)

Figure 11-3 Percentage of items named correctly in probes. (From Wambaugh JL: A comparison of relative effects of phonologic and semantic cueing treatments, *Aphasiology* 17:433–441, 2003. Reprinted by permission of Taylor & Francis Ltd.)

Although these features of single-subject designs (e.g., extended and stable baselines; changes of behavior with changes of phase) are desirable, adaptations may be made for clinical use, which may decrease the internal validity of the study but substantially improve the outcomes compared with a case report. For example, the intervention may be introduced to subsequent patients before the preceding patient's performance is stabilized. In Broach and Datillo's[16] study on the effects of aquatic therapy on lower-extremity strength of persons with multiple sclerosis, they introduced the intervention for all subjects without any of the immediately preceding subjects first achieving criterion levels in their intervention phase, as is illustrated in Figure 11-4. In this figure, the first subject, Dorothy, did not begin to show an effect of the aquatic therapy until about session 40, approximately 27 sessions after the introduction of the intervention, and plateaued at about session 47. By comparison, the second subject, Teresa, began the intervention at session 17, well before Dorothy's performance plateaued, and even before she began to show an effect of the intervention. Although it might be argued that the intervention for the third subject, Anita, began after Teresa's performance plateaued at about session 25, the intervention for the fourth subject, Margo, began before Anita's performance plateaued. Indeed, it might be argued that Margo's baseline performance was on the rise before her aquatic therapy began, although it is readily evident that Margo's hamstring strength stabilized at about 45 lb before the intervention was introduced.

In addition, not all patients may begin the baseline phase on the same date. Sullivan and Hedman[17] used a nonconcurrent multiple-baseline design across subjects in an investigation of the effects of sensory and motor electrical stimulation of 10 adults with chronic arm hemiparesis following a stroke. Their subjects experienced a randomly selected baseline length of 3, 4, or 5 weeks. The authors also indicated the baseline was extended where necessary to achieve baseline stability. The threat of history is assumed controlled in nonconcurrent multiple-baseline design because it is unlikely that the historical event would occur across the different participants during their random length baseline.[18] Thus, this design included both ways of varying the baselines—by having baselines occur at different times and for different durations.

Alternating-Treatments Designs

Alternating-treatments designs, sometimes referred to as simultaneous treatments designs,[6] include the use of different treatments, each administered independently of the other, within the same phase. These designs answer the clinical question, "Which of two (or sometimes more) treatments is better?" The treatments are rapidly alternated based on a random pattern. Because the effects of the interventions are short lived and rapidly presented in an alternating manner, a direct comparison of the treatments may be made, and a baseline phase becomes optional. This design is well suited to treatments that are expected to have short-lived effects, and it may be conducted without a baseline phase. In describing such designs, the letters B, C, D, E, and so on are used to represent the different treatments; A continues to represent the baseline phase or phases.

When presenting the different interventions, a pattern of presentation must be avoided in order to rule out that pattern as the cause of change. For example, we may want to see if treatment A (TxA) is more effective than treatment B (TxB). We are concerned that if we use a strict every-other-session sequence, we will have an order or pattern effect on the performance. Yet we want to be certain the participant receives an equal number of sessions of each treatment. Thus, we may use a sequence shown in Table 11-1 to deliver TxA and TxB.

In this example we see the participant receives each treatment for an equal number of sessions (TxA 1, 3, 6, 7, 8, 12 and TxB 2, 4, 5, 9, 10, 11). In addition, we note the participant receives an equal number of the couplet sequences of A preceding B and the opposite couplet sequences of B preceding A (AB sequence 1,2; 3,4; 8,9; and BA sequence 2,3; 5,6; 11,12). However, we must note the participant will receive TxB for a two-consecutive session sequence and a three-consecutive session sequence, but only a three-consecutive session sequence for TxA.

Presentation patterns may not only be found in the exposure to the interventions, but other factors that are part of the intervention context, such as different therapists delivering the intervention, or time of day the intervention is delivered, potentially influence the effect. In the example below is a sequence of implementing TxA and TxB to eliminate a pattern sequence by session and by time of day. The participant receives the intervention twice a day, once in the morning and once in the afternoon. To control for order effects, we might use the sequence in Table 11-2 to deliver the different treatments.

In this example, we have TxA delivered four times in the morning (sessions 1, 3, 7, 15) and four times in the afternoon (sessions 6, 8, 12,14). Similarly, TxB is delivered four times in the morning (sessions 5, 9, 11, 13) and four times in the afternoon (sessions 2, 4, 10, 16). In addition, we have TxA delivered for two consecutive sessions (14,15) and three consecutive sessions (6–8) and TxB delivered for two consecutive sessions

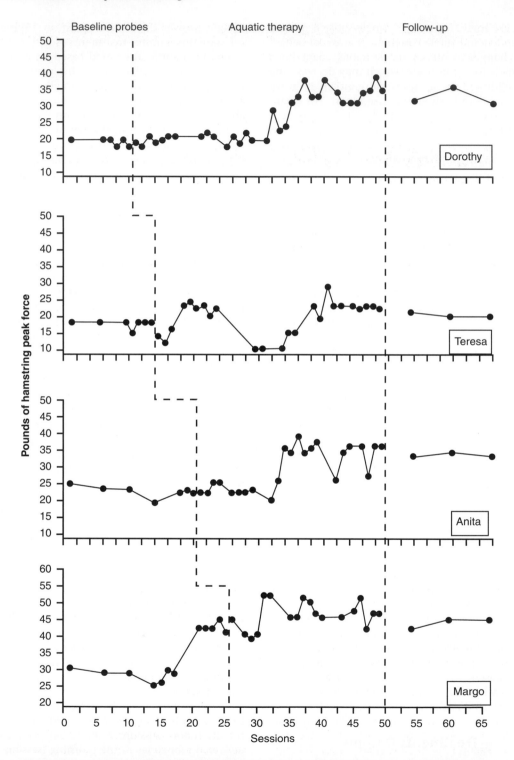

Figure 11-4 Multiple-baseline design indicating the effect of aquatic therapy on the peak hamstring force for persons with multiple sclerosis. (From Broach EM, Dattilo J: The effect of aquatic therapy on strength of adults with multiple sclerosis, *Ther Recreation J* 37:224–239, 2003.)

Table **11-1**

Sequence of Treatment A (TxA) and Treatment B (TxB) Offerings by Session

Session	1	2	3	4	5	6	7	8	9	10	11	12
Tx type	A	B	A	B	B	A	A	A	B	B	B	A

Table **11-2**

Sequence of Treatment A (TxA) and Treatment B (TxB) Offerings by Session and Time of Day

Session	1	2	3	4	5	6	7	8	9	10	11	12	13	14	15	16
Time of day	AM	PM	AM	PM	AM	PM	AM	PM	AM	PM	AM	PM	AM	PM	AM	PM
Tx type	A	B	A	B	B	A	A	A	B	B	B	A	B	A	A	B

(4,5) and three consecutive sessions (9–11). Thus, each treatment is delivered an equal number of morning and afternoon sessions, and each treatment is delivered an equal number of two and three consecutive sessions. If we examine how many sequences for which A precedes B, and the reverse, as we did previously, we have nearly an equal number of sequences.

Hains and Baer[19] suggested that the random assignment of patients to different interventions, as well as settings or other environmental or contextual factors (e.g., locations, different therapists, time of day), may reduce the pattern effects of these factors, individually or in combination.

Lewis and associates[20] controlled for combined and individual pattern effects of intervention and time of day by randomly assigning the patient, a 21-year-old man with traumatic brain injury, to two different intervention lengths of negative practice (i.e., short [SNP] and long [LNP]) across twice-daily practice sessions. In addition, the authors controlled for therapist effects by counterbalancing the number of LNP and SNP sessions, which were delivered by six different therapists, so each therapist delivered the same number of LNP and SNP sessions.

Using combined alternating-treatments designs and multiple-baseline designs across sets of word retrieval opportunities, Wambaugh[15] examined the effects of two different interventions—phonological and semantic cueing—on word retrieval by a 44-year-old man with chronic anomic aphasia. In her study, both treatments were administered in each session, with a 15- to 20-minute break between treatments; however, the order of treatment presentation was alternated as opposed to a random presentation order. Thus, notation for the order of presentation was as follows: BC,CB,BC,CB,BC, where BC was the order of presentation for the first session, CB was the presentation order for the second session, BC for

the third session, CB for the fourth session, and so on, with the comma separating each session for which the two conditions were used within the same session. Here, an alternating pattern of presentation, BCCBBBCCBB, may be perceived as a threat to the internal validity of the study's outcomes, even though Wambaugh used random ordering of the word sets with the change of conditions.

Washington and associates[21] used a different variation of the alternating-treatments design to study the impact of a contoured foam seat on sitting alignment and upper-extremity function of infants with neuromotor impairments. Alignment and upper-extremity function were measured with the children seated in a standard highchair during the baseline phase. During the intervention phase, two different interventions were presented each day: use of a thin foam liner within the highchair and use of a contoured foam seat within the highchair. Notation for this study might be "A-B,C" with the comma indicating that the two conditions (B and C) were alternated within a single phase. Another interesting design element of this particular study was the random reintroduction of the standard highchair at some point during the intervention phase for all children to determine whether maturation could be an explanation for any changes in status. Figure 11-5 shows these various elements for all four infants with whom the single-subject design was replicated. The alternating-treatments design works particularly well when the status of an individual is expected to fluctuate from day to day, as may be the case with infants who can be cranky and distracted on one day and cheery and focused on another day without any true change in status. The alternating-treatments design lets the researcher evaluate each condition in light of the performance exhibited on a given day. Thus, day-to-day

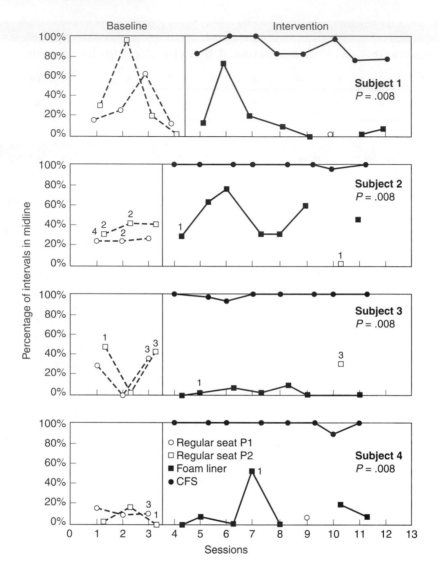

Figure 11-5 Example of data presentation for an alternating-treatments study. The authors tested the postural alignment of infants with neuromotor impairments under one baseline condition in a standard highchair and two alternating conditions (a thin foam liner in a standard highchair and a contoured foam seat in the highchair). (From Washington K, Deitz JC, White OR, Schwartz IS: The effects of a contoured foam seat on postural alignment and upper-extremity function in infants with neuromotor impairments, *Phys Ther* 82:1064–1076, 2002.)

variability is controlled because the measure of interest is not absolute performance, but rather the difference in performance between conditions for a given day. The authors reported that when the infants received the contour foam cushion condition, their postural alignment improved, but there was no improvement in bimanual play. Freeing of an arm from support role was variable across conditions.

Interaction Designs

Interaction designs are used to evaluate the effect of different combinations of treatments. They answer the clinical question, "Which aspect(s) of a treatment program is/are the agent(s) of therapeutic change?" Assume that a multimodal speech-language therapy program, such as that documented by Murray and Ray,[22] has been designed for individuals with aphasia. Two important components of this program are traditional syntax stimulation (B) and nontraditional relaxation training (C). Researchers might wish to differentiate the effects of these components to determine whether a single component or the combination of components is most effective.

The following design could separate these effects: B-C-B-BC-B-BC-C-BC-C, where the effectiveness of the traditional syntax is evaluated against the nontraditional relaxation training in the B-C-B sequence; the effectiveness of the traditional syntax to the combination of the two interventions is evaluated by B-BC-B-BC sequence; and the nontraditional relaxation training to the combination is evaluated by BC-C-BC-C.

Embrey and associates'[23] examination of the effects of neurodevelopmental treatment and orthoses on knee flexion during gait is another example of a design examining interaction effects. The design of this study is A-B-A-BC-A, with neurodevelopmental treatment (NDT) as the B intervention and BC the combination of NDT and orthoses treatments. In this study, the researchers apparently were not interested in the effect of the orthoses alone, hence the absence of an isolated C treatment.

Changing-Criterion Designs

This set of single-subject designs may be considered as a design that has great utility for clinical practice. In common clinical practice, we often attempt to help our clients achieve complex behaviors in partial steps. We reinforce those partial steps (or they are intrinsically reinforcing) and then attempt to have the patient accomplish a somewhat more difficult step. The changing-criterion design answers the clinical question, "Does changing the criterion for success lead to improved performance?" Thus, the question is critical for rehabilitation therapies that include reinforcement for desired behaviors at defined levels so that the desired behavior is likely to continue.

Unlike the withdrawal design, the changing-criterion design does not remove the intervention, and unlike the multiple-baseline design, it does not apply the intervention to just one setting, behavior, or person before being applied to another. The changing-criterion design begins with a baseline phase (A), followed by the intervention phase (B). The distinguishing feature of the changing-criterion design is that the participant's performance level is pre-established, and then the intervention is conducted with the purpose of achieving the pre-established criterion. Once that criterion is achieved, the participant's performance level is reset to a more stringent level, and once again the intervention is implemented with the purpose of

achieving the newly preset criterion. Thereafter, in subsequent sessions, the performance criterion continues to be reset, and the intervention is implemented with the purpose of achieving the criterion. The effectiveness of the intervention is determined by how closely the participant achieves or exceeds the preset criterion. If the participant fails to achieve the criterion, we assume the intervention is ineffective or that the criterion level has been set too high. If the participant overachieves the criterion by a large difference, we assume there are influences other than the intervention affecting the performance. Thus, determining where to set the criterion level can affect interpretation of the effectiveness of the intervention.

There does not appear to be a preferred method of determining the level at which to set the criterion sessions. One method for determining the criterion level uses an average of the previous sessions' performance, assuming the previous sessions' performance exceeded the previously preset criterion. Another method sets the next session's criterion at the highest performance level of the previous session. Still another approach is to simply rely on the therapist's clinical judgment.[24] Figure 11-6 presents an example of how the average performance of a subject's previous session, baseline, or intervention may be used to set the next session's criterion level. In this example, the intervention consists of a subject's walking three trials of 100 steps per session. The dependent variable is the proportion of steps with heel-strike gait on the involved foot. Thus, for a trial of 100 steps, there are 50 opportunities for the subject to exhibit a heel-strike gait on the involved side. The first

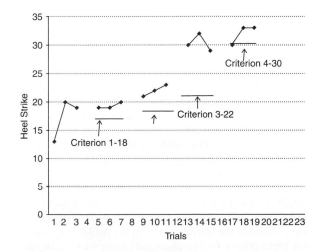

Figure 11-6 Changing-criterion design illustrating number of involved side heel-strike occurrences in trials of 50 steps as a result of changing-criterion intervention.

three trials are the baseline performance. The patient demonstrated a heel-strike gait for 13 of 50 steps on the first trial, 20 of 50 steps in the second trial, and 19 of 50 steps in the third trial for an average of 17.3 steps with a heel-strike gait.

Assuming the baseline is stable, the first intervention session's criterion level (17) is the average of the subject's baseline performance. The criterion for the second intervention session is the average of the subject's performance on the first intervention session (19). As we see in Figure 11-6, the subject had 19 heel strikes in each of the first two 50-step trials of the first criterion or intervention and 20 heel strikes in the third 50-step trial, for an average of 19.3 heel strikes. This pattern is then repeated for subsequent sessions until the subject plateaus. Remember, if during any session the subject greatly exceeds the criterion, a conservative interpretation of that session's data assumes there is something in addition to the intervention that has affected the performance. Continuing with the example, if we assume for the next session of three trials that the criterion is 22 steps with a heel-toe gait, but the patient is able to obtain 30, 32, and 29 heel-toe steps, then the assumption is that something other than the intervention may have influenced the patient's performance (see Fig. 11-6, criterion 3). If on the subsequent criterion the patient performs close to the criterion (see Fig. 11-6, criterion 4), then the previous performance may be considered an aberration.

In addition, McDougall[24] has suggested setting both minimum and maximum criterion levels for each session as a method to determine when a performance underachieves or overachieves the criterion level, even though the only guidance given for determining the criterion levels was the therapist's best clinical judgment.

Although this design appears to have great applicability to clinical practice, few studies have used it.

GRAPHING SINGLE-SUBJECT DATA

Generally, single-subject data are visually analyzed from graphed data, as opposed to statistically analyzed (see Chapter 22). The availability of computer-based spreadsheet software readily allows the graphing of patient data as they are collected. Typically, single-subject data are graphed while they are collected, enabling the scientist-practitioner to use the data in his or her clinical decision making. For example, consider the patient who lacks heel strike of the right foot during ambulation. Let's assume the physical therapist walks the patient for three trials of 20 steps each (10 steps with the right foot, 10 steps with the left foot) during the baseline or assessment phase to determine how significant the lack of heel strike is. In the first trial of 10 steps with the right

leg, the patient demonstrated right heel-strike steps for 3 out of 10 steps, 5 out of 10 steps for the second trial, and 4 out of 10 steps for the third trial, for an average of 4 heel-strike steps out of 10 steps with the right foot. If the physical therapist kept individual right-foot step data during this assessment, the raw data collection sheets might appear as shown in Table 11-3.

These three data collection sheets provide more information than just an average of 4 heel-strike steps out of 10 steps with the right foot or even the number of heel-strike steps for each of the three trials. The data sheets afford examination of individual patterns of heel-strike and non-heel-strike steps. Of note is the apparent randomness of heel-strike steps in the first trial, two sequences of 2 sequential heel-strike steps in the second trial, and the loss of sequential heel strikes in the third trial. The data, when graphed as a cumulative record, afford a visual perspective of the baseline data (Fig. 11-7).

In this cumulative record example, the X-axis is the number of steps the patient takes with the right leg, and the Y-axis is the number of heel-strike steps obtained on the right leg. Beginning with the first step in the first trial, the patient fails to give a heel strike; however, the patient does demonstrate a heel-strike step for the second step. For the third, fourth, and fifth steps, the patient fails to give a heel-strike step. A heel-strike step occurs in step 6, but not for steps 7 and 8. The next heel strike occurs at step 9, and that is the end of heel strikes for the first trial of 10 steps. Thus, on the X-axis, the graphed line encompasses steps 1 through 10, and the heel strikes for this first trial are a total of 4, as we can see on the Y-axis. In addition, from this graph we know in what step sequence the heel strikes occurred. For illustration purposes, we have provided a break between trials; thus, the first step of the second trial of 10 corresponds to step 12. In the second trial of 10 steps, heel strike occurs for the first 2 steps. Thus, we see that the first data point of the second trial is at the level of number 4 on the Y-axis, and the second data point is at the level of 5. From this graphed data, we can see a likely pattern emerging, that consecutive or only 1 non-heel-strike step between heel strikes occurs in the middle of the trials of 10 steps, suggesting the patient needs a few attempts before being successful with a heel strike and that the patient fatigues after step 8.

As a result of this apparent pattern, we decide our patient's intervention is going to emphasize getting the patient "ready" to take the first steps, in an effort to avoid the "warm-up steps," and have heel-strike steps at the beginning of each trial of 10 steps. Thus, we implement our intervention and record the heel strikes and steps we see our patient take after our intervention of getting her

Table **11-3**

Baseline Assessment of Involved Side Heel-Strike Step-by-Step Occurrence Data

TRIAL 1, BASELINE		TRIAL 2, BASELINE		TRIAL 3, BASELINE	
No. of Steps	**No. of Heel Strikes**	**No. of Steps**	**No. of Heel Strikes**	**No. of Steps**	**No. of Heel Strikes**
1	0	1	X	1	X
2	X	2	X	2	0
3	0	3	0	3	0
4	0	4	0	4	0
5	0	5	0	5	X
6	X	6	X	6	0
7	0	7	X	7	X
8	0	8	0	8	0
9	X	9	0	9	X
10	0	10	X	10	0
	Total 3/10		Total 5/10		Total 4/10

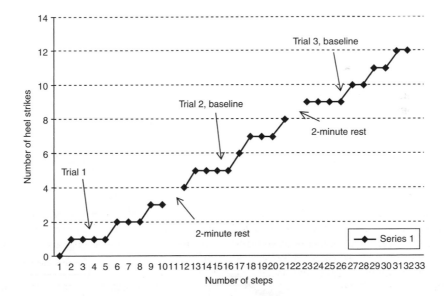

Figure 11-7 Cumulative record of three trials of 10 steps per trial of involved side heel-strike step-by-step occurrences.

"ready." The raw data collection sheets for this first day of intervention might appear as shown in Table 11-4.

From the data collection sheets in Table 11-4 for the first intervention session for this patient, her heel-strike data, with the baseline data, would appear as in Figure 11-8, if graphed.

Based on Figure 11-8, it is evident that the intervention emphasizing being "ready" for the first steps resulted in an increase in heel-strike steps for each of the three intervention trials, but especially during the first 3 steps in each of the trials. Trial 1 had a total of 6 heel-strike steps, trial 2 had a total of 7 heel-strike steps, and trial 3 had a total of

Table 11-4

Intervention Day 1: Involved Side Heel-Strike Step-By-Step Occurrence Data

TRIAL 1, BASELINE		TRIAL 2, BASELINE		TRIAL 3, BASELINE	
No. of Steps	No. of Heel Strikes	No. of Steps	No. of Heel Strikes	No. of Steps	No. of Heel Strikes
1	X	1	X	1	X
2	X	2	X	2	X
3	X	3	X	3	X
4	0	4	0	4	0
5	X	5	X	5	X
6	0	6	X	6	X
7	X	7	X	7	X
8	X	8	X	8	0
9	0	9	0	9	0
10	0	10	0	10	0
	Total 6/10		Total 7/10		Total 6/10

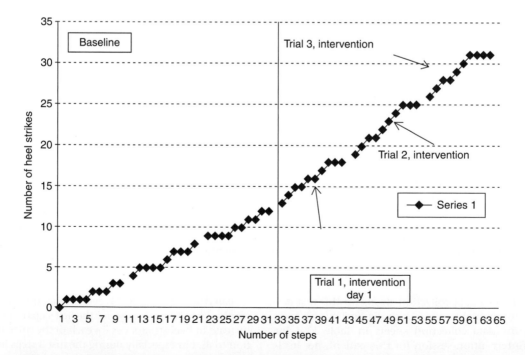

Figure 11-8 Cumulative record of 10 step trials of involved side heel-strike step-by-step occurrences for baseline and intervention.

6 heel-strike steps. Of interest is the "falling off" of heel-strike steps in the last several trials, suggesting that fatigue may be a factor in obtaining heel strike through the whole trial. Thus, a cumulative record graphing of data can be used to assist in clinical decision making.

Graphing Data for Alternating-Treatments Designs

The cumulative record method of graphing is the basis for generating graphs for all of the single-subject designs. Dixon and colleagues[25] describe the simple adjustments necessary to make to a data spreadsheet in order to produce a graph that corresponds to the single-subject design used by the scientist-practitioner. Included in their article are adjustments necessary for creating an alternating-treatments design. The following example describes the sequence for implementing an alternating-treatments design, presenting the resulting graphs for this design. Let's consider a case in which our patient has difficulty swallowing fluids. We want to determine whether thickened fluids (TxA), consumed by a person who has a tendency to choke on liquids, is a more effective intervention than an intervention that teaches the person

to "visualize" controlling the liquid's movement through the oral cavity (TxB). For this example, the measure is the number of choking/aspirating episodes per opportunities to swallow a liquid during a feeding session. Each of the interventions is implemented twice daily. To avoid "order effects," interventions TxA and TxB will be implemented in the sequence as presented in Table 11-5.

Table 11-6 shows recording sheets for baseline and two interventions (TxA and TxB) on swallowing opportunities and choking episodes for our patient. Baseline data collection was initiated the morning of Day 1. After seven swallowing attempts baseline data collection ceased because the patient had significant difficulty swallowing, choking on five of seven attempts (see Table 11-6, Baseline Data: Day 1), whereupon Intervention TxA commenced immediately after Baseline. During Intervention TxA the patient choked during swallowing attempts 4, 6, and 7 (see Table 11-6, Intervention TxA Session 1, Day 1). Intervention TxB commenced immediately after termination of Intervention TxA. Intervention TxB ceased after the patient's five consecutive attempts at swallowing resulted in choking. The next intervention session occurred in the afternoon of Day 1, beginning with Intervention TxB (see Table 11-5). Table 11-7 presents the raw date for Session 2, Day 1.

Table **11-5**

Sequence of Treatment A (TxA) and Treatment B (TxB) Offerings by Session

Session	1	2	3	4	5	6	7	8	9	10	11	12
Tx type	A	B	A	B	B	A	A	A	B	B	B	A

Table **11-6**

Baseline and Intervention Data for Number of Choking Episodes per Number of Swallowing Attempts for Day 1

BASELINE DATA: DAY 1		INTERVENTION TxA SESSION 1, DAY 1		INTERVENTION TxB SESSION 1, DAY 1	
No. of Swallowing Attempts	No. of Choking Episodes	No. of Swallowing Attempts	No. of Choking Episodes	No. of Swallowing Attempts	No. of Choking Episodes
1	X	1	0	1	X
2	0	2	0	2	X
3	X	3	0	3	X
4	X	4	X	4	X
5	X	5	0	5	X
6	X	6	X		
7	X	7	X		

Because the patient choked on all four attempts at swallowing under condition Intervention TxB in Session 2, Day 1, the intervention was terminated and Intervention TxA was initiated (see Table 11-7, Intervention TxA Session 2, Day 1). As we can see by the data, choking occurred on only one of the six swallowing attempts under Intervention TxA. The next day, Day 2, the feeding session (Session 3) commenced with Intervention TxA (see Table 11-8). As with the patient's performance under Intervention TxA in Session 2, Day 1, the patient had only one episode of choking. Intervention TxB commenced following the 8 attempts under Intervention TxA. Choking occurred with all

four swallowing attempts under Intervention TxB (see Table 11-8, Intervention TxB Session 3, Day 2). Because the data from Sessions 1, 2 and 3 provided evidence that Intervention TxA resulted in far fewer choking episodes during feeding with our patient than with Intervention TxB, Intervention TxA was reinstated as the intervention of choice.

Figure 11-9 shows the graphed data from this alternating-treatments design example. The graph illustrates a clear separation of treatment effects for the two interventions: TxA and TxB. With this evidence, the scientist-practitioner proceeded with TxA as the best intervention to be used with this specific patient.

Table 11-7

Intervention Data for Number of Choking Episodes per Number of Swallowing Attempts for Day 1, Session 2

INTERVENTION TxB SESSION 2, DAY 1		INTERVENTION TxA SESSION 2, DAY 1	
No. of Swallowing Attempts	No. of Choking Episodes	No. of Swallowing Attempts	No. of Choking Episodes
1	X	1	0
2	X	2	0
3	X	3	X
4	X	4	0
		5	0
		6	0

Table 11-8

Intervention Data for Number of Choking Episodes per Number of Swallowing Attempts for Day 2, Session 3

INTERVENTION TxA SESSION 3, DAY 2		INTERVENTION TxB, SESSION 3, DAY 2	
No. of Swallowing Attempts	No. of Choking Episodes	No. of Swallowing Attempts	No. of Choking Episodes
1	0	1	X
2	0	2	X
3	0	3	X
4	X	4	X
5	0		
6	0		
7	0		
8	0		

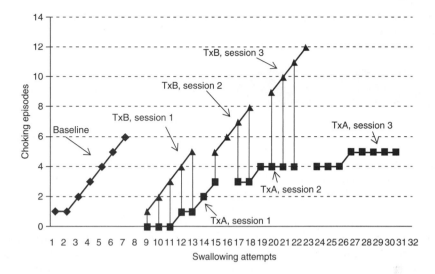

Figure 11-9 Alternating-treatments graph of choking episodes per swallow attempts under two different interventions: TxA and TxB.

CONSIDERATIONS WHEN USING SINGLE-SUBJECT DESIGNS

The duration of each intervention and the frequency with which to alternate the intervention sessions or phases are two considerations with which scientist-practitioners, as well as researchers, struggle. Determining when to change interventions is logically based on the patient's performance and is done as the intervention is ongoing. Although there is no "hard rule" for determining when to change interventions or study phases, the "soft rule" for changing sessions or phases may be when data are stable and a pattern has emerged.[2] With the exception of those cases in which a deteriorating behavior is detrimental to a patient's immediate or nearly immediate safety, when a single data point may suffice to indicate a change of phases, a minimum of three data points is necessary to determine a trend but may be insufficient to determine stability. Thus, it is likely that the length of an intervention session will occur for more than three data points. In the case of alternating-treatments designs, then, each intervention might be conducted for five or possibly more consecutive sessions. Alternatively, when there is a concern for "order effects" on a patient's performance, and the behaviors are highly responsive to the intervention, the intervention session length may be less than three data points.

To more objectively determine when data are stable, we may borrow from methods of single-subject data analysis, as presented in Chapter 22. For withdrawal designs, a phase change decision may use the 2 standard deviations width band method, whereby the band is based on a line determined from the previous phase's mean score, making a phase change rule when a preset percentage or number of data points exceed the 2 standard deviations limits. Earlier, for the changing-criterion designs, we described a method of determining intervention session duration when the data exceeded the previous session's average, or highest, performance.

As with the duration of an intervention phase, there is no objective method for determining the number of changes of interventions necessary to demonstrate treatment effects, whether withdrawing a treatment as in a withdrawal design, or substituting one intervention for another as in an alternating-treatments design. In the case of alternating designs, alternating the interventions may be continued until there is a distinct separation in the patient's performance for one intervention. Determining that "distinct separation" may be left to the scientist-practitioner's judgment. For withdrawal designs, three phases (i.e., two withdrawal phases and one intervention phase) are considered the minimum number of phases. Of course, it is unethical to end a study by removing an effective intervention; hence, most withdrawal studies have two withdrawal and two intervention phases, ending the study with the effective intervention. For changing-criterion and multiple-baseline designs, the general rule is to end the study when the preset criteria are achieved. In those instances in which the patient makes very slow progress, or ceases progress toward the criteria, continuation of the study is left to the judgment of the scientist-practitioner. Practically, the scientist-practitioner's judgment may be influenced by third-party payers.

LIMITATIONS OF SINGLE-SUBJECT DESIGNS

Just as with group designs, many authors and researchers are enthusiastic about the information that can be gleaned from carefully constructed single-subject designs, and others are sharply critical of this form of inquiry for at least four reasons.[26,27] In this chapter, we have presented alternative designs for each of the concerns. For example, one concern is that single-subject designs may create ethical dilemmas because the need for an extended baseline leads to a delay in treatment, because researchers may withdraw effective treatments during the course of the study, and because of the increased cost of care related to data collection during baseline and withdrawal phases. We have presented different designs that do not require the extended baselines (e.g., nonconcurrent multiple-baseline designs, alternating-treatments designs, withdrawal designs in which two interventions are compared) or withdraw effective treatments (e.g., multiple-baseline designs, changing-criterion designs). Because there are designs that address this concern, the concern for increased costs for these designs is similarly addressed.

A second concern is the amount of control single-subject designs have over internal validity threats, such as history or maturation, that might be responsible for changes in the dependent variables. In addition, there is the possibility that apparent improvements may reflect either familiarity with, or a treatment effect from, the repeated testing. As we presented in this chapter, certain designs address the control of internal validity threats better than other designs, just as do different group designs. We have noted that the stability of an extended baseline and the change of the behavior with the introduction of the intervention represent a powerful display of control of history and maturation threats, especially when repeated over behaviors, subjects, or settings. Similarly, the repeated withdrawal and reinstatement of an intervention, with a corresponding change in performance, is a strong statement of control over history. In addition, we have indicated that the differentiating performance of the subject under different conditions in the alternating-treatments designs is another example of controlling for history threats. The concern for the effects of repeated testing is mitigated when we consider that the intent of interventions is to obtain a change in performance of specified behaviors. If the test is the same as the intervention, the concern of repeated testing is unfounded.

A third concern, generalizability of results, may be low in single-subject designs, despite the position, as advanced by Sim,[5] that case-by-case generalizability of single-subject designs is as valid as the sample-to-population of group designs and that group designs are unable to determine which subgroups of subjects responded best and which subgroups failed to respond to the intervention. Group-design proponents argue that single-subject designs vary too greatly on subject features and on interventions, even though group designs deliver a set intervention not tailored to the individual needs of the subjects, and that subject features are "averaged." The issue of generalizability of results to a single patient will require a determination of how well the patient's features and the intervention are matched to that of the study, regardless of design.

The fourth reason for concern advanced by critics of single-subject designs relates to the theory and practice of statistical analysis of single-subject designs. Critics argue that statistical analysis of single-subject designs is in its infancy. We have indicated that historically statistical analyses of single-subject designs are largely rejected because single-subject designs are concerned with clinically significant changes, not statistical changes, and that this position of clinically important changes is the direction in which evidence-based practice is proceeding. Some authors believe that the common methods of analysis that are reported in the literature frequently violate a variety of statistical tenets. A more complete discussion of statistical analysis of single-subject designs is presented in Chapter 22.

Single-subject designs have great utility for the scientist-practitioner. Single-subject designs have great flexibility to afford adaptation to changes in the clinical care of patients. Other features of the designs, such as the frequent data taken to adjust interventions to the changing performance of the individual, as well as the emphasis on using reliable measures in the clinical practice, make these designs clinically applicable for the scientist-practitioner. Furthermore, the designs use features that afford the clinician the opportunity to make cause-and-effect statements. Thus, these designs have been recognized by the American Academy for Cerebral Palsy and Developmental Medicine for their research rigor in that their own separate and distinct hierarchy of levels of evidence has been adopted, as well as for their clinical applicability.[28,29]

SUMMARY

Group research designs are often limited because too few participants are available for powerful statistical analysis and because the impact of the treatment on individuals is obscured by the group results. Single-subject designs overcome these limitations with controlled initiation and withdrawal of individualized treatments for a single participant, with repeated measurements of the dependent variables across time, and by analysis methods designed for use with data from only one participant. Broad categories of single-subject designs include A-B designs, withdrawal designs, multiple-baseline designs, alternating-treatments designs, and interaction designs. In addition, single-subject designs are readily adapted for clinical use. Despite the advantages of single-subject designs, some find them to be limited because of ethical concerns, lack of control of extraneous variables, limited generalizability, and violation of statistical assumptions.

REFERENCES

1. Hislop HJ: Tenth Mary McMillan lecture: The not-so-impossible dream, *Phys Ther* 55:1069–1080, 1975.
2. Kazdin AE: *Single-Case Research Designs: Methods for Clinical and Applied Settings*, New York, NY, 1982, Oxford University Press.
3. Morgan DL, Morgan RK: Single-participant research design: Bringing science to managed care, *Am Psychol* 56:119–127, 2001.
4. Suen HK, Ary D: *Analyzing Quantitative Behavioral Observation Data*, Hillsdale, NJ, 1989, Lawrence Erlbaum.
5. Sim J: The external validity of group comparative and single system studies, *Physiotherapy* 81:263–270, 1995.
6. Kazdin AE: The case study and single-case research designs. In Kazdin AE, editor: *Research Design in Clinical Psychology*, 4th ed, Boston, Mass, 2003, Allyn & Bacon.
7. Ottenbacher KJ: *Evaluating Clinical Change: Strategies for Occupational and Physical Therapists*, Baltimore, Md, 1986, Williams & Wilkins.
8. Backman CL, Harris SR, Chisholm JAM, Monette AD: Single-subject research in rehabilitation: A review of studies using AB, withdrawal, multiple baseline, and alternating treatments designs, *Arch Phys Med Rehabil* 78:1145–1153, 1997.
9. Zhan S, Ottenbacher K: Single subject research designs for disability research, *Disabil Rehabil* 23:1–8, 2001.
10. Marklund I, Klässbo M: Effects of lower limb intensive mass practice in poststroke patients: Single-subject experimental design with long-term follow-up, *Clin Rehabil* 20:568–576, 2006.
11. Cross J, Tyson SF: The effect of a slider shoe on hemiplegic gait, *Clin Rehabil* 17:817–824, 2003.
12. Miller EW: Body weight supported treadmill and overground training in a patient post cerebrovascular accident, *Neurorehabilitation* 16:155–163, 2001.
13. Deitz J, Swinth Y, White O: Powered mobility and preschoolers with complex developmental delays, *Am J Occup Ther* 56:86–96, 2002.
14. Hayes SD, Barlow DH, Nelson-Gray RO: *The Scientist Practitioner: Research and Accountability in the Age of Managed Care*, Boston, Mass, 1999, Allyn & Bacon.
15. Wambaugh JL: A comparison of relative effects of phonologic and semantic cueing treatments, *Aphasiology* 17:433–441, 2003.
16. Broach EM, Dattilo J: The effect of aquatic therapy on strength of adults with multiple sclerosis, *Ther Recreation J* 37:224–239, 2003.
17. Sullivan JE, Hedman LD: Effects of home-based sensory and motor amplitude electrical stimulation on arm dysfunction in chronic stroke, *Clin Rehabil* 21:142–150, 2007.
18. Watson PJ, Workman EA: The non-concurrent multiple baseline across-individuals design: An extension of the traditional multiple baseline design, *J Behav Ther Exp Psychol* 12:257–259, 1981.
19. Hains AH, Baer DM: Interaction effects in multi-element designs: Inevitable, desirable, and ignorable, *J Appl Behav Anal* 22:57–69, 1989.
20. Lewis FD, Blackerby WF, Ross JR, et al. Duration of negative practice and the reduction of leg pounding of a traumatically brain-injured adult, *Behav Residential Treat* 1:265–274, 1986.
21. Washington K, Deitz JC, White OR, Schwartz IS: The effects of a contoured foam seat on postural alignment and upper-extremity function in infants with neuromotor impairments, *Phys Ther* 82:1064–1076, 2002.
22. Murray LL, Ray AH: A comparison of relaxation training and syntax stimulation for chronic nonfluent aphasia, *J Commun Disord* 34:87–113, 2001.
23. Embrey DG, Yates L, Mott DH: Effects of neuro-developmental treatment and orthoses on knee flexion during gait: A single-subject design, *Phys Ther* 70:626–637, 1990.
24. McDougall D: The range-bound changing criterion design, *Behav Intervent* 20:129–137, 2005.
25. Dixon MR, Jackson JW, Small SL, et al: Creating single-subject design graphs in Microsoft Excel™ 2007, *JABA* 41:277–293, 2008.
26. Bithell C: Single subject experimental design: A case for concern? *Physiotherapy* 80:85–87, 1994.
27. Reboussin DM, Morgan TM: Statistical considerations in the use and analysis of single-subject designs, *Med Sci Sports Exerc* 28:639–644, 1996.
28. Logan LR, Hickman RR, Harris SR, Heriza CB: Single-subject research design: Recommendations for levels of evidence and quality rating, *Dev Med Child Neurol* 50:99–103, 2008.
29. Darragh J, Hickman R, O'Donnell M, et al: *AACPDM Methodology to Develop Systematic Reviews of Treatment Interventions (rev 1.2)*, 2008. Available at: http://www.aacpdm.org/UserFiles/file/systematic-review-methodology.pdf. Accessed February 10, 2015.

CHAPTER

12

Overview of Nonexperimental Research

CHAPTER OUTLINE

Description
  Retrospective Descriptive Research
  Prospective Descriptive Research
    Observation
    Examination
    Interview
    Questionnaire

Analysis of Relationships
  Retrospective Analysis of
    Relationships
  Prospective Analysis of Relationships

Analysis of Differences
  Retrospective Analysis of Differences
  Prospective Analysis of Differences
Summary

Thus far, we have concentrated on experiments—that is, types of research designed to answer cause-and-effect questions. However, the scientist-practitioner will also engage in nonexperimental research. These research endeavors are often referred to as "descriptive," although we offer a particular and narrower use of that term. Many of these research behaviors are common to the practitioner, such as observation, interview, and questionnaires. Keeping in mind principles of research, the clinical activity can qualify in the research category, making nonexperimental research vital for the scientist-practitioner.

In contrast to experimental research, nonexperimental research does not involve manipulation of variables. In nonexperimental studies, then, the researcher examines records of past phenomena, documents existing phenomena, or observes new phenomena unfolding. Although investigators do not manipulate variables in the nonexperimental paradigm, they can—and quite often do—select variables or levels of variables for observation, comparison, or other nonexperimental study. Investigators undertake those studies understanding that they will not produce cause-and-effect data.

However, in at least some descriptive methods, such as comparison, descriptive research employs quantitative methods to analyze data. For example, one of the most common types of research in rehabilitation is a comparison of typically developing participants with participants having some clinical diagnostic category. An investigator may wish to compare a group of children having autism with a typically developing group on ability to draw inferences from a story. Any differences found could easily be subjected to statistical analysis of the types used for true experiments. At the same time, many types of nonexperimental studies are qualitative in nature, relying on nonquantitative descriptions of results.

The label "nonexperimental" may imply an unfavorable comparison with research that meets the controlled-manipulation criterion for "experimental" research. This is an unfortunate implication, in that nonexperimental research is exceedingly important within the rehabilitation literature. Law and colleagues[1] articulate four situations in which more exploratory, generally nonexperimental, designs may be appropriate: (1) when little is known about the topic, (2) when outcomes are not easily quantified, (3) when ethical issues preclude experimental approaches, and (4) when the purpose of the research is something other than determination of treatment effectiveness.

We may imagine a continuum of research questions or development of knowledge that would necessitate beginning with nonexperiments and proceeding to experiments. It is not, then, that experiments are more valuable or more important in the scheme of science, but only that experiments answer different questions than do nonexperiments.

When clinicians and scientists are faced with a new or little-studied phenomenon, it is necessary to first learn all that is possible about it. The subject of autism provides a good example for the rehabilitation professions. Although identified some years ago, the epidemic proportion of autism in the United States in recent years has spurred a great deal of recent research. It has first been necessary to learn the characteristics of autism. What are the dimensions of the disability in terms of physical, communicative, and emotional manifestations? What common characteristics seem to be in the histories of people with autism? These are questions for description, rather than the cause-and-effect questions posed of experiments. After we have learned a good deal about autism, we can begin to ask some "what-if" questions, primarily aimed at determining the effectiveness of therapeutic routines. That is, what *effect* does a particular treatment have on certain behaviors of autistic people? This is a question for experiment.

The purpose of this chapter is to provide the reader with an overview of the diversity of nonexperimental research designs. Because nonexperimental research does not have to fit a rigid definition of controlled manipulation, the variety of nonexperimental designs is greater than that of experimental designs. In fact, there are nonexperimental research designs to fit every research type in the design matrix in Figure 12-1. Therefore, this chapter is organized by providing examples of nonexperimental research articles that fit into each of the six cells of the matrix of research types. As in earlier chapters, the pertinent portion of each study is reviewed; readers who go to the literature will find that some of the articles are more involved than would be assumed just from reading this chapter. A factor that complicates discussion of nonexperimental research is that there are many different terms that are used to describe certain types of nonexperimental studies. Table 12-1 provides a brief description of these forms of research. Because some of these forms of nonexperimental research are extremely important within the rehabilitation literature, they are presented in more detail in later chapters: case reports (Chapter 13),

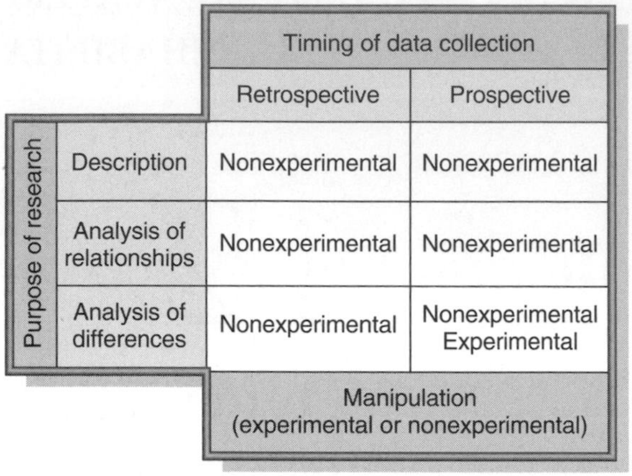

Figure 12-1 Matrix of research types showing three design dimensions: purpose of the research (rows), timing of data collection (columns), and manipulation (cells).

qualitative research (Chapter 14), epidemiological research (Chapter 15), outcomes research (Chapter 16), survey research (Chapter 17), and methodological research (Chapter 19).

DESCRIPTION

The purpose of descriptive research (as we use the term in this book) is to document the nature of a phenomenon through the systematic collection of data. In this text, a study is considered descriptive if it either provides a snapshot view of a single sample measured once or involves measurement and description of a sample several times over an extended period. The former approach is said to be cross-sectional; the latter is referred to as longitudinal.

In a typical descriptive study, many different variables are documented. For the most part, however, there is no presumption of cause or effect. Thus, the distinction between independent and dependent variables is not usually made in reports of descriptive research. As is the case with all three research purposes that make up the matrix of research types, a distinction can be made between prospective and retrospective descriptive research designs.

Retrospective Descriptive Research

The purpose of retrospective descriptive research is to document the past. The description of the past may be of inherent interest, may be used to evaluate the present against the past, or may be used to make decisions in the present based on information from the past.

Table 12-1	

Types of Nonexperimental Research

Case report	Systematic documentation of a well-defined unit; usually a description of an episode of care for an individual, but sometimes an administrative, educational, or other unit
Case-control design	An epidemiological research design in which groups of individuals with and without a certain condition or characteristic (the "effect") are compared to determine whether they have been differentially exposed to presumed causes of the condition or characteristic
Cohort design	An epidemiological research design that works forward from cause to effect, identifying groups of participants thought to have differing risks for developing a condition or characteristic and observing them over time to determine which group of participants is more likely to develop the condition or characteristic
Correlational research	Research conducted for the purpose of determining the interrelationships among variables
Developmental research	Research in which observations are made over time to document the natural history of the phenomenon of interest
Epidemiological research	Research that documents the incidence of a disease or injury, determines causes for the disease or injury, or develops mechanisms to control the disease or injury
Evaluation research	Research conducted to determine the effectiveness of a program or policy
Historical research	Research in which past events are documented because they are of inherent interest or because they provide a perspective that can guide decision making in the present
Meta-analysis	Research process by which the results of several studies are synthesized in a quantitative way
Methodological research	Research conducted to determine the reliability and validity of clinical and research measurements
Normative research	Research that uses large, representative samples to generate norms on measures of interest
Policy research	Research conducted to inform policymaking and implementation
Qualitative research	Research conducted to develop a deep understanding of the particular, usually using interview and observation
Secondary analysis	Research that reanalyzes data collected for the sole purpose of answering new research questions
Survey research	Research in which the data are collected by having participants complete questionnaires or respond to interview questions

The common denominator among research studies of this type is the reliance on archival data. Archival data may be found in medical records, voter registration rosters, newspapers and magazines, telephone directories, meeting minutes, television news programs, and a host of other sources. The information found in archival records must be systematically analyzed by the researcher for its relevance. Content analysis is the painstaking process that involves applying operational definitions and decision rules to the records to extract the data of interest.

Examples of the decisions that might need to be made can be seen in a study by Marmura and colleagues,[2] in which they used electronic medical records (EMRs) to evaluate physician prescription use and dosing patterns of topiramate in a headache clinic. First, the authors note, "EMRs vary widely in their structure, capacity, and extent of data capture."[(p. 770)] Thus, the most basic decision was whether EMRs available would suit their purposes. The same would be true of any archival data. Next, Marmura and colleagues needed to define their patient populations. In this case, it seemed fairly simple: those who had a record of receiving topiramate treatment and those who did not. However, the investigators sought a more complex analysis and, so, further subdivided patients treated with topiramate into dosing patterns. Thus, another decision to be made is how complex the investigators wish the analysis to be. Although a complex analysis of objective data may be tedious, when moving away from numerical data the picture becomes even more complicated. Marmura and colleagues note that "Subjective or complex variables can be more challenging to measure and document." Investigators need to consider this difficulty if the goal of research is some analysis of, for example, attitude change.

When using archival data, decision rules would be established to enable the researchers to determine which of the charts or records they reviewed fit all the parts of the definition. Because it is difficult to anticipate every possible variation within the medical records, the operational definitions are usually established with the help of a pilot data extraction project. Based on the pilot study, definitive decision rules and operational definitions are made before the study is begun.[3]

Medical record data are not the only type of retrospective work that may be of interest to the profession of rehabilitation. Censuses and surveys are commonly used sources of retrospective data. Some recent examples can be found in (1) a survey of ear and hearing disorders in four Chinese provinces[4] and (2) an analysis, based on census data, of the distribution of physiotherapists in Ontario.[5]

Evaluation research is another type of descriptive nonexperimental research that is typically conducted retrospectively. Polit and Beck[6] note that "Evaluation research focuses on developing information needed by decision makers about whether to adopt, modify, or abandon a program, practice, procedure, or policy."[(p. 260)] The research can lead to formative evaluations, in which evaluation during the course of a program or practice can lead to program improvements. The research can also be summative, which takes place after a program or practice has been completed and a decision needs to be made about continuation.

Sometimes evaluation research looks at the outcomes of a program at a single entity, facility, or institution. Such was the case in Spalding and Killet's[7] evaluation of an adapted approach to problem-based learning (labeled placement PBL) in a single master's degree course in occupational therapy at one university in England. The evaluation purpose was to determine the students' views of the efficacy of placement PBL for facilitating their learning in the final 3 months of their preregistration (i.e., before beginning professional practice) education. Evaluation was based on questionnaires and focus groups. Overall, students were very satisfied with the placement PBL, and the authors note its value in preprofessional education.

In other cases, evaluation research looks at services delivered to (often) large numbers of patients and across several institutions. The evaluation of Project Home[8] is a good example. Here, the authors identified barriers to home return for 60 nursing home residents across nine facilities in central New York State. Another possible retrospective approach is epidemiological research. Epidemiology is the study of disease, injury, and health in a population, and epidemiological research encompasses a broad range of methods (not all of them retrospective) that are used to study population-based health issues. Lu-Yao and associates[9] used retrospective methods to study the treatment of elderly Americans with hip fractures. In this study, a sample of the Medicare claims database was used to determine the characteristics of patients with hip fracture, the surgical procedure used to repair the fracture, and the survival rate up to 3 years after the fracture. The very large sample size (26,434 cases), which is likely to be representative of the larger population of elderly Americans with hip fractures, is one thing that differentiates epidemiological research from smaller studies that use samples of convenience from one or just a few hospitals. See Chapter 15 for additional information on epidemiological research.

Another research approach that uses retrospective descriptive methods is historical research. The purpose of historical research is to document past events because they are of inherent interest or because they provide a perspective that can guide decision making in the present. One type of historical research documents the accomplishments of prominent individuals within a profession, as in a report based on information found in unpublished archival documents of Nicholas Taptas's[10] development of the artificial larynx. Another form of historical research documents trends in clinical care across time, as in the description of changes in physical therapy practice over the period from 1945 through 2010.[11] Still another form is policy research, which analyzes the history or impact of public policy, as in Reed's[12] review of the history of federal legislation in the United States for persons with disabilities.

Another form of research that often rests on retrospective description is the case report or case study.

Although the terms are often used interchangeably, they are sometimes differentiated. When they are, the case report is described as the less controlled, less systematic of the two forms of inquiry.[13] Readers should also note the differentiation of (qualitative) case studies with (experimental) studies using single-subject designs (see Chapter 11). One example of a retrospective case report is Norén, Svensson, and Telford's[14] report of their work using a voice-output communication aid (VOCA) for one 13-year-old with cerebral palsy and his adult communication partner. The investigators found that the use of the VOCA altered several pragmatic aspects of conversation. This study is retrospective because the investigators did not know in advance what kinds of data they would be analyzing. Case reports and case studies are discussed in more detail in Chapters 13 and 14.

Prospective Descriptive Research

Prospective descriptive research enables the researcher to control the data that are collected for the purpose of describing a phenomenon. The prospective nature of data collection often makes the results of such research more believable than the results of purely retrospective studies. There are four basic methods of data collection in prospective descriptive research: observation, examination, interview, and questionnaire.

Observation

The processes of observation are more fully presented in Chapter 14. However, as an introduction, it is important for the scientist-practitioner to understand that there is more than one type of observation and that observation can be quite structured, as well as less structured.

A good example is the study by Johnson and colleagues,[15] in which they observed the effects of internal and external focus of attention on gait rehabilitation in patients who had had a stroke. Rather than instructing the physical therapists involved to direct patients' attention one way or another, the investigators videotaped what transpired in the natural rehabilitation setting. This study is prospective in that the investigators knew before the analysis what kinds of data (i.e., focus of attention) they would be looking at.

Examination

In these studies, investigators examine patients to analyze predefined sources of information. In a study by McCarthy and colleagues,[16] two physiotherapists performed standard clinical evaluations on a series of 301 patients with nonspecific low back pain. The purpose was to determine the ability of the clinical examination to form homogeneous patient subgroups. In this case, the investigators knew in advance they wanted to analyze results such as interrater reliability and cluster formation.

Another variation on prospective descriptive research is seen in the methodological study of Rosa and associates,[17] who examined the ability of therapeutic touch practitioners to detect the human energy fields they claim to be able to detect and manipulate. The goals of methodological research are to document and improve the reliability and validity of clinical and research measures. This study, published in the *Journal of the American Medical Association*, was received with a great deal of interest because a portion of the article reported on the fourth-grade science project of one of the authors. To determine the ability of the practitioners to detect a human energy field, each practitioner placed his or her hands palm up through a screen that kept the practitioner from seeing the experimenter. The experimenter then conducted 10 trials with each practitioner in which the experimenter hovered one of her hands over one of the hands of the practitioner. The practitioner was asked to indicate which of his or her hands was closest to the examiner's hands for each trial. Most practitioners were not able to reliably detect the correct hand. More detail about methodological research is presented in Chapters 18 and 19.

Interview

An interview is a structured conversation between a researcher/clinician and a participant/patient. It is not the same as an ordinary conversation between friends or acquaintances or even between business associates. Its purpose is primarily to gather information, and both parties have roles to carry out: the scientist-practitioner to obtain information and the participant/patient to provide it. The scientist-practitioner can use various interview techniques or procedures to help the participant provide information, some more effective than others. These will be further explained in Chapter 14.

Focus-group interviews were used by Holland, Middleton, and Uys[18] in their analysis of sources of professional confidence among South African occupational therapy students. The researchers interviewed 19 final-year students as well as five lecturers and six clinical supervisors. It is interesting and important to note that the students represented a spectrum of ethnic, religious, educational, and socioeconomic backgrounds representative of South Africa's population. All students had taken at least one semester of isiZulu language and Zulu culture as preparation for professional practice. The researchers found that both external (e.g., clinical experiences) and internal (e.g., personality traits) sources contributed (or not) to the students' confidence.

The interview method is not without hazards, however. Without the anonymity of a mailed questionnaire, participants may give what they believe to be socially acceptable answers. In this study, they might have exaggerated the importance of being confident or accepting of diversity if they believed that the interviewers themselves placed a great deal of importance on those qualities. Further, the investigators in this study used focus groups rather than individual interviews, allowing each participant to hear other participants' responses. Interviewing is discussed in more detail in Chapter 14.

Questionnaire

In a questionnaire, or survey, questions and the types of responses to questions are determined in advance: Typically, the researcher does not depart from the predetermined questions or statements, and typically respondents are not asked to depart from the predetermined answer style. For example, questions in a survey might ask respondents to rate their degree of agreement/disagreement with several statements. At other times, respondents might be asked to rate the degree of importance of several topics on a numerical scale. Quite often, questionnaires are administered in a written format (now often electronic), although "live" questionnaires are certainly possible; most of us have received telephone calls asking us to respond to a survey.

Questionnaires and surveys are extremely prevalent in rehabilitation research. A search in CINAHL using the search terms "survey" OR "questionnaire" with no specific fields (e.g., author or title), but limited to peer-reviewed research articles in English from 2010 to 2013 (searching in November of 2013), yielded 37,195 references.

A very popular variant in survey research is the Delphi method. The CINAHL search above, including AND "Delphi method," yielded 24,362 references. The Delphi technique uses a series of questionnaires to elicit a consensus from a group of experts. Each round of questionnaires builds on information collected in the previous round and generally asks participants to indicate their levels of agreement or disagreement with group opinions from the previous round. Chapter 17 provides guidelines for survey research.

ANALYSIS OF RELATIONSHIPS

The second major group of nonexperimental research consists of the designs in which the primary purpose is the analysis of relationships among variables. The general format for this research is that a single group of participants is tested on several different variables and the mathematical interrelationships among the variables

are studied. This type of research is sometimes called *correlational research*. The term *correlation* also refers to a specific statistical technique. Therefore, there is a temptation to consider as correlational research only those studies in which the statistical correlation technique is used. As is seen in the examples, however, analysis of relationships entails more than just statistical correlation techniques. For example, epidemiological researchers often use a variety of ratios to express the association between subject characteristics and the presence or absence of disease. Therefore, in this text, the term *correlation* is reserved for the specific statistical analysis, and the longer, but more accurate, *analysis of relationships* is used to describe a general type of research.

There are several reasons one would want to identify relationships among variables. The first is that establishing relationships among variables without researcher manipulation may suggest fruitful areas for future experimental study. Research of this type is said to have heuristic value, meaning that the purpose of the study is to discover or reveal relationships that may lead to further enlightenment. The value of such heuristic research is not necessarily in its immediate results but rather is in the direction in which it moves the researcher.

The second specific purpose for the analysis of relationships among variables is that it allows scores on one variable to be predicted based on scores on another variable. In clinical practice, a strong relationship between certain admission and discharge characteristics in a group of patients who recently completed their course of treatment might allow better prediction of discharge status for future patients.

The third specific purpose of the analysis of relationships is to determine the reliability of measurement tools. Reliability is the extent to which measurements are repeatable. In clinical practice, we plan intervention based on certain measurements or observations. If, for example, a prosthetist cannot reliably determine whether the pelvis is level when a patient with an amputation is fitted with a new prosthesis, she might elect to shorten the prosthesis on Monday, lengthen the prosthesis on Tuesday, and leave it alone on Wednesday! The statistical determination of the reliability of measurements provides an indication of the amount of confidence that should be placed in such measures.

A fourth reason to analyze relationships among variables is to determine the validity of a measure. By comparing scores on a new test with those on a well-established, or criterion, test, the extent to which the tests are in agreement can be established. Reliability and validity of measurements are discussed in detail in Chapters 18 and 19.

Retrospective Analysis of Relationships

Relationships can be analyzed retrospectively through use of medical records or through secondary analysis of data collected for other purposes. The well-known Framingham Study collected a variety of health status measures on residents of this Massachusetts town every 2 years beginning in 1948. Kimokoti and colleagues[19] used data from an 8-year period of the Framingham study. Specifically, they looked at the nutritional intake over time to determine the stability of the Framingham Nutritional Risk Score (FNRS). They studied the 3-day dietary records of 1734 participants, men and women, over a wide adult age range at baseline (1984 to 1988) and at follow-up (1992 to 1996). Their findings indicated only modest changes in diet over time, modest indices of stability. The FNRS was directly associated with body mass index in women ($p < .01$) and high-density lipoprotein cholesterol among both women ($p < .001$) and men ($p < .01$). Because scores did not change over time, one can conclude that risk for diet-related conditions (e.g., cardiovascular disease) did not improve. The authors noted that their results could be used to guide further, prospective, research. Thus, this study fulfilled two of the purposes mentioned above: assessing reliability of measures and suggesting areas for future studies.

Prospective Analysis of Relationships

Analysis of relationships is often accomplished prospectively, with concomitant control over selection of subjects and administration of the measuring tools. A good recent example of a prospective analysis of relationships is found in the study by Phonthee and associates.[20] The investigators wished to analyze the relationship of predetermined factors, for example, demographic categories and spinal cord injury (SCI) characteristics, on likelihood of falling in 89 adult participants with SCI. Participants were first interviewed and assessed for baseline data and functional ability. They then were interviewed by telephone once per week for 6 months to report on falls. Participants with an educational level of high school graduate or greater, an American Spinal Injury Association Impairment Scale C (AIS-C) classification, and a fear of falling (FOF) significantly increased their risk for falls approximately four times more than those who graduated primary education, had an AIS-D classification, and did not have FOF."[(p. 1061)] Readers should note that the characteristics to be correlated with the falls were determined in advance, making the study prospective.

One of the reasons mentioned above for the value of analysis of relationships is to determine the validity of various measures. Morton and colleagues[21] assessed the validity of the Proficiency in Oral English Communication Screening (POEC-S), a tool commonly used to assess speakers of accented English. The authors note that validity had not been previously established. The investigators administered the POEC-S and also collected a spontaneous speech sample from 28 nonnative adult speakers of English, all graduate students at George Washington University. The speakers had previously scored well on the Test of English as a Foreign Language (TOEFL), often used to determined English proficiency of foreign university students. The speech samples were rated on several parameters by 20 linguistically naïve listeners (undergraduate students) and by 20 professional speech-language pathologists. Overall, there were significant correlations between ratings and POEC-S scores. The authors concluded that the POEC-S had satisfactory construct, criterion, and social validity, at least for accent speakers who had scored well on TOEFL.

Normative research is another form of descriptive research. In normative studies, large representative groups are examined to determine typical values on the variables of interest. Burger and McCluskey[22] updated normative data on handwriting speed for 120 adults aged 60 to 99 years. To gather data, they administered the Handwriting Speed Test and Handwriting Assessment Battery and also had participants write a shopping list. To further analyze their results, the authors separated the participants into four age categories and grouped them by sex. Overall, they found that handwriting speed had increased since the last collection of normative data in 1992.

ANALYSIS OF DIFFERENCES

The general purpose of research in which differences are analyzed is to focus on whether groups or treatments are different in some reliable way. Although analysis of differences is often accomplished experimentally, there are many ways to analyze differences nonexperimentally. Nonexperimental analysis of differences among groups or treatments is called ex post facto (after the fact) or causal-comparative research. The independent variables in such studies are not manipulated but are the presumed cause of differences in the dependent variable. The ex post facto designation refers to the fact that assignment to groups is not under the control of the investigator but rather is determined by existing characteristics of the individuals within the study. Note that ex post facto does not mean questions are developed after data collection; ex post facto designs may use either retrospective or prospective data collection.

Retrospective Analysis of Differences

Medical records provide a vast source of information about patient treatment and outcomes. When groups of patients can be identified from the medical records as having undergone certain courses of treatments or sharing certain characteristics, it is possible to study the relationship of treatment or characteristic to outcome in a retrospective manner. Four articles illustrate four different ways of developing groups in the retrospective ex post facto designs.

One way of developing groups is through an analysis of medical records of a total group to determine how groups of interest may have been formed. Such an analysis was the basis of the retrospective research by Bailes and Succop.[23] They were interested in finding factors that predicted the total physical therapy units received in 1 year in a group of patients with cerebral palsy in one pediatric medical center. To do so, they examined the medical records of 425 individuals with cerebral palsy. They determined that the records included patients in four levels of the Gross Motor Function Classification System. They also determined age, race, sex, and type of insurance. From the data, they were able to determine which factors were strong predictors of amount of therapy received.

In a second retrospective ex post facto study, successive cohorts were studied to determine whether a change in policy on the use of physical restraints for institutionalized older adults had an impact on number of falls and severity of injuries associated with falls. To do so, Dunn[24] studied incident reports in one long-term care facility before and after a restraint-free policy was adopted, finding that the number of falls remained the same but the severity of injury decreased under the restraint-free policy. The difference in patient selection between this study and Bailes and Succop's[23] study of postoperative knee rehabilitation is that answering this study question required sampling of patients from two different points in time. The study by Bailes and Succop is strengthened by its use of patients treated in a single time frame.

A third example of subject grouping within the retrospective ex post facto designs follows what is called the case-control design. In this design, a group of patients with the investigated effect (cases) is identified, and then a group without the effect (controls) is identified. Presumed causes for the effects are then sought, and the proportions of patients with the causes in the two groups are compared. One example of a case-control design is Highman and colleagues'[25] investigation of prelinguistic communication development as a factor possibly related to development of childhood apraxia of speech (CAS). Case participants were nine children aged 38 to 52 months whose speech and language the investigators evaluated. All had previously taken part in the Community Health Branch of the Health Department of Western Australia's implementation of the WILSTAAR/Baby Talk program and were recruited from speech-language pathology clinics and Language Development Centers in the metropolitan Perth, Western Australia area. Referred children did not necessarily have CAS. On evaluation, all exhibited delayed language, and five had features of CAS. The controls were 21 age-matched children with typically developing speech and language. The authors then did a retrospective study of assessments at 9 months of age and related the results to present functioning. Overall, they found a variety of patterns but were able to conclude that some children with features of suspected CAS have a selective deficit originating within speech motor development.

A fourth example of subject grouping within the retrospective ex post facto designs follows what is called the cohort design. Sometimes viewed as the "opposite" of a case-control study, cohort studies follow a group across time, starting with "presumed causes" and looking for "effects." This is in contrast to the case-control study, in which an "effect" is identified and presumed causes are explored. In a retrospective cohort study, all of the data have already been collected at the time the research question is developed; the researcher extracts the appropriate data, groups participants based on the variable or variables of interest, and looks for differences in a variety of predictor variables. This approach was used by Cushman and associates[26] in their study of readmissions to inpatient pediatric rehabilitation. Their retrospective review of records identified children who had required oxygen or ventilator support during an inpatient pulmonary rehabilitation admission and then grouped the children according to whether they had subsequent readmissions. The children with readmissions were found to need more ventilator support, nursing care, and acute-care transfers than children without readmissions.

A final example of retrospective analysis of differences among groups is a specialized research technique called *meta-analysis*. This technique is one of three general approaches to synthesizing research results across several different studies: narrative reviews, systematic reviews, and meta-analysis. Narrative reviews of the literature are subject to the biases of the author, as noted rather humorously, but perhaps truthfully, by Glass:

> A common method of integrating several studies with inconsistent findings is to carp on the design or analysis deficiencies of all but a few studies—those remaining frequently being one's own work or that of one's students and friends—and then advance the one or two "acceptable" studies as the truth of the matter.[27(p. 7)]

Systematic reviews, which require documented search strategies and explicit inclusion and exclusion criteria for studies used in the review, reduce the sorts of biases noted in the quote above. See Chapter 26 for more information on conducting and critiquing systematic reviews.

Meta-analysis provides a quantitative way of synthesizing the results of different research studies on the same topic. The basic concept behind meta-analysis is that the size of the differences between treatment groups (the effect size) is mathematically standardized so that it can be compared between studies with different, but conceptually related, dependent variables. It has become a commonly used tool in rehabilitation, particularly in physical therapy. A search on the term "meta-analysis" in CINAHL from 2010 through October 2013 yielded 213 references when paired with the term "physical therapy," 34 references when paired with "occupational therapy," and 37 references when paired with "speech." Because meta-analysis requires specialized knowledge and techniques, we refer readers to some recent helpful sources.[28–30]

Prospective Analysis of Differences

Prospective analysis of differences is the final cell of the six-cell matrix of research types. It is the only cell that is shared between the experimental and nonexperimental designs. By definition, the experimental designs must be prospective, and their purpose is to determine the effects of some intervention on a dependent variable by analyzing the differences in groups that were and were not exposed to a manipulation or the differences within a single group exposed to more than one experimental treatment. Differences between groups or within a group can also be analyzed in the absence of controlled manipulation.

An example of a study in which independent variables could have been manipulated but weren't is seen in the research by Robinson and associates.[31] The authors wished to examine the factors that either facilitated or inhibited community walking in a group of 30 patients who had had a stroke. Rather than prospectively assign the participants to groups based on facilitative or inhibitory factors (independent variables), their study was observational, and grouping was done post hoc. However, they did choose the factors prospectively.

There are many examples of nonexperimental analyses of differences in which the independent variable is inherently nonmanipulable. For example, some research questions focus on differences between groups of people with different attributes. Quite commonly, the comparison is between participants with some clinical condition and participants who are "typical," or "normal." For example, Koehlinger and colleagues[32] compared language outcomes between 3- and 6-year-old children who either had impaired hearing or normal hearing. Prospective comparisons of individuals with

and without a particular condition may be referred to as a cross-sectional case-control design.[33] This design is similar to the classic case-control design described earlier in that researchers must identify cases and then search for controls that are matched on important characteristics such as age. It differs from the classic case-control design in that there is no backward search for presumed causes. Rather, researchers collect prospective cross-sectional data to determine whether those with and without the condition differ on other variables. Likewise, the retrospective cohort design described earlier has a prospective counterpart. Paans and colleagues[34] used a prospective cohort design to examine the effects of an 8-month regimen of exercise and weight loss in 35 adult participants who had osteoarthritis of the hip and who were overweight or obese. Outcome measures included self-reported function as well as quantitative measures of pain and walking ability. The authors considered the 32.6% improvement in self-reported function to be clinically significant, and they also found significant improvements in their quantitative measures. The authors correctly note the lack of a control group as a limitation, but withholding treatment in a control group would have raised ethical concerns.

SUMMARY

Unlike experimental research, nonexperimental research does not require controlled manipulation of variables. Because of this permissive definition, there are a great variety of nonexperimental research designs. Descriptive studies use retrospective or prospective data collection to characterize a phenomenon of interest. In studies that involve the analysis of relationships, researchers use prospective or retrospective data collection to measure variables, which they then analyze to make predictions, establish odds, or determine reliability or validity of the measures. Nonexperimental analysis of differences can take many forms, including case-control and cohort designs.

REFERENCES

1. Law M, Stewart D, Pollack N, et al. Guidelines for critical review form: Quantitative studies. Available at: http://www.cotfcanada.org/documents/critical_reviews/quantguide.pdf. Accessed May 25, 2015.
2. Marmura MJ, Hopkins M, Andrel J, et al: Electronic medical records as a research tool: Evaluating topiramate use at a headache center, *Headache J Head Face Pain* 50(5):769–778, 2010.
3. Findley TW, Daum MC: Research in physical medicine and rehabilitation. III. The chart review, or how to use clinical data for exploratory retrospective studies, *Am J Phys Med Rehabil* 68:150–157, 1989.

4. Bu X, Liu C, Xing G, et al: WHO Ear and Hearing Disorders Survey in four provinces in China, *Audiol Med* 9(4):141–146, 2011.

5. Holyoke P, Verrier MC, Landry MD, Deber RB: The distribution of physiotherapists in Ontario: Understanding the market drivers, *Physiother Can* 64(4):329–337, 2012.

6. Polit DF, Beck CT: *Nursing Research*, 9th ed, Philadelphia, Pa, 2012, Lippincott Williams & Wilkins.

7. Spalding N, Killett A: An evaluation of a problem-based learning experience in an occupational therapy curriculum in the UK, *Occup Ther Int* 17(2):64–73, 2010.

8. Meador R, Chen E, Schultz L, et al: Going home: Identifying and overcoming barriers to nursing home discharge, *Care Manage J* 12(1):2–11, 2011.

9. Lu-Yao GL, Baron JA, Barrett JA, Fisher ES: Treatment and survival among elderly Americans with hip fractures: A population-based study, *Am J Public Health* 84:1287–1291, 1994.

10. Lascaratos JG, Trompoukis C, Segas JV, Assimakopoulos DA: Professor Nicolas Taptas (1871-1955): A pioneer of post-laryngectomy voice rehabilitation, *Laryngoscope* 113:702–705, 2003.

11. Wiles L, Matricciani L, Williams M, Olds T: Sixty-five years of physical therapy: Bibliometric analysis of research publications from 1945 through 2010, *Phys Ther*, 92(4):493–506, 2012.

12. Reed KL: History of federal legislation for persons with disabilities, *Am J Occup Ther* 46:397–408, 1992.

13. McEwen I: *Writing Case Reports: A How-To Manual for Clinicians*, 3rd ed, Alexandria, Va, 2009, American Physical Therapy Association.

14. Norén N, Svensson E, Telford J: Participants' dynamic orientation to folder navigation when using a VOCA with a touch screen in talk-in-interaction, *AAC Augment Altern Commun* 29(1):20–36, 2013.

15. Johnson L, Burridge JH, Demain SH: Internal and external focus of attention during gait re-education: An observational study of physical therapist practice in stroke rehabilitation, *Phys Ther* 93(7):957–966, 2013.

16. McCarthy CJ, Roberts C, Gittins M, Oldham JA: A process of subgroup identification in non-specific low back pain using a standard clinical examination and cluster analysis, *Physiother Res Int* 17(2):92–100, 2012.

17. Rosa L, Rosa E, Sarner L, Barrett S: A close look at therapeutic touch, *JAMA* 279:1005–1010, 1998.

18. Holland K, Middleton L, Uys L: The sources of professional confidence in occupational therapy students, *S Afr J Occup Ther* 42(3):19–25, 2012.

19. Kimokoti RW, Newby PK, Gona P, et al: Stability of the Framingham Nutritional Risk Score and its component nutrients over 8 years: The Framingham Nutrition Studies, *Eur J Clin Nutr* 66(3):336–344, 2012.

20. Phonthee S, Saengsuwan J, Siritaratiwat W, Amatachaya S: Incidence and factors associated with falls in independent ambulatory individuals with spinal cord injury: A 6-month prospective study, *Phys Ther* 93(8):1061–1072, 2013.

21. Morton ES, Brundage SB, Hancock AB: Validity of the proficiency in oral English communication screening, *Contemp Issues Commun Sci Disord* 38:153–166, 2010.

22. Burger D, McCluskey A: An investigation of normative handwriting speed in healthy older adults. Occupational Therapy Australia, 24th National Conference and Exhibition, 29 June– 1 July 2011, *Aust Occup Ther J* 58(Suppl):66, 2011.

23. Bailes AF, Succop P: Factors associated with physical therapy services received for individuals with cerebral palsy in an outpatient pediatric medical setting, *Phys Ther* 92(11):1411–1418, 2012.

24. Dunn KS: The effect of physical restraints on fall rates in older adults who are institutionalized, *J Gerontol Nurs* 27:40–48, 2001.

25. Highman C, Leitao S, Hennessey N, Piek J: Prelinguistic communication development in children with childhood apraxia of speech: A retrospective analysis, *Int J Speech Lang Pathol* 14(1):35–47, 2012.

26. Cushman DG, Dumas HM, Haley SM, et al: Re-admissions to inpatient paediatric pulmonary rehabilitation, *Pediatr Rehabil* 5:133–139, 2002.

27. Glass GV: Primary, secondary and meta-analysis of research, *Educ Res* 5:3–9, 1976.

28. Borenstein M: *Introduction to Meta-Analysis*, Chichester, UK, 2009, John Wiley & Sons.

29. Littell JH, Corcoran J, Pillai V: *Systematic Reviews and Meta-Analysis*, Oxford, UK, 2008, Oxford University Press.

30. Pigott PD: *Advances in Meta-Analysis*, New York, NY, 2012, Springer.

31. Robinson CA, Noritake Matsuda P, Ciol MA, Shumway-Cook A: Participation in community walking following stroke: The influence of self-perceived environmental barriers, *Phys Ther* 93(5):620–627, 2013.

32. Koehlinger KM, Owen Van Horne AJ, Moeller MP: Grammatical outcomes of 3- and 6-year-old children who are hard of hearing, *J Speech Lang Hear Res* 56(5):1701–1714, 2013.

33. Kazdin AE: Observational research: Case-control and cohort designs. In Kazdin AE, editor: *Research Design in Clinical Psychology*, 4th ed, Boston, Mass, 2003, Allyn & Bacon.

34. Paans N, van den Akker-Scheek I, Dilling RG, et al: Effect of exercise and weight loss in people who have hip osteoarthritis and are overweight or obese: A prospective cohort study, *Phys Ther* 93(2):137–146, 2013.

13

Clinical Case Reports

CHAPTER OUTLINE

Contributions of Case Reports to Theory and Practice
Purposes of Case Reports
  Sharing Clinical Experiences
  Illustrating Evidence-Based Practice

Developing Hypotheses for Research
Building Problem-Solving Skills
Testing Theory
Persuading and Motivating

Helping to Develop Practice Guidelines and Pathways
Format of Case Reports
Summary

Clinical case reports are the means by which clinicians explore their practice through thoughtful description and analysis of clinical information from one or more cases. Sometimes dismissed as "not research," several authors consider clinical case reports to be important forms of inquiry in the health sciences. In 1993, Rothstein, in an editor's note in the journal *Physical Therapy*, noted that case reports are "too rare in this journal and in the rehabilitation literature in general."[1(p. 492)] He believes that case reports are useful because they "clarify clinical terminology, concepts, and approaches to problem solving"[1(p. 493)] through the careful documentation of practice. Despite their low status on the evidence-based medicine (EBM)/evidence-based practice (EBP) hierarchy of evidence, case reports continue to be recognized as contributing to the pantheon of valuable scholarship, especially that which is applicable to clinical practice, with emphasis on the richness of detail of clinical practice.[2-4] A review of the case reports published in *Physical Therapy* between 2007 and 2009 continues to support Rothstein's position that case reports clarify clinical concepts and problem-solving approaches.

Sometimes the terms *case report* and *case study* are used interchangeably as labels for systematic descriptions of practice. However, the term *case study* is also used, particularly by qualitative researchers, to describe a more complex analysis of "the particularity and complexity of a single case"[5(p. xi)] within its organizational, social, or environmental context. For the purpose of this text, the term "case report" refers to descriptions of clinical practice (described in this chapter), and "case study" refers to the more complete descriptions typical of research in the qualitative tradition (see Chapter 14). Case reports, which are nonexperimental descriptions

of practice, should also be clearly differentiated from single-subject experimental designs, which are discussed in detail in Chapter 11.

Case reports can be developed either retrospectively or prospectively. Retrospective case reports are developed when a practitioner realizes that there are valuable lessons to be shared from a case in which the rehabilitation episode has been completed. Prospective case reports are developed when a practitioner, on initial contact with a patient or sometime early in the course of treatment, recognizes that the case is likely to produce interesting findings that should be shared. When a case report is developed prospectively, there is the potential for excellent control of measurement techniques and complete description of the treatments and responses as they unfold. Kazdin[6] observed that case reports could be greatly improved by simply adding good practice elements, such as use of objective measures of functional behaviors as well as those of impairments, and frequent assessments. For example, Chatham and colleagues[7] presented a case report in which objective measures of peak inspiratory muscle power were documented weekly over a 5-month period, as evidence of influence of inspiratory muscle training for diaphragmatic paralysis, with and without the patient taking statins.

The remainder of this chapter examines the ways in which case reports can contribute to theory and practice, cites examples of case reports that fulfill different purposes within the literature, and briefly outlines the format of case reports. Although this chapter focuses on clinical case reports, readers should recognize that case reports can also be used to document educational or administrative practices, such as the report from Noonan and colleagues[8] on the implementation and outcomes of a program to improve retention of physical therapy students in a DPT program and a report by Boissonault and associates[9] on the development and implementation of direct-access to hospital-based outpatient physical therapy services, respectively.

CONTRIBUTIONS OF CASE REPORTS TO THEORY AND PRACTICE

The potential value of case reports is illustrated by reviewing the relationships between theory, research, and practice presented in Chapter 2. Figure 13-1, a modification of Figure 2-1 to include case reports, shows these relationships visually. Reflection on experience and logical speculation, which contribute to the development of theory, can be documented or developed in clinical case reports. Theories are put into action in practice, and careful documentation of this practice within case reports can help test the theories. The information presented in case reports may be used directly to change practice, to revise theories, and to suggest areas for future research. This figure suggests, then, that case reports can contribute to the development of knowledge in rehabilitation by contributing to theory development, by testing theory, by leading to the revision of theory, and by suggesting areas for further research. This figure also suggests that the information gleaned from case reports can contribute directly or indirectly

to changes in practice. This suggestion, however, is not supported by everyone.

Haynes,[10] a physician and epidemiologist, identified several purposes of various forms of scholarly communications and presented a thoughtful analysis of the usefulness of clinical case reports. His analysis is shown in the matrix in Figure 13-2. Research reports of basic science research (sometimes called "bench research") and preliminary reports of clinical research ("field trials") are viewed as communications between scientists because their results are not yet applicable enough or rigorous enough to be applied in routine practice. Research reports of rigorous clinical trials are viewed as communications from scientists to practitioners because the findings within these definitive clinical studies are ready for application to practice. Articles that synthesize the findings of others are seen as communications between practitioners because they can help clinicians identify and rectify gaps in their knowledge base. Finally, case reports are viewed as communications from practitioners to scientists. This view, which differs from the common perception of case reports as valuable contributions to practice, is supported as follows:

> Clinicians who use case reports and case series as guidance for management of their own patients are at risk for deceiving themselves and hurting their patients.... Some case reports eventually prove to

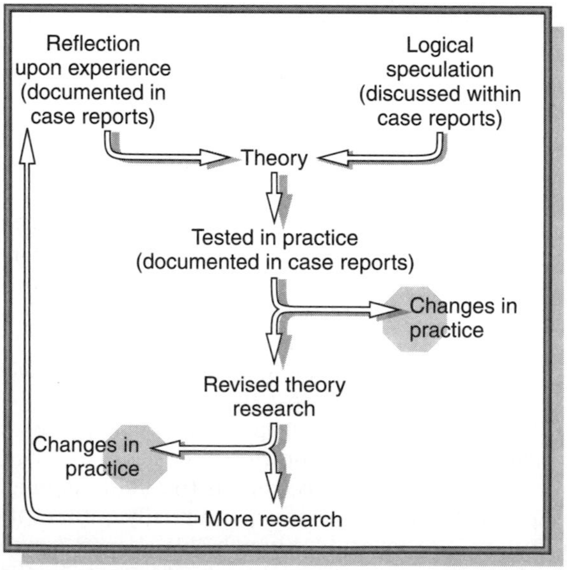

Figure 13-1 Modified version of Figure 2-1 showing the contribution of case reporting to the relationship between theory, practice, and research.

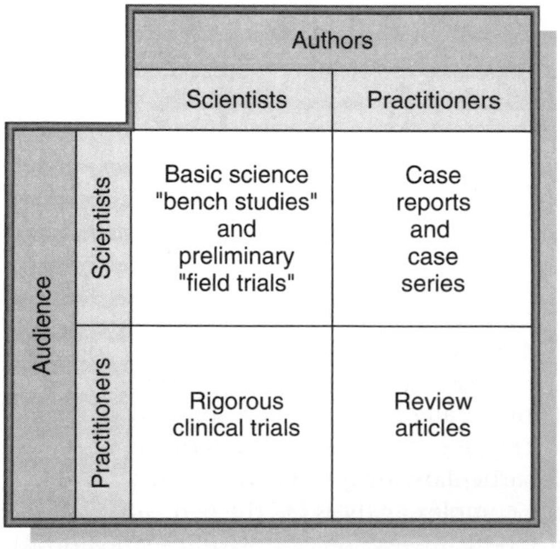

Figure 13-2 Matrix showing the purposes of various scholarly communications, delineated by the author and the audience for the communication. (Generated from information presented in Haynes RB: Loose connections between peer-reviewed clinical journals and clinical practice, *Ann Intern Med* 113:724-728, 1990.)

be important; most do not. Unfortunately, their methods do not permit discrimination of the valid from the interesting but erroneous, and they cannot provide a sound basis for clinical action. Case reports are, however, a fertile source of hypotheses that could lead to systematic observation.[10(pp. 725–726)]

Thus, Haynes believes that the primary value of case reports is in their contributions to theory and research, rather than their direct contributions to practice. This view of case reports is not presented to discourage practitioners from reading and learning from case reports. Rather, this alternative view is presented to remind practitioners that they need to thoughtfully critique the findings of case reports, just as they would assess the validity of more traditional research reports. In addition, because case reports are presented in the familiar language of practice rather than the sometimes foreign language of research, clinicians may find that their reading habits gravitate toward case reports. Haynes's matrix of scholarly communications reminds us to broaden our reading habits to include review articles and the reports of rigorous clinical trials.

PURPOSES OF CASE REPORTS

Although the general purpose of case reports is to carefully describe practice, the case reports that are presented in the literature show that there are many ways in which this general purpose can be fulfilled. McEwen,[11] in her manual on writing case reports, identifies seven functions of case reports: (1) sharing clinical experiences, (2) illustrating evidence-based practice, (3) developing hypotheses for research, (4) building problem-solving skills, (5) testing theory, (6) persuading and motivating, and (7) helping to develop practice guidelines and pathways. Recent examples of case reports that fulfill these seven functions are presented.

Sharing Clinical Experiences

One clinical experience that is commonly shared through a case report is that of the diagnostic enigma. For example, Hong and associates[12] presented a brief report on a patient who was diagnosed with primary progressive aphasia, a rare condition to diagnose. In making their diagnosis, they used behavioral (e.g., present premorbid language, gradual progression of word-finding impairment) and pathology (e.g., absence of tumor or stroke) criteria, as well as video imaging of central nervous system functions. In another case report of a diagnostic enigma, Diers[13] reported on a difficult-to-diagnose case of heel pain using several different musculoskeletal tests in his examination to

narrow the cause of foot pain to a neurogenic origin. This was later confirmed by an orthopedic physician.

Another common clinical experience that is shared through case reports is the presentation of unusual patients. Pidcoe and Burnet[14] described their rehabilitation of a young elite gymnast who incurred a manubriosternal dislocation. The rehabilitation program used a biomechanical hierarchy that focused on a progressive cycle of tensile and compressive loading activities, resulting in the successful return of the gymnast to the sport.

The clinical experiences documented in case reports do not, however, need to focus on the odd or the unusual in clinical practice. Careful documentation and discussion of commonplace cases can also be instructive. For example, Page and colleagues[15] combined constraint-induced therapy and botulinum toxin A to treat an individual with residual upper limb spasticity following a stroke, and Bruce and colleagues[16] reported on the use of a voice recognition system as a writing aid for a man with aphasia. In both cases, neither the diagnosis nor the treatments were particularly unusual. However, in both cases, unique combinations or applications of treatments were documented with the common diagnosis.

Illustrating Evidence-Based Practice

Some case reports may be used to illustrate how a practitioner used evidence-based practice principles to manage the case. Mohamed and Wong[17] did just this in a report showing the literature-based decision-making process and reflection used to revise the plan of care for the management of nonphysical pain and preventative complex regional pain syndrome of a chronic ankle sprain in an adolescent girl. Likewise, Whitman and associates[18] reviewed the literature related to nonsurgical management of lumbar spinal stenosis, noting the inconsistency of radio imaging and presence of symptoms, the use of different skills to assist in diagnosing the condition, and a review of conservative management methods before documenting a case series using techniques supported in the literature.

Using hypothetical patients, while also using the American Speech-Language-Hearing Association (ASHA) recommended process for implementing the EBP process, Brackenbury and associates[19] described three case studies in which systematic reviews and individual research studies were separately sought using databases typically available to academicians versus those available to the general public (e.g., Google Scholar) or the professional association (ASHA). They found that the length of time to conduct the evidence-based practice process, regardless of databases, was longer than what would likely be available to clinicians.

Developing Hypotheses for Research

Although most case reports have the potential to help develop hypotheses for research, some authors include an explicit discussion of the research applications of their work. For example, Barlow and Gierut[20] describe the application of a linguistic approach with word pairs for a child with a phonological delay. This approach included development of a series of treatment options with different levels of hypothesized effectiveness. This pattern of hypothesized effectiveness can form the basis for further research.

Another case with an explicit connection to future research is the report by Fritz and colleagues[21] of the results of a nonsurgical treatment approach for patients with lumbar spinal stenosis (LSS). They provided readers with a clear indication of the line of research that needs to flow from the case report:

> In our view, experimental studies can be performed only after an approach to evaluation, treatment, and outcome assessment has been defined for the population being studied. This case report of two patients with short-term follow-up needs to be followed by reports describing larger series of patients with LSS treated with this approach with longer follow-up periods. If the treatment approach we are recommending produces favorable long-term outcomes in larger series of patients, then a randomized clinical trial would be warranted to compare this approach with the present "standard of care," which consists of the use of medications and nonspecific exercises. Only a randomized clinical trial could produce experimental evidence for the efficacy of the treatment approach we suggest.[21(p. 971)]

Note that the sequence of events they described corresponds closely to the types of research described in the matrix of communication presented earlier in this chapter. The first research approach that is recommended—a larger descriptive series—is a limited "field trial." If the field trial is promising, a formal randomized clinical trial is recommended to compare this new treatment with existing ones.

Building Problem-Solving Skills

Some clinical case reports contribute to practice by presenting frameworks for problem solving by clinicians. Helgeson and Smith[22] described the use of the International Classification of Functioning, Disability, and Health (ICF) to diagnose and develop a plan of care for a 23-year-old woman who had experienced a patellar dislocation. Following a brief description of the

ICF model, the patient, and the examination results, the authors then categorized their examination results according to the different ICF components, followed by an evaluation of the relationships of the different components. This allowed them to determine a physical therapy diagnosis. Their clinical reasoning at determining the patient's plan of care was then illustrated by their prioritizing the impairments and limitations of the patient according to the components of body structure and function and activity, respectively.

Problem-solving skills in relation to teaching children who are congenitally deaf-blind was the topic of Bruce's[23] case report on the impact of an inservice training program on the teaching practices of teachers without formal preparation for working with these children. This case report used qualitative methods to document the process by which the teachers learned to implement the principles presented in the inservice program.

Testing Theory

Case reports can provide preliminary tests of various theories about patient management. For example, Moyers and Stoffel[24] presented a case report of a client with a work-related injury and alcohol dependence. A theoretical model of behavior change was presented, and this theory was applied to the client described in the report. Likewise, Ross[25] described the evaluation and treatment of a patient with foot dysfunction using a tissue stress model. The patient history and physical therapy examination determined which tissues were being stressed as a result of the patient's activities. The subsequent interventions focused on reducing the pain, inflammation, and stresses on the tissues, resulting in recovery of the patient at 7 weeks' postinitial examination.

Persuading and Motivating

Although some are uncomfortable with the idea of immediate application of the results of case reports, others find it appealing that "case reports can help practitioners deal with change, influence administrators, and persuade physicians and insurers of the value of services for particular patients."[11(p. 11)] One example of a case report with persuasion potential is Schindler and colleagues'[26] report on the functional effect of bilateral tendon transfers on a person with quadriplegia. Rather than reporting on a new technique, this case report extended the findings of almost 20 years of experience with tendon transfers for persons with quadriplegia. The authors of this case indicated that, although previous reports had documented improvements in hand function tests and some activities of daily living after tendon transfer, none had examined the impact of the surgeries on the amount of assistance needed with various tasks or the amount of equipment needed to accomplish the tasks. For individuals with quadriplegia who are considering tendon transfer surgery, it is exceedingly important to answer the question of whether the well-documented improvements in hand function lead to any meaningful changes in independence. Although this single case report does not provide a definitive answer to that question, the data in the case report, coupled with the well-documented experiences of the 20 years before it, may assist with the decision-making process.

Other examples of the role of case reports in persuading and motivating include Wills's[27] report on the role of physical therapists in skin cancer screening. Wills described a patient who was referred for cervical stenosis. When several skin lesions were noted during the initial examination, Wills used the ABCD checklist to screen the lesions for skin cancer. On completion of the screening, Wills counseled the patient to contact her physician for closer examination of the lesions. Subsequently, the patient did follow up with her physician, who then excised the lesion; the biopsy confirmed the presence of basal cell carcinoma. In this report, the author used the case to illustrate what the author believes is an important role for rehabilitation professionals.

Helping to Develop Practice Guidelines and Pathways

McEwen's[11] final purpose for presenting case reports is that they may help develop practice guidelines and pathways. An excellent example of a case report that accomplishes this purpose is Fritz's[28] report on the application of a classification approach to the treatment of three patients with low back syndrome. This approach to care of patients with low back pain classifies patients according to clusters of signs and symptoms and then provides treatment that "matches" the classification. If adequate testing demonstrates the validity of the classification and the effectiveness of the matched treatments, classification approaches can be the basis for developing practice guidelines or preferred clinical pathways.

Fritz[28] contributed to these efforts by describing three patients who appeared to have similar pathology but fell into three different classifications and were successfully treated three different ways with treatments that matched their classifications. This case-based evidence is not sufficient to conclude that this classification approach is valid but, combined with the positive results of a similar field trial,[29] suggests that this approach may be appropriate to study with rigorous randomized clinical trials.

In a variation that applies guidelines rather than develops them, Rhon and associates[30] reported employing the Ottawa Ankle Rule to screen a combat military person for a fracture.

FORMAT OF CASE REPORTS

Case reports that appear in peer-reviewed journals typically follow the format—or a modified format—of more traditional research reports. First there is an introduction, critical review of the literature, and purpose statement to place the case into the context of what is already known about the phenomenon. This section of a case report will make an argument for why the case report is being presented. For example, Pidcoe and Burnet[14] described the biomechanical basis for the types of injuries that must occur for a manubriosternal dislocation to occur and then described the nature of the injury as well as the paucity of literature addressing the rehabilitation of such an injury. Scheets and colleagues[31] argued how an appropriate diagnostic system would greatly assist physical therapists in determining the appropriate interventions for persons with different kinds of neuromuscular conditions, affording less "trial and error" in the clinical reasoning process.

Next, the equivalent of the methods section describes the subject, analyzes the presenting problem, presents examination data, outlines the conclusions drawn from the examination data (often illustrating the authors' clinical decision-making process), and describes the intervention.

The equivalent of the results section presents the outcomes of care. As is the case with a traditional research report, the results are then placed into context in a discussion and conclusion section in which the authors discuss the meaning and application of the case, including possibilities for future research. Detailed instructions for writing case reports, regardless of profession, can be found in McEwen's[11] "how-to" manual.

SUMMARY

Case reports are systematic descriptions of practice. It is clear that the information in case reports can be used to contribute to the development of theory and the design of research. There are differing opinions about the extent to which the information in case reports should be used directly to change practice. The written format of case reports is analogous to traditional research reports, with introduction, methods, results, and discussion sections.

REFERENCES

1. Rothstein JM: The case for case reports [Editor's Note], *Phys Ther* 73:492–493, 1993.
2. McEwen I: Editorial, *Phys Ther* 84:126–127, 2004.
3. Fitzgerald GK: Editorial, *Phys Ther* 87:494–495, 2007.
4. Craik RL: Editorial, *Phys Ther* 89:626–627, 2009.
5. Stake RE: *The Art of Case Study Research*, Thousand Oaks, Calif, 1995, Sage.
6. Kazdin AE: *Single-Case Research Designs: Methods for Clinical and Applied Settings*, New York, NY, 1982, Oxford University Press.
7. Chatham K, Gelder CM, Lines TA, Cahalin LP: Suspected statin-induced muscle myopathy during long-term inspiratory muscle training in a patient with diaphragmatic paralysis, *Phys Ther* 89:257–266, 2009.
8. Noonan AC, Lundy M, Smith AR Jr, Livingston BP: A successful model for improving student retention in physical therapist education programs: A case report, *J Phys Ther Ed* 26:74–80, 2012.
9. Boissonault WG, Badke MB, Powers JM: Pursuit and implementation of hospital-based outpatient direct access to physical therapy services: An administrative case report, *Phys Ther* 90:100–109, 2010.
10. Haynes RB: Loose connections between peer-reviewed clinical journals and clinical practice, *Ann Intern Med* 113:724–728, 1990.
11. McEwen I: *Writing Case Reports: A How-To Manual for Clinicians*, 3rd ed, Alexandria, Va, 2009, American Physical Therapy Association.
12. Hong FS, Sinnappu RN, Lim WK: Primary progressive aphasia, *Age Aging* 36:700–702, 2007.
13. Diers DJ: Medial calcaneal nerve entrapment as a cause for chronic heel pain, *Physiother Theory Pract* 24:291–298, 2008.
14. Pidcoe PE, Burnet EN: Rehabilitation of an elite gymnast with a type II manubriosternal dislocation, *Phys Ther* 87:468–475, 2007.
15. Page SJ, Elovic E, Levine P, Sisto SA: Modified constraint-induced therapy and botulinum toxin A: A promising combination, *Am J Phys Med Rehabil* 82:76–80, 2003.
16. Bruce C, Edmundson A, Coleman M: Writing with voice: An investigation of the use of voice recognition system as a writing aid for a man with aphasia, *Int J Lang Commun Disord* 38:131–148, 2003.
17. Mohamed M, Wong CK: More than meets the eye: Clinical reflection and evidence-based practice in an unusual case of adolescent chronic ankle sprain, *Phys Ther* 91:1395–1402, 2011.
18. Whitman JM, Flynn TW, Fritz JM: Nonsurgical management of patients with lumbar spinal stenosis: A literature review and case series of three patients managed with physical therapy, *Phys Med Rehabil Clin North Am* 14:77–101, vi–vii, 2003.
19. Brackenbury T, Burroughs E, Hewitt LE: A qualitative examination of current guidelines for evidence-based practice in child language intervention, *Lang Speech Hear Serv Sch* 39:78–88, 2008.
20. Barlow JA, Gierut JA: Minimal pair approaches to phonological remediation, *Semin Speech Lang* 23:57–68, 2002.
21. Fritz JM, Erhard RE, Vignovic M: A nonsurgical treatment approach for patients with lumbar spinal stenosis, *Phys Ther* 77:962–973, 1997.
22. Helgeson K, Smith AR Jr: Process for applying the *International Classification of Functioning, Disability and Health* model to a patient with patellar dislocation, *Phys Ther* 88:956–964, 2008.
23. Bruce SM: Impact of a communication intervention model on teachers' practice with children who are congenitally deaf-blind, *J Visual Impairment Blindness* 96:154–168, 2002.
24. Moyers PA, Stoffel VC: Alcohol dependence in a client with a work-related injury, *Am J Occup Ther* 53:640–645, 1999.
25. Ross M: Use of the tissue stress model as a paradigm for developing an examination and management plan for a patient with plantar fasciitis, *J Am Podiatr Med Assoc* 92:499–506, 2002.
26. Schindler L, Robbins G, Hamlin C: Functional effect of bilateral tendon transfers on a person with C-5 quadriplegia, *Am J Occup Ther* 48:750–757, 1994.
27. Wills M: Skin cancer screening, *Phys Ther* 82:1232–1237, 2002.
28. Fritz JM: Use of a classification approach to the treatment of 3 patients with low back syndrome, *Phys Ther* 78:766–777, 1998.
29. Delitto A, Cibulka MT, Erhard RE, et al: Evidence for use of an extension-mobilization category in acute low back syndrome: A prescriptive validation pilot study, *Phys Ther* 73:216–222, 1993.
30. Rhon DI, Deyle GD, Gill NW: Clinical reasoning and advanced practice privileges enable physical therapist point-of-care decisions in the military health care system: 3 Clinical cases, *Phys Ther* 93:1234–1243, 2013.
31. Scheets PL, Sahrmann SA, Norton BJ: Use of movement system diagnoses in the management of patients with neuromuscular conditions: A multiple-patient case report, *Phys Ther* 87:654–669, 2007.

CHAPTER 14

Qualitative Research

CHAPTER OUTLINE

Assumptions of the Qualitative Paradigm
Qualitative Designs
Case Study
Ethnography
Phenomenology
Grounded Theory

Qualitative Methods
Sampling
Data Collection
Interview
Observation
Artifacts

Data Analysis
Data Management
Generating Meaning
Verification
Summary

Qualitative research is a long-standing methodology of the social sciences, although it has not been used as much in rehabilitation professions. That is changing, and some rehabilitation professionals make qualitative research the focus of their research endeavors. However, there are aspects of qualitative research that might make one wonder if a clinician or student would ever take part in such an endeavor. For one, qualitative research is quite time consuming. For another, training in qualitative research is typically very limited in rehabilitation educational programs.

That said, there are good reasons for students and clinicians to understand qualitative research and become familiar with its methods. Obviously, one is to be able to understand professional literature that includes it. Another is that a student who is intrigued, and needs to complete a long-term research project such as a dissertation or thesis, may well wish to carry out a qualitative project. Finally, many of the methods of qualitative research are also the methods of everyday clinical practice, especially skills in interviewing and observation.

Research conducted in the tradition of the qualitative paradigm is of growing importance to rehabilitation literature. As health care practitioners begin to conceptualize what they do according to biopsychosocial models

of care rather than focusing solely on disease-based biomedical models of care, so too must health care researchers embrace research methods that capture the complexity of these new models of care. The qualitative research paradigm and the methods that flow from that paradigm provide a means by which researchers can match their research methods to the complex phenomena they wish to study.

Thus, the methods of qualitative research are highly consistent with the model of functioning, disability, and health in the classification system of the World Health Organization (WHO).[1] This is especially true in the sense of considering a person's degree of participation rather than just the disease or disability and in the sense of the importance of the role of multiple and complex environmental factors (including personal) that have an impact on a person's overall function. An example from the speech-language pathology literature is offered by Yorkston and associates, who noted, "If we are to understand communicative participation or the restrictions in participation that accompany chronic neurologic conditions, we must understand communication as occurring in context."[2(p. 126)]

This chapter reviews the assumptions of the qualitative research paradigm (originally presented in Chapter 6), introduces the various research designs associated with the qualitative tradition, and discusses a variety of methods and issues related to qualitative research.

ASSUMPTIONS OF THE QUALITATIVE PARADIGM

Five central assumptions of the qualitative paradigm are introduced in Chapter 6 and are reviewed here. The first assumption is that the world consists of multiple constructed realities. There are always several versions of reality, and the meaning that participants construct from events is an inseparable component of the events themselves. The second assumption is that the investigator and the subject (or participant or "informant") are interdependent and that the process of inquiry changes both. The third assumption is that knowledge is dependent on time and context. As a consequence, qualitative research is idiographic, meaning that it pertains to a particular case in a particular time and context. The fourth assumption is that it is impossible to distinguish causes from effects. Researchers who adopt the qualitative paradigm believe it is more useful to describe and interpret events than to attempt to control them to establish oversimplified causes and effects. The fifth assumption is that inquiry is value bound. This value-laden quality is exemplified in the type of questions qualitative researchers ask, the way they define and measure constructs, and the way they interpret the results of their research.

QUALITATIVE DESIGNS

The qualitative research paradigm encompasses a wide range of designs that flow from the five basic assumptions previously outlined. In fact, the boundaries between different types of qualitative research are far less clear than the boundaries between different quantitative designs. Carpenter and Suto[3] offer an explanation, noting that qualitative research "cuts across disciplines, subject matters and practice areas. Qualitative research is an umbrella term for the concepts, assumptions and methods shared by a complex and interconnected family of research traditions and it has meant different things at different points in its history."[p. 2]

Whereas there is relatively well-standardized terminology for the different classifications of quantitative designs, the terminology for the different types of qualitative research is far less universally accepted. Four sometimes overlapping design strategies are discussed in this section of the chapter. Although it is useful to categorize the design strategies into a manageable number of approaches, readers should recognize that there

is disagreement about what defines each approach and that there is considerable overlap among the methods used in the approaches.

To illustrate the similarities and differences between the methods, a single hypothetical research problem is developed in different ways using the four design strategies. Table 14-1 introduces this problem, which focuses on shifts in how the rehabilitation team is conceptualized and implemented in the United States.

Case Study

Case study, rather than being a complete design strategy or method, is one way of structuring a qualitative research project. By nature, a case has boundaries that define the limits of the inquiry. The boundaries may not be as limited as one might think. In the rehabilitation context, case studies usually present the characteristics, treatments, and outcomes of a single person. However, Holloway and Wheeler[4] refer to case study research as "research in a unit, a location, a community, or an organization"[p. 249] as well as in a single clinical case. In the context of the hypothetical problem defined in Table 14-1, the case is identified as the rehabilitation team at one inpatient rehabilitation facility. The purpose of such a study would be to gain an in-depth perspective on the evolution of rehabilitation team roles in the contemporary health care environment. Having identified the case, the qualitative researcher still has a choice of studying the case through any single or combination of the remaining designs, which are discussed in subsequent sections of this chapter. The researcher who studies a case chooses to emphasize the idiographic nature of qualitative research and recognizes that the results of the study will be particularly time and context dependent. Another researcher might choose to study the same problem, also guided by the qualitative paradigm, by studying rehabilitation teams at several different inpatient rehabilitation centers. The purpose of this research would be to understand the phenomenon of rehabilitation teams, rather than gaining an in-depth view of the evolution of a single rehabilitation team.

The previous paragraph identifies what is and is not a case study by contrasting the study of a single rehabilitation team with the study of several rehabilitation teams at different centers. This example leaves open the possibility of two ways of identifying what is and what is not a case: the number of elements and the relationship among the elements. The relationship among the elements is the key. If several different rehabilitation teams at one facility were studied, the "case study" would be of the evolution of rehabilitation teams at

Table **14-1**

Hypothetical Research Problems That Match Different Qualitative Design Strategies

Given:	During the 1980s and 1990s, comprehensive rehabilitation teams were used routinely to plan, implement, and manage the care of individuals being treated in inpatient rehabilitation centers. All of the members of the team routinely evaluated each new admission, made management recommendations, and participated in regular team meetings about each patient.
However:	As widespread health care cost-containment efforts became the norm in the late 1990s and into the 2000s, the routine, comprehensive rehabilitation team approach came under scrutiny from health care insurers and facility administrators. Rehabilitation professions are being asked to reduce the number of different professionals involved in each case, to eliminate services perceived to be duplications of effort, and to reduce the amount of time spent in team meetings. The simultaneous demand to provide quality, comprehensive care while reducing costs has required rehabilitation teams to redefine themselves and the roles of the individual professionals who constitute the team.
Therefore:	(Case Study) We did an in-depth case study of the evolution of rehabilitation team roles at one inpatient rehabilitation facility.
Therefore:	(Ethnography) We used participant observation to develop an understanding of the functioning of a contemporary rehabilitation team at an inpatient rehabilitation center.
Therefore:	(Phenomenology) The purpose of our study was to describe the experience of being a member of a contemporary rehabilitation team in an inpatient rehabilitation center.
Therefore:	(Grounded Theory) The purpose of our study was to develop a preliminary theory to explain how members of contemporary rehabilitation teams work to provide high-quality, cost-effective care.

that particular facility. The researchers would seek information about each team's story, but would also find out about how facility-wide change was accomplished. Because of the facility boundary, different things would be learned from this case than would be learned in a qualitative study of several rehabilitation teams at different, unaffiliated facilities.

There are several good examples of qualitative case studies in rehabilitation. In a study of a single individual, Neville-Jan,[5] an occupational therapist, documented her own experiences with chronic pain. In a multiple case study with very clear boundaries—both in identifying the activity of interest and the people to study—Garza Lozano[6] examined the ways in which radiation oncologists within one organization developed training methods to enhance patient safety. Yet another unit as "case" was chosen by Motley and associates[7] in their study of one community's capacity to address obesity. These three articles illustrate three different ways of defining the "case" or "cases" of interest. Examples abound. A search in CINAHL in November 2013 using the terms "case study" AND "qualitative," without limiting fields, from 2010 to 2013 yielded 1426 results.

Ethnography

The purpose of ethnography is to describe a culture. Broadly, *culture* can be defined as the knowledge, beliefs, and behaviors that define a group. The group can be a societal group such as "Americans," "French-Canadians," or "Southeast Asian immigrants." The group can also be a small, specialized unit such as "burn therapists," "members of a wheelchair basketball team," or "physical medicine and rehabilitation faculty members at a particular institution."

The ethnographic approach requires that the researcher, usually an outsider to the culture, describe the culture from the perspective of an insider. Spradley, in his classic text, indicated that "rather than studying people, ethnography means learning from people."[8(p. 3)] The way that one learns from people is often described as *participant observation*. Participant-observers immerse themselves in a new culture so that they can participate in and experience, in part, what it means to be within this culture. Rather than being complete insiders, however, participant-observers maintain a level of detachment that enables them to analyze, reflect on, and place the happenings within the observed culture into a broader framework. The concept of the researcher as both observer and participant illustrates clearly the qualitative research assumption that the investigator and subject are interdependent. Table 14-1 includes a purpose statement for an ethnographic study consistent with the background information on evolution of rehabilitation team roles. Whereas the purpose statement for the case study identifies only who is to be studied, the purpose statement for the ethnographic study also includes information about the methods to be used as well as the interest in the broader culture surrounding the person being studied.

Clinicians who undertake ethnographic research are required to shift their "gaze" from being the expert professional observer to being a different kind of observer. Lawlor[9] has described this shift as involving vulnerability (entering into someone else's unfamiliar world rather than controlling the familiar clinical environment), being present (watching attentively rather than doing), human sociality and social graces (establishing social connections rather than maintaining professional distance), and self-consciousness and reflexivity (focusing on the role of self as researcher rather than on the client).

The nature of ethnography can be illustrated by contrasting quantitative and ethnographic approaches to studying the rehabilitation team. A quantitative approach to studying these teams might focus on the cost of services provided by each member of the team, the average number of different professionals involved in the care of patients with different diagnoses, the amount of time spent in team meetings by each professional, and scores on a written questionnaire seeking patient and family opinions about the effectiveness of the team. The ethnographic approach would require observation and documentation of some of the same activities explored by the quantitative approach but would also focus on the factors that define the "culture" of the team: their language, interactive style (among themselves and with patients), biases, and even dress, for example. To do so, the ethnographer needs to request this information from the participants in the culture being studied. To become a participant-observer, the ethnographer would spend a great deal of time with the team members being studied, participating in the team for a period of time. For example, the researcher might participate by eating lunch with team members who dine together regularly, by attending a softball game in the recreational league in which staff members participate, and by accompanying team members to professional meetings where the researcher could observe interactions of team members with other members of their own profession.

As an observer, the researcher might privately note how much spontaneous conversation is focused on defining team roles, how the heroes and villains of a team are depicted in conversations in which all members are not present, or how much conversation focuses on past team functions versus contemporary realities. As a participant, the researcher would ask direct questions about what had been observed: "One member of the team seems to dominate during team meetings and nobody challenges her—why is that?" "Today you saw your physician, three therapists, and a social worker—how well do you think they are working together to help you meet your goal of returning home?" "I noticed today that you and the occupational therapist came to a quick resolution about which one of you would focus on treating Mrs. Henry's shoulder—what factors go into making decisions about the division of labor when more than one professional is qualified to implement certain interventions?" In addition to asking questions of the team members being studied, the ethnographic researcher would likely question other important members of the "culture": patients and their families, facility administrators, outside vendors, and colleagues outside of the facility. As a participant, the researcher would recognize that his or her presence changed things in some way—people would say things for the researcher's benefit or would fail to do or say things they might have otherwise done or said if the researcher were not present. In addition, reflecting on and articulating feelings and concerns might change the way that the participants deal with those concerns.

An example from rehabilitation literature is Burgon's[10] study of equine-assisted therapy for seven at-risk youngsters, aged 11 to 16 years. In this "participative ethnography," the author sought to examine the young people's experiences as they participated in a program of therapeutic horsemanship for a period of 2 years. Data analysis revealed themes "related to the risk and resilience literature such as self-confidence, self-esteem, self-efficacy and a sense of mastery, empathy and the opening of positive opportunities."[10(p. 165)]

Besides studies using ethnographic approaches in single studies, a growing body of literature is applying the principles of meta-analysis to develop meta-ethnographies. An example from health literature is a meta-ethnography of older people's views about the risk for falls.[11] For this analysis, the authors searched seven electronic databases from 1999 to 2009, as well as the reference lists of all relevant papers. They found 11 articles they felt met their standards for quality. From those, they extracted themes they thought related to the topic.

A review of references in a search in November 2013 combining CINAHL, PsycARTICLES, and PsycINFO shows only moderate use of ethnography in rehabilitation research. Using the terms "ethnography" AND "physical therapy" (with no field definers and allowing related terms) and searching for articles from 2010 to 2013 yielded 5 results, and "ethnography" AND "occupational therapy" yielded 18 citations. The case seems to be different in communication disorders, where "ethnography" AND "speech" yielded 85 results. As the rehabilitation professions further incorporate broader perspectives of health, for example, from the WHO classification system,[1] we may see increased access in rehabilitation to this very rich source of valuable clinical information.

Phenomenology

A phenomenological approach to research asks "[q]uestions about what is the 'essence' that all persons experience about a specific phenomenon?"[3(p. 43)] Referring back to Table 14-1, the distinction between the phenomenological and ethnographic approaches, as defined here, can be seen if the ethnographic study of the culture of rehabilitation teams is recast as a phenomenological study. The purpose of the ethnography was to develop an understanding of the functioning of a contemporary rehabilitation team, and the methods included participant observation of team members in work and leisure settings as well as interviews with patients and families. As observers as well as participants, ethnographers interpret the many sources of data to provide a unique combination of insider and outsider insights into the situation. Phenomenological research "gives voice" to the people being studied and requires that the researcher present the participants' view of their world. In a phenomenological study of rehabilitation teams, the only informants would be members of the team. For example, what patients think of the level of teamwork among the rehabilitation professionals would not be relevant to a phenomenological study. However, team members' perceptions of how patients are affected by teamwork would be of great importance in describing the experience of being a member of a rehabilitation team. Table 14-1 lists a sample purpose statement that would be consistent with a phenomenological approach.

The case study described earlier regarding radiation oncologists[6] serves as an example of using a phenomenological approach. The authors wished to determine the experiences of the members of the oncology team and, so, interviewed them—and only them—individually. Among the experiences the authors probed were the physicians' values and philosophies of care. An example from speech-language pathology is the phenomenological study of children with speech-sound disorders by McCormack and colleagues.[12] The authors wished to examine the everyday experience of having a speech impairment. To complete the study, they interviewed 13 preschool children identified with speech-sound disorders. Because significant others were intimately bound up in this everyday experience, the authors also interviewed 21 family members or teachers. Analysis revealed two themes: the problems experienced by the children who could not "speak properly," and the problems experienced by the others who could not "listen properly."

A third example, from the physical therapy literature, is the study by Tasker and associates[13] of the relationships between physiotherapists and their community-based adult clients. The authors wished to explore the "lived experience of relationships that developed between five participating physiotherapists and their 'family care teams.'"[(p. 5)] The authors gathered data via semistructured interviews and a focus group. Results revealed that physiotherapeutic relationships evolved as the clients, families, and carers allowed their therapists to learn about them.

Thus, it can be seen that the scope of the "life world" described within a phenomenological study can vary greatly—from children to adults and from the confines of a medical practice to a community at large.

Grounded Theory

The grounded theory approach was developed by Glaser[14] in the 1960s. This method departs from almost everything we have discussed about research methods thus far. An explanation from the Grounded Theory Institute[15] indicates that grounded theory "... is the systematic generation of theory from systematic research." It is designed as "a *research method* that will enable [researchers] to develop a *theory* which offers an explanation about the main concern of the population of [the] substantive area and how that concern is resolved or processed."[16]

A critical point is that the grounded theory researcher has "no preconceptions," that is, no *a priori* hypotheses or theories. Classic grounded theory does not even have an investigator perform a literature review before data collection, although Calman[17] contests this notion. Following the grounded theory protocols, researchers identify an area of concern and begin their investigations. Data are analyzed while they are being collected, and theory is derived only *after* data are collected and analyzed; any theories developed are thus "grounded" in the data. Because of the absence of theories and hypotheses, grounded theory has a good deal of "intuitive appeal," especially for new investigators.[18] Because of this interplay between data collection and analysis, grounded theory is often referred to as a constant comparative method. Although initially viewed as a means of generating new theory, contemporary writers also allow that grounded theory approaches may be used to elaborate and modify existing theories, although they caution that relying on previous theories may generate preconceptions.[18]

Grounded theory research uses familiar qualitative data collection procedures: interviews, focus groups, observation, and questionnaires. As the data are collected, they are analyzed and "coded." The coding is complex, and we refer readers to the sources cited for more information. Ultimately, "[t]he theory that emerges is a set of relationships that offer a plausible explanation of the phenomenon under study."[18]

Although the grounded theory approach shares interview and observational methods with other qualitative approaches, the goal of the research is different. Ethnography and phenomenology are distinguished from grounded theory research in that the goals of the former are to describe the phenomenon of interest, whereas the goal of the latter is to explain the phenomenon through the analysis of the relationships among concepts. In the hypothetical example of the changing role of rehabilitation teams, a purpose consistent with a grounded theory approach would focus on the development of a theory to explain how members of rehabilitation teams work together to balance high-quality care with cost effectiveness (see Table 14-1).

Holloway and Wheeler[4] note that grounded theory "has been used in healthcare research and particularly in nursing for decades and is still popular."[(p. 173)] This seems still to be the case. Thomson and Hilton[19] used grounded theory to examine students' perceptions of a university program to better prepare them for professional life. The program, which had been running for 2 years, involved patients, caregivers, and service users as facilitators of learning. Data collection methods were focus groups and semistructured interviews. Students' responses were analyzed according to their "level" or years in the physiotherapy program. The investigators concluded that students "appeared to value the programme as part of their development as physiotherapists and in particular the involvement of the clinicians who they perceived guided them in their insights."[(p. 45)] Grounded theory is an excellent analysis choice for a case like this because nothing would have been known about the topic of concern (the students' perceptions) before the study began and the researchers did not need an *a priori* hypothesis.

In some other examples, Dodds and Herkt[20] used grounded theory to examine the return of occupational therapists after a career break, and Merrick and Roulsone[21] examined the experiences of young children receiving speech-language pathology services. Thus, we can see that grounded theory can be used with a variety of cases (e.g., students, professionals, clients) and with a variety of data collection procedures.

As noted previously, the boundaries between the qualitative approaches are not clear. Some studies may not fit any of the categories; others may fit more than one of the categories. Labels such as "case study," "grounded theory," "ethnography," and "phenomenology" are important because they provide a way to organize what we know about qualitative research. However, arguments about which definition is the "one true definition" tend to be counterproductive in that they violate one of the basic tenets of qualitative research—the acceptance of multiple realities. Thus, readers should use this classification of qualitative research as one way to organize information and recognize that others may use equally useful alternative classification systems.

QUALITATIVE METHODS

The methods of qualitative research are consistent with the assumptions presented earlier in the chapter and often cross the lines between the various research designs associated with qualitative research. This section of the chapter introduces sampling, data collection, and data analysis procedures commonly used by qualitative researchers. More detail about these procedures can be found in several excellent textbooks devoted to qualitative research.[4,22,23]

Sampling

Qualitative researchers use nonprobability sampling methods, originally described in Chapter 9, to identify the individuals who participate within their studies. These individuals are typically referred to as *informants* rather than *subjects*, reflecting the emphasis on gaining access to their point of view rather than on manipulating them in some way, as would be typical in quantitative experimental studies.

In the broadest sense, the sampling method is one of convenience because researchers often study informants they know who meet their study criteria or facilities or organizations with which they have connections. Beyond the initial convenient selection of sites or subjects, qualitative researchers often use a combination of purposive sampling and snowball sampling techniques. Recall that purposive sampling involves

In the participant-as-observer model, the researcher assumes limited membership roles within a community for the purpose of conducting the research. This role has generated controversy in past research, mostly in sociological studies of illegal or socially unacceptable behavior, when researchers inserted themselves into a community without disclosing their role as a researcher. In today's electronic world, this issue has arisen anew in conjunction with the use of Internet communities, such as mailing lists and chat rooms, for qualitative research.[34] This model of observation can be accomplished, however, with the knowledge and consent of the members of the community. If, for example, a speech-language pathologist researcher wished to gain an insider perspective on the work of rehabilitation teams, he or she might work as a clinician within the facility for several hours a day and assume a visible role as researcher for the rest of each day.

In the observer-as-participant model, the researcher does not assume membership roles within the community. Rather, the researcher is available for relatively brief periods during which interviews and observations take place. Despite the relatively brief contact, the researcher recognizes that the very process of implementing the study changes the environment. The concept of the participant-observer, discussed earlier in the chapter, is generally broad enough to include both the observer-as-participant and participant-as-observer levels along this continuum.

In the complete observer model, the researcher assumes the role of the "objective observer" who does not change the situation being observed. Qualitative researchers generally believe that this end of the continuum is not possible to achieve because the mere presence of the investigator changes the dynamics of the situation.

The kinds of observations that one makes are dependent on the purpose of the research. In general, observations relate to the nonverbal behaviors of individual informants, interpersonal exchanges among informants, and the physical setting associated with the problem. In the study of the evolution of rehabilitation teams, the researcher might note posture, hand gestures, and the tone of voice of individual informants; might note that Informants A, E, and G not only share similar views of the situation but also tend to sit together at team meetings; and might observe that an old schedule of team meetings is posted on one ward with two scrawled notes in different handwriting reading "the good old days" and "the bad old days." Some of these observations may confirm information gained in the interviews, and other observations may require follow-up in interviews. For example, a researcher might ask the following: "I notice that an old schedule of team meetings, with graffiti added, is still posted on the ward—what are your views on the impact of fewer routine team meetings?"

There are several ethical issues involved with observation in qualitative research. When one interviews informants, there is a formal opportunity to discuss the study and gain the informed consent of the informant. Observation, however, may result in the inclusion of information about the behavior of members of the community who did not specifically agree to participate in the research. Even if observation occurs in public places, people who are observed may feel that their privacy has been violated. If descriptions of observations are sufficiently detailed, readers of the research results may be able to identify the participants, even if an attempt has been made to disguise the identity of the setting or of the particular informants. As discussed earlier, researchers who assume increasingly legitimate membership roles within the communities they study will likely interact with many people who are unaware of their research role—even if key members of the community have given informed consent to the project.

Techniques and Processes of Observation As with interviewing, the processes of observation learned for clinical purposes are essentially those used for qualitative research. We cannot overemphasize the importance of good observation in qualitative research and so offer some critical points.

Lichtman[25] offers several useful suggestions and guidelines for observation, divided into stages of planning, conducting the observation, and considering additional issues. For planning, Lichtman recommends (1) identifying a specific aspect of human interaction to study; (2) within that aspect, identifying three to five areas; (3) deciding on a recording method (e.g., notes, video); (4) deciding on a time frame; and (5) choosing public spaces where the interactions will occur. For the study of rehabilitation teams, the investigator might choose to observe personal interaction among team members and might identify terms of address, turn-taking, and conversational dominance as specific areas. The investigator might choose to take notes in the hospital cafeteria, allowing 3 hours per week, 1 hour at a time, for 6 weeks.

For conducting the observations, Lichtman suggests first finding an appropriate vantage point for observation. She then suggests looking at and describing the surroundings. If the study is about individuals, describe the "main characters." Finally, focus on the areas chosen during the preparation phase. Lichtman also raises collateral issues. One is deciding on the role, for example, observer-participant. Remember that having an observer present changes the situation dynamics. Decide whether or not to reveal yourself as an observer. Decide when to stop.

Data are often recorded categorically. That is, what the researchers expects to observe is defined in advance. Categories should be mutually exclusive and should exhaust the domain of interest. Often a category of "other" or "miscellaneous" is created to have exhaustive categories. For example, if observing for patterns of leadership, the researcher may wish to have categories for sharing leadership, reluctance to assume leadership, grabbing of leadership, other, and so on. Data can then be analyzed in terms of frequency of occurrence, perhaps with some explanatory notes. Data might also be analyzed with rating scales when appropriate.

Researchers should be familiar with a few forms of narrative recording for observation. One type is a journal, which is useful for observations over an extended period. Typically, journals include not only observations of events but also personal reflections, thoughts, and so forth. Another narrative tool is the *critical incident report,* which is used to illustrate a particular point (e.g., that one rehabilitation team member is resentful whenever anyone else appropriates leadership). A third is the *running record,* in which everything possible is recorded in sequence. In the last, it is best to make some mechanical recording and transcribe and analyze later.

Researchers will often need to observe several factors at once. For example, any time the researcher observes personal interactions, he or she will need to account for (1) sociocultural factors, (2) participants' physical characteristics, (3) the physical setting, (4) language factors, and (5) emotional factors. One of the authors had an assignment for his speech-language pathology students to observe conversation, accounting for these factors. The students used the outline reproduced in Box 14-1.

Artifacts

Artifacts are sometimes known as the "material traces" associated with the research or as the "material culture" of the setting.[35] Artifacts include any physical evidence that contributes to the understanding of the problem at hand. Some artifacts are readily available and observable to the researcher; others require that the researcher inquire about their existence or look in archives or public document depositories to locate them. Artifacts can be broadly divided into written documents, written records, objects, and the environment.

Although the terms *documents* and *records* are often used interchangeably, Hodder[35] believes that it is useful to

---

Box 14-1

Outline of Factors to Account for in Observation of Conversation

The following are factors that often contribute to successful or unsuccessful communication. The first of each pair generally supports successful communication. The list is probably not exhaustive.

Social/Cultural Factors
Familiar vs. unfamiliar setting
Familiar vs. unfamiliar people
Casual vs. formal setting
Same culture vs. different culture (ethnicity, age, gender)
Correct vs. incorrect suppositions about communicative partner

Participants' Physical Characteristics
Adequate vs. impaired hearing
Adequate vs. inadequate vision
Intelligible vs. unintelligible speech
    Speed. Loudness. Prosody. Dialect.
Good vs. poor language skills
    Vocabulary. Grammar. Sequence. Cohesion.

Physical Setting
Quiet vs. noise
Adequate vs. inadequate lighting
No reverberation vs. reverberation
Shared vs. separate activity
Close (but not too close) vs. far interpersonal distance
Multiple sensory cues (e.g., lip-reading) available vs. not available

Language
Familiar vs. unfamiliar topic
Simple vs. complex sentence structure
Short vs. long segments
Low-level vs. high-level vocabulary
Simple vs. complex response requirement
Ability vs. inability to recognize communication breakdown and to use repair strategies
Conversational rules followed vs. violated (e.g., topic maintenance, turn taking, distance, attention, new information, eye contact, and other nonverbal communication)

Emotion
High vs. low interest in topic and partner
Friendly vs. unfriendly attitude
Sharing/cooperating vs. dominating
Focus on partner vs. self-centered

distinguish between them. He defines written *documents* as unofficial or personal writings. For our hypothetical study of the evolving role of rehabilitation teams, one set of relevant documents might include informal correspondence on the job—perhaps a trail of e-mail messages between members of a team or working papers of a reorganization committee. Personal writings might include a journal that a therapist keeps or a letter to the team from a former coworker who moved out of state.

Records are then defined as official documents. In our hypothetical study, records that are relevant might include licenses of the practitioners involved, annual performance reviews, and transcribed notes documenting team meetings. Some records, such as birth, death, marriage, and professional licensure, are public and can be obtained by the researcher, or anyone else. Other records, including medical records, are private and require the cooperation and permission of those who have access to the private records.

Objects can send powerful qualitative messages. Think about the gift that might be given by coworkers to a team member moving to another job. A carefully wrapped memory book of photos and letters from coworkers says one thing; a gift basket with cheeses and jams says another; and an unwrapped gift that everyone recognizes as coming from the facility gift shop says another! Clearly, the researcher would not conclude that the relationship between team members was close, distant, or dysfunctional based on the gift alone, but the gift would be a part of the pattern of evidence that would describe team relationships. Other common objects to be studied include photographs and personal effects in the offices or homes of informants.

The environment offers other artifactual evidence that may be important to the research. For example, the retention of memos on the bulletin board, described earlier as an observation, might also be considered an artifact. Whether they are considered to be artifacts or observations, they can provide evidence that supplements the data gathered directly from informants.

Artifacts, then, provide material evidence that contributes to the breadth and depth of information collected by the qualitative researcher. Unlike archaeologists or criminal forensic investigators, qualitative researchers rarely base their conclusions on the analysis of artifacts alone. Rather, they use artifacts to supplement the data they collect through interview and observation.

Data Analysis

Data analysis in qualitative research is a process that differs greatly from data analysis in quantitative research.

Whereas quantitative researchers typically describe their conclusions in statistical, probabilistic terms, qualitative researchers typically describe their conclusions in interpretive narratives that provide "thick description" of the phenomenon being studied. Generating this narrative rests on three general steps in the data analysis process: data management, generating meaning, and verification.

Data Management

Data management relates to the collection, storage, and retrieval of information collected within the study. One of the consequences of seeking depth and breadth of information from multiple sources is that the amount of data becomes voluminous. A 30-minute interview with one informant might yield 20 pages of verbatim transcript based on an audio recording of the interview, 12 marginal notes on the transcript to remind the researcher of things to follow up on with future informants, and two pages of hand-written observations. If one does three interviews with each of 10 informants, this could easily result in more than 600 pages of data! Clearly, the qualitative researcher needs to develop a system for organizing and storing the information collected throughout the study.

One of the keys to the organization of data is the identification of the source of the data. Researchers come up with an identification code that enables them to determine where a piece of data came from originally. For example, a code of JP/I/02/07 might refer to the seventh page of the transcript of the second interview conducted with an informant with the code initials JP. A code of MM/R/12/02 might refer to the second page of the 12th record that was authored by an informant with the code initials MM.

A second key to the organization and reduction of data is use of a code-and-retrieve system. A coding system is the means by which the researcher labels the themes that emerge as the data are amassed. We have mentioned coding briefly in the discussion of grounded theory. Based on Glaser's early work in grounded theory, Holloway and Wheeler[4] provide the "six Cs" of coding: causes, context, covariance, conditions, contingency, and consequences.[(p. 180)]

Holloway and Wheeler also provide some common coding strategies. Line by line, for example, "identifies information which both participant and researcher consider important." *In vivo* involves actual informant quotes. *Open coding* names specific pieces of data. All these (and there are others) are reduced to yield units of meaning, which are then linked as concepts.[(pp. 286–287)]

We can see an example of coding and concept formation in the work by Moyson and Roeyers.[36] These authors completed a qualitative study of self-reported quality of life as a sibling of someone with intellectual disability. Data collection was completed by in-depth individual interviews. The interviews were analyzed and coded according to the means of grounded theory. From a technical standpoint, qualitative researchers used to (and some still do) generate hundreds, sometimes thousands, of index cards in the course of a study. Each card would include a coded snippet of interview, observation, or reflection, cross-referenced to the original source of the data. The researchers would sort and re-sort the cards, seeking to understand the relationships among the various themes that emerged. Today, qualitative researchers can use word processing or relational database programs with search-and-sort properties to manage this process. In addition, several commercial software products have been designed to help qualitative researchers with the code-and-retrieve process, as well as the process of identifying relationships among concepts.[37]

Generating Meaning

After the data are coded, the researcher's job is to generate meaning from the data by noting themes, patterns, and clusters within the data, as well as by identifying relationships among the themes and clusters. This is a reflective process that requires that the researcher "try on" ideas based on a portion of the data, test them against other portions of the data, and modify them as needed. After analyzing coded data, Moyson and Roeyers[36] were able to generate nine distinct themes. Some examples are "mutual understanding," "acceptance," and "dealing with the outside world." Generating meaning from qualitative data, then, involves an interpretive process in which data are reduced into small components (coding), reorganized into larger components (themes), and then displayed in ways that illustrate the relationships among components. This process is an iterative one, meaning that the researcher goes back and forth among the steps several times, making modifications along the way until the final analysis of relationships among themes fits with the data.

This sequence of steps is illustrated nicely in a diagram of the determinants of adherence to anterior cruciate ligament rehabilitation, from the research of Pizzari and colleagues.[26]

Reproduced here as Figure 14-1, the ellipses represent the codes, the boxes represent the themes, and the placement of arrows connecting the many codes to the three themes that feed into the core concept of adherence indicates the relationships between concepts. Several texts provide detailed guidance on the process of generating meaning from qualitative data. In

addition to the text by Holloway and Wheeler,[4] readers may also wish to view other helpful texts.[37,38]

Verification

A final step in data analysis is the process of verifying the conclusions that have been drawn.[37] Without some verification process, qualitative research results remain open to the criticism that the researcher found what he or she was hoping to find. One form of verification is the triangulation of results. This is done by comparing multiple sources of information to determine whether they all point to similar conclusions.

A second form of verification is the use of multiple researchers to code data independently. Typically, two or more researchers independently code a small amount of data at the beginning of the study, compare their results, discuss discrepancies, and code another small set of data until they are satisfied that they have a common understanding of what the codes mean. If they then divide the data so that each researcher codes just a portion of the data, they may complete periodic reliability checks to ensure that they remain consistent throughout the course of the study.

A third form of verification is called *member checking*. In this process, informants review the interpretive "story" that the researcher has generated and have the opportunity to correct technical errors or take issue with ways in which the researcher has interpreted their situation. The researcher uses this information to revise the story or, at least, to indicate points of departure between his or her views and the views of the informants.

A fourth way of verifying the data analysis process is to have an outside researcher audit the analysis. Through this process, the outsider does a detailed "walk through" of the data analysis to determine whether the steps the researcher took and the conclusions that were drawn at each step make logical sense and appear to fit the data. Comments from the auditor are carefully considered and, as is the case with member checks, used to either revise the results or indicate points of departure between the researcher and the auditor.

A final way of enhancing the quality of qualitative research is to present reflexive accounts of ways in which the subjectivity of the researcher had an impact on all phases of the study, from the conceptualization of the research problem to the analysis of data. In a reflexive account, researchers reflect on the ways in which they affected and were affected by the qualitative research process. Primeau,[39] for example, both describes reflexive analysis and presents a reflexive account of her role in a qualitative study of work and play in families.

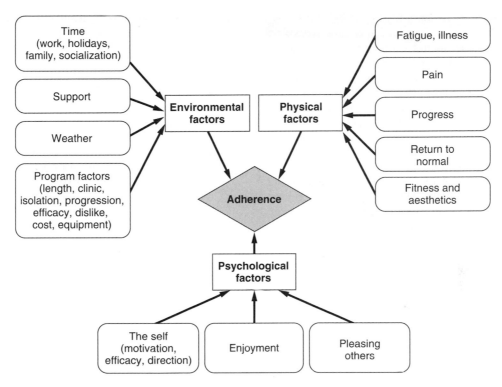

Figure 14-1 Flowchart representing factors influencing adherence to anterior cruciate ligament rehabilitation. The ellipses correspond to codes, the boxes to themes, and the arrangement of arrows to the relationship among codes, themes, and the core concept of adherence. (From Pizzari T, McBurney H, Taylor NF, Feller JA: Adherence to anterior cruciate ligament rehabilitation: A qualitative analysis, *J Sport Rehabil* 11:90–102, 2002.)

The various pieces of qualitative research that have been cited throughout this chapter illustrate, in the aggregate, all of the first four classes of verification techniques. Garza Lozano,[6] and Motley[7] and McCormack[12] and their respective colleagues, gathered data from multiple sources. Motley[7] and Pizzari[26] and associates developed themes using multiple coders. Garza Lozano[6] and Burgon[10] used participants in a member-check role. Finally, McCormack and associates[12] had colleagues audit their coding and theme formation.

By implementing these verification steps, qualitative researchers help to establish the credibility of qualitative findings by subjecting themselves to external review and demonstrating to skeptics that "qualitative" is not synonymous with "arbitrary."

For final thoughts on data analysis in qualitative research, the words of Dickie, an occupational therapist and anthropologist, say it well:

Qualitative research data analysis should not be easy. Ultimately it takes an enormous amount of intellectual "sweat" by the humans who are trying to make sense out of a situation, a setting, or a culture they thought was interesting enough to study.... Different research traditions and methodologies require different sorts of data analysis activities and call them by different names even when they are essentially the same.... Coding of some sort lays the foundation for most analytical processes,... but the nature of the coding process is specific to the researcher(s). The development and explication of the categories that are defined through reading and coding the data can become the "secret world" of the researcher, where magic does indeed take place but is never shared. But it shouldn't be that way. We need to learn what the labels and the jargon mean, then throw out the terms and describe what we do. We need to tell the research story, including the challenges of data analysis and how we resolved them, to support our interpretations. Researchers must be present in the stories they tell.[40(pp. 50–51)]

SUMMARY

Qualitative research includes a broad group of designs that generally follow five assumptions: that reality is constructed by participants, that researchers and subjects are interdependent, that research results are time and context dependent, that differentiating between causes and effects is not generally possible, and that research is a value-laden process. Although many different terms are used to describe qualitative design strategies, major approaches include case studies, ethnography, phenomenology, and grounded theory. Sampling in qualitative research generally includes convenience sampling, often selecting informants purposively through snowball sampling procedures. Common data collection methods include interviews, observation, and collection and review of artifacts. The data analysis process includes methods for managing large volumes of data from different sources; ways of generating meaning from codes, themes, and relationships among themes; and techniques to verify the conclusions.

REFERENCES

1. World Health Organization. International Classification of Functioning, Disability, and Health (ICF). Available at: www.who.int/classifications/icf/en/. Accessed December 2, 2014.
2. Yorkston KM, Klasner ER, Swanson KM: Communication in context: A qualitative study of the experiences of individuals with multiple sclerosis, *Am J Speech Lang Pathol* 10:126–137, 2010.
3. Carpenter C, Suto M: *Qualitative Research for Occupational and Physical Therapists*, Oxford, UK, 2008, Blackwell.
4. Holloway I, Wheeler S: *Qualitative Research in Nursing and Healthcare*, 3rd ed, Chichester, UK, 2010, Wiley Blackwell.
5. Neville-Jan A: Encounters in a world of pain: An autoethnography, *Am J Occup Ther* 57:88–98, 2003.
6. Garza Lozano R: Characterizing a culture of training and safety: A qualitative case study in radiation oncology, *Radiat Ther* 22(2):139–153, 2013.
7. Motley M, Holmes A, Hill J, et al: Evaluating community capacity to address obesity in the Dan River region: A case study, *Am J Health Behav* 37(2):208–217, 2013.
8. Spradley JP: *The Ethnographic Interview*, New York, NY, 1979, Holt, Rinehart & Winston.
9. Lawlor MC: Gazing anew: The shift from a clinical gaze to an ethnographic lens, *Am J Occup Ther* 57:29–39, 2003.
10. Burgon HL: "Queen of the world": Experiences of "at-risk" young people participating in equine-assisted learning/therapy, *J Soc Work Pract* 25(2):165–183, 2011.
11. McInnes E, Seers K, Tutton L: Older people's views in relation to risk of falling and need for intervention: A meta-ethnography, *J Adv Nurs* 67(12):2525–2536, 2011.
12. McCormack J, McLeod S, McAllister L, Harrison LJ: My speech problem, your listening problem, and my frustration: The experience of living with childhood speech impairment, *Lang Speech Hear Serv Sch* 41(4):379–392, 2010.
13. Tasker D, Loftus S, Higgs J: Head, heart and hands: Creating mindful dialogues in community-based physiotherapy, *N Z J Physiother* 40(1):5–12, 2012.
14. Glaser BG, Strauss AL: *The Discovery of Grounded Theory: Strategies for Qualitative Research*, Chicago, Ill, 1967, Aldine Publishing.
15. Andrews T, Scott H: What Is Grounded Theory? Grounded Theory Online. Available at: http://www.groundedtheoryonline.com/what-is-grounded-theory. Accessed December 2, 2014.
16. Grounded Theory Institute. What Is Grounded Theory? Available at: http://www.groundedtheory.com/what-is-gt.aspx. Accessed December 2, 2014.
17. University of Manchester. What Is Grounded Theory? Available at: http://www.methods.manchester.ac.uk/resources/categories/theoretical/grounded/. Accessed February 16, 2015.
18. El Hussein M, Hirst S, Salyers V, Osuji J: Using grounded theory as a method of inquiry: Advantages and disadvantages. *The Qualitatvie Report*, 19, *How-to Article* 13, 1–15, 2014. Available at: http://www.nova.edu/ssss/QR/QR19/el-hussein13.pdf. Accessed February 17, 2015.
19. Thomson D, Hilton R: An evaluation of students' perceptions of a college-based programme that involves patients, carers and service users in physiotherapy education, *Physiother Res Int* 17(1):36–47, 2012.
20. Dodds K, Herkt J: Exploring transition back to occupational therapy practice following a career break, *N Z J Occup Ther* 60(2):5–12, 2013.
21. Merrick R, Roulstone S: Children's views of communication and speech-language pathology, *Int J Speech Lang Pathol* 13(4):281–290, 2011.
22. Denzin NK, Lincoln YS, editors: *The Sage Handbook of Qualitative Research*, 4th ed, Thousand Oaks, Calif, 2011, Sage.
23. Bourgeault I, Dingwall R, DeVries RG: *The SAGE Handbook of Qualitative Methods in Health Research*, Los Angeles, 2010, Sage.
24. Gustafsson L, Hodge A, Robinson M, et al: Information provision to clients with stroke and their carers: Self-reported practices of occupational therapists, *Aust Occup Ther J* 57(3):190–196, 2010.
25. Lichtman M: *Qualitative Research in Education: A User's Guide*, 3rd ed, Los Angeles, 2013, Sage.
26. Pizzari T, McBurney H, Taylor NF, Feller JA: Adherence to anterior cruciate ligament rehabilitation: A qualitative analysis, *J Sport Rehabil* 11:90–102, 2002.
27. Johansson C, Isaksson G: Experiences of participation in occupations of women on long-term sick leave, *Scand J Occup Ther* 18(4):294–301, 2011.
28. Froelich RE, Bishop FM: *Medical Interviewing*, 2nd ed, St Louis, Mo, 1972, CV Mosby.
29. Haynes WO, Pindzola RH: *Diagnosis and Evaluation in Speech Pathology*, 7th ed, Boston, Mass, 2008, Allyn & Bacon.
30. Westby C, Burda, A, Mehta Z. Asking the right questions in the right ways: Strategies for ethnographic interviewing. Available at: http://www.asha.org/Publications/leader/2003/030429/f030429b.htm. Accessed December 2, 2014.

31. Kwan-Gett T. Collecting ethnographic data: The ethnographic interview. Available at: http://ethnomed.org/about/contribute/collecting-ethnographic-data-the-ethnographic-interview?searchterm=collecting+ethnographic+data. Accessed December 2, 2014.

32. Angrosino MV, Rosenberg J: Observations on observation: Continuities and challenges. In Denzin NK, Lincoln YS, editors: *Sage Handbook of Qualitative Research*, 4th ed, Thousand Oaks, Calif, 2011, Sage.

33. Letts L: Occupational therapy and participatory research: Partnership worth pursuing, *Am J Occup Ther* 57:77–87, 2003.

34. Palys T: Qualitative research in the digital era: Obstacles and opportunities, *Int J Qualitat Meth* 11(4):352–367, 2012.

35. Hodder I: The interpretation of documents and material culture. In Denzin NK, Lincoln YS, editors: *Handbook of Qualitative Research*, 2nd ed, Thousand Oaks, Calif, 2000, Sage.

36. Moyson T, Roeyers H: "The overall quality of my life as a sibling is all right, but of course, it could always be better." Quality of life of siblings of children with intellectual disability: The siblings' perspectives, *J Intell Disabil Res* 56(1):87–101, 2012.

37. Miles MB, Huberman AM, Saldana J: *Qualitative Data Analysis: A Methods Sourcebook*, 3rd ed, Thousand Oaks, Calif, 2014, Sage.

38. Dey I: *Qualitative Data Analysis: A User-Friendly Guide for Social Scientists*, New York, NY, 1993, Routledge.

39. Primeau LA: Reflections on self in qualitative research: Stories of family, *Am J Occup Ther* 57:9–16, 2003.

40. Dickie VA: Data analysis in qualitative research: A plea for sharing the magic and the effort, *Am J Occup Ther* 57:49–56, 2003.

CHAPTER 15

Epidemiology

CHAPTER OUTLINE

Ratios, Proportions, and Rates
Ratios
Proportions
Rates
Prevalence
Incidence
Relationship Between Incidence and
Prevalence
Crude, Specific, and Adjusted Rates

Relative Risk: Risk Ratios and Odds
Ratios
Screening and Diagnosis
Some Concepts from Psychophysics
Sensitivity and Specificity
*Receiver-Operating Characteristic
Curves*
Likelihood Ratios
Predictive Value

**Nonexperimental Epidemiological
Designs**
Cross-Sectional Studies
Case-Control Studies
Cohort Studies
Summary

Epidemiology has been defined as the "branch of science that investigates the risk factors responsible for the causation of diseases through retrospective and prospective observation, a complete history of disease, and the frequency of occurrence or transmission mechanisms of disease in populations and explores preventive and therapeutic control measures."[1(p. 1)] The definition covers many aspects—causation, methods of study, descriptive statistics, prevention, and rehabilitation. However, as Saracci[2] notes, "The population aspect is the distinctive trait of epidemiology."[(p. 2)] This definition articulates a descriptive role for epidemiological research (studying distributions of health and illness), as well as an analytical role (studying determinants of health and illness). At first, epidemiology might not seem an appropriate topic for the rehabilitation researcher or scientist-practitioner because its descriptive nature is not typically useful in the rehabilitation of a particular patient. However, rehabilitation research will include any research important to the rehabilitation professions. There is an implied element of diagnosis and screening in this definition, in that both are necessary for distinguishing between those who are healthy and those who are ill.

Another element is that the study of epidemiology can assist rehabilitation professionals in prevention of disability, an essential function of physical, occupational, and speech-language therapists and other rehabilitation professionals. The other critical component of this definition is the emphasis on populations—epidemiological research tends to focus on large groups of people. Although Hayes

and colleagues note that psychotherapists (and, we would add, other rehabilitation professionals) "tend to address and treat ... problems as they occur at the level of the individual,"[3(p. 76)] they add, "the alternative in prevention is a public health model"[3(p. 76)] (i.e., dealing with large populations). The World Health Organization, in its projection for the International Classification of Health Interventions, indicates, "The envisaged International Classification of Health Interventions aims to cover a wide range of measures taken for curative and *preventive* purposes by medical, surgical and *other health-related care services* [emphasis added]."[4] It becomes clear, then, that epidemiology has important applications in public and community health and that these are important for rehabilitation professionals. With its emphasis on the study of large groups, epidemiological research tends to focus on describing the characteristics of existing groups of people or analyzing the relationships among various health and demographic factors as they unfold within certain subgroups or across time. Both of these foci are nonexperimental in nature because they document existing health and illness states rather than attempting to change these states by introducing a controlled treatment. Despite this predominantly nonexperimental focus, some epidemiological research may be experimental in nature and follow the principles outlined in Chapter 10.

This chapter is organized around three major sections. The first section examines the use of ratios, proportions, and rates to describe various health and illness phenomena. The second section presents a variety of concepts that are important to the understanding of screening and diagnostic processes. The third section presents nonexperimental epidemiological designs that compare health and illness in different naturally occurring groups.

RATIOS, PROPORTIONS, AND RATES

Researchers and practitioners are often interested in documenting "how many" cases of particular diseases or injuries occur in different groups, regions, or time frames. However, raw frequency counts of cases are rarely valuable because they are not directly comparable across groups of different sizes or across varied time frames. For example, knowing the total number of cases of sport-induced brain concussion in a very large population is of limited utility. Much more useful would be the number of cases in athletes of different ages, or wearing different brands or types of head protection, or even in which sport the athletes were engaged.

Changing frequencies into meaningful epidemiological data depends on the calculation of various ratios, proportions, and rates. The discussion of these concepts is accompanied by a hypothetical example related to ankle sprains on a college campus (Table 15-1).

Ratios

A ratio expresses the relationship between two numbers by dividing the numerator (top number) by the denominator (bottom number). The numerator of a ratio is not necessarily a subset of the denominator. The simple formula for a ratio is therefore:

Table **15-1**

Hypothetical Data on Ankle Sprains, University A, 2012–2013

Number at risk during the year	12,237
Athletes	1216
Nonathletes	11,021
Number surveyed at beginning of year	9857
Number of ankle sprains at beginning of year	61
Total new ankle sprains during year	436
Distribution by type of sprains	
Inversion sprains	401
Eversion sprains	35
Distribution by activity level of individual	
Athletes	170
Nonathletes	266

$$\text{Ratio} = a/b$$

(Formula 15-1)

An example is the ratio of inversion to eversion ankle sprains. The hypothetical data shown in Table 15-1 show that, of a total of 436 new ankle sprains documented during the 2012–2013 academic year, 401 were inversion sprains ("a" in Formula 15-1) and 35 were eversion sprains ("b" in Formula 15-1). This divides out to a ratio of 11.46 to 1 (401/35 = 11.46). The notation for ratios is that a colon (:) is used for the "to" so that the ratio of inversion to eversion ankle sprains would be expressed as 11.46:1. The interpretation of this ratio is that there were almost 11½ inversion ankle sprains for every eversion ankle sprain reported on the campus of University A during the 2012–2013 academic year.

Proportions

A proportion is a fraction in which the numerator is a subset of the denominator. The formula for a proportion is:

$$\text{Proportion} = a/a + b$$

(Formula 15-2)

If we wish to know what proportion of ankle sprains are inversion sprains, we must divide the number of inversion sprains (a) by the total number of ankle sprains, equal to the sum of the inversion sprains (a) and the eversion sprains (b). Thus, the proportion of inversion sprains is 401/(401 + 35) = .9197. Proportions are often converted to percentages by multiplying by 100. Thus, we find that 91.97% of ankle sprains at University A are inversion sprains. Sometimes very small proportions are multiplied by constants larger than 100 in order to express them as whole numbers rather than decimals.

Rates

A rate is a proportion expressed over a particular unit of time. In epidemiology, rates are used to express the change in a health variable in the population at risk over a certain period. Because rates often describe fairly rare events in large populations, the number that is calculated is often a decimal beginning with one or more zeros. At University A, the rates of new inversion and eversion ankle sprains in a year are as follows:

Rate of new inversion sprains per year
= 401/12,237 = .03277

Rate of new eversion sprains per year
$$= 35/12{,}237 = .00286$$

Because it is difficult to conceptualize these small decimal values, rates are multiplied by a constant to obtain values that are whole numbers. To use the same constant to express both inversion and eversion ankle sprain rates as whole numbers, multiply each rate by 1000, as follows:

Rate of new inversion sprains
$$= [401/12{,}237] \times 1000$$
$$= 32.77 \text{ per 1000 people per year}$$

Rate of new eversion sprains
$$= [35/12{,}237] \times 1000$$
$$= 2.86 \text{ per 1000 people per year}$$

When rates are multiplied by a constant, it is important to include the constant when listing the rate so that readers know whether the rate is, for example, for 1000 people or 1 million people.

Epidemiologists use ratios, percentages, and rates to express many important concepts. Two of the most common are prevalence and incidence. Each of these can be expressed in crude, specific, and adjusted forms.

Prevalence

Prevalence expresses the proportion of a population that exhibits a certain condition at a given point in time.

Prevalence = Existing cases/Population examined
at a given point in time

(Formula 15-3)

Because the proportion is often small, it is usually multiplied by an appropriate constant. Because prevalence is a value at a given time, rather than a value calculated over a given period of time, it is a proportion rather than a rate. To determine prevalence, one must consider which individuals to count in the numerator and denominator of Formula 15-3.

The numerator contains all of the cases of the condition of interest at the time of measurement. Consider the example of multiple sclerosis. Because the symptoms of multiple sclerosis come and go and may resemble symptoms of other disorders, at any one point in time there are many individuals who have the disease but have not been diagnosed. Once diagnosed, however, the condition is presumed to exist for a lifetime. Therefore, the difficulty in defining cases of multiple sclerosis is in knowing when the disease begins, not when it ends.

Contrast this with the case of acute conditions that have more distinct beginnings but less clear end points. An ankle sprain might be defined as posttraumatic pain, swelling, bruising, or instability that results in an inability to participate fully in desired activities. With this definition, one would count all of the following as cases: an individual who sprained her ankle 2 days ago and is still walking gingerly, an intercollegiate athlete who sprained her ankle 3 weeks ago and is now practicing with the team but is not yet back on the game roster, and a recreational athlete who sprained her ankle 3 years ago and gave up racquetball because of chronic instability. One would not count an individual who "twisted" his ankle but did not experience swelling, bruising, or functional difficulties, nor would one count an individual who sustained a sprain in the past but has no residual swelling or instability and has returned to full function.

The denominator contains all of the people "examined" to determine whether they have the condition. Sometimes this number represents an actual examination of the individuals in the population; other times the number is determined from responses to a survey or numbers of cases within a large health care system or health insurer database.

To determine the prevalence of ankle sprains at University A, researchers need to pick a reporting date and a mechanism to obtain the information. Knowing that all members of the community need to renew parking permits during the first week of September, the researchers might set up shop at the parking permit window and administer a brief survey to all members of the campus who are willing to participate. If they administered 9857 questionnaires and identified 61 cases of ankle sprain, prevalence would be calculated as follows:

Prevalence of ankle sprains at the beginning
of the academic year $= [61/9857] \times 1000 = 6.19$

When reporting the prevalence, it is important to include the constant and the point in time in which the data were collected. In a report about ankle sprains at University A, the researchers might, after presenting their definition of what constituted an ankle sprain, write that "the prevalence of ankle sprains in the academic community at the beginning of the academic year was 6.19 sprains per 1000 people."

The "point in time" used to define prevalence can vary, yielding "point prevalence" and "period prevalence." When determining the point prevalence, the point in time is literally the time of measurement, for example, if a researcher asks study participants, "Do you currently have low back pain?" When determining period prevalence, the point in time is a longer time frame defined by the researcher. For example, the 1-year period prevalence could be calculated if a researcher asks study participants, "Have you had low back pain any time in the past 12 months?"

Because of the complexities in defining the numerator and denominator to determine prevalence, it is not always feasible to provide definitive estimates of prevalence for any number of common conditions seen by rehabilitation professionals. For example, Hill and Keating[5] provided a meta-analysis of the literature on prevalence (and incidence) of low back pain (LBP) in children 7 to 18 years old. Their table listing definitions of LBP among the 35 studies reviewed shows 4 different definitions as well as 2 studies providing no details [of LBP definition] and 4 studies in which LBP was, in their opinion, not clearly defined.[(p. 278)] Given differing definitions, it is not surprising to find different values of incidence.

Incidence

Incidence is the rate of new cases of a condition that develop during a specified period of time. The numerator represents the number of new cases, and the denominator represents the number in the population at risk:

Incidence = New cases during time period/
Population at risk during time period

(Formula 15-4)

As with other values, the incidence is often multiplied by a constant so that it can be expressed as a whole number rather than as a decimal.

To determine the incidence of ankle sprains at University A, researchers would need to set up a monitoring system to ensure good reporting of ankle sprains among members of the university community. In this example, the following (unrealistic) assumptions are made: (1) all members of the community will seek care for sprained ankles, (2) all will seek care at the campus health center or the athletic training center, and (3) all the professionals providing the care will use the same operational definition of ankle sprain and will report the number of new cases accurately. In the real world, determining incidence is complicated because people do not always seek medical care for new conditions, the care they receive occurs in many different places, and the providers they see define conditions differently and report them inconsistently. In our ideal world, we have already established the number of new cases of ankle sprain at University A to be 436 during the 2009–2010 academic year (see Table 15-1). Thus, 436 is the numerator of the incidence formula.

The denominator for incidence is the population at risk during the time period being measured. Determining this number is harder than it seems. First, one must determine the number in the "population." However, the number of individuals in a population usually varies over the course of the time period being studied. One common way to handle this is to use the number in the population at the midpoint of the period of study. For this ankle sprain example, the 2009–2010 academic year could be defined as September 1, 2009 to August 31, 2010, with a midpoint at March 1, 2010. This is probably a good date in the academic calendar because it avoids the peak enrollment time of early September as well as the valley of summer enrollments. Incidence studies frequently use the calendar year as the reporting period, with July 1 as the midpoint for determining the denominator.

The second difficulty in determining the denominator for an incidence calculation is in determining who is "at risk." If some conditions affect only one sex, or are virtually unheard of in certain age groups, then the population at risk should include only those of the appropriate sex or age. If having the condition means that one is no longer at risk for developing a new case of the disease (e.g., multiple sclerosis), then individuals with the condition at the start of the reporting period should be excluded from the denominator. In contrast, if the condition of interest can occur multiple times in the same individuals, then even those with the condition at the start of the reporting period remain at risk for new events. In the example of ankle sprains, the 61 people with ankle sprains during the first week of September 2009 remain at risk for a new ankle sprain during the academic year and are not excluded from the denominator. Therefore, the incidence of ankle sprains at University A would be calculated as follows:

Incidence of ankle sprains during 2009–2010
$= [436/12{,}237] \times 1000 = 35.63$

Note that the constant of 1000 is used, even though we could have multiplied by a constant of 100 to get a value that was a whole number. Because incidence and prevalence are often reported together, it is helpful to express them in terms of the same multiple of the population. Because the constant of 1000 was used to express the prevalence, it was also used to express the incidence. When reporting incidence rates, it is important to include the time period studied and the population multiplier. In a report about ankle sprains at University A, researchers would indicate that the "incidence of ankle sprains during the

2009–2010 academic year was 35.63 per 1000 people in the academic community."

Like prevalence, incidence estimates for a particular condition can vary greatly based on differences in how the numerator and denominator are defined. The study by Hill and Keating,[5] cited above, provides evidence again of the importance of definition of conditions in estimating incidence.

Relationship Between Incidence and Prevalence

The relationship between incidence and prevalence depends on the nature of the condition being examined. For diseases or injuries that are of short duration (either rapidly resolving or quickly fatal), the incidence is often greater than the prevalence. Consider the common cold—during the course of a year, most people get a new cold at some point (high incidence), but far fewer have colds at the same time (lower prevalence). This general statement is complicated by the seasonal nature of colds; it sometimes seems like everyone has them at once. The hypothetical ankle sprain example in this chapter exhibits this relationship between incidence and prevalence: the incidence is high (35.63 per 1000 people during the 2012–2013 academic year) compared with the prevalence (6.19 sprains per 1000 people at the beginning of September 2012).

For conditions that are of long duration, incidence is often lower than prevalence. Consider Parkinson's disease (PD). Reports of crude prevalence range from approximately 65 to 187 cases per 100,000 population, depending on geographical region.[6] In fact, Bronstein and colleagues[7] note, "As the U.S. population ages, prevalence of this disabling disorder is expected to rise dramatically" and also cite data "suggesting that underestimation of PD prevalence is common."[(p. 117)] The annual incidence is much lower, ranging from approximately 4 to 20 new cases per 100,000 population across the same regions.[6] Similar patterns can be expected with conditions such as multiple sclerosis, spinal cord injury, cerebral palsy, and diabetes.

Even though "incidence" and "prevalence" have the specific meanings outlined here, sometimes the terms are used inaccurately as general measures of frequency. The following mnemonic device, based on the first three letters of each word, helps readers remember which is which:

Incidence = **N**ew **C**ases (**INC**idence)

PRevalence = **E**xisting cases (**PRE**valence)

Crude, Specific, and Adjusted Rates

Although rates are sometimes calculated for purely descriptive purposes, researchers often wish to compare the rates with one another. They may wish to compare their sample with established population norms, they may wish to determine whether the rate within their population has changed over time, or they may wish to see whether their rates are approaching some desirable target rate. Making valid comparisons, however, depends on comparing the rates for similar populations. To generate the data appropriate for these "apple-to-apple" comparisons, researchers often modify their rates in several different ways.

Crude rates are calculated using the entire population at risk or of interest (see, e.g., the study by Tanner and Goldman[6] cited above). Generating a crude rate is usually the starting point for the researcher's calculations. The incidence rate of 35.63 ankle sprains per 1000 people during the 2012–2013 academic year is a crude rate. In certain circumstances, crude rates are systematically modified to become specific and adjusted rates.

Specific rates are rates for specified subgroups of the population. In the ankle sprain example, we might wonder whether athletes and nonathletes had different rates of ankle sprains. To determine this, we would first need an operational definition of athlete (perhaps someone who participates in recreational or intercollegiate team sports or individual physical activities an average of two times per week). Next, we would need to determine the number of athletes and nonathletes for the denominators of our specific rates. Finally, we would need to know how many of our 436 new cases occurred in athletes versus nonathletes. Figure 15-1, which presents a 2×2 matrix containing this hypothetical information, shows that the specific incidence for athletes appears to be much higher (139.80 per 1000 athletes) than it is for the nonathletes (24.14 per 1000 nonathletes).

If we wished, we could get even more specific. Among athletes, we might generate sport-specific incidence rates to determine whether there is a higher incidence among basketball, volleyball, and soccer players than among swimmers, golfers, and baseball or softball players. We also might determine competition-specific rates to look at incidence in recreational versus intercollegiate athletes. In addition, we might suspect that there are age or gender differences in ankle sprain incidence and calculate age- and sex-specific rates as well.

Adjusted rates are used when one wishes to compare rates across populations with different proportions of various subgroups. Let us assume that the injury

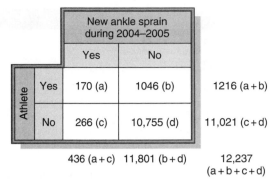

Figure 15-1 Crude and specific incidence rates of ankle sprain at University A during the 2009–2010 academic year.
Crude incidence rate: $[(a+c)/(a+b+c+d)] \times \text{constant} = [436/12,237] \times 1000 = 35.63$ per 1000 people
Specific incidence rate for athletes: $[a/(a+b)] \times \text{constant} = [170/1216] \times 1000 = 139.80$ per 1000 athletes
Specific incidence rate for nonathletes: $[c/(c+d)] \times \text{constant} = [266/11,021] \times 1000 = 24.14$ per 1000 nonathletes

statistics for University B report that their ankle sprain incidence for the year was only 100.8 sprains per 1000 athletes. Initially concerned because University A's incidence for athletes seems so much higher, the researcher realizes that the rates must be adjusted before a valid comparison can be made. Table 15-2 shows the specific, unadjusted rates for each university. A much higher proportion of athletes are soccer players at University A than at University B. Furthermore, soccer players at both universities have a high incidence of ankle sprains. To compare "apples to apples," the researcher needs to mathematically adjust the proportion of athletes in each sport at one university so that it matches the

proportion at the other university, and then adjust the presumed number of injuries and the incidence rates in light of the new proportions. Table 15-3 shows how this is done, by adjusting the University A data to match the proportions at University B. For example, at University B, only 1.6% of the athletes are soccer players. If University A, with 1216 athletes overall, had only 1.6% soccer players, then they would have 19 soccer players $(1216 \times .016 = 19.456)$. If these 19.46 players sustained ankle injuries at the same rate that the original 92 players did (532.6 per 1000 players), they would be expected to have sustained roughly 10.36 injuries during the year $(19.46 \times .5326 = 10.36)$. First, the University B subgroup proportions are used to adjust the proportions in the University A population. Then, the University A incidence rates are applied to the new proportions to calculate the adjusted injury numbers.

This adjustment is done for each subgroup within the population, as shown in Table 15-3. If University A had the same distribution of athletes as University B, then University A would expect to have 139.35 ankle sprains among its 1216 athletes for an adjusted incidence of 114.60 sprains per 1000 athletes. This process shows that the adjusted incidence rates are more similar to those of University B (114.60 compared with 100.82) than the original unadjusted rates (139.80 compared with 100.82).

Relative Risk: Risk Ratios and Odds Ratios

Epidemiologists often wish to move beyond describing groups to compare the probability that different groups with different characteristics will be affected by disease or injury in some way. That is, they seek to determine the relative risk for disease or injury of two different groups. There are two important ways in which relative

Table **15-2**

Hypothetical Sport-Specific Incidence Rates at Universities A and B

	UNIVERSITY A			UNIVERSITY B		
Category	No. of Sprains	No. (%) in Group	Incidence of Sprains (per 1000)	No. of Sprains	No. (%) in Group	Incidence of Sprains (per 1000)
Recreational	109	968 (79.6)	112.6	81	821 (84.5)	98.7
Intercollegiate						
Soccer	49	92 (7.6)	532.6	9	16 (1.6)	562.5
Baseball, softball	8	74 (6.1)	108.1	5	68 (7.0)	73.5
Swimming	4	82 (6.7)	48.7	3	67 (6.9)	44.8
Total	170	1216 (100.0)	139.8	98	972 (100.0)	100.82

Table **15-3**

Adjusted Hypothetical Sport-Specific Incidence Rates at University A

Category	UNIVERSITY A			UNIVERSITY A—ADJUSTED		
	No. of Sprains	No. (%) in Group	Incidence of Sprains (per 1000)	No. of Sprains	No. (%) in Group	Incidence of Sprains (per 1000)
Recreational	109	968 (79.6)	112.6	115.70	1027.52 (84.5)	112.6
Intercollegiate						
Soccer	49	92 (7.6)	532.6	10.36	19.46 (1.6)	532.6
Baseball, softball	8	74 (6.1)	108.1	9.20	85.12 (7.0)	108.1
Swimming	4	82 (6.7)	48.7	4.09	83.90 (6.9)	48.7
Total	170	1216 (100.0)	139.8	139.35	1216 (100.0)	114.60

risk is calculated: using risk ratios and using odds ratios. The distinction between the two is important and warrants careful consideration of the examples that follow.

The risk ratio is calculated by creating a ratio of the incidence rate for one subgroup and the incidence rate for another subgroup. In the example of ankle sprain, athletes sustained ankle sprains at a rate of 139.8 per 1000 people and nonathletes sustained ankle sprains at a rate of 24.14 per 1000 people (see Fig. 15-1). If we create a ratio out of these two numbers (139.8/24.14), we find that the athletes are 5.79 times as likely to sustain ankle sprains as nonathletes. Earlier, a 2×2 matrix was used to organize the data. The formula for determining the risk ratio is often given with a standard form of this table in mind (Fig. 15-2). The risk ratio is defined as:

$$\text{Risk ratio} = [a/(a+b)]/[c/(c+d)]$$

(Formula 15-5)

Note that this is calculated by "working" the table horizontally—determining the incidence of ankle sprains for the row that represents athletes and then

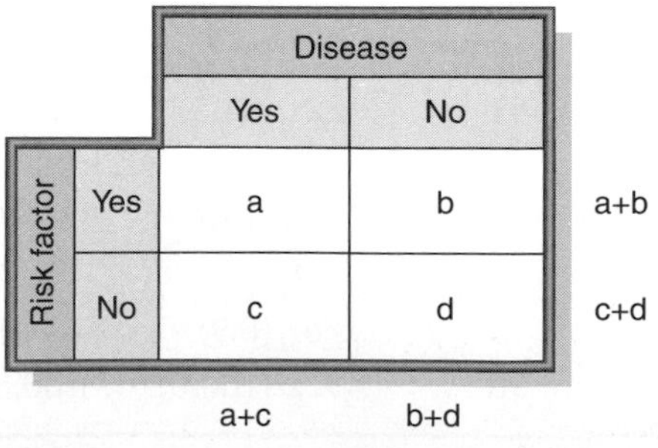

determining the incidence for the row that represents nonathletes. We can compute relative risks this way because we have measured the entire population of interest, and the totals for each row [(a+b) and (c+d)] give us meaningful information about the number of athletes and nonathletes in the population.

Relative risk is actually a familiar concept in everyday life. One common occurrence is to compute how much more likely people who do not exercise are to experience stroke than are people who do exercise. In a recent examination of this risk, Diep and colleagues[8] performed a meta-analysis of the relative risk for having a stroke in people who are physically active (PA) compared with people who are not. Not surprisingly, they found, compared with low PA, moderate PA caused an 11% reduction in risk for stroke outcome and high PA a 19% reduction.

Many epidemiological researchers, however, do not have access to an entire population of interest. Instead of measuring the entire population of interest, the researcher identifies a number of individuals who have the condition or risk factor of interest. The researchers then seek out matched controls without the condition or risk factor in order to create a comparison group. Figure 15-3 shows two new sets of hypothetical data used to determine the relative risk of ankle sprains in athletes and nonathletes. In Figure 15-3A, the researchers identified one control for each case; in Figure 15-3B, they identified three controls for each case. In both parts of Figure 15-3, the numbers for those with ankle sprains remain constant. In addition, the distribution of athletes and nonathletes without ankle sprains remains the same even though the absolute numbers change from part A to part B. Watch what happens mathematically if we apply the risk ratio formula to these tables. Figure 15-3 shows that the risk ratio is different for the two parts of the figure. This is because the totals in the margin

Figure 15-2 Standard table for determining relative risk.

A

		Ankle sprains September 2012		
		Yes	No	
Athlete	Yes	18 (a)	6 (b)	24 (a + b)
	No	32 (c)	44 (d)	76 (c + d)
		50 (a + c)	50 (b + d)	

B

		Ankle sprains September 2012		
		Yes	No	
Athlete	Yes	18 (a)	18 (b)	36 (a + b)
	No	32 (c)	132 (d)	164 (c + d)
		50 (a + c)	150 (b + d)	

Figure 15-3 Relative risk for sustaining an ankle sprain for athletes and nonathletes. The two parts of the figure demonstrate the problem of calculating risk ratios when the total population of interest has not been studied. Because the totals in the row margins reflect the sampling design rather than the proportion of injury in the population, the risk ratio changes from A to B. The odds ratio, which does not depend on the totals in the margins, remains the same.
A, Hypothetical study in which one control subject is identified for each case.
Proportion of athletes with ankle sprains = a/(a + b) = 18/24 = .75
Proportion of nonathletes with ankle sprains = c/(c + d) = 32/76 = .42
Risk ratio = [a/(a + b)]/[c/(c + d)] = .75/.42 = 1.79
Odds of someone with an ankle sprain being an athlete = a/c = 18/32 = .5625
Odds of someone without an ankle sprain being an athlete = b/d = 6/44 = .1364
Odds ratio = (a/c)/(b/d) = .5625/.1364 = 4.124
B, Hypothetical study in which three controls are identified for each case.
Proportion of athletes with ankle sprains = a/(a + b) = 18/36 = .500
Proportion of nonathletes with ankle sprains = c/(c + d) = 32/164 = .195
Risk ratio = [a/(a + b)]/[c/(c + d)] = .500/.195 = 2.56
Odds of someone with an ankle sprain being an athlete = a/c = 18/32 = .5625
Odds of someone without an ankle sprain being an athlete = b/d = 18/132 = .1364
Odds ratio = (a/c)/(b/d) = .5625/.1364 = 4.124

change as the number of control subjects changes. Because the totals in the margins reflect the sampling design and not the actual totals in the population, it is not valid to use the risk ratio in this situation.

When computing risk ratios is not valid, a value known as the *odds ratio* is used to estimate relative risk. To understand the difference between these two ratios, the difference between proportions and odds must be clarified. To use an everyday example,[9(p. 91)] consider a baseball player who has one hit (and three outs—we'll call them "misses") in four times at bat in a game. A hit is represented by "a," and a miss is represented by "b." The formula for a proportion is a/(a + b), which in this case means that the proportion of hits is 1/4, or .25. The proportion divides the "part" by the "whole." In contrast, odds are determined by creating a ratio between hit and misses, or a/b. The odds ratio divides one "part" by the other "part." In this baseball example, the proportion of hits is one out of four (.25), and the proportion of misses is three out of four (.75); thus, the odds of getting a hit are 1:3 or .333.

Returning to the ankle sprain example, the totals in the margins of the rows in Figure 15-3 are not meaningful because they do not represent the "whole" population of interest; instead, they reflect the sampling design of the researchers. When this is the case, researchers use an odds ratio, rather than a risk ratio based on proportions, to estimate relative risk among subgroups.

The odds ratio uses only the numbers found within the table (not those in the margin) and works the table "vertically." In Figure 15-3A, the odds of a person with an ankle sprain being an athlete are 18/32, or .5625. The odds of a person without an ankle sprain being an athlete are 6/44, or .1364. The odds ratio is simply the ratio of these two odds. The conceptual formula for the odds ratio is given below, along with a common algebraic simplification:

$$\text{Odds ratio} = (a/c)/(b/d) = ad/bc$$

(Formula 15-6)

In contrast to the changing value of the risk ratio between parts A and B of Figure 15-3A, the odds ratio remains the same whether the researcher selects one or three controls for each case. That is, for the nonsprains in B, the odds ratio is 18/132, or .1364, the same as in A.

Epidemiologists use measures such as incidence, prevalence, risk ratios, and odds ratios to describe the distribution of disease and injury within populations and population subgroups. Epidemiological studies frequently report these measures or variations on these measures. Readers who encounter a rate, proportion, or ratio with which they are unfamiliar should be able to apply the general principles in this section to gain a general understanding of the unfamiliar measure.

SCREENING AND DIAGNOSIS

A common function of epidemiological research is to evaluate the usefulness of various screening and diagnostic tests. Four key proportions are used to compare the usefulness of the test being evaluated to a criterion test that is considered the "gold standard." These four proportions are the sensitivity, specificity, positive predictive value, and negative predictive value. They are generally represented by a standard 2×2 table, as shown in Figure 15-4.

Some Concepts from Psychophysics

The discussion of epidemiological concepts below relies heavily on some concepts taken from areas of experimental psychology, especially psychophysics, or the measurement of human reactions to physical stimuli. We think it will be useful then to introduce some of these concepts.

Let us consider the simple task of detecting an auditory signal in a noisy background. There are two forces at work. One is the listener's physical ability of hearing acuity. The other is how sure the listener feels she must be to report having heard a signal. The latter is called the listener's "response criterion" and can be "strict" (i.e., must be very sure a signal was or was not present), or "lax" (i.e., is willing to report presence or absence of a signal even if not

sure), or somewhere in between. There are four possible conditions: (1) a signal is presented and a listener indicates hearing it (also known as a HIT), (2) a signal is presented but the listener does not report hearing it (a MISS), (3) a signal is *not* presented but the listener reports hearing it anyway (a false alarm, or FA), and (4) a signal is *not* presented and the listener reports no signal was present (a correct rejection, or CR). Typically, these four values are reported as proportions, or percentages—for example, the proportion of HIT responses out of some number of trials.

Translating to epidemiological constructs, we can think of a clinical condition of interest (ankle sprain in our example) as the signal. In Figure 15-4, box (a) is the HIT rate, (b) is the FA, (c) is the MISS, and (d) is the CR. We will now see how epidemiological concepts are then derived.

Sensitivity and Specificity

Sensitivity and specificity compare the conclusions of the new test with the results on the criterion test. They are determined by "working" the 2×2 table vertically. The sensitivity of a test is the proportion or percentage of individuals with a particular diagnosis who are correctly identified as positive by the test. It is the HIT rate. The specificity is the proportion or percentage of individuals without a particular diagnosis who are correctly identified as negative by the test—that is, the rate of correct rejections.

$$\text{Sensitivity} = a/(a+c)$$

(Formula 15-7)

$$\text{Specificity} = d/(b/d)$$

(Formula 15-8)

Continuing with the ankle injury examples already presented, these two epidemiological concepts are illustrated in Figure 15-5, which uses data from Clark and associates'[10] study of ankle joint effusion and occult ankle fractures. A series of patients with severe ankle sprains, but without apparent fractures on plain radiographs, were studied with plain radiographs and computed tomography (CT). The gold standard for identifying ankle fractures was CT of the ankle. The new test involved measuring the extent of ankle joint effusion on the plain radiographs. The researchers found that an ankle effusion of 15 mm or more on plain radiography had a sensitivity of 83.3% for detecting occult ankle fractures. This means that 83.3% of patients with fractures also had an effusion of 15 mm or more. When testing patients without occult fractures, they found

		Condition according to gold standard		
		Present	Absent	
Condition according to test being evaluated	Present	a	b	(a+b)
	Absent	c	d	(c+d)
		(a+c)	(b+d)	

Figure 15-4 Illustration of traditional epidemiological concepts.
Sensitivity = a/(a+c)
Specificity = d/(b+d)
Positive predictive value = a/(a+b)
Negative predictive value = d/(c+d)

	Fracture found with computed tomography		
	Yes	No	
Ankle effusion found on plain radiograph ≥15 mm	10 (a)	2 (b)	12
<15 mm	2 (c)	12 (d)	14
	12	14	

Figure 15-5 Calculation of sensitivity, specificity, positive predictive value, and negative predictive value.
Sensitivity=a/(a+c)=10/12=.833=83.3%
Specificity=d/(b+d)=12/14=.857=85.7%
Positive predictive value=a/(a+b)=10/12=.833=83.3%
Negative predictive value=d/(c+d)=12/14=.857=85.7%
In this example, the sensitivity and the positive predictive value are the same, and the specificity and negative predictive value are the same. This is because the number of false-positive results and the number of false-negative results are the same in this example. In most examples, this is not the case and all four of the proportions take different values. (From data in Clark TWI, Janzen DL, Logan PM, Connell DG: Improving the detection of radiographically occult ankle fractures: Positive predictive value of an ankle joint effusion, *Clin Radiol* 51:632–636, 1996.)

	Computed tomography results	
	Fracture	No fracture
Size of effusion (mm)	21	
	19,19,19	
	18,18,18	
		17,17
	16,16	
	15	
	14	14,14
	12	12
		11,11,11,11
		10
		9,9
		6
		5

Figure 15-6 Illustration of how changing the cutoff score influences sensitivity and specificity. If the cutoff is between 11 and 12 mm, sensitivity is maximized. If the cutoff is between 17 and 18 mm, specificity is maximized.
Sensitivity if cutoff is set at 12 mm or more:
(12/12)×100=100.0%
Specificity if cutoff is set at 12 mm or more:
(9/14)×100=64.3%
Sensitivity if cutoff is set at 18 mm or more:
(7/12)×100=58.3%
Specificity if cutoff is set at 18 mm or more:
(14/14)×100=100.0%
(From data in Clark TWI, Janzen DL, Logan PM, Connell DG: Improving the detection of radiographically occult ankle fractures: Positive predictive value of an ankle joint effusion, *Clin Radiol* 51:632–636, 1996.)

that an effusion of less than 15 mm had a specificity of 85.7%. This means that 85.7% of the patients without occult fractures had effusions of less than 15 mm.

When test results can take more than two values, as in this study, the researchers need to determine the "cutoff" score for differentiating between positive and negative results. Figure 15-6 shows an approximate reconstruction of the results of the two tests for all 26 patients in the series. If the criterion for a positive result were set at 12 mm or more of effusion, the sensitivity of the test would be 100% because all 12 patients with fractures visualized by CT had an effusion of 12 mm or more. However, the specificity would be only 64.3% because this permissive criterion would result in many false-positive (or false alarm [FA]) results. Mathematically, the proportion of FA is 100 minus the specificity because the proportions of all subjects without sprain must equal 100.

$$pFA = 100 - [d/(b+d)]$$

(Formula 15-9)

in which "d" is the correct rejection rate and "b" is the FA rate. That is, all subjects without sprain are either correctly identified as not sprained (specificity) or incorrectly identified as being sprained (FA). If the criterion

for a positive result were set at 18 mm or more of effusion, the specificity of the test would be 100% because all 14 patients without fractures had effusions of less than 18 mm.

Using a criterion of 18 mm or more, however, the sensitivity would be only 58.3% because this stringent criterion would result in many false-negative results (i.e., high MISS rate). Mathematically, the sensitivity (HIT) is 100 minus the MISS rate because the summed proportions of all subjects with sprain must equal 100. That is, all subjects with sprain are either correctly identified as being sprained (sensitivity) or incorrectly identified as not being sprained (MISS rate). Test developers work to determine an intermediate cutoff score that results in a desirable balance between the sensitivity and specificity of the test.

Receiver-Operating Characteristic Curves

The notion of the receiver-operating characteristic (ROC) curve is also derived from psychophysics, using the concepts described previously. Typically, it is a plot of HIT

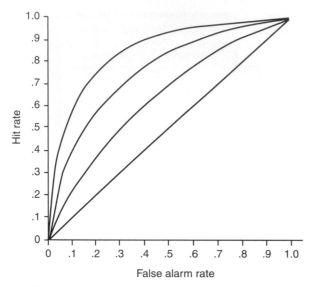

Figure 15-7 A "family" of three typical ROC curves.

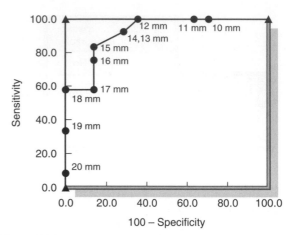

Figure 15-8 Receiver-operator curve illustrating how changing the cutoff score influences the sensitivity and specificity of a test. In general, the ideal cutoff score is the one closest to the upper left-hand corner of the graph.

versus FA rates. What makes ROC curves useful is that they incorporate both forces at work in a psychophysical decision—physical ability and response criterion—into one curve. Figure 15.7 shows a typical family of ROC curves. The metric on each of the curves is called d-prime (d'; for background, see the classic text by Green and Swets[11]; for readings in applications to diagnostics, see Swets[12]). There are two critical points to note. First is that, on each curve, the ability of interest (e.g., detection) is equal everywhere along the curve. Data points that generated any single curve varied only in the response criterion. Data points on the lower left result from a strict criterion, so, even though HIT rate might be low, FA rate is also low. Data points moving toward the upper right result from more lax criteria; even though HIT rates may be high, FA rates are also high. The second aspect to notice is that curves move toward the upper left when the ability of interest is better.

Data about sensitivity and specificity may also be visualized through an ROC curve. In this conception, the diagnostic capability of the test is the "ability of interest." Clark and associates[10] related their data to ROC curves, as shown in Figure 15-8. Axes are still HIT and FA rates but are reconceptualized as sensitivity and 100 minus the specificity. The heavy line with the triangles for data points represents a test with an ideal cutoff point—at 100% sensitivity and 100% specificity (the upper left-hand corner of the graph). In practice, tests generally deviate from this ideal, as is the case with the use of the extent of ankle effusion to predict occult ankle fractures (the circular points on the graph). These points demonstrate visually that cutoff

scores of 20, 19, and 18 mm result in perfect specificity. These scores represent a strict criterion yielding low FA rate or low specificity; the cutoff will not identify any nonsprains as sprains. The same scores also yield a low HIT rate, or low sensitivity; the cutoff will miss identifying sprains correctly. The cutoff scores of 12, 11, and 10 mm result in perfect sensitivity (high HIT rate; the cutoffs will perfectly identify those with sprains) but low specificity (high FA rate; the cutoffs will identify nonsprains as sprains). The cutoff score of 15 mm results in the best balance between sensitivity and specificity; it is the point closest to the ideal point in the upper left-hand corner. When two points are approximately equidistant from this ideal point, researchers consider the impact of false-positive results (needlessly worrying the healthy) or false-negative results (falsely reassuring the ill) in determining which cutoff score to select. If the disease being screened for were serious but treatable in early stages, the researchers would probably choose the cutoff score with somewhat lower specificity and higher sensitivity so that the probability of false-negative results would be lower. If the disease being screened for were less serious and could be effectively treated even at later stages of the disease, the researchers would probably choose a cutoff score with lower sensitivity and higher specificity so that the probability of false-positive results would be lower.

Likelihood Ratios

Simply put, "The [likelihood ratio] LR of any clinical finding is the probability of that finding in patients with disease divided by the probability of the same finding in patients without disease.... LRs may range from 0 to infinity. Findings with LRs greater than 1 argue for the diagnosis of interest; the bigger the number, the more convincingly the finding suggests that disease."[13]

The following is an important way that sensitivity and specificity are used in the calculation of likelihood ratios:

$$\text{Likelihood ratio of a positive test} = \text{Sensitivity}\%/(100-\text{Specificity}\%)$$

(Formula 15-10)

$$\text{Likelihood ratio of a negative test} = (100-\text{Sensitivity}\%)/\text{Specificity}\%$$

(Formula 15-11)

A likelihood ratio of a positive test of 1.0 does not help to rule in disease because the false-positive results (100−specificity) are as likely as true-positive results (sensitivity). The higher the likelihood ratio of a positive test, the more information the test gives for ruling in a disease or injury. A likelihood ratio of a negative test of 1.0 also does not help to rule out disease because the false-negative results (100−sensitivity) are as likely as the true-negative results (specificity). The lower the likelihood of a negative test, the more information the test gives for ruling out a disease or injury.[14] Likelihood ratios are also a good way to determine the information provided by tests that have multiple levels of cutoff points.[9(p. 92)]

One important characteristic of sensitivity and specificity is that they are unaffected by the proportion of individuals with the disease or injury of interest. Because they are each calculated from one column of the 2×2 table, the number of individuals in the other column does not affect their value. Thus, ankle effusion measurement should yield similar sensitivity and specificity whether it is applied to a group with minor ankle sprains with few fractures or to a group with severe sprains and many fractures.

Predictive Value

Although sensitivity and specificity are useful concepts, they only tell half the story about diagnostic and screening tests. The other half of the story is told by the positive and negative predictive values. The positive predictive value is the percentage of individuals identified by the test as positive who actually have the diagnosis. The negative predictive value is the percentage of those identified by the test as negative who actually do not have the diagnosis. These values are found by "working" the table horizontally:

$$\text{Positive predictive value} = a/(a+b)$$

(Formula 15-12)

$$\text{Negative predictive value} = c/(c+d)$$

(Formula 15-13)

A

		Computed tomography		
		Fracture	No fracture	
Ankle effusion	≥15 mm	5 (a)	20 (b)	25 (a+b)
	<15 mm	1 (c)	120 (d)	121 (c+d)
		6 (a+c)	140 (b+d)	

B

		Computed tomography		
		Fracture	No fracture	
Ankle effusion	≥15 mm	100 (a)	1 (b)	101 (a+b)
	<15 mm	20 (c)	6 (d)	26 (c+d)
		120 (a+c)	7 (b+d)	

Figure 15-9 Changing the prevalence of fractures influences the predictive values, but not the sensitivity and specificity.
A, Illustration with prevalence of 4%.
Sensitivity = a/(a+c) = 5/6 = 83%
Specificity = d/(b+d) = 120/140 = 86%
Positive predictive value = a/(a+b) = 5/25 = 20%
Negative predictive value = d/(c+d) = 120/121 = 99%
B, Illustration with prevalence of 94%
Sensitivity = a/(a+c) = 100/120 = 83%
Specificity = d/(b+d) = 6/7 = 86%
Positive predictive value = a/(a+b) = 100/101 = 99%
Negative predictive value = d/(c+d) = 6/26 = 23%

Because the table is worked horizontally, the predictive values vary greatly depending on the proportion of individuals with and without the disease or injury. This is illustrated in Figure 15-9, which maintains the sensitivity and specificity values of the original study. What is varied, however, is the proportion of total cases with and without an ankle fracture. In the original study, 46% of the cases had an ankle fracture identified through CT. In Figure 15-9A, only 4% (6 of 146) of the cases have an ankle fracture; in Figure 15-9B, 94% (120 of 127) of cases have an ankle fracture. When dealing with a population with only a 4% probability of having a fracture, the predictive value of a positive test is only 20%, which means that 80% of positive test results would be false positive. Although this sounds bad, the upside is that the predictive value of a negative test is 99%; there would be very few false-negative results. Conversely, when dealing with a population with a 94% probability of having a fracture, the predictive value of a positive test is 99%, and the predictive value of a negative test is only 23%. Because the positive and negative predictive values are dependent on the proportion of diseased or injured individuals within the population studied, this proportion should always be specified when the predictive values are reported.

This characteristic of the predictive values has a great deal of impact for clinicians who are performing diagnostic or screening tests. To know how to interpret the predictive value of a test, the clinician should estimate the "pretest" probability of the patient having the condition. If an asymptomatic individual is being screened, the probability of having the condition is low. In this instance, the predictive value of a positive test is likely to be low, but the predictive value of a negative test is likely to be high. If an individual with a history and physical examination that is highly suggestive of the condition is tested, the predictive value of a positive test is likely to be high, and the predictive value of a negative test is likely to be low. Applying this information to the example of ankle effusion, a clinician who notes a 15-mm ankle effusion on the plain radiograph of a patient experiencing an uncomplicated recovery from ankle sprain would likely not order a CT to look for an occult fracture. The assumption would be that the patient belongs to a population similar to the one in Figure 15-9A, and the positive ankle effusion has a high probability of being a false-positive finding. In contrast, if a clinician notes a 15-mm ankle effusion on the radiograph of a patient with a great deal of swelling and discoloration, malleolar tenderness, and inability to bear weight 72 hours after injury, a follow-up CT would likely be ordered to look for an occult fracture. The assumption would be that the patient belongs to a population similar to the one in Figure 15-9B, and the positive ankle effusion has a high probability of being a true indication of an occult fracture.

This section of the chapter has only introduced the complex interrelationships among sensitivity, specificity, likelihood ratios, prevalence, and predictive values. Several excellent texts and articles present a fuller description of these topics.[1,14-16]

A number of contemporary articles in the rehabilitation literature use these concepts to examine screening and diagnostic tests of importance to rehabilitation professionals. Schneiders and colleagues[17] included use of sensitivity, specificity, positive likelihood ratio, and negative likelihood ratio in their meta-analysis of tuning fork and ultrasound testing to identify lower-limb stress fractures. Strand and associates[18] employed epidemiologic diagnostic concepts, including likelihood ratios, sensitivity, and specificity in their evaluation of the Dynamic Evaluation of Motor Speech Skill, a new test to help diagnose childhood apraxia of speech. Eyssen and colleagues[19] employed ROC curve analysis to help evaluate the responsiveness of the Canadian Occupational Performance Measure, "an individualized, client-centered outcome measure for the identification and evaluation of self-perceived occupational performance problems." Page, Fulk, and Boyne[20] also employed ROC curves to help determine "the amount of change in UE-FM [upper extremity portion of the Fugl-Meyer scale] scores that can be regarded as important and clinically meaningful."[(p. 791)] Literature searches using the terms "specificity," "ROC curve," or "likelihood ratio" will yield many more examples.

NONEXPERIMENTAL EPIDEMIOLOGICAL DESIGNS

Three common nonexperimental designs are used to implement epidemiological research: cross-sectional, case-control, and cohort designs. Figure 15-10 shows

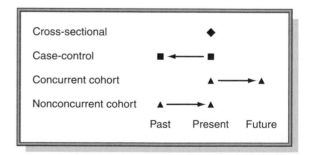

Figure 15-10 The epidemiological designs can be characterized by the timing of measurements, as well as the direction in which the logic of the design proceeds. Data are collected at one point in time for cross-sectional studies; researchers work from effects to causes in case-control designs and work from causes to effects in two variations on cohort designs.

how each design is related to the timing of various elements of the design. *Cross-sectional* studies are used to document the status of a group at a particular point in time. With *case-control studies*, researchers identify individuals with the condition of interest (the cases) and individuals without the condition of interest (the controls). They then look into the past for the presence or absence of risk factors that might explain the presence or absence of the condition. In effect, in case-control studies, the researchers start with an effect and go looking for a cause. With *cohort studies* (also termed *concurrent cohort studies*), researchers identify individuals with various risk factors and look into the future to see if the condition of interest develops. In a variation on cohort studies, sometimes termed *historical cohort studies* or *nonconcurrent cohort studies*, the researchers identify a group of interest, identify risk factors from the past, and then determine whether a condition of interest is present or absent. In both variations of cohort studies, the researchers start with the cause and look for the effect.

Recall from Chapter 9, the terms "prospective" and "retrospective" are defined in terms of the timing of data collection in relation to the development of the research problem. It is also noted that alternative definitions of these two terms are sometimes used to describe the "direction" in which the research proceeds. According to these alternative definitions, a prospective study proceeds from cause to effect, as do the cohort designs. A retrospective study proceeds from effect to cause, as do the case-control designs. In this text, the terms refer to the timing of data collection (versus the time of establishing the hypothesis), as recommended by Friedman.[21] When referring to the direction in which the research proceeds, the terms *cohort* and *case-control* are used.

Cross-Sectional Studies

Cross-sectional studies are used to document health status at a single point in time for each participant within the study. In some instances, the point in time may be a range of calendar dates (e.g., a study in which fitness levels of top executives in a particular company are collected between January and March of one year); in other instances, the point in time may be a particular event (e.g., a study of fitness levels of top executives as they turn 60 years old). In studies that document health status, the point in time is often the point of entry into a health system. For example, Resnik and Borgia[22] examined the application of Veterans' Administration guidelines for implementing rehabilitation services to 12,599 military personnel who underwent major lower-limb amputation. The "point in time" was their first amputation, and Resnik and Borgia limited their

analysis to subjects only at the time of their first amputation: their entry into the health care system of interest. Even though the study used data collected from the beginning of 2005 until the end of 2010, there was only one point in time of interest for each subject. Thus, the study is considered cross-sectional.

Many reports of case-control and cohort research include a cross-sectional component that describes the patient groups at a single point in time. For example, O'Reilly and colleagues[23] completed a case-control study of adults 55 to 80 years of age, comparing those who had sustained a fall and subsequent wrist fracture within the 12 months before the study (cases) with those who had not (controls). The study had a cross-sectional component in that several health measures were used to describe the entire population.

Case-Control Studies

The defining characteristic of a case-control study is that the researchers start with "effects" and look for "causes." First, the researchers identify individuals with the effect of interest (the cases). Second, they identify appropriately matched individuals without the effect of interest (the controls). Third, they evaluate all the participants (cases and controls alike) to determine the presence or absence of various factors hypothesized to cause the effect of interest. This evaluation may involve review of records to determine previous health status, collection of new information that asks subjects to recall past behaviors or events, or observation of characteristics that were presumed to have existed before the effect of interest occurred. Finally, they conduct statistical analyses to determine whether individuals with the presumed causes have a higher relative risk for being a case than a control. One very common example is studies that examine people with lung cancer (the effect) and determine how many of them were smokers as opposed to those who did not smoke. Another common example is studies of people with diabetes and determining how many were obese as opposed to how many were not. Higher numbers of smokers and obese people, respectively, would make those two conditions suspect as causes for the outcomes. Although describing case-control studies as "inexpensive and relatively quick to complete,"[24(p. 92)] Curley and Vitale offer some cautions. First, because subjects in the groups are not randomly assigned, "associations found in the analysis may be the result of another, unknown variable."[(p. 92)] Additionally, Curly and Vitale state that data, often abstracted from medical records, often were not designed to be collected for research purposes and, so, "may not provide adequate or accurate information on exposures."[(p. 92)]

An example of a classic case-control study is that of Ratnapradipa and associates.[25] These investigators looked into the history of environmental exposures of preschool children with asthma ($N=279$) and without asthma ($N=412$). The design was a "nested" case-control study, which Saracci[2] describes as a "case-control study within a cohort" and further notes that nested case-control studies "may be advantageously used in every situation in which assessing an exposure is very cumbersome or costly."[(p. 74)] The cohort consisted of preschool children in a local health program providing nutritional and other services to income-eligible mothers. The local health department had noted potentially poor air quality. Through detailed interviews, the investigators gained information about prior environmental exposures. Ultimately, they found that children with asthma had significantly higher exposure to wood or oil smoke, soot, exhaust, or cockroaches.

Given the current very high prevalence of autism spectrum disorder (ASD), investigators are in the process of examining correlations between many potential causes and later findings of ASD. Hendrix and colleagues[26] posited a link between maternal prenatal body mass index (BMI), gestational weight gain (GWG), and later findings of ASD in their children. In an uncommon variation, the controls in this study were the siblings of the children with ASD. The authors collected prenatal data for 140 mothers, each of whom had one child with ASD and one without. Ultimately, the authors found, "There was no difference in BMI category between pregnancies nor was a weight gain different from the IOM recommendations by BMI category associated with ASD."[(p. 81)]

The study by O'Reilly and colleagues,[23] cited earlier, is an example of a case-control study. They were interested in finding factors that predicted falls in 41 older (55 to 80 years) adults. As noted, their cases were adults who had fallen and sustained low-trauma wrist fracture within the last year, and controls were 41 age-matched adults who had not fallen. All participants were also community dwelling and mobile (with or without aid). Patients (cases) were assessed on the same day they were referred to physiotherapy. Controls were recruited through convenience sampling. Health information was collected on all participants, with special notation about the history of falls. The investigators also administered several tests. Results indicated that the cases scored had impaired gait and balance and scored lower on the Timed Up-and-Go (TUG) test; the Modified Clinical Test of Sensory Integration and Balance (M-CTSIB); knee flexor strength; and cognition. After falls and wrist fracture, the cases also had higher levels of health care demands and medical interventions and need for further physical therapy.

Aram and colleagues[27] determined the ability of a group of hearing-impaired children in alphabetic and language skills. They then videotaped each child-mother dyad in joint storytelling and joint writing sessions. The mothers were equated for educational level and other variables and had no particular training in storytelling or joint writing and were encouraged to tell the story of an unfamiliar illustrated book, "in your regular, everyday way." The mothers were also asked to help their children write out the names of drawings. No other instructions were given. The authors found that higher scores in storytelling were predictive of more advanced phonological awareness, general knowledge, and receptive vocabulary, all known to be prevalent in better reading ability. More complex maternal writing mediation was correlated with higher skills in word writing, letter recognition, and word recognition.

Readers need to be alert to some limitations in the studies by O'Reilly and associates[23] and Aram and colleagues[27] because they vary from the classic case-control design. In the instance of the study of falls, the measures differentiating cases from controls were applied at the time of evaluation; the investigators did not delve into participants' medical histories. Thus, for example, they could not prove that fallers had slower TUG times than nonfallers before the study, and it is possible that the slower TUG times resulted from, rather than increased the risk for, falls.

Although the study by Aram and colleagues[27] was described by them as a case-control study, again be aware of the difference from a classic case-control study and of a possible flaw in the study. In the classic case-control study, the researcher relies on already established data (e.g., medical records) to draw conclusions. In this study, the authors did not and instead relied on concurrent measures of storytelling and writing support. Thus, the authors had no way of knowing the true past patterns of the mothers' storytelling and writing support as well as to what extent the mother-child interactions during the study were actually representative of past practices. We included these studies here to indicate that (1) variations of classic designs are possible and (2) even studies published in peer-reviewed journals merit critical review.

These four studies illustrate some of the positive and negative features of case-control methods. In the study of the association between preexisting environmental conditions and asthma, the case-control methods enabled the researchers to study a large number of asthma cases cost effectively. If the researchers had tried to implement this study with a cohort design, they would have had to enroll a much larger cohort of patients and follow them for years until enough of the subjects developed asthma. This illustrates one of the chief advantages of the case-control design over other designs—the ability to study a reasonable number of individuals with relatively rare or concerning conditions without needing to observe the entire population at risk for long periods. A second advantage of the case-control design is that it enables researchers to study things that might not otherwise be ethical to study. In the study of asthma, one would clearly not be able to study this experimentally by randomly placing patients into hazardous and nonhazardous home environments. One would not even be able to study this ethically with a nonexperimental cohort design. To do so would involve identifying a group of at-risk children to study, evaluating their homes for hazards, and then doing nothing about those hazards until observing who did and who did not develop the disease. Ethical practice would demand that subjects at least be given advice about how to remedy the hazards that were identified—and, if enough patients took that advice, the level of hazards across the homes would become much more uniform, and one of the variables of interest would be nearly eliminated. Therefore, the case-control method, in which hazards that were presumed to exist before the onset of disease are identified after the return home, provides an ethical way to study this potential relationship.

One of the chief concerns about case-control designs is the manner in which the presumed causes are documented or identified. In the asthma study,[24] risk factors were identified through interviews with mothers; this is good, but not foolproof. In the ASD study,[25] data on BMI and GWG were obtained from medical records; this is a much better approach. We have already indicated some limitations in the data collection of the studies by O'Reilly and associates[23] and Aram and colleagues.[27]

However, in all fairness, these studies also showed that it is often difficult to obtain accurate historical data. One must be careful of assuming that an observed behavior or condition is a continuation of, or is indicative of, past behaviors or conditions.

Cohort Studies

Cohort designs are characterized by their progression from cause to effect. In a cohort study, individuals are selected because they do not have the disease or injury of interest, and they can be classified as to their status on a risk factor or factors of interest. The "healthy" individuals (at least with respect to the disease or injury of interest) in the different risk categories are followed for a period of time to compare their relative risks for developing the disease or injury of interest.

There are several variants of the cohort design. In the first, the subjects are identified in the present and

followed into the future to see who does and does not develop the outcome of interest. This variant is known either simply as a cohort design or as a prospective or concurrent cohort design. In the second variant, the subjects are placed into risk factor groupings based on data collected in the past. Then they are measured in the present or future to determine who develops the outcome of interest. This variant is known as either a historical cohort design or a nonconcurrent cohort design. In the third variant, the retrospective cohort design, all of the data have already been collected at the time the research question is developed; the researchers extract the appropriate data, group participants based on a variable or variables of interest, and look for differences in a variety of predictor variables. In all of the variants, the researcher establishes the presence or absence of the risk factor first and then determines the presence or absence of the outcome of interest. This is the reverse of the case-control design, in which the outcome is established before the risk factors are identified.

A concurrent cohort design was used by Karver and associates[28] to study "the effects of age at injury on the persistence of behavior problems and social skill deficits in young children with complicated mild to severe traumatic brain injury (TBI)."[(p. 256)] The cohort consisted of children 3 to 7 years with a history of either severe ($N=19$) or moderate ($N=49$) TBI or orthopedic injury (OI; $N=75$). All were equated for similar histories of hospitalization and preexisting factors that might make them vulnerable to either TBI or OI. Approximately 1 to 2 months after injury, through parental retrospective rating, the investigators gained baseline information about the children's preinjury behavior problems, executive function, and social competence. The assessments were repeated no less than 24 months after the injury. Overall, with increasing time since injury, children who sustained severe TBI reported significantly higher levels of problematic behavioral symptoms than did children with OI. Symptoms included greater incidence of anxiety, attention deficit hyperactivity disorder, and executive dysfunction. The younger the children were at the time of injury, the greater the likelihood of these outcomes. Karver and associates[28] alerted rehabilitation professionals to the possible need for follow-up behavioral monitoring or treatment after TBI in children, most especially in younger children.

Zubrick and associates completed a prospective cohort study whose purpose was to "determine the prevalence of late language emergence (LLE) and to investigate the predictive status of maternal, family, and child variables."[29(p. 1562)] Noting mixed evidence regarding the predictive power of maternal educational and other socioeconomic factors and maternal talkativeness on language development in 24- to 36-month-old children, they recruited newborn children (1995–1996), ultimately ending with a random sample of 1766 children. After a 3-month follow-up, they converted the study to a longitudinal one and collected data by mailing a questionnaire at each child's birthday up to 8 years. The 2007 article reports on data obtained at years 1 and 2 with an 85% completion rate. The authors determined that 13.4% of the sample had LLE. Looking for characteristics related to the child, the mother, and the family at large, they found that the risk for late language emergence at 24 months was "not associated with particular strata of parental educational level, socioeconomic resources, parental mental health, parenting practices, or family functioning." They did find that family history of LLE was predictive, as were male sex and delayed early neurobiological growth.

A nonconcurrent cohort design was used in a study of return to work (RTW) among 323 Chinese laborers for a locomotive manufacturer, all of whom had sustained work-related injuries. He and colleagues[30] used company archival records to categorize workers injured from October 2004 through June 2008 and examined RTW rates after that period. Females who were included were 55 years or younger and males were 60 years or younger. Categories included demographic characteristics, clinical status (e.g., nature and extent of injuries), education level, salary history, and compensation for injury among others. Postinjury information was obtained through structured interviews. Ultimately, 93% of the workers returned to their jobs. Through univariate and multivariate analyses, the authors found that factors from sociodemographic, clinical, economic, and psychological domains affected RTW. Specifically, they found that "returning to the original job, full-time work, high satisfaction with RTW, and active asking for RTW were associated with shorter absenteeism."[(p. 380)] Workers 46 years or older had lower RTW rates. Less serious injuries were associated with higher RTWs. Higher pre-RTW salary was the only economic factor positively related to higher RTW rate.

Brennan, Parent, and Cleland[31] employed a retrospective cohort design to investigate the role of post-(shoulder) surgical physical therapy in predicting clinical outcomes. The retrospective data consisted of hospital records describing and classifying types of shoulder surgery in 856 adult patients. The patients were categorized into four surgical categories: repair of a unidirectional instability, rotator cuff repair, rotator cuff repair with a subacromial decompression, or subacromial decompression alone. Additionally, data were available describing scores on shoulder disability and pain at both initial and final physical therapy visits, as well as number of physical therapy sessions and length of hospital stay (LOS). Results indicated significant differences in outcomes between men and women. Women had greater disability than men in every surgical category except subacromial decompression alone. Both men and women improved in both pain and ability ratings. The authors point to the usefulness of their findings in considering prognoses for men and women undergoing shoulder repair.

SUMMARY

Epidemiology is the study of the distribution and determinants of disease and injury in populations. Common measures used in epidemiology include ratios, proportions, and rates. Prevalence is the proportion of existing cases of a disease or injury in a population at a particular point of time. Incidence is the rate of development of new cases of a disease or injury in a population at risk. Relative risk for disease or injury in different groups is expressed with risk ratios and odds ratios. Screening and diagnostic tests are evaluated by measures of sensitivity (the proportion of patients with the condition who test positive), specificity (the proportion of patients without the condition who test negative), and the likelihood ratios (usefulness for ruling in and ruling out diagnoses). In addition, predictive values for positive and negative tests can be calculated for populations with different proportions of individuals with disease or injury. Common epidemiological research designs include cross-sectional studies (subjects measured at one point in time), case-control studies (researchers work backward from effect to cause), and cohort studies (researchers work forward from cause to effect).

REFERENCES

1. Macha K, McDonough JP: Epidemiology and its progress. In Macha K, McDonough JP, editors: *Epidemiology for Advanced Nursing Practice*, Sudbury, Mass, 2012, Jones & Bartlett Learning, pp 1–26.
2. Saracci R: *Epidemiology: A Very Short Introduction*, Oxford, UK, 2010, Oxford University Press.
3. Hayes SC, Barlow DH, Nelson-Gray R: *The Scientist Practitioner*, Boston, Mass, 1999, Allyn & Bacon.
4. World Health Organization. International Classification of Health Interventions (ICHI). Available at: http://www.who.int/classifications/ichi/en/. Accessed December 3, 2014.
5. Hill JJ, Keating JL: A systematic review of the incidence and prevalence of low back pain in children, *Phys Ther Rev* 14(4):272–284, 2009.
6. Tanner CM, Goldman SM: Epidemiology of Parkinson's disease, *Neurol Clin* 14:317–335, 1996.

7. Bronstein J, Carvey P, Chen H, et al: Meeting report: Consensus statement. Parkinson's disease and the environment: Collaborative on Health and the Environment and Parkinson's Action Network (CHE PAN) Conference, June 26–28, 2007, *Environ Health Perspect* 117(1):117–121, 2009.

8. Diep L, Kwagyan J, Kurantsin-Mills J, et al: Association of physical activity level and stroke outcomes in men and women: A meta-analysis, *J Womens Health* 19:1815–1822, 2010.

9. Jekel JF, Elmore JG, Katz DL: *Epidemiology, Biostatistics, and Preventive Medicine*, 2nd ed, Philadelphia, Pa, 2001, WB Saunders.

10. Clark TW, Janzen DL, Logan PM, et al: Improving the detection of radiographically occult ankle fractures: Positive predictive value of an ankle joint effusion, *Clin Radiol* 51:632–636, 1996.

11. Green DM, Swets JA: *Signal Detection Theory and Psychophysics*, Huntington, NY, 1974, Krieger.

12. Swets JA: *Signal Detection Theory and ROC Analysis in Psychology and Diagnostics: Collected Papers*, Mahwah, NJ, 1996, Lawrence Erlbaum.

13. McGee S: Simplifying likelihood ratios, *J Gen Intern Med* 17(8):647–650, 2002. Also available at http://www.ncbi.nlm.nih.gov/pmc/articles/PMC1495095/ Accessed December 3, 2014.

14. Riegelman RK: *Studying a Study and Testing a Test: Reading Evidence-Based Health Research*, 6th ed, Philadelphia, Pa, 2013, Wolters Kluwer Health/Lippincott Williams & Wilkins.

15. Gerstman BB: *Epidemiology Kept Simple: An Introduction to Classic and Modern Epidemiology*, 2nd ed, New York, NY, 2003, Wiley-Liss.

16. Fletcher RH, Fletcher SW: *Clinical Epidemiology: The Essentials*, 4th ed, Philadelphia, Pa, 2005, Lippincott, Williams & Wilkins.

17. Schneiders AG, Sullivan SJ, Hendrick PA, et al: The ability of clinical tests to diagnose stress fractures: A systematic review and meta-analysis, *J Orthop Sports Phys Ther* 42:760–771, 2012.

18. Strand EA, McCauley RJ, Weigand SD, et al: A motor speech assessment for children with severe speech disorders: Reliability and validity evidence, *J Speech Lang Hear Res* 56:505–520, 2013.

19. Eyssen ICJM, Steultjens MPM, Oud TAM, et al: Responsiveness of the Canadian Occupational Performance Measure, *J Rehabil Res Dev* 48:517–528, 2011.

20. Page SJ, Fulk GD, Boyne P: Clinically important differences for the upper-extremity Fugl-Meyer scale in people with minimal to moderate impairment due to chronic stroke, *Phys Ther* 92(6):791–798, 2012.

21. Friedman GD: *Primer of Epidemiology*, 5th ed, New York, NY, 2004, McGraw-Hill Medical.

22. Resnik LJ, Borgia ML: Factors associated with utilization of preoperative and postoperative rehabilitation services by patients with amputation in the VA System: An observational study, *Phys Ther* 93(9):1197–1210, 2013.

23. O'Reilly C, Keogan F, Breen R, et al: Falls risk factors and healthcare use in patients with a low-trauma wrist fracture attending a physiotherapy clinic, *Int J Ther Rehabil* 20(10):480–486, 2013.

24. Curley ALC, Vitale PA: Applying epidemiological methods in population-based nursing practice. In Curley ALC, Vitale PA, editors: *Population-Based Nursing: Concepts and Competencies for Advanced Practice*, New York, NY, 2012, Springer, pp 75–98.

25. Ratnapradipa D, Robins AG, Ratnapradipa K: Preschool children's environmental exposures: A case-control epidemiological study of the presence of asthma-like symptoms, *J Environ Health* 76(4):12–17, 2013.

26. Hendrix R, Rohrer JE, Danawi H, Refaat A: Autism spectrum disorders: A sibling case-control study of maternal prenatal body mass index, *Int J Childbirth Educ* 27(4):79–83, 2012.

27. Aram D, Most T, Mayafit H: Contributions of mother-child storybook telling and joint writing to literacy development in kindergartners with hearing loss, *Lang Speech Hearing Serv Sch* 37:209–223, 2006.

28. Karver CL, Wade SL, Cassedy A, et al: Age at injury and long-term behavior problems after traumatic brain injury in young children, *Rehabil Psychol* 57:256–265, 2012.

29. Zubrick SR, Taylor CL, Rice ML, Slegers DW: Late language emergence at 24 months: An epidemiological study of prevalence, predictors, and covariates, *J Speech Lang Hear Res* 50:1562–1592, 2007.

30. He Y, Hu J, Yu ITS, et al: Determinants of return to work after occupational injury, *J Occup Rehabil* 20:378–386, 2010.

31. Brennan GP, Parent EC, Cleland JA: Description of clinical outcomes and postoperative utilization of physical therapy services within 4 categories of shoulder surgery, *J Orthop Sports Phys Ther* 40:20–29, 2010.

CHAPTER 16

Outcomes Research

CHAPTER OUTLINE

Purpose of Outcomes Research
Efficacy
Effectiveness
Frameworks for Outcomes Research
Nagi Model
International Classification of Impairments, Disabilities, and Handicaps
International Classification of Functioning, Disability, and Health
Measurement Tools for Outcomes Research

Self-Assessment and Other Rating Scales
Quality of Life
Health-Related Quality of Life
Short Form-36
PROMIS
Condition-Specific Tools
Patient-Specific Instruments
Satisfaction
Design Issues for Outcomes Research
Database Research
Review of Existing Medical Records
Abstracts of Medical Records

Administrative Databases
In-House Databases
National Outcomes Databases
Analysis Issues
Case Mix Adjustments
Techniques for Dealing with Missing Data
Survival Analysis
Comparisons Across Scales
Multivariate Statistics
Summary

For years, the randomized clinical trial (RCT) was the gold standard as a research paradigm for health care. RCTs were promoted as the standard of proof for drug trials and generalized to other types of therapies, including those for rehabilitation. The RCT has its basis as the pretest–posttest control group design, including assumption of true randomization—that is, groups representing the entire population of interest.

Over time, researchers and clinicians recognized some serious shortcomings of RCTs. For example, Hegde notes, "A researcher using the randomized group design usually cannot select participants [truly] randomly from a defined clinical population."[1(p. 125)] Thus, and perhaps even more important, the generalizability of RCTs to populations at large is questionable.[1] That is because, even when the sample in an RCT is large, there is little predictability of results to an individual receiving treatment. As Hicks[2] also indicates, RCTs are "often criticized for being reductionist and losing sight of the whole person or the real nature of the clinical condition."[(p. 8)] Another reason is that treatments in RCTs must adhere to strict protocols and uniform conditions in order to maximize internal validity. Although having some scientific merit, uniform conditions are not found in everyday clinical practice.

Another factor to consider is that RCTs, at least historically, concentrated on physiological changes as outcome measures per the influence of drug treatment trials. Over time, this focus has been realized as being inadequate to measure several important outcomes of value to patients, especially their emotional, occupational, communicative, and other outcomes that describe the totality of an individual's environment and his or her interactions in it. As the importance of these latter outcomes became recognized, the field of "outcomes research" emerged.

The outcomes movement in health care policy, practice, and research received widespread recognition during the 1990s and 2000s. Most writers attribute the emergence of the outcomes movement to (1) the need for cost containment in the health care sector, (2) the need to examine outcomes other than mortality, such as "health-related quality of life," when dealing with the increasingly prevalent chronic diseases of an aging society, and (3) the need to determine "best practices" and thereby reduce the great variations in health care that occur for reasons apparently unrelated to the characteristics of the group receiving care.[3–5]

Some early thinkers and writers about outcomes research[6,7] credit the conceptual basis for outcomes assessment to Avedis Donabedian, whose "structure, process, outcomes" framework influenced the design of the Medical Outcomes Study (MOS), an important outcomes project initiated in the late 1980s.[8]

As with many developing movements, there is neither widespread agreement about the definitions of various components related to health care outcomes nor agreement as to the boundaries of the outcomes movement. For example, as the incorporation of outcomes research has grown, the outcomes examined have expanded as well, such as quality of life beyond "health related."[9,10]

Consequently, the terms "outcomes" and "outcomes research" are used in different ways by the many participants in and observers of the health care system.[11,12] One area of commonality, however, is the shift in emphasis from looking for narrow biological effects of treatments delivered under highly controlled conditions to assessing the broad biopsychosocial impact of treatments implemented in typical clinical settings.[13] This shift, from what is termed "efficacy" to what is characterized as "effectiveness," has profound implications for the conduct of outcomes research. These implications extend from the nature of the overall research design to the selection of the dependent measures of interest. A general text that addresses many of these issues is *Conducting Health Outcomes Research* by Kane and Radosevich.[14]

The purpose of this chapter is to present an overview of the outcomes movement in rehabilitation research. First, the purpose of outcomes research is explored by contrasting the concepts of efficacy and effectiveness. Second, broad frameworks for outcomes research are presented. Third, several measurement tools consistent with these frameworks are described. Finally, design and implementation issues related to outcomes research are addressed.

PURPOSE OF OUTCOMES RESEARCH

One thing that has consistently been used to characterize the outcomes movement is the differentiation of "efficacy" and "effectiveness." Although he does not use these words, Kane identified the tension between these two concepts and between-the-research models that support each concept:

> If the practice of medicine (including rehabilitation) is to become more empiric, it will have to rely on epidemiological methods. Although some may urge the primacy of randomized clinical trials as the only path to true enlightenment, such a position is untenable for several reasons. First, the exclusivity of most trials is so great that the results are difficult to extrapolate to practice. Such trials may be the source of clinically important truths, but these findings will have to be bent and shaped to fit most clinical

situations. Second, researchers do not have the time or resources to conduct enough trials to guide all practice. Instead, we need a more balanced strategy that combines targeted trials with well-organized analysis of carefully recorded clinical practice.[15(p. JS22)]

As noted earlier in the text, RCTs have been considered the gold standard for health research because of their strict protocols, including randomized groupings, leading to high internal validity. Previously, however, we have also mentioned objections to RCTs brought forth by Hegde.[1] Primarily, because experimental participants usually self-select for clinical trials, the participant pool is not truly a random representation of the population of interest. Hegde also notes limited generalizability (external validity), stating, "generality of treatment effect is always a matter of replications, not of experimental designs. The sample size is irrelevant to generality."[1(p. 126)] For that reason, we also need a research paradigm in which results are generated under more "everyday" conditions, with high numbers of replications to establish external validity.

This duality emphasizes the importance of studying health care under ideal conditions through highly controlled experimental studies (e.g., RCTs) as well as through well-organized analysis of clinical practice as it actually occurs (outcomes research). In short, we need a balanced strategy that combines targeted trials with well-organized analysis of carefully recorded clinical practice.[15]

Efficacy

Efficacy is usually defined as the effect of treatment delivered under carefully controlled conditions. The research method that is best suited to determining efficacy is the randomized controlled trial, in which researchers control for a variety of factors that would interfere with an understanding of the impact of the treatment of interest. Thus, participants are selected to be relatively homogeneous, treatments are implemented in uniform ways, and dependent variables are selected because they are objective and relate directly to the expected biological effect of the treatment (see also the discussion of RCTs in Chapter 10). Research to determine efficacy focuses on the "does it work?" and "is it safe?" questions and does not often examine issues of cost, feasibility, and acceptability to practitioners and patients.

Effectiveness

In contrast, *effectiveness* is defined as the usefulness of a particular treatment to the individuals receiving it under typical clinical conditions. Nonexperimental research methods are often used to determine effectiveness. Rather than manipulating the treatment patients receive, as well as the conditions under which they receive it, researchers implementing nonexperimental designs examine the effectiveness of actual treatment that has already occurred or observe actual treatment as it is delivered. This is a messy process that usually results in heterogeneous groups of subjects, treatments that are implemented in various ways by different clinicians and patients, and dependent variables that focus on broader outcomes of interest to patients, payers, and practitioners. However, effectiveness can also be studied with experimental paradigms, especially those of single-subject research (see Chapter 11).

FRAMEWORKS FOR OUTCOMES RESEARCH

The shift from looking at narrow efficacy to broader effectiveness has required that practitioners develop broad-based frameworks to guide the way that they think about disease and injury, as well as the consequences of disease and injury. Three frameworks that have received widespread discussion within the rehabilitation literature include the Nagi model,[16] the World Health Organization (WHO) original International Classification of Impairments, Disabilities, and Handicaps (ICIDH),[17] and the revised WHO International Classification of Functioning, Disability, and Health (ICF).[18] Each of the three frameworks is presented here, followed by a summary of issues and refinements that have been articulated by others.

Nagi Model

Saad Nagi, a sociologist, first presented his model in 1964.[19] He revisited this original model as an appendix to a report of the Committee on a National Agenda for the Prevention of Disabilities,[16] a group appointed jointly by the Centers for Disease Control and Prevention and the National Council on Disability. His scheme, rooted in "disability," describes active pathology, impairment, functional limitation, and disability, as shown in the top row of Figure 16-1. For example, a man with osteoarthritis experiences inflammation (the active pathology, manifested at the cellular level), which contributes to muscle weakness and valgus deformity at the knees (the impairments, at the tissue, organ, or system level). He has difficulty walking long distances or climbing stairs (the functional impairment, at the level of the person), and he gives up his position as a field-based police officer because it involves more walking and stair climbing than is tolerable (the disability, at the level of social functioning).

International Classification of Impairments, Disabilities, and Handicaps

The WHO published its initial ICIDH in 1980.[17] This classification, a supplement to the International Classification of Diseases, Ninth Revision (ICD-9), was needed because of the inadequacies of the ICD-9 in addressing the long-term impact of chronic diseases. The ICIDH, as can be inferred from its name and as shown in the middle row of Figure 16-1, conceptualized the long-term sequelae of disease as impairments, disabilities, and handicaps; thus, this is also essentially a "disability"-based classification. For example, a man with osteoarthritis experiences inflammation (the disease, manifested at the cellular level) that leads to muscle weakness and valgus deformity at the knees (the impairments, at the tissue, organ, or system level). The person has difficulty walking long distances or climbing stairs (the disability, at the level of the person), and he changes from a field position as a police officer to a desk job because the demands of and architectural barriers in the field involve more walking and stair climbing than is tolerable (the handicap, at the level of society and the environment). Although the ICIDH has been replaced by the newer ICF described in the following section, it remains an important framework for rehabilitation professionals because much of the rehabilitation literature from the 1980s and 1990s uses ICIDH concepts and terminology.

International Classification of Functioning, Disability, and Health

A major reformulation of the ICIDH occurred with the endorsement of the ICF by the WHO Assembly in 2001.[18] Seen by some as a synthesis of the Nagi and ICIDH frameworks,[20] the ICF uses a different set of terms for key concepts (see bottom row of Figure 16-1). The concept of impairment is known in the ICF by "changes in body functions or structures." The terms "functional limitation" (Nagi), "disability" (Nagi and ICIDH), and "handicap" (ICIDH) are either not used or are used differently. The new terms are "activities," "participation," and "disability"; thus we see a change in emphasis from what people cannot do to what they can do. There are also other changes in emphasis. For one, there is recognition that disability is a "universal human experience."[21] Additionally, the framework sees disability/ability in its social context and, so, includes a list of "environmental factors."[21,22] Activities refer to functioning at an individual level and participation to functioning at a societal level. Disability is seen as the consequence of either activity limitations or

Nagi

Active Pathology	Impairment	Functional Limitation	Disability
Interruption or interference with normal processes and efforts of the organism to regain normal state	Anatomical, physiological, mental, or emotional abnormalities or loss	Limitation in performance at the level of the whole organism or person	Limitation in performance of socially defined roles and tasks within a sociocultural and physical environment

ICIDH

Disease	Impairment	Disability	Handicap
Intrinsic pathology or disorder	Loss or abnormality of psychological, physiological, or anatomical structure or function at organ level	Restriction or lack of ability to perform an activity in a normal manner	Disadvantage resulting from impairment or disability that limits or prevents fulfillment of a normal role (depends on age, sex, sociocultural factors for the person)

ICF

Body Functions and Structures	Activities	Participation
Changes in body functions (physiological) or structures (anatomical). When these changes are positive, they result in functional and structural integrity; when these changes are negative, they result in impairment	Functioning at an individual level Both activities and participation can be viewed in terms of capacity (ability to execute a task in a standard environment) and performance (executing tasks in the current environment) Disability occurs when activities are limited or participation in societal roles is restricted. Disability is modified by the environmental and personal context in which the individual functions.	Functioning at a societal level

Figure 16-1 Frameworks for Outcomes Research: Nagi Model; the International Classification of Impairments, Disabilities, and Handicaps (ICIDH); and the International Classification of Functioning, Disability, and Health (ICF). (The verbal descriptions of the Nagi and ICIDH models are from Jette AM: Physical disablement concepts for physical therapy research and practice, *Phys Ther* 74:380–386, 1994. Their presentation has been modified to show how the categories are related across the models. Used with permission of the American Physical Therapy Association. ICF descriptions are from World Health Organization. *International Classification of Functioning, Disability, and Health.* Available at: www.who.int/classification/icf. Accessed December 4, 2014.)

participation restrictions. Both activities and participation can be viewed in terms of "capacity" (the ability to execute a task in a standard environment) and performance (executing tasks in the current environment). Disability is seen as modifiable by the environment and personal context in which the individual functions. In ICF language, the same man with osteoarthritis of the knees would have impairments related to inflammation (a change in body function) and joint space narrowing (a change in body structure). Although he can walk

more than a mile and climb stairs if the terrain is level and there is only one flight of stairs (he retains walking and stair-climbing capacity in standard environmental contexts), he rarely performs these tasks in his daily life (his performance is indicative of an activity limitation, which is a disability at the individual level). He changes from a field position as a police officer to a desk job because the demands of as well as the architectural barriers in the field involve more walking, running, and stair climbing than is tolerable (this restriction in a societal job role is also a disability). His work disability is modified by environmental and personal contexts. For example, the field environment cannot change to accommodate his activity limitations, but an alternative administrative environment that meets his activity needs is available. This particular police officer has the personal attributes and abilities—organizational and computer skills, for example—to make the transition from field to desk work possible; others would not have these skills, and the disability would be much greater because the personal context would be a barrier to changing job roles.

The ICF appears to have addressed many of the concerns that individuals and groups had identified with either or both of the other frameworks. For example, Jette[23] was critical of the ICIDH scheme because it mingled both attribute (individual level) and relational (societal level) concepts within the "disability" category and because the "handicap" category did not clearly differentiate among individual characteristics and the social and environmental circumstances that place an individual with a disability at a disadvantage. The ICF clearly separates attribute (activities) and relational (participation) concepts, redefines disability to reflect limitations or restrictions at either level, and adds the modifying concepts of personal and environmental factors. Personal and environmental factors are critical to consider in the WHO ecological framework. A personal factor such as high motivation to succeed can optimize activity participation, whereas lack of motivation can contribute to lack of participation. An environmental factor such as the presence or absence of readily available and competent health care can maximize or minimize participation.

Another criticism of the earlier frameworks was the lack of differentiation between capacity and performance. For example, in a 1994 article, Verbrugge and Jette[24] discussed the importance of distinguishing between intrinsic disability (difficulty experienced when external assistance, either equipment or personnel, is not available) and actual disability (difficulty experienced when external assistance is available). Similarly, in 1997, Liang[25] identified three domains that enter into function: capacity (the level of impairment), will (psychological factors such as motivation and self-confidence), and need (the social and environmental context). The ICF tries to capture the complex interplay among these factors by differentiating between capacity (the ability to execute a task in a standard environment) and performance (executing tasks in the current environment).

Despite the differences among the frameworks, the complexity of the disablement process, and the difficulties with measurement within any of the models, these frameworks convey a central message that has shaped outcomes research in rehabilitation. The message is that simply measuring changes in body structures and functions is insufficient for the study of person-level concepts such as activity, participation, and disability. Rehabilitation professionals have received this message and have changed the ways in which they measure outcomes in both clinical and research settings. The next section of this chapter highlights measures that reflect the person-level categories within the disablement models.

MEASUREMENT TOOLS FOR OUTCOMES RESEARCH

Clinicians and researchers have long used measures of pathology (e.g., laboratory values and imaging techniques) and measures of changes in body functions and structures (e.g., range of motion, muscle performance) to guide their practice and to serve as dependent measures in research studies. Outcomes research, or an outcomes focus to practice, generally means that researchers and practitioners supplement these measures of pathology and bodily changes with person-level measures of activity, participation, or disability. This section of the chapter is designed to provide an overview of these person-level measures.

Similarities are evident between topics presented here and the principles of qualitative research discussed in Chapter 14. Outcomes research takes into account, for example, the multiple realities constructed by individuals as they are faced with clinical conditions. Outcomes research is largely nonexperimental and integrates the value systems of patients/clients. There may also be more similarity in methodology than seems immediately apparent. Kennedy,[26] for example, makes the case that adaptation of rating scales and ethnographic research overlap to a large extent. In addition, Alpiner and Schow note, "Self-assessment [using rating scales] is really a form of case history interview."[27(p. 309)]

Self-Assessment and Other Rating Scales

A major feature of outcomes research is the use of rating scales as dependent measures. The construction and use of a rating scale is inherently subjective and therefore quite different from a more standardized measure, such as range of motion or mean length of utterance. For that reason, researchers should be aware of design issues in creating scales for outcomes research.

Demorest and DeHaven[28] provided an overview of the necessary psychometric components in the development of self-assessments and other types of rating scales. As researchers contemplate using a scale of any kind for outcomes research, they should account for three broad issues defined by these authors: (1) construct definition, (2) target population, and (3) anticipated use of the scale.

Any self-assessment or other rating scale must meet criteria for validity, as discussed in Chapter 8. That is, the concepts or "constructs" used in the scale must be relevant to the clinical or other research questions raised. Demorest and DeHaven indicate, "It is important for a test developer to state explicitly how each construct is conceptualized."[28](p. 315) Later writers have used Demorest and DeHaven's recommendations to advantage. For example, Ivarsson and colleagues needed to be explicit about terms in validating the construct validity of the Global Quality of Life scale.[29] If the researcher is satisfied that constructs have been delineated and are appropriate, he or she should next look at content validity—that is, how the scale's authors determined that test items (1) exhaust the domains of the constructs and (2) are all relevant to the constructs. He or she should also look for whether the authors used any other measures as criterion measures—that is, how they determined criterion validity.

Demorest and DeHaven stated, "Identification of the target population is important because it has an impact on decisions regarding administration format, response options, reading level, and even test content."[28](p. 315) Scale items then should be pertinent to that population, and the researcher should note how the authors determined the relevance. Demorest and DeHaven are careful to note, "It cannot be assumed that instruments developed within and for one population will maintain their psychometric characteristics in another population."[28](p. 315)

Scales may be for different purposes and should note the authors' intention. For example, many scales are intended only as screening instruments, to be followed up with more complete diagnosis if necessary. In outcomes research, the scales will be for the purpose of comparing behavior before and after treatment. In this case, Demorest and DeHaven[28] note implications for test content.

Pay careful attention to how a scale was developed. Demorest and DeHaven noted, "Instruments intended for widespread clinical and research use should be developed and refined in a series of stages."[28](p. 316) That is, test development should have occurred by more than a BOPSAT ("bunch of people sitting around a table," even if they are experts). After defining a measurement's object and content domain, test items are written. Test items may be developed by recourse to experts, existing scales, and even focus groups of the target population (remember qualitative research?). The authors should describe a trial or pilot period using a large sample representative of the target population and then refine the scale. Authors should describe item response frequencies, means, standard deviations, skewness, item-total correlations, factor analysis, and measurements of reliability.

These psychometric descriptions should guide administration and scoring, recalling that the psychometric properties were developed typically under one set of conditions. Although researchers might vary from these to meet some clinical need, it is probably not advisable when using a scale for research.

Quality of Life

Quality of life is a global concept that can include elements as diverse as perceptions of health, satisfaction with the work environment, quality of family and social relationships, satisfaction with schools and neighborhoods, productive use of leisure time, connections with one's spiritual nature, and financial well-being. Although problems in many of these areas can lead to health-related problems associated with stress, poor eating habits, sedentary lifestyles, and tobacco, alcohol, and drug use, global measures of quality of life are so broad as to have limited use in health care research and practice settings.

Health-Related Quality of Life

Because quality of life, as a global concept, is limited in its usefulness in health care research, a variety of measures of health-related quality of life (HRQL) have been developed. These measures have also been termed "health status" and "outcomes" measures. They may also be referred to as "generic" tools because they are designed for use with individuals with health conditions of all types, although their suitability for use with some populations has been questioned. For example, Lefebvre and associates described several barriers to the use of HRQL measurements in cardiac physical therapy rehabilitation.[30] However, Hefford and colleagues[31] noted, "In the clinical setting, outcome measurement may be used in clinical audit to inform patients, therapists, managers, and health care funding agencies whether relevant goals are being met (or not) in an efficient and timely manner. In research, outcome measures (OMs) may be used, for example, in controlled trials to determine whether one type of intervention is superior to another."(p. 155)

There is no doubt that HRQL is being used increasingly. A search on Cumulative Index to Nursing and Allied Health Literature (CINAHL) for the period

January 2009 to December 2013 revealed 117 journal articles using HRQL in occupational therapy, physical therapy, and speech-language pathology/audiology. Topics included such diverse foci as HRQL related to aphasia, specific language impairment in childhood, hemiparesis following stroke, multiple sclerosis, anterior cruciate ligament reconstruction, quality and quantity of interests in older persons, and occupational proficiency in people with schizophrenia. Age range of research subjects spanned from early childhood to nonagenarians. Many of the reports were studies of the HRQL outcomes associated with various therapies, such as qigong,[32] exercise training for patients with multiple sclerosis,[33] progressive resistance with counseling,[34] cochlear implantation,[35] and client-centered occupational therapy.[36]

There is general agreement that measures of HRQL should include elements related to physical, social, psychological/emotional, and cognitive functioning.[14,37] Because many of these measures have been well described by others,[14,37] only two currently in widespread use are described here.

Short Form-36

The Medical Outcomes Study (MOS), begun in the late 1980s, was designed to develop patient outcome tools and to monitor variations in outcome based on differences in health care systems, clinician styles, and clinician specialties.[8] One of the major tools to come out of this study is the Short Form-36, commonly known as the SF-36. The self-report includes 36 items covering eight domains of functioning: (1) role limitation caused by physical problems, (2) role limitation caused by emotional problems, (3) social functioning, (4) mental health, (5) pain, (6) energy, (7) fatigue, and (8) general health perceptions. The SF-36 is scored to produce a profile of the eight domains, each with scores ranging from 0 to 100, with higher scores representing better health. The eight scores are used to derive two summary scales: the physical component summary (PCS) and the mental component summary (MCS). Although this tool takes only about 10 minutes to complete, the desire for an even briefer tool has led to its modification into a shorter tool known as the SF-12. This 12-item tool includes one or two items from each of the eight components of the SF-36.[38] Melville and associates[39] found the SF-12 to be as reliable and sensitive as the SF-36 in distinguishing symptom severity in myocardial infarction survivors. Further, in a large health interview survey, Cunillera and colleagues[40] found that the SF-12 "showed a good capacity to distinguish between groups defined by socio-demographic and health variables,"[(p. 858)] although they noted that the scale "did,

however, generally show poorer discriminative capacity for chronic physical conditions [than two other scales used]."[(p. 858)]

The SF-36 has been used as one of the major health status measures in many rehabilitation research studies, including randomized controlled trials, outcomes research as defined in this chapter, and many descriptive and relationship analysis studies. For example, Angst and colleagues[41] found that the SF-36 "can be recommended as a responsive instrument for measurement of pain and function in chronic whiplash syndrome."[(p. 142)] Cabral and associates[42] found the SF-36 to be a useful measure of for the assessment of quality of life of chronic stroke subjects. In addition, they found that the SF-36 yielded better results and appeared to be more appropriate than the Nottingham Health Survey.

Jones and associates[43] used it as a measure of global function in a study that determined preoperative predictors of function after total knee arthroplasty. The SF-36 has also recently been adapted for use in telehealth. Turner-Bowker and associates[44] modified the SF-36 to be used as an adaptive, computerized version (the DYNHA SF-36). They examined its usefulness in 100 patients with HIV who could participate in face-to-face interviews and 100 who could not. They concluded, "The DYNHA SF-36 may be a promising tool for measuring the impact of HIV and its treatment on HRQOL outcomes."[(p. 893)]

We should make a particular note regarding the SF-36 (and probably every other scale) when used with populations whose native language is not English (or not the language in which the scale was developed). Bennett and Riegel[45] compared the U.S. Spanish version of the SF-36 to normed scores of the standard English version in 65 elderly Mexican participants (78% female). Although they found that the scales were largely equivalent in this case, they caution, "It is difficult to determine whether measured health disparities are the result of actual differences or due to measurement error resulting from translation or conceptual differences." On the other hand, we should note that Cunillera and colleagues[40] successfully used a Spanish version of SF-12 with their participants (whose first language was actually Catalan) and that Cabral and associates[42] employed a previously validated Portuguese version of the SF-36.

PROMIS

In the early 2000s, the National Institutes of Health (NIH) wanted to promote the development of health outcomes measures that would "use modern measurement theory to assess patient-reported health status for physical, mental, and social well-being to reliably and validly measure patient-reported outcomes (PROs) for clinical research and practice."[46] In 2004, the NIH granted funding to six research centers to develop the instruments. The result was the Patient Reported Outcome Measurement Information System, or PROMIS. In 2010, the number of participating research centers was increased to 12. PROMIS was to have uniqueness in four areas: (1) comparability with other scales, (2) high reliability and validity, (3) flexibility, and (4) inclusiveness (different languages and ages). The result is "measures ... available for use across a wide variety of chronic diseases and conditions and in the general population."[46] Thus, PROMIS measures cover physical, mental, and social health and can be used across chronic conditions, rather than for a specific condition. The PROMIS instruments can also be used for research. Its Web site states that PROMIS "can be used in clinical, observational, comparative effectiveness, health services and health policy research."[46]

PROMIS has three areas of development: (1) PRO (patient-reported outcomes) Measure Development Standards to develop instruments; (2) PRO Measures, that is, the instruments themselves, which are available for both adults and children 8 to 17 years in several languages; and (3) administrative software.

Item Response Therapy and Computer Adaptive Testing PROMIS aims to improve PRO measurement quality and precision and does this in part through item response theory (IRT). IRT has been used extensively in educational research and has more recently been applied to health outcomes research. "Statistical models based on IRT produce scores (that is, calibrations) associated with answers to questions. These calibrations provide computer software with the information it needs to select the most informative follow-up question to an initial question. This computer software is called Computer Adaptive Testing (CAT) because the content of the assessment, that is the questions that are asked, adapts to the patient based on his or her responses to the previous question."[46] Using IRT and CAT, the questions asked of a patient or research participant are narrowed down to the most salient, thus saving time and energy of both the patient and the clinician/researcher. Highly informative questions are selected so that test administrators may estimate scores that represent a person's standing on a domain (e.g., physical functioning, depression) with the minimal number of questions and without a loss in measurement precision. Because of the use of IRT and CAT, PROMIS scales can be used in short forms as well as longer forms.

Instruments, Current and Under Development Measurement in all PROMIS instruments is guided by "domains" of inquiry for both adults and children.

Broad domains for adults are (1) global health, (2), physical health, (3) mental health, and (4) social health. Each is composed of subdomains scores that constitute a profile for that domain. In physical health, for example, subdomains relate to pain, fatigue, sleep, and physical function. Mental health includes depression and anxiety. Social health includes satisfaction with participation in social roles. There are also additional domains for each. One of the main objectives of PROMIS is to compile a core set of questions to assess the most common or salient dimensions of patient-relevant outcomes for the widest possible range of chronic disorders and diseases.

There are three types of PROMIS instruments. Short forms are a fixed set of items administered in their entirety. Short forms typically include 4 to 10 items per domain. Profiles are full scales, a fixed collection of short forms measuring multiple concepts such as physical function. The third type of instrument, CAT, must be administered by computer and is highly reliant on IRT.

With a broad-ranging bank of items and forms, the PROMIS system contains many item banks associated with many health concepts or domains. In selecting an instrument, the user must first determine the subset of domains to measure. Thus, the scientist-practitioner can validly select subsets to suit the clinical or research questions of interest.

Several scales are currently available in Spanish and some are in German; scales in other languages are planned.[47] A complete list of instruments is available on the NIH Web site.[48]

Validation PROMIS instruments have been subjected to rigorous validation testing. A summary of the process is available online.[49] Several of the scales have been the subject of disorder- or disease-specific validation testing.[50] Hinchcliff and colleagues[51] determined good construct validity of PROMIS when used to assess health status and dyspnea outcomes in patients with systemic sclerosis. Fries, Rose, and Krishnan[52] found PROMIS to be more sensitive than the SF-36 to changes in patients with arthritis.

Condition-Specific Tools

In addition to generic health status instruments, a variety of condition-specific tools have been developed. Atherly[53] provides an overview of differences between condition-specific and generic measures. Hundreds of condition-specific tools exist, ranging from well-tested tools that have been translated into many languages and used widely in research to little-tested tools that are never used by researchers other than the instrument developer. Table 16-1 presents a synopsis of several condition-specific tools that are relevant to rehabilitation research, providing basic information about each tool, one or more references about the measurement characteristics of the tool, and one or more references to research using the tool as an outcome measure.[43,54-89] Note that the "conditions" to which the tools are "specific" range from specific primary diagnoses (e.g., stroke and hearing loss), to general primary diagnoses (e.g., low back pain and osteoarthritis), to secondary conditions seen in rehabilitation (e.g., fatigue and depression), and to body regions (e.g., arm, shoulder, and hand).

The profession of audiology has generated literally dozens of condition-specific (i.e., hearing disability) self-assessment scales and similar instruments. Typically, these scales have items in three domains: (1) difficulty of various listening situations, (2) emotional reactions of both the hearing-impaired person and those around her, and (3) adjustments to the disability by either the hearing-impaired person or those around her. Two well-known scales are included in Table 16-1. Many of the scales are reproduced in Alpiner and McCarthy[90] and Hull.[91]

Condition-specific rating scales have also been developed in speech-language pathology. There are, for example, scales for stroke,[92,93] voice disorders,[94,95] and stuttering.[96] Eadie and colleagues[97] examined the ability of various rating scales in measuring "communicative participation," attempting to incorporate concepts from the ICF. At that time, Eadie and colleagues concluded none of the scales examined provided an adequate measure, but this was an important step in integrating outcomes research concepts. Later work by Baylor and associates[98] helped develop a scale that better measured "communicative participation."

Patient-Specific Instruments

Although the use of generic and condition-specific outcomes measures for research with groups of individuals has ballooned over the past two decades, many of the tools are not very responsive to individual changes in functional status, thereby limiting their clinical utility. The patient-specific class of outcome measures is a group of tools designed to identify individualized goals and detect individual changes in status related to those goals.[99]

Generic patient-specific instruments can be used with patients or clients with any type of problem. One scale with a long history of use in psychotherapy and more recent use in rehabilitation is Goal Attainment Scaling (GAS).[100,101] With GAS, individualized problems are identified, and a continuum of five possible outcomes related to each problem is developed. Scoring is standardized, with the most unfavorable outcome

scored as $\simeq 2$, less than the expected outcome as $\simeq 1$, the expected outcome as 0, a greater than expected outcome as +1, and the most favorable outcome likely as +2.[100] The same highly individualized approach, but with a different scoring system, is found in the Canadian Occupational Performance Measure (COPM)[99,102] and the Patient-Specific Functional Scale (PSFS).[99,103] The GAS approach is still often used. It has been used for measuring outcomes in autism.[101] Hale[104] used GAS to measure progress in a home program of stroke rehabilitation. Using GAS, Steenbeek and colleagues[105] measured progress toward parents' goals for their children with cerebral palsy.

In a variation of generic patient-specific instruments, providers and clients choose from a menu of goal statements rather than generating highly individualized problems and goals.[106,107] For example, in Beurskens and colleagues'[107] study of a patient-specific approach to measuring functional status in individuals with low back pain, they presented patients with a list of 36 activities that are often limited by low back pain. Patients could, however, identify problematic activities not on the list.

Patient-specific tools that are also disorder specific are available. The McMaster Toronto Arthritis (MACTAR) scale includes a list of activities expected to be affected by arthritis. Five priority items are selected, and changes in status are scored on the 3-point scale of worse, no change, and improved.[99] The American Speech-Language-Hearing Association (ASHA) uses a disorder-specific, patient-specific tool as the outcome measure in its National Outcomes Measurement System.[108] A large set of Functional Communication Measures (FCMs), with subsets specific to different communication disorders, has been developed by ASHA, with each measure scored on a 7-point scale appropriate to the item and disorder. FCMs are categorized either for adults or for pre-kindergarten children. In 2008, 8 of the FCMs from the Adult National Outcomes Measurement System (NOMS) were submitted to the National Quality Forum for review. All 8 were endorsed and subsequently became part of the public domain. To provide ease of access, all 15 adult NOMS FCMs are now available for download.[108] It is important to note that the FCMs are only one component of NOMS.

Satisfaction

Satisfaction is seen as an important outcome of treatment as well as an indicator of the effectiveness of various structures and processes within the health care system. The health status measures described in the previous section may demonstrate changes in status

Table 16-1

A Sampler of Condition-Specific Tools for Rehabilitation

Tool	Characteristics	Research About the Tool	Research Using the Tool
Stroke-Adapted Sickness Impact Profile	30-item, 8-scale version of the Sickness Impact Profile, adapted for individuals with stroke	van Straten et al, 1997[54] Van de Port et al, 2004[55] Buck et al, 2000[56]	van Straten et al, 2000[57] Zedlitz et al, 2012[58] Huijbregts et al, 2009[59]
Oswestry Disability Index	Measures 10 areas of perceived disability related to low back pain: pain intensity, changing pain status, personal hygiene, lifting, walking, sitting, standing, sleeping, social activity, and traveling. Scoring is converted to a percentage, with a higher score representing a higher percentage of disability.	Fairbank & Pynsent, 2000[60] Lochhead & MacMillan, 2013[61]	Flynn et al, 2003[62] Nunn, 2012[63]
Western Ontario and McMaster University Osteoarthritis Index (WOMAC)	24-item tool with 3 subscales: joint pain, physical joint function, and joint stiffness. Available in 60 alternative language forms.	Bellamy, 2002[64] Kennedy et al, 2003[65] Baron et al, 2007[66] McKay et al, 2013[67]	Jones et al, 2003[43] Wagenmakers et al, 2008[68] Elbaz et al, 2011[69]
Disabilities of the Arm, Shoulder, and Hand (DASH)	30-item scale measuring self-reported upper-extremity disability and symptoms. Scores on individual items are summed and converted to a scale with a range from 0 to 100, with higher scores representing greater disability.	Gummesson et al, 2003[70] Mousavi et al, 2008[71] Franchignoni et al, 2010[72]	Østlie et al, 2011[73] Thormodsgard et al, 2011[74] Rostami et al, 2013[75]
Fatigue Questionnaire	14 items assessing physical and mental fatigue and duration and extent of fatigue. Maximum score of 33, with physical and mental fatigue subscores.	Chalder et al, 1993[76]	Jahnsen, 2003[77]
Hearing Handicap Inventory for the Elderly	A scale of 25 questions answered on a 3-point yes/no/not applicable scale. Has an "emotional" scale and a "social/situational" scale.	Ventry & Weinstein, 1982[78] Newman & Weinstein, 1989[79] Jupiter & Delgado, 2003[80] Deepthi & Kasthuri, 2012[81]	Jupiter, 2009[85] Saito et al, 2010[86] Silverman et al, 2011[87]
Communication Profile for the Hearing Impaired (CPHI)	A scale of 145 questions examining 25 scales. Divided into three parts asking about (1) communication situations, (2) communication management skills, and (3) attitudes and feelings.	Demorest & Erdman, 1987[82] Erdman, 2006[83] Mokkink et al, 2009[84]	Chisolm et al, 2004[88] Lewis et al, 2005[89]

over the course of treatment yet still fail to indicate whether the extent of change met the expectation of the patient. Conversely, some patients may be satisfied with only little improvement in health status.

Measurements of patient satisfaction provide this important perspective. In addition to satisfaction with the outcomes of care, patients' opinions may be sought on other structural and process dimensions of the health care system: accessibility and convenience of care, availability of resources, continuity of care, efficacy/outcomes of care, finances, humaneness, information gathering, information giving, pleasantness of surroundings, and quality of caregivers. Input into the structure and process of health care is seen as important because it can help health care entities organize themselves more effectively. For example, a survey of patients who had received nursing services in a community health center found only moderate levels of satisfaction.[109] The authors used the results to recommend reforming community health nursing care policies to place more attention on increasing the level of coordination and the interpersonal aspects of the provided care to increase their satisfaction.

Satisfaction is also important because it may be related indirectly to clinical outcomes if it affects appointment keeping and adherence to treatment recommendations. In a review article about satisfaction research, Di Palo[110] discussed several national efforts to collect satisfaction data. As is the case with health status tools, both global and condition-specific satisfaction tools have been developed. In addition, many tools are developed by individual facilities for their own use each year. In contrast to the health status tools, a few of which enjoy widespread popularity for clinical and research use, there seem to be, as yet, no clear "winners" in the satisfaction instrument sweepstakes. Similarly, in a systematic review of satisfaction studies in residential centers for care of elderly residents, Yun-Hee and colleagues[111] found a wide range of domains used, most often reflecting the particular needs of the study or organization. The authors were able to identify seven domains that seemed to be common among studies but indicated that further work is needed to develop a single more widely usable satisfaction instrument, at least for that population. Kane and Radosevich[14(pp. 159–198)] and Smith and colleagues[112] provide an overview of many of the issues related to measurement of satisfaction in health care settings.

DESIGN ISSUES FOR OUTCOMES RESEARCH

Although research of any type can have person-level outcomes as dependent measures, outcomes research, as defined by the focus on effectiveness, is about much more than simply broadening the measurement tools used in research. It also involves a commitment to studying care as it actually occurs, rather than under the ideal, controlled conditions of experimental research. Therefore, for the purpose of this chapter, outcomes research is also assumed to imply a set of methods related to the assessment of care as it occurs in the real world. The design elements that characterize outcomes research, as they are presented here, include nonexperimental design and the analysis of information contained in various health care databases.

Database Research

The databases used in outcomes research can be medical records themselves, computerized abstracts of medical records, health care insurance claims databases, databases generated within one's own facility or within a network of facilities associated with a large health care conglomerate, or participation in national databases that combine data from clinical entities from many regions. In the United States and the United Kingdom, recent changes to health care privacy regulations have presented outcomes researchers with new challenges related to gaining access to these databases, as noted in Chapters 5.[113–115]

Review of Existing Medical Records

Medical records themselves may be used as sources of data in outcomes projects. The biggest advantage to using medical records is that they contain a great deal of information that can be evaluated in context. However, this advantage is balanced by at least two disadvantages. First, reviewing records is a time-consuming process that requires the personnel extracting the data to make judgment calls about which of the many pieces of information is relevant to the questions at hand. Second, the information in medical records is often inconsistent and incomplete. Kane and Radosevich note that clinical data "are not collected systematically."[14(p. 281)] Both of these disadvantages have the impact of reducing the available sample size that can be generated for a given project.

Abstracts of Medical Records

The various reporting mechanisms required for billing, reporting, and accreditation processes mean that records of hospitalization are routinely abstracted, summarized on a "facesheet," and computerized at discharge. Use of this computerized information is time efficient for the researcher and generally ensures that there is a common data set on all patients of interest. One problem with the abstracted information is that there may be errors in coding the information, including diagnoses, comorbidities, and complications. A study that compared facesheet information with information in the medical chart of patients with hip fracture found that there was an error rate of 12% related to diagnoses, 17% related to complications, and 16% related to surgical procedures.[116] It is clear, though, that use of electronic medical records will significantly increase. "As of January 1, 2014, all public and private healthcare providers and other eligible professionals (EP) must have adopted and demonstrated 'meaningful use' of electronic medical records (EMR) in order to maintain their existing Medicaid and Medicare reimbursement levels."[117] However, Kern and associates,[118] examining electronic reports of quality, found wide measure-by-measure variations in accuracy, threatening the validity of electronic reporting.

In addition to this concern about the accuracy of the data, the information in the abstract is often less specific than desired by the researcher, so "proxy" measures are used instead of the real measures of interest. For example, researchers who wish to eliminate chronically depressed patients from their sample might screen out patients taking antidepressant medication. If antidepressant medications are used for conditions other than chronic depression, or if many patients receive antidepressants for a short period after an acute health care event, then many relevant patients may be excluded from the study. Conversely, if depression is prevalent but often untreated, many depressed patients may not be screened from the analysis.

Administrative Databases

Administrative data include information from the federal government (e.g., Medicare), state governments (e.g., Medicaid), private insurers, and regulatory agencies.[14] All but the last of these refer essentially to billing and/or insurance. Chan and colleagues[119] and Freburger and Konrad[120] summarized specific issues in using the Medicare database. Kane and Radosevich[14] note several advantages to using administrative data: (1) large numbers of study subjects, (2) highly representative data, (3) linkable records that facilitate tracking individuals over time, (4) standardized data content and formats, and (5) use of preexisting data so that no additional data collection is required. At the same time, these authors note several limitations: (1) inability to include subjects who do not have medical insurance, (2) variations in coding among agencies, (3) lack of unique identifiers for combining and merging patient data sets, and (4) lack of insurance coverage (leading to lack of data) for procedures that the insurer does not cover (and these commonly include measures of HRQL).(p. 291) Despite the

limitations, Cullen and colleagues[121] found insurance claims databases to be a valuable source for research.

In-House Databases

To solve many of the problems with the use of medical records, abstracts of medical records, and administrative databases, facilities may choose to develop and manage their own outcomes databases. Experience in developing such databases was described by Shields and colleagues[122] and, more recently, by Hordacre and associates.[123]

Developing one's own database is a time-consuming, expensive venture. For example, the project reported by Hordacre and associates[123] took place over a 15-year period. In the project described by Shields and colleagues,[122] staff at the University of Iowa Hospitals and Clinics began the development process in 1986, began collecting data in 1991, and began retrieving data in 1993. This long-term commitment was feasible for a teaching hospital with a research mission and access to university resources in instrument development, computer systems, and research design and analysis. Hospitals in large systems, extended care and rehabilitation facilities that are part of a nationwide system, or outpatient clinics that are affiliated with a national corporation may also have the resources to pursue this type of a database and may find competitive business reasons to collect this information even if they do not have primary research missions.

Despite the time and money involved in creating an in-house database, there are many benefits to doing so. In-house outcomes systems may have high levels of use by staff members who participate in the development process, have local control of the training process for staff members who contribute information to the database, and have staff who are able to design data collection tools to answer specific questions of interest within the setting.

National Outcomes Databases

Clinical leaders who wish to involve their facilities in outcomes research may not believe that developing an in-house database is the best solution. They may not have the resources to develop and maintain a system, and they may wish to be able to compare the care at their facilities with that delivered in other centers. Participating in a national outcomes database gives clinics access to the needed resources and allows them to "benchmark" their practices against other similar clinics in the database. In addition, in comparison to in-house databases, the pooling of data from many clinics may increase sample size, enhance statistical power, and improve the generalizability of research results generated from the database.

National databases in the United States exist as government, professional, and commercial enterprises. For example, the National Institute on Disability and Rehabilitation Research (NIDRR) sponsors three model systems in burn, spinal cord injury (SCI), and traumatic brain injury (TBI) care. One component of each model system is an outcomes database.[124-126] As of December, 2011, the National Spinal Cord Injuries Database (established in 1973) associated with the Model Spinal Cord Injury Systems contained data on 28,450 individuals with SCI.[127] Despite the promise of such a database, the National Spinal Cord Statistical Center reported that the database captures data from an estimated 13% of new SCI cases in the United States.[127] Longitudinal data are spotty because treatment centers have moved in and out of the model system, HRQL data have only been collected for the last few years, and there are large gaps in the economic data within the database.[128] Despite these limitations, the SCI model system database has been used for outcomes research about individuals with SCI, as in Lysack and colleagues' study examining self-rated health in SCI survivors.[129]

The Uniform Data System for Medical Rehabilitation (UDSMR), with relationships with more than 1400 facilities worldwide, sponsors outcomes databases that currently house more than 13 million patient assessments that include scores on its well-known Functional Independence Measure (FIM) and WeeFIM (the FIM instrument adapted for children and adolescents) instruments and several other FIM adaptations. The UDSMR was established in the 1980s with government funding from the NIDRR and co-sponsorship from the American Congress of Rehabilitation Medicine, the American Academy of Physical Medicine and Rehabilitation, and several other national professional organizations.[130]

The NOMS of ASHA is an example of an association-sponsored national outcomes database.[108] As noted earlier in this chapter, the outcomes measures used in this database are a set of ASHA-developed FCMs selected for each patient according to their individual conditions and needs and their communication or swallowing disorder. As described by ASHA, "Based on an individual's treatment plan/IEP, FCMs are chosen and scored by a certified speech-language pathologist on admission and again at discharge to depict the amount of change in communication and/or swallowing abilities after speech and language intervention." By examining the scores from admission and discharge, clinicians can assess the amount of change and, thus, the benefits of treatment. Speech-language pathologists in health care facilities, preschools, and schools can participate in NOMS and can contribute data after they are trained and registered in the use of the FCMs.

Focus on Therapeutic Outcomes, Inc. (FOTO), is a widely used commercial outcomes database for rehabilitation.[131] Developed in 1993 through a grant from several national rehabilitation companies, it is now privately owned. Subscribers collect a number of standard outcomes measures (such as the SF-36 and Oswestry scales) on their patients and submit them to FOTO for inclusion in the database. FOTO provides benchmarking reports to subscribers that enable them to compare their outcomes against national norms.

Although participation in national outcomes databases, such as those just outlined, has the advantages of access to resources and benchmarking information, there may be considerable reluctance on the part of rehabilitation professionals to participate in the process. For example, several national outcomes projects in prosthetics and orthotics did not garner the necessary participation from prosthetists and orthotists in the field,[132] and Russek and colleagues[133] were disappointed by the level of therapist participation in data collection for a database for a multisite corporation with 71 clinics nationwide. These investigators explored these participation issues by surveying therapists who should have been able to participate in their data collection effort. Five major factors concerning attitudes about standardized data collection were identified: inconvenience of the data collection tool, lack of acceptance of the operational definitions used for the data collection effort, lack of automation of the process, the paperwork load within the clinic in general, and training issues. They also found that clinics with a staff member responsible for the organization and management of the data collection effort tended to have higher levels of participation. Together, these factors seem to indicate that administrators who wish for their facilities to participate in national outcomes databases should attend to the convenience of doing so for individual staff members and should also work to enhance "buy-in" by providing local support to the effort and improving the training of staff for the data collection effort.

However, not all investigators have found the same obstacles. The National Athletic Trainers' Association completed an early high school athletics injury surveillance project with a database of 23,566 injuries documented by athletic trainers at more than 250 different schools nationwide.[134] In its series of NOMS reports of the period 2006 to 2010, ASHA summarized data in its adult section alone of more than 81,000 cases.[135] Consistent with recent data, Loan and associates[136] found a high degree of participation in developing their outcomes database for military nurses (although their military status may have had an impact on participation rate). Richardson and colleagues[137] examined some of the barriers to implementing the NIH Stroke Scale linked to an outcomes database and found, through an education program, an increase from 12% to 69% over the course of their project. It seems that, as notions of outcome measures continue to gain use, overall participation has increased in recent years.

Analysis Issues

The design of outcomes research studies has a major impact on the way in which the data are analyzed. Because the foundation needed to understand statistical analysis issues has not yet been laid, these statistical issues are introduced briefly here and followed up in more detail in Section Seven (see Chapters 20 through 24).

Case Mix Adjustments

Because outcomes research studies tend to be nonexperimental, the researcher has little or no control over which patients are placed into which groups within the study. Thus, there are often important differences among study groups, some of which occur because there are systematic biases in the way that clinical decisions are made. For example, older adults with more active lifestyles may seek total knee replacement as a treatment for osteoarthritis, whereas less active patients may choose more conservative care. Differences in outcomes between these two groups, then, might be the result of preoperative lifestyles rather than the treatment of interest. In addition, if the outcomes reported are to be compared with outcomes in other facilities or regions, researchers need to ensure that they are "benchmarking" themselves against comparable groups.[14,138]

There are two general ways to deal with case mix problems in outcomes research. The first is to stratify the groups and compare only those subgroups that have, for example, similar ages, comorbidities, or disease or condition severity. The second way of managing case mix problems is to mathematically adjust the data so that two groups with, for example, different average ages are equalized in some way. Sometimes this is done by "weighting" subgroups within the analysis, much as epidemiological rates are adjusted for valid comparisons between groups (see Chapter 15). Kane[14] and Smith and colleagues[138] provide guidance about case mix adjustment for severity and comorbidity. Rockwood and Constantine[139] provide the same for demographic and psychosocial factors.

Techniques for Dealing with Missing Data

Kane Radosevich[14] describe background on missing data and several methods in some detail for dealing with it. First, Kane Radosevich note that prevention (of missing data) should be the overriding priority and is largely accomplished by careful attention to study design and quality control. However, they allow that "data will always be missing."[(p. 308)] They also caution, "It is always best to use available data rather than discarding study variables or cases."[(p. 308)] Researchers should look at the types of missing data; if data are missing randomly, no systematic bias should result. If data are missing selectively (common, e.g., in special populations such as elderly), they may not be able to provide baseline or risk factor information. Investigators may wish to drop some variables from analysis altogether, particularly if a good deal (i.e., more than about 2%) of the data are missing. Kane Radosevich note that dropping variables is often a better course than dropping subjects. But one needs to look carefully; "If the data being dropped makes [*sic*] no material contribution to the outcomes study, dropping it is of little consequence."[(p. 309)] If dropping subjects seems the better course, investigators have recourse to computerized statistical packages that provide analysis, although attrition bias is still a serious problem if more than 2% of subject data are missing. If studies are correlational, pairwise dropping of subjects is a reasonable approach in which like subjects are dropped from each group.

One way to actually treat missing data or actually include them in the analysis (data from dropped variables or subjects are not actually included) is to use a "dummy" variable code, which flags the variable as missing and is used in the place of the missing variable value. "This strategy has the effect of creating an additional variable for the missing factor and quantifying potential bias introduced by the absence of a value for that variable."[14(p. 310)]

Another way to treat missing data is by interpolation of data, and Kane Radosevich provide strategies for accomplishing the interpolation. Yet one more way to treat missing data is "mean substitution," based on the assumption that the best predictor for a missing value is the other values for the same individual. This may be the method of choice if the investigation instrument is a multi-item scale.

Survival Analysis

Because the data in existing databases often include events such as death, readmission, and discharge, outcomes research reports often use a technique called *survival analysis* to analyze the timing of these events. In general, survival analysis involves creating a graph that indicates the cumulative proportion of individuals for whom an event has or has not occurred (Y-axis) against time (X-axis). There are several different ways of creating survival analysis graphs, some of which result in smooth curves and some of which result in stair-step graphs (Kaplan-Meier method).[140(pp. 154–158)] Survival analysis can be used to show the pattern of achievement of the milestone for a single group, or it can be used to compare patterns across groups. Figure 16-2 shows the survival curves generated in Hoenig and colleagues'[141] study of the timing of surgery and rehabilitation care after hip fracture. In this study, most of the surviving patients regained ambulation ability after hip fracture. Therefore, the outcome of "ambulation," per se, was not a good indicator of differences between treatment regimens. However, the time it took until ambulation occurred turned out to be a useful measure. The survival curves, for example, show that those receiving high-frequency physical therapy (PT), occupational therapy (OT), or both (more than five visits per week) ambulated earlier than those who received low-frequency PT or

OT, regardless of whether the surgical repair was done early (within 2 days of hospitalization) or late.

Comparisons Across Scales

Outcome studies often involve several different dependent variables, and some of these dependent variables contain multiple subscales. Often, the different tools are scored differently and have different scales of measurement. In addition, the groups being studied may show more or less variability on the different measures, which also influences the interpretation of changes in scores. If a researcher wishes to know which of the many different variables changed the most, then the changes need to be expressed on a common scale that captures both the size of the change and the variability within the group. The

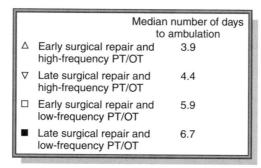

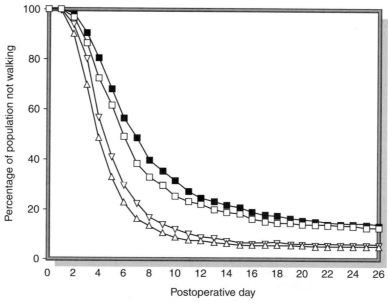

Figure 16-2 Illustration of the use of survival curves. The curves show the probability and timing of ambulation according to timing of surgical repair and the frequency of physical and occupational therapy (PT/OT). (From Hoenig H, Rubenstein LV, Sloane R, et al: What is the role of timing in the surgical and rehabilitative care of community-dwelling older persons with acute hip fracture? *Arch Intern Med* 157:513–520, 1997. Used with permission of the American Medical Association.)

usual scale that is used is a measure of effect size, which expresses the difference between two means in terms of the amount of variability within the data. An effect size of 1.0 indicates that the difference between the means of two groups is the same size as the standard deviation, a measure of variability within each group. Effect sizes less than 1.0 indicate that the difference between the means is smaller than the standard deviation, and effect sizes larger than 1.0 indicate that the difference is greater than the standard deviation. The conceptual basis for effect size becomes clearer after a review of the statistics chapters, which lay the statistical foundation needed for a full understanding of effect sizes. For now, it is enough to know that the use of effect sizes enables the researcher to compare the magnitude of change across many different variables. Jette and Jette[142] used effect sizes to evaluate changes in SF-36 scores and Lysholm Knee Rating Scale scores over an episode of physical therapy for patients with knee impairments. Figure 16-3 shows a radar graph of their results. In a radar graph, each dependent variable is displayed as a "spoke" coming from a common center. The scale on each spoke is the same and in this example represents effect size, marked in increments of

one tenth of a standard deviation. It is readily apparent from this graph that the biggest changes were seen in Lysholm scores and in the bodily pain and physical function subscales of the SF-36.

Multivariate Statistics

The final analysis issue covered here also stems from the multiple dependent variables that are often measured in outcomes studies. Because of these many variables, researchers often use statistical tools that enable them to analyze many dependent variables simultaneously. The general term for these types of statistical tools is multivariate. Although the descriptions of multivariate results often appear intimidating, they rest on many of the same statistical foundations as do the simpler univariate statistics that handle one dependent variable at a time (see Chapters 22 and 24).

SUMMARY

Outcomes research refers to a broad group of research designs that evaluate the overall effectiveness of clinical care as it is delivered in actual practice, rather

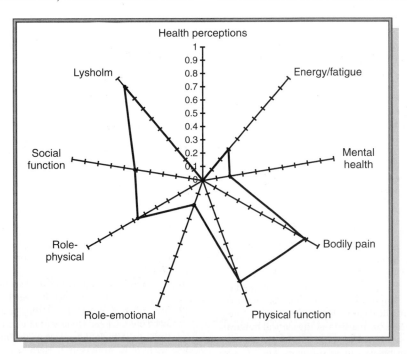

Figure 16-3 Use of effect sizes in a radar graph format to display changes in SF-36 and Lysholm scores over a physical therapy episode for patients with knee impairments. Changes are presented as effect sizes for each outcome and are represented by a point on an arm of the radar graph. The center of the graph is no change. Each hatch mark represents a change of one tenth of a standard deviation. (From Jette DU, Jette AM: Physical therapy and health outcomes in patients with knee impairments, *Phys Ther* 76:1178–1187, 1996. Used with permission of the American Physical Therapy Association.)

than the physiological efficacy of treatments given under tightly controlled circumstances to narrowly defined groups of subjects. Evaluations of effectiveness in rehabilitation are often guided by one of three widely used frameworks: the Nagi model, the WHO's original International Classification of Impairments, Disabilities, and Handicaps (ICIDH), or its newer International Classification of Functioning, Disability, and Health (ICF). These frameworks add the ecological concepts of activity, participation, and disability to traditional measures of changes in bodily functions or structures. Elements of this broader conceptualization of health status can be measured by a number of generic, condition-specific, person-specific, or satisfaction tools. Outcomes research studies generally rely on databases that are generated by review of medical records, computerized abstracts of medical records, insurance claims data, in-house data collection efforts, or national databases that provide standardized data collection forms and analysis services. Statistical analysis of outcomes research is often complex and must address issues of case mix, missing data, survival analysis, comparisons across different scales, and analysis of many dependent variables simultaneously.

REFERENCES

1. Hegde MN: *Clinical Research in Communicative Disorders*, 3rd ed, Austin, Tex, 2003, Pro-Ed.
2. Hicks CM: *Research Methods for Clinical Therapists*, 5th ed, Edinburgh, UK, 2009, Churchill Livingstone.
3. Hayes SC, Barlow DH, Nelson-Gray R: *The Scientist Practitioner*, Boston, Mass, 1999, Allyn & Bacon.
4. Calvert MJ, Freemantle N: Use of health-related quality of life in prescribing research. Part 1: Why evaluate health-related quality of life? *J Clin Pharm Ther* 28:513–521, 2003.
5. Bowman J, Llewellyn G: Clinical outcomes research from the occupational therapist's perspective, *Occup Ther Int* 9:145–166, 2002.
6. Birkmeyer JD: Outcomes research and surgeons, *Surgery* 124:477–483, 1998.
7. Jette AM: Outcomes research: Shifting the dominant research paradigm in physical therapy, *Phys Ther* 75:965–970, 1995.
8. Tarlov AR, Ware JE, Greenfield S, et al: The Medical Outcomes Study: An application of methods for monitoring the results of medical care, *JAMA* 262:925–930, 1989.
9. Tessier P, Lelorain S: A comparison of the clinical determinants of health-related quality of life and subjective well-being in long-term breast cancer survivors, *Eur J Cancer Care* 21:692–700, 2012.
10. Mccabe C: Issues for researchers to consider when using health-related quality of life outcomes in cancer research, *Eur J Cancer Care* 20:563–569, 2011.
11. Faust HB, Mirowski GW, Chuang T-Y, et al: Outcomes research: An overview, *J Am Acad Dermatol* 36:999–1006, 1997.
12. Rothermel C: What is health economics and outcomes research? A primer for medical writers, *AMWA J* 28:98–104, 2013.
13. Kane RL, editor: *Understanding Health Care Outcomes Research*, 2nd ed. Sudbury, Mass, 2006, Jones & Bartlett.
14. Kane RL, Radosevich DM: *Conducting Health Outcomes Research*, Sudbury, Mass, 2011, Jones & Bartlett.
15. Kane RL: Improving outcomes in rehabilitation: A call to arms (and legs), *Med Care* 35(Suppl):JS21–JS27, 1997.
16. Nagi SA: Disability concepts revisited: Implications for prevention. In Pope AM, Tarlov AR, editors: *Disability in America: Toward a National Agenda for Prevention*, Washington, DC, 1991, National Academy Press.
17. World Health Organization: *International Classification of Impairments, Disabilities, and Handicaps*, Geneva, Switzerland, 1980, World Health Organization.
18. World Health Organization: *International Classification of Functioning, Disability, and Health*, Geneva, Switzerland, 2001, World Health Organization.
19. Nagi SZ: A study in the evaluation of disability and rehabilitation potential: Concepts, methods, and procedures, *Am J Public Health Nations Health* 54:1568–1579, 1964.
20. Stucki G, Ewert T, Cieza A: Value and application of the ICF in rehabilitation medicine, *Disabil Rehabil* 24:932–938, 2002.
21. World Health Organization. International Classification of Functioning, Disability, and Health (ICF). Available at: http://www.who.int/classifications/icf/en/. Accessed December 4, 2014.
22. World Health Organization. ICF Browser. Available at: http://apps.who.int/classifications/icfbrowser/. Accessed December 4, 2014.
23. Jette AM: Disablement outcomes in geriatric rehabilitation, *Med Care* 35(Suppl):JS28–JS37, 1997.
24. Verbrugge LM, Jette AM: The disablement process, *Soc Sci Med* 38:1–14, 1994.
25. Liang MH: Comments on: Jette AM: Disablement outcomes in geriatric rehabilitation, *Med Care* 35(Suppl):JS28–JS37, 1997.
26. Kennedy DP: Scale adaptation and ethnography, *Field Meth* 17:412–431, 2005.
27. Alpiner JG, Schow RL: Rehabilitative evaluation of hearing-impaired adults. In Alpiner JG, McCarthy PA, editors: *Rehabilitative Audiology: Children and Adults*, 3rd ed, Philadelphia, Pa, 2000, Lippincott, William & Wilkins, pp 305–331.
28. Demorest ME, DeHaven GP: Psychometric adequacy of self-assessment scales, *Semin Hear* 14:314–325, 1993.
29. Ivarsson B, Malm U, Lindström L, Norlander T: The self-assessment Global Quality of Life scale: Reliability and construct validity, *Int J Psychiatry Clin Pract* 14:287–297, 2010.
30. Lefebvre K, Anderson T, Herbertson K, et al: The use of Health Related Quality of Life Measurement in cardiovascular and pulmonary physical therapy practice: An exploratory study, *Cardiopulm Phys Ther J* 21:5–13, 2010.
31. Hefford C, Abbott JH, Baxter GD, Arnold R: Outcome measurement in clinical practice: Practical and theoretical issues for health related quality of life (HRQOL) questionnaires, *Phys Ther Rev* 16:155–167, 2011.

32. Lansinger B, Carlsson JY, Kreuter M, Taft C: Health-related quality of life in persons with long-term neck pain after treatment with qigong and exercise therapy respectively, *Eur J Physiother* 15(3):111–117, 2013.

33. Latimer-Cheung AE, Pilutti LA, Hicks AL, et al: Effects of exercise training on fitness, mobility, fatigue, and health-related quality of life among adults with multiple sclerosis: A systematic review to inform guideline development, *Arch Phys Med Rehabil* 94:1800–1828.e3, 2013.

34. Brovold T, Skelton DA, Bergland A: The efficacy of counseling and progressive resistance home-exercises on adherence, health-related quality of life and function after discharge from a geriatric day-hospital, *Arch Gerontol Geriatr* 55:453–459, 2012.

35. Olze H, Gräbel S, Haupt H, et al: Extra benefit of a second cochlear implant with respect to health-related quality of life and tinnitus, *Otol Neurotol* 33:1169–1175, 2012.

36. Eyssen ICJM, Steultjens MPM, de Groot V, et al: A cluster randomised controlled trial on the efficacy of client-centred occupational therapy in multiple sclerosis: Good process, poor outcome, *Disabil Rehabil* 35:1636–1646, 2013.

37. Maciejewski M: Generic measures. In Kane RL, editor: *Understanding Health Care Outcomes Research*, 2nd ed, Sudbury, Mass, 2006, Jones & Bartlett, pp 123–164.

38. Ware JE, Kosinski M, Keller SD: A 12-item short form health survey: Construction of scales and preliminary tests of reliability and validity, *Med Care* 34:220–223, 1996.

39. Melville MR, Lari MA, Brown N, et al: Quality of life assessment using the short form 12 questionnaire is as reliable and sensitive as the short form 36 in distinguishing symptom severity in myocardial infarction survivors, *Heart* 89:1445–1446, 2003.

40. Cunillera O, Tresserras R, Rajmil L, et al: Discriminative capacity of the EQ-5D, SF-6D, and SF-12 as measures of health status in population health survey, *Qual Life Res* 19:853–864, 2010.

41. Angst F, Verra ML, Lehmann S, et al: Responsiveness of the cervical Northern American Spine Society questionnaire (NASS) and the Short Form 36 (SF-36) in chronic whiplash, *Clin Rehabil* 26:142–151, 2012.

42. Cabral DL, Laurentino GE, Damascena CG, et al: Comparisons of the Nottingham Health Profile and the SF-36 health survey for the assessment of quality of life in individuals with chronic stroke, *Rev Brasil Fisioter* 16:301–308, 2012.

43. Jones CA, Voaklander DC, Suarez-Alma ME: Determinants of function after total knee arthroplasty, *Phys Ther* 83:696–706, 2003.

44. Turner-Bowker DM, Saris-Baglama RN, DeRosa MA, et al: A computerized adaptive version of the SF-36 is feasible for clinic and Internet administration in adults with HIV, *AIDS Care* 24:886–896, 2012.

45. Bennett JA, Riegel B: Brief report. United States Spanish Short-Form-36 Health Survey: Scaling assumptions and reliability in elderly community-dwelling Mexican Americans, *Nurs Res* 52:262–269, 2003.

46. National Institutes of Health (NIH). PROMIS®. Available at: http://www.nihpromis.org/. Accessed December 4, 2014.

47. National Institutes of Health (NIH). PROMIS®. Translations. Available at: http://www.nihpromis.org/measures/translations. Accessed December 4, 2014.

48. National Institutes of Health (NIH). PROMIS®. Instruments Available for Use in Assessment Center. Available at: http://www.assessmentcenter.net/documents/InstrumentLibrary.pdf. Accessed December 4, 2014.

49. National Institutes of Health (NIH). PROMIS®. Instrument Development and Psychometric Evaluation Scientific Standards. Available at: http://www.nihpromis.org/Documents/PROMISStandards_Vers2.0_Final.pdf. Accessed February 20, 2015.

50. National Institutes of Health (NIH). PROMIS®. Validity Studies. Available at: http://www.nihpromis.org/science/validitystudies.aspx. Accessed December 4, 2014.

51. Hinchcliff M, Beaumont JL, Thavarajah K, et al: Validity of two new patient-reported outcome measures in systemic sclerosis: Patient-Reported Outcomes Measurement Information System 29-Item Health Profile and Functional Assessment of Chronic Illness Therapy-Dyspnea Short Form, *Arthritis Care Res* 63:1620–1628, 2011.

52. Fries J, Rose M, Krishnan E: The PROMIS(R) of better outcome assessment: Responsiveness, floor and ceiling effects, and Internet administration, *J Rheumatol* 38:1759–1764, 2011.

53. Atherly A: Condition-specific measures. In Kane RL, editor: *Understanding Health Care Outcomes Research*, 2nd ed, Sudbury, Mass, 2006, Jones & Bartlett, pp 53–66.

54. van Straten A, de Haan RJ, Limburg M, et al: A stroke-adapted 30-item version of the Sickness Impact Profile to assess quality of life (SA-SIP30), *Stroke* 28:2155–2161, 1997.

55. Van de Port IGL, Ketelaar M, Schepers VPM, et al: Monitoring the functional health status of stroke patients: The value of the Stroke-Adapted Sickness Impact Profile-30, *Disabil Rehabil* 26:635–640, 2004.

56. Buck D, Jacoby A, Massey A, Ford G: Evaluation of measures used to assess quality of life after stroke, *Stroke* 31:2004–2010, 2000.

57. van Straten A, de Haan RJ, Limburg M, van den Bos GA: Clinical meaning of the Stroke-Adapted Sickness Impact Profile-30 and the Sickness Impact Profile-136, *Stroke* 31:2610–2615, 2000.

58. Zedlitz AM, Rietveld TC, Geurts AC, Fasotti L: Cognitive and graded activity training can alleviate persistent fatigue after stroke: A randomized, controlled trial, *Stroke* 43:1046–1051, 2012.

59. Huijbregts MPJ, McEwen S, Taylor D: Exploring the feasibility and efficacy of a telehealth stroke self-management programme: A pilot study, *Physiother Can* 61:210–220, 2009.

60. Fairbank JC, Pynsent PB: The Oswestry Disability Index, *Spine* 25:2940–2952, 2000.

61. Lochhead LE, MacMillan PD: Psychometric properties of the Oswestry Disability Index: Rasch analysis of responses in a work-disabled population, *Work* 46:67–76, 2013.

62. Flynn TW, Fritz JM, Wainner RS, Whitman JM: The audible pop is not necessary for successful spinal high-velocity thrust manipulation in individuals with low back pain, *Arch Phys Med Rehabil* 84:1057–1060, 2003.

63. Nunn N: Practical challenges and limitations using the Oswestry Disability Low Back Pain Questionnaire in a private practice setting in New Zealand: A clinical audit, *N Z J Physiother* 40:242–248, 2012.

64. Bellamy N: WOMAC: A 20-year experiential review of a patient-centered self-reported health status questionnaire, *J Rheumatol* 29:2473–2476, 2002.

65. Kennedy D, Stratford PW, Pagura SMC, et al: Exploring the factorial validity and clinical interpretability of the Western Ontario and McMaster Universities Osteoarthritis Index (WOMAC), *Physiother Can* 55(3):160–168, 2003.

66. Baron G, Tubach F, Ravaud P, et al: Validation of a short form of the Western Ontario and McMaster Universities Osteoarthritis Index function subscale in hip and knee osteoarthritis, *Arthritis Care Res* 57(4):633–638, 2007.

67. McKay C, Prapavessis H, McNair P: Comparing the Lower Limb Tasks Questionnaire to the Western Ontario and McMaster Universities Osteoarthritis Index: Agreement, responsiveness, and convergence with physical performance for knee osteoarthritis patients, *Arch Phys Med Rehabil* 94:474–479, 2013.

68. Wagenmakers R, Stevens M, van den Akker-Scheek I, et al: Predictive value of the Western Ontario and McMaster Universities Osteoarthritis Index for the amount of physical activity after total hip arthroplasty, *Phys Ther* 88(2):211–218, 2008.

69. Elbaz A, Debbi EM, Segal G, et al: Sex and body mass index correlate with Western Ontario and McMaster Universities Osteoarthritis Index and quality of life scores in knee osteoarthritis, *Arch Phys Med Rehabil* 92:1618–1623, 2011.

70. Gummesson C, Atroshi I, Ekdahl C: The disabilities of the arm, shoulder and hand (DASH) outcome questionnaire: Longitudinal construct validity and measuring self-rated health change after surgery, *BMC Musculoskelet Disord* 4:11, 2003.

71. Mousavi SJ, Parnianpour M, Abedi M, et al: Cultural adaptation and validation of the Persian version of the Disabilities of the Arm, Shoulder and Hand (DASH) outcome measure, *Clin Rehabil* 22(8):749–757, 2008.

72. Franchignoni F, Giordano A, Sartorio F, et al: Suggestions for refinement of the Disabilities of the Arm, Shoulder and Hand outcome measure (DASH): A factor analysis and Rasch validation study, *Arch Phys Med Rehabil* 91:1370–1377, 2010.

73. Østlie K, Franklin RJ, Skjeldal OH, et al: Assessing physical function in adult acquired major upper-limb amputees by combining the Disabilities of the Arm, Shoulder and Hand (DASH) outcome questionnaire and clinical examination, *Arch Phys Med Rehabil* 92(10):1636–1645, 2011.

74. Thormodsgard TM, Stone K, Ciraulo DL, et al: An assessment of patient satisfaction with nonoperative management of clavicular fractures using the disabilities of the arm, shoulder and hand outcome measure, *J Trauma* 71(5):1126–1129, 2011.

75. Rostami HR, Arefi A, Tabatabaei S: Effect of mirror therapy on hand function in patients with hand orthopaedic injuries: A randomized controlled trial, *Disabil Rehabil* 35(19):1647–1651, 2013.

76. Chalder T, Berelowitz G, Pawlikowska T, et al: Development of a fatigue scale, *J Psychosom Res* 37:147–153, 1993.

77. Jahnsen R, Villien L, Stanghelle JK, Holm I: Fatigue in adults with cerebral palsy in Norway compared with the general population, *Dev Med Child Neurol* 45:296–303, 2003.

78. Ventry IM, Weinstein BE: The Hearing Handicap Inventory for the Elderly: A new tool, *Ear Hear* 3:128–134, 1982.

79. Newman CW, Weinstein BE: Test-retest reliability of the Hearing Handicap Inventory for the Elderly using two administration approaches, *Ear Hear* 10:190–191, 1989.

80. Jupiter T, Delgado DF: Outcome measures comparing two tools for identifying audiological needs in the elderly homebound population, *J Acad Rehabil Audiol* 36:11–22, 2003.

81. Deepthi R, Kasthuri A: Validation of the use of self-reported hearing loss and the Hearing Handicap Inventory for elderly among rural Indian elderly population, *Arch Gerontol Geriatr* 55:762–767, 2012.

82. Demorest ME, Erdman SA: Development of the communication profile for the hearing impaired, *J Speech Hearing Disord* 52:129–143, 1987.

83. Erdman SA: Clinical interpretation of the CPHI: Communication Profile for the Hearing Impaired, *Perspect Aural Rehabil Instrum* 13:3–18, 2006.

84. Mokkink LB, Knol DL, Zekveld AA, et al: Factor structure and reliability of the Dutch version of seven scales of the Communication Profile for the Hearing Impaired (CPHI), *J Speech Lang Hear Res* 52:454–464, 2009.

85. Jupiter T: Screening for hearing loss in the elderly using distortion product otoacoustic emissions, pure tones, and a self-assessment tool, *Am J Audiol* 18:99–107, 2009.

86. Saito H, Nishiwaki Y, Michikawa T, et al: Hearing handicap predicts the development of depressive symptoms after 3 years in older community-dwelling Japanese, *J Am Geriatr Soc* 58:93–97, 2010.

87. Silverman S, Cates M, Saunders G: Is measured hearing aid benefit affected by seeing baseline outcome questionnaire responses? *Am J Audiol* 20:90–99, 2011.

88. Chisolm TH, Abrams HB, McArdle R: Short- and long-term outcomes of adult audiological rehabilitation, *Ear Hear* 25:4644–4677, 2004.

89. Lewis MS, Valente M, Horn JE, Crandell C: The effect of hearing aids and frequency modulation technology on results from the communication profile for the hearing impaired, *J Am Acad Audiol* 16:250–261, 2005.

90. Alpiner JG, McCarthy PA: *Rehabilitative Audiology: Children and Adults*, Baltimore, Md, 2000, Lippincott, Williams & Wilkins.

91. Hull RH: Appendices materials and scales for assessment of communication for the hearing impaired. In Hull RH, editor: *Introduction to Aural Rehabilitation*, San Diego, Calif, 2010, Plural Publishing.

92. Doyle P, McNeil M, Hula W, Mikolic J: The Burden of Stroke Scale (BOSS): Validating patient-reported communication difficulty and associated psychological distress in stroke survivors, *Aphasiology* 17:291–304, 2003.

93. Duncan PW, Bode RK, Lai SM, Perera S: Rasch analysis of a new stroke-specific outcome scale: The Stroke Impact Scale, *Arch Phys Med Rehabil* 84:950–963, 2003.

94. Jacobson BH, Johnson A, Grywalski C, et al: The Voice Handicap Index (VHI): Development and validation, *Am J Speech Lang Pathol* 6(3):66–70, 1997.

95. Evans E, Carding P, Drinnan M: The Voice Handicap Index with post-laryngectomy male voices, *Int J Lang Commun Disord* 44:575–586, 2009.

96. Huinck W, Rietveld T: The validity of a simple outcome measure to assess stuttering therapy, *Folia Phoniatr Logop* 59:91–99, 2007.

97. Eadie TL, Yorkston KM, Klasner ER, et al: Measuring communicative participation: A review of self-report instruments in speech-language pathology, *Am J Speech Lang Pathol* 15:307–320, 2006.

98. Baylor C, Yorkston K, Eadie T, et al: The Communicative Participation Item Bank (CPIB): Item Bank Calibration and Development of a Disorder-Generic Short Form, *J Speech Lang Hear Res* 56:1190–1208, 2013.

99. Donnelly C, Carswell A: Individualized outcome measures: A review of the literature. *Can J Occup Ther* 69:84–94, 2002.

100. Ottenbacher KJ, Cusick A: Goal attainment scaling as a method of clinical service evaluation, *Am J Occup Ther* 44:519–525, 1990.

101. Ruble L, McGrew J, Toland M: Goal attainment scaling as an outcome measure in randomized controlled trials of psychosocial interventions in autism, *J Autism Dev Disord* 42:1974–1983, 2012.

102. Knecht-Sabres L: The Canadian Occupational Performance Measure: An outcome measure, *Communique* 2011:4–11, 2011.

103. Kowalchuk Horn K, Jennings S, Richardson G, et al: The Patient-Specific Functional Scale: Psychometrics, clinimetrics, and application as a clinical outcome measure, *J Orthop Sports Phys Ther* 42(1):30–42, 2012.

104. Hale LA: Using Goal Attainment Scaling in physiotherapeutic home-based stroke rehabilitation, *Adv Physiother* 12:142–149, 2010.

105. Steenbeek D, Gorter JW, Ketelaar M, et al: Responsiveness of Goal Attainment Scaling in comparison to two standardized measures in outcome evaluation of children with cerebral palsy, *Clin Rehabil* 25(12):1128–1139, 2011.

106. Smith A, Cardillo JE, Smith SC, Amezaga A: Improvement scaling (rehabilitation version): A new approach to measuring progress of patients in achieving their individual rehabilitation goals, *Med Care* 36:333–347, 1998.

107. Beurskens AJ, de Vet HC, Koke AJ, et al: A patient-specific approach for measuring functional status in low back pain, *J Manipulative Physiol Ther* 22:144–148, 1999.

108. American Speech-Language-Hearing Association. National Outcomes Measurement System. Available at: http://www.asha.org/NOMS/. Accessed December 4, 2014.

109. Ahmed M, Shehadeh A, Collins M: Quality of nursing care in community health centers: Clients' satisfaction, *Health Sci J* 7:229–236, 2013.

110. Di Palo MT: Rating satisfaction research: Is it poor, fair, good, very good, or excellent? *Arthritis Care Res* 10:422–430, 1997.

111. Yun-Hee J, Fethney J, Ludford I: Measuring client satisfaction in residential aged care settings: A narrative review of instruments, *Internet J Healthc Adm* 8:1, 2012.

112. Smith MA, Schüssler-Fiorenza C, Rockwood T: Satisfaction with care. In Kane RL, editor: *Understanding Health Care Outcomes Research*, 2nd ed, Sudbury, Mass, 2006, Jones & Bartlett, pp 185–216.

113. Durham ML: How research will adapt to HIPAA: A view from within the healthcare delivery system, *Am J Law Med* 28:491–502, 2002.

114. Cassell J, Young A: Why we should not seek individual informed consent for participation in health services research, *J Med Ethics* 28:313–317, 2002.

115. Hoffmann DE, Fortenberry JD, Ravel J: Are changes to the common rule necessary to address evolving areas of research? A case study focusing on the human microbiome project, *J Law Med Ethics* 41:454–469, 2013.

116. Fox KM, Reuland M, Hawkes WG, et al: Accuracy of medical records in hip fracture, *J Am Geriatr Soc* 46:745–750, 1998.

117. University of South Florida: Morsani College of Medicine. January 1, 2014. Federal Mandates for Healthcare: Digital Record-Keeping Will Be Required of Public and Private Healthcare Providers. Available at: http://www.usfhealthonline.com/news/healthcare/electronic-medical-records-mandate-january-2014/#.Us746Z5dXL8. Accessed December 4, 2014.

118. Kern LM, Malhotra S, Barrón Y, et al: Accuracy of electronically reported "meaningful use" clinical quality measures, *Ann Intern Med* 158:77–83, 2013.

119. Chan L, Houck P, Prela CM, MacLehose RF: Using Medicare databases for outcomes research in rehabilitation medicine, *Am J Phys Med Rehabil* 80:474–480, 2001.

120. Freburger JK, Konrad TR: The use of federal and state databases to conduct health services research related to physical and occupational therapy, *Arch Phys Med Rehabil* 83(6):837–845, 2002.

121. Cullen MR, Vegso S, Cantley L, et al: Use of medical insurance claims data for occupational health research, *J Occup Environ Med* 48(10):1054–1061, 2006.

122. Shields RK, Leo KC, Miller B, et al: An acute care physical therapy clinical practice database for outcomes research, *Phys Ther* 74:463–470, 1994.

123. Hordacre B, Birks V, Quinn S, et al: Physiotherapy rehabilitation for individuals with lower limb amputation: A 15-year clinical series, *Physiother Res Int* 18:70–80, 2013.

124. COMBI: The Center for Outcome Measurement in Brain Injury. Available at: www.tbims.org/combi. Accessed December 4, 2014.

125. UCHSC Burn Model System Data Coordination Center (BMS/DCC). Available at: http://burndata.washington.edu/. Accessed December 4, 2014.

126. National Spinal Cord Injury Statistical Center. NSCISC home. Available at: https://www.nscisc.uab.edu/. Accessed February 20, 2015.

127. National Spinal Cord Injury Statistical Center. Spinal Cord Injury Facts and Figures at a Glance. Available at: https://www.nscisc.uab.edu/PublicDocuments/fact_figures_docs/Facts%202012%20Feb%20Final.pdf. Accessed December 4, 2014.

128. Meyers AR, Andresen EM, Hagglund KJ: A model of outcomes research: Spinal cord injury, *Arch Phys Med Rehabil* 81(Suppl 2):S81–90, 2000.

129. Lysack C, Neufeld S, Machacova K: Self-rated health among spinal cord injury survivors: Directions for future research, *Int J Ther Rehabil* 17:648–653, 2010.

130. Uniform Data System for Medical Rehabilitation. Available at: http://www.udsmr.org/. Accessed December 4, 2014.

131. Focus on Therapeutic Outcomes, Inc. (FOTO). Available at: www.fotoinc.com. Accessed December 4, 2014.

132. Jerrell ML: Revisiting outcomes research in O & P, *O & P Bus News* 12:18–19, 21, 22, 24, 2003.

133. Russek L, Wooden M, Ekedahl S, Bush A: Attitudes toward standardized data collection, *Phys Ther* 77:714–729, 1997.

134. Powell JW, Barber-Foss KD: Injury patterns in selected high school sports: A review of the 1995-1997 seasons, *J Athl Train* 34:277–284, 1999.

135. American Speech-Language-Hearing Association. NOMS Data Reports and Fact Sheets. Available at: http://www.asha.org/content.aspx?id=8589940108&LangType=1033. Accessed January 16, 2014.

136. Loan LA, Patrician PA, McCarthy M: Participation in a national nursing outcomes database: monitoring outcomes over time. *Nurs Adm Q* 35:72–78, 2011.

137. Richardson J, Murray D, House CK et al: Successful implementation of the National Institutes of Health Stroke Scale on a stroke/neurovascular unit, *J Neurosci Nurs* 38(Suppl):309–314, 2006.

138. Smith MA, Nitz NM, Stuart SK: Severity and comorbidity. In Kane RL, editor: *Understanding Health Care Outcomes Research*, 2nd ed, Sudbury, Mass, 2006, Jones & Bartlett, pp 219–263.

139. Rockwood T, Constantine M: Demographic, psychological, and social. In Kane RL, editor: *Understanding Health Care Outcomes Research*, 2nd ed, Sudbury, Mass, 2006, Jones & Bartlett, pp 265–303.

140. Jekel JF, Elmore JG, Katz DL: *Epidemiology, Biostatistics, and Preventive Medicine*, 2nd ed, Philadelphia, Pa, 2001, WB Saunders.

141. Hoenig H, Rubenstein LV, Sloane R, et al: What is the role of timing in the surgical and rehabilitative care of community-dwelling older persons with acute hip fracture? *Arch Intern Med* 157:513–520, 1997.

142. Jette AM, Jette DU: Physical therapy and health outcomes in patients with knee impairments, *Phys Ther* 76:1178–1187, 1996.

CHAPTER 17

Survey Research

CHAPTER OUTLINE

Scope of Survey Research
Types of Information
Types of Items
  Open-Format Items
  Closed-Format Items
    Multiple Choice
    Likert Type
    Semantic Differential
    Q-Sort
Implementation Overview
  Need for Rigor

Sample Size and Sampling
Mailed Surveys
  Access to a Sampling Frame
  Researcher-Developed Versus
    Existing Instruments
  Questionnaire Development
    Drafting
    Expert Review
    First Revision
    Pilot Test
    Final Revision

Motivating Prospects to Respond
  Implementation Details
Internet Surveys
Interview Surveys
  Access to Prospective Participants
  Development of Interview
    Schedules
  Motivating Prospects to Participate
  Implementation Details
Summary

Survey research is a form of inquiry that rests on the assumption that meaningful information can be obtained by asking the parties of interest what they know, what they believe, and how they behave. This chapter defines the scope of survey research, identifies the type of information that can be gleaned from survey research, presents a variety of types of items that are used within questionnaires, and addresses a variety of implementation details for mailed surveys, Internet surveys, and in-person or telephone interviews.

SCOPE OF SURVEY RESEARCH

A survey has been defined as a "system for collecting information from or about people to describe, compare, or explain their knowledge, attitudes, and behavior."[1(p. 1)] More specifically, survey research relies on self-reported information from participants, rather than on observations or measurements taken by the researcher. For example, consider ways of studying the extent to which patients adhere to a prescribed regimen. One way to study this topic would be to ask patients how often they are taking their medications or performing a home therapy regimen or to ask questions to determine their recall of important details about the regimen. This self-report information could be collected with survey methods in a face-to-face interview, by administering a questionnaire over the telephone, or with a mailed or Internet questionnaire. An assumption of the survey approach is that patients would provide accurate information about their activities.

In contrast, this topic could also be studied by having researchers score patients in some way as they observe them demonstrating the prescribed regimen. An assumption of the observational approach is that patients who were adherent to the regimen would, for example, set up a week's worth of medications correctly without prompting, and those who were not adherent would set up the medications incorrectly or would require prompting from the researcher. Neither the survey approach nor the observational approach is inherently superior for studying this topic. Each rests on assumptions that will not be met in all cases—some patients would exaggerate their adherence if surveyed, and some patients who faithfully take their medications may become flustered in front of the researcher and require prompting to demonstrate the regimen. Researchers need to consider which of the potential problems to avoid when they make decisions among the approaches that could be taken with a given topic.

To place survey research into the context of other forms of research, recall the six-celled matrix of research types presented in Chapter 12 (see Fig. 12-1). One dimension of the matrix is the purpose of the research. Survey techniques can be used for all three purposes: describing phenomena, analyzing relationships among variables, and analyzing differences among groups or across time.

The second dimension of the matrix is the timing of data collection. Clearly, surveys can be prospective, with self-reported information collected to answer specific research questions developed by the researchers. It is equally clear that self-reported information may be used retrospectively—that is, data collected for one purpose might be extracted and reanalyzed to meet another research need. For example, Chevan and Chevan[2] used U.S. Bureau of the Census data to develop a profile of physical therapists. However, most would not label this study "survey research." Instead, they would refer to it as a secondary analysis. The term *survey research* is generally used to describe original, prospective collection of self-reported data, whereas analysis of data sets collected by someone else, such as the U.S. Census data, is known as *secondary analysis*.

The third dimension of the matrix is whether the research is experimental or nonexperimental in nature. Clearly, survey research can be nonexperimental, with no controlled manipulation of independent variables. It is equally clear that self-reported information can be used as a method of data collection in experimental research—as was the case when Balogun and associates[3] studied the impact of educational programs on physical therapist and occupational therapist student attitudes toward working with individuals with acquired immunodeficiency syndrome. This project was experimental in that there was controlled manipulation of the type of education received. Researchers surveyed participants to determine self-reported attitudes across time (preeducation, mideducation, and posteducation). However, most would not label this study as "survey" research; they might label it as an experimental, educational research project. Thus, although survey research can be experimental in nature, the term is often reserved for nonexperimental studies using self-reported information.

In summary, survey research can be used to meet the purposes of description, analysis of relationships, or analysis of differences. The term "survey research" is generally reserved for nonexperimental research with prospective collection of self-reported data. It is important to recognize that although all survey research projects use self-reported information, not all research projects that use self-reported information are considered survey research.

TYPES OF INFORMATION

The scope of information that can be obtained through self-report instruments is vast. Surveys can document (1) concrete facts about respondents, (2) their knowledge, and (3) behavior, as well as (4) their abstract opinions and (5) personal characteristics. The rehabilitation literature contains many examples of each of the five types of survey information just mentioned; one example of each follows. Hagberg and Brånemark[4] collected factual information about prosthetic use from individuals with transfemoral amputation, and Nadler and associates[5] collected factual information from athletic trainers about complications encountered when delivering therapeutic modalities.

To examine respondent knowledge, Wagner and Stewart[6] did preprogram and postprogram surveys of college students enrolled in a physical medicine and rehabilitation internship to determine whether their knowledge of physical medicine and rehabilitation increased after completing the internship. To collect data about respondent behavior, Tepe and associates[7] and Carter and Stoecker[8] used survey methods to determine the vocal habits and hygiene of young choir singers and the professional reading practices of American Physical Therapy Association (APTA) physical therapist members, respectively.

Surveys can also ask about opinions and personal and setting characteristics. Brown and colleagues[9] examined the opinions of occupational therapists from Australia, the United Kingdom, and Taiwan toward research use. In a study of utilization of speech and language services for postextubation dysphagia, Macht and associates[10] surveyed the practices, setting characteristics, and staffing patterns of inpatient speech-language pathologists.

TYPES OF ITEMS

Although the format of interview and questionnaire items is limited only by the creativity of the researcher, several standard item formats exist. The broadest distinction among item types is open-format versus closed-format items.

Open-Format Items

Open-format items permit a flexible response. Interviews frequently include open-format items, and it is these open-format items that allow for the greater breadth of response that is a major advantage of using the interview in survey research. Suppose that a researcher is interested in identifying the sources of job satisfaction and dissatisfaction for rehabilitation professionals. An open-format interview question might be, "What about your job is satisfying to you?" Respondents would be free to structure their responses as desired. Some might emphasize aspects of patient care, others might focus on working with a respected leader, others might discuss the quality of interactions among coworkers, and others might list several different satisfying aspects of their work.

Questionnaires may also include open-format items, although the depth of response depends on the respondents' ability to communicate in writing and their willingness to provide an in-depth answer in the absence of an interviewer who can prompt them and provide encouragement during the course of their response.

The major difficulty with open-format items is their analysis. The researcher must sift and categorize the responses into a relatively small number of manageable categories. The literature on the qualitative research paradigm provides guidelines for the classification of responses from open-format items, as discussed in Chapter 14. The categorization of responses from open-format items is sometimes used to generate the fixed alternatives needed for closed-format items.

Closed-Format Items

Closed-format items restrict the range of possible responses. Mailed and Internet delivered questionnaires often include a high proportion of closed-format responses. In addition, highly structured interviews may use closed-format responses. In such a case, the interview becomes nothing more than an orally administered questionnaire, and the breadth of response characteristic of most interview formats is lost. Four types of closed-format items are discussed below: multiple choice, Likert type, semantic differential, and Q-sort items.

Multiple Choice

Multiple-choice items can be used to measure knowledge, behavior, opinions, or personal characteristics. Some researchers design closed-format items that allow some flexibility of response by including "other" as a possible response category and permitting respondents to write in a response of their choice. The multiple-choice question is known as the "stem" of the question, and the possible responses are known as response options.

In a variation of the multiple-choice item, a vignette may be used as the stem of the item. A vignette is a short story or scenario that sets a scene. Employing a Web-based survey, Archer and colleagues[11] used vignettes to measure the likelihood of surgeons referring patients who had traumatic lower-extremity injuries to physical therapy. Vignettes permit researchers to evaluate responses to a complex circumstance that may better approximate clinical settings than do traditional multiple-choice items.

Likert Type

Likert-type items, named for their originator, Rensis Likert, are used to assess the strength of response to a declarative statement. The most typical set of responses includes "strongly agree," "agree," "undecided," "disagree," and "strongly disagree." Many others are available, a few of which are "very important" to "very unimportant," "strongly encourage" to "strongly discourage," and "definitely yes" to "definitely no."[12] Likert-type items (with ratings from "negative effect" to "positive effect") were used by Rozier and colleagues[13] to determine the perceived impact of various factors (e.g., age, family responsibilities) on the career success of physical therapists.

Semantic Differential

Semantic differential items are based on the work of Osgood and colleagues[14] in the 1950s. Semantic differential items consist of adjective pairs that represent different ends of a continuum. The members of the pair are separated by a line, representing a continuum. If semantic differential items were used to study rehabilitation professionals' opinions about their department, word pairs such as "cohesive–fragmented," "invigorating–dull," and "organized–disorganized" might be used to elicit their opinions. The respondent indicates the place on the continuum that best represents the item or person being described. Semantic differential items were used by Streed and Stoecker[15] to assess the levels of stereotyping in physical therapy and occupational therapy students.

Q-Sort

A Q-sort is a method of forced-choice ranking of many alternatives.[16] It could be used, for example, to study job satisfaction of rehabilitation professionals. To do so, the researcher would generate a set of, say, 50 items about the job that might be important to rehabilitation professionals, such as "chance to rotate among services," "collegial team relationships," and "availability of support staff." Each item would be written on a single card. Each clinician in the study would be asked to sort the cards into categories based on a preset distribution. For example, for our 50-card sort, there might be five categories with the following forced distribution: exceedingly important (4 cards), very important (10 cards), moderately important (22 cards), minimally important (10 cards), and of negligible importance (4 cards). This distribution would force clinicians to differentiate among a set of job-satisfaction items by identifying the very few that are most important as well as the very few that are least important. Responses could be quantified by assigning numerals to each category (exceedingly important=5; of negligible importance=1) and adding the scores for each item across therapists. Items with the highest scores would be those that were consistently placed in the more important categories. Kovach and Krejci[17] used Q-sort methodology to determine the factors that staff members in long-term care facilities perceived were most important in improving care for residents with dementia.

IMPLEMENTATION OVERVIEW

There are four methods of collecting survey data: personal interviews, telephone interviews, mailed questionnaires, and Internet-delivered questionnaires. Each of these four methods has its advantages and disadvantages, as indicated in Table 17-1.

Need for Rigor

Survey research is sometimes viewed as an "easy" approach to research—write a few questions, interview participants, mail out questionnaires, or post a survey using the Internet, and wait for the information to come pouring in. Unfortunately, this view sometimes leads to surveys that are conducted casually and lead to a superficial or distorted understanding of a topic based on the responses of a few. In contrast, well-designed and well-implemented survey research involves meticulous attention to the details of sampling, interview, or questionnaire design; interview implementation or questionnaire distribution; and follow-up. Dillman and associates'[18] text on the "tailored design method" of implementing surveys, Fink's[19] overview text on conducting surveys, and the Survey Kit[20] (a set of 10 slim volumes covering different aspects of survey research) provide prospective researchers with the information needed to implement survey research in rigorous ways to produce valid and reliable information. Information on designing surveys may be obtained from Internet sources, as well.[21,22] Most of the proprietary Internet survey software also offers guidance on developing quality surveys. In addition, survey researchers, just like researchers who study health care interventions,[23] need to attend to the ethical implications of their research, including issues of informed consent, anonymity of responses, and psychological impact of answering sensitive questions. Procedural guidelines for conducting mailed surveys, Internet surveys, and interviews are discussed in the next three main sections of this chapter.

Sample Size and Sampling

One task common to all surveys is the sampling process. First, the population of interest is defined (e.g., pediatric physical therapists). Second, the sampling frame is created (e.g., physical therapists who belong to the Pediatric Section of the APTA or physical therapists who are board-certified pediatric clinical specialists). Either one of these sampling frames is limited because it will not contain all physical therapists who work with children.

In addition, the two sampling frames differ, and researchers need to consider which sampling frame best meets their needs—one is larger and includes therapists with an interest in pediatrics, but who may not have much experience or expertise in the area; the other is smaller and includes only those who have undergone a certification process in pediatric physical therapy. In some instances, the population and the sampling frame are the same, and the researcher wishes to study the entire population of interest; in these cases, the sampling process is complete after just two steps. This was the case with Sneed and colleagues'[24] study of pediatric physiatrists and training programs, with Domholdt and colleagues'[25] study of physical therapist program directors, and with Sim and Adams's[26] study of therapeutic approaches of occupational therapists and physical therapists in the United Kingdom for individuals with fibromyalgia syndrome. In most instances, however, the sampling frame is much larger than is needed or than is practical, and the researcher must determine how to sample from among the many elements within the sampling frame.

The third step, then, is determining how many responses to the survey are desired. To do so for questionnaires that will result in proportions (e.g., what proportion of pediatric physical therapists work in school systems), the researchers need to determine the level of confidence they wish to have in their results (typically 95%, which corresponds to a z score of approximately 2), the proportion they expect to answer "yes" to the questions of interest (often simplified to $p=.50$, which maximizes the sample size estimate), and the amount of error they are willing to tolerate in their results.[27] The formula for determining sample size with these factors is:

$$n = \frac{Z^2(p)(1-p)}{error^2}$$

(Formula 17-1)

Inserting "2" for the Z and ".05" for the p yields a simplified formula of:

$$n = \frac{1}{error^2}$$

(Formula 17-2)

A researcher, then, who wishes to estimate a proportion with a 5% error in either direction would require a sample size of 400:

$$n = \frac{1}{.05^2} = 400$$

(Formula 17-3)

Table 17-1

Advantages and Disadvantages of Interviews and Questionnaires

Characteristics	METHOD			
	Personal Interviews	Telephone Interviews	Mailed Questionnaires	Internet Questionnaires
Time	Very time consuming	Time consuming	Time efficient	Time efficient
Cost	Personnel to conduct interviews, clerical or data entry personnel, travel	Personnel to conduct interviews, clerical or data entry personnel, long-distance telephone	Clerical or data entry personnel, printing and mailing	Internet and e-mail access, survey software
Geographic distribution	Greatly limited unless very well funded	Somewhat limited by long-distance telephone costs	Broad geographic distribution feasible because mailings can reach long distances at low cost	Very broad geographic distribution feasible because of quick world-wide Internet availability
Depth of response	Can be extensive	Somewhat limited	Limited	Limited
Anonymity	Difficult to achieve	Difficult to achieve	Easily achieved	Easily achieved
Literacy of respondents	Can sample those unable to read/write	Can sample those unable to read/write	Respondents must be able to read/write	Respondents must be able to read/write
Ability to clarify questions	Possible	Possible	Difficult, depends on respondent initiative	Difficult, depends on respondent initiative
Scheduling	Must coordinate researchers' and respondents' schedules	Must coordinate researchers' and respondents' schedules	Completed at respondents' convenience	Completed at respondents' convenience
Data entry	By researcher or assistant	By researcher or assistant	By researcher or assistant	By respondents as they complete the questionnaire

A researcher who wants considerably more precision, within 2% in either direction, would require a much larger sample of 2500:

$$n = \frac{1}{.02^2} = 2500$$

(Formula 17-4)

When the sample size exceeds 5% to 10% of the size of the population, the sample size can be reduced from these estimates. More detail on sample size determination for surveys can be found in other texts.[7,28]

The fourth step is determining the number of surveys to distribute. After the desired number of respondents is determined, the researchers must estimate what proportion of individuals will respond to the survey to determine how many surveys must be distributed. If, for example, 400 responses from pediatric physical therapists are desired and a 50% response rate is expected, then 800 surveys must be distributed. The expected response rate is affected by the length of the questionnaire, the connection between researchers and respondents, and the level of interest respondents are expected to have in the topic. A survey on a "hot" topic, studied with a brief questionnaire, by researchers who are known to the respondents, with incentives for respondents, may yield a response rate of 90%. A lengthy, unsolicited survey on an obscure topic from researchers not known to respondents may yield a response rate of 10%.

The final step is determining how to select the prospective respondents from the larger sampling frame. If, for example, there are 4000 pediatric physical therapists in the Pediatric Section of the APTA and we wish to send surveys to 800 of them, then we need to determine how to select the 800 from the 4000. The various probability and nonprobability sampling methods described in Chapter 9 are all possible methods of selecting the sample. When working with organizations that sell mailing lists to researchers, it is often possible to request a random or systematic sample so that the researchers do not have to undertake the sampling process themselves. For example, the researcher for our hypothetical study of pediatric physical therapists could purchase a systematic sample of 800 mailing labels or Internet addresses for members of the Pediatric Section of the APTA. Clearly, researchers will tailor these general sample size and sampling guidelines to fit the needs of their particular survey.

MAILED SURVEYS

Compared with interviews, mailed surveys cost less and permit a broader sampling frame and larger numbers of participants. Despite these advantages, mailed surveys may also have the disadvantages of unavailability of appropriate mailing lists of participants, low response rates, inability to gain information from individuals who cannot read, and lack of control over who actually responds to the questionnaire. Borque and Fielder[29] present the details of conducting mailed surveys in one volume of the Survey Kit. This section presents an overview of details related to the following: access to a sampling frame, deciding between researcher-developed and existing self-report instruments, questionnaire development, motivating prospects to respond, and implementation details.

Access to a Sampling Frame

When survey data are collected through a mailed questionnaire, potential participants can often be identified from the mailing lists of various groups. Mailing labels or directories of member addresses are available from sources such as professional associations. For example, when Carter and Stoecker[8,28] conducted their study of the reading of professional journals practices

of physical therapists, they used membership lists of several specialty sections as well as the general membership list from the APTA. A researcher interested in surveying rehabilitation directors at acute care hospitals across the United States might purchase American Hospital Association labels as a route to the appropriate people. When labels are ordered, the researcher can often specify several inclusion and exclusion criteria, as well as ask for a random sampling of labels meeting those criteria. In one step, then, the researcher can define the population, sample from that population, and obtain the labels needed to do the mailing. More details about sampling procedures are provided in Chapter 9.

Researcher-Developed Versus Existing Instruments

Researchers who wish to collect data through survey methods are faced with the question of whether to develop their own questionnaire or use an existing self-report instrument. A literature review should be done to determine what instruments have been used in related studies. Existing instruments that are commercially available and frequently cited in the literature can be identified from references such as the *Mental Measurements Yearbook*[30] and *Tests in Print*.[31] The text *Instruments for Clinical Health Care Research*[32] includes descriptions of existing measures for constructs such as quality of life, coping, hope, self-care, and body image. An instrument that was developed for a single study can often be obtained by writing to the researcher. Even if an instrument has been used only once before, there is a base of information about the tool on which subsequent research can build. We encourage researchers to use or adapt existing self-report tools that meet their needs before they develop their own.

Questionnaire Development

When researchers determine that they require unique information for their study, they must develop their own questionnaire. There are five basic steps to questionnaire development: drafting, expert review, first revision, pilot test, and final revision.

Drafting

The first step in developing a questionnaire is to draft items for consideration for inclusion in the questionnaire. In some cases, researchers may conduct focus groups or other interview studies to assist with this first step, as was the case in a report by Koopman[33] on the use of a small focus group to help identify needs of individuals with multiple sclerosis. These needs, along with information found in the literature, were then used as the basis for the development of a written needs assessment questionnaire. Before writing any items, the researcher must reexamine the purposes of the study and outline the major sections the questionnaire needs to include to answer the questions under study. Researchers seem to have an almost irresistible urge to ask questions because they seem interesting, without knowing how the answers will be used. This lengthens the questionnaire and may decrease the number of participants who respond. Several authors have provided specific suggestions for questionnaire design and format.[13,18,34]

Even for the first draft, the researcher must begin to consider issues of format and comprehensibility. The items in a questionnaire are often divided into topical groups to break the questionnaire into more easily digestible parts. In addition, because different topics may require items with different formats, the section headings provide a transition between different types of items. Some recommend that easier items be placed first on the questionnaire, with more difficult items presented later. The thought behind this is that the easy initial questions will get respondents interested in the questionnaire so that they will follow through with the more difficult questions that come later. For similar reasons, some recommend that demographic questions come last. It is thought that completing the demographic questions first will either bore respondents or offend them with questions about sensitive areas such as salary.

The readability of the type used in the questionnaire is important. The smallest readable type is generally considered to be 10-point type. Twelve-point type is more readable and is probably preferable for most questionnaires. If the population is expected to have difficulty with vision or if reading skills are likely to be low, 14-point type may be useful.

The type font is also important; researchers should not use atypical fonts that may be difficult to read. With the widespread availability of personal computers and low-cost desktop publishing services, any researcher should be able to produce an attractive, inviting questionnaire at a reasonable cost.

A second aspect of readability is the reading level required to understand the questionnaire. College-educated researchers are so accustomed to reading and writing that they forget that their writing is likely to be at an academic level that many will not be able to comprehend. To increase readability, researchers should write clearly and avoid jargon.

The instructions on how to complete the survey must also be clear and specific (e.g., "Check one box," "Circle as many items as apply," and "Write in your age in years at your last birthday"). If the same format of questions is used throughout a questionnaire, the instructions need to be given only once. If the format of questions changes from item to item, instructions should be provided for each item.

Researchers designing questionnaires must decide whether to include space for data coding on the questionnaire itself. Data coding is used to turn answers into numbers suitable for statistical analysis. Figure 17-1 shows an example of a questionnaire page, with a data coding column completed, based on a survey conducted by Bashi and Domholdt.[35] Some researchers do not like to include a data-coding column on questionnaires because they believe it is distracting to the respondent and takes up unnecessary space.

The researcher must also consider format and printing decisions such as the color of paper, the size and arrangement of pages, and the amount of white space on the questionnaire. The color of paper should be fairly light to ensure good readability. Good-quality paper should be used because it is the first means by which the potential respondent determines whether the questionnaire is worth answering. One format that has been recommended is a booklet.[18] A four-page questionnaire could be made by printing on both sides of a single sheet of 11-×17-inch paper and folding it in half to make an 8½-×11-inch booklet. In such a booklet, because multiple sheets of paper are not needed, none are inadvertently separated from one another. Another benefit is that the familiar booklet form should lead to fewer skipped questions; if single pages are printed front and back and stapled together, the reverse side of one sheet may be omitted by some respondents. The booklet may also have the appearance of being more professional, thereby increasing the return rate for the study.

Expert Review

Once the draft is written, the researcher needs to undertake the second step in questionnaire development: subjecting the questionnaire to review by a colleague or colleagues knowledgeable about the topic under study. This is essentially a check for content validity. Did the colleagues think that all the important elements of the constructs under study were addressed? Were questions understandable? Were terms defined satisfactorily? In addition to providing feedback on the content of the questionnaire, colleagues can also assess the format of the questionnaire.

First Revision

After the expert review, the researcher makes revisions in the questionnaire based on the feedback. If the selected colleagues make no recommendations for change, the

27. At some point during my professional career, utilization of support personnel for patient treatment has presented me with ethical dilemmas. (Circle appropriate letter)

    a. Strongly agree
    b. Agree
    c. Disagree
    (d.) Strongly disagree
    e. Unable to decide

28. I am comfortable with support personnel involvement in patient treatment at my current job. (Circle appropriate letter)

    a. Strongly agree
    (b.) Agree
    c. Disagree
    d. Strongly disagree
    e. Unable to decide

29. I am satisfied with professional association guidelines regarding utilization of support personnel in patient treatment. (Circle appropriate letter)

    a. Strongly agree
    b. Agree
    c. Disagree
    d. Strongly disagree
    (e.) Unable to decide

This column for researcher use only

1. _4_

2. _2_

3. _5_

Figure 17-1 Questionnaire excerpt, with coding column. The circled letters are converted to numbers before data entry. (Items modified from a survey described in Bashi HL, Domholdt E: Use of support personnel for physical therapy treatment, *Phys Ther* 73:421–436, 1993.)

researcher probably needs to identify other colleagues who are willing to be more critical.

Pilot Test

The next step is to pilot test the instrument on the types of participants who will complete the questionnaire. When pilot testing, it is useful to have participants indicate the time it took them to complete the questionnaire. The final item on the pilot questionnaire should be a request for the participants to review the questionnaire and write any comments they might have about the nature and format of the items.

When the pilot surveys are returned, the researcher should determine the return rate of the questionnaires and look for troublesome response patterns. For example, if only 40% of the pilot participants return questionnaires, then the researcher should not expect a better return rate from actual participants. The researcher should attempt to determine the reasons for

nonresponse to the pilot survey so that corrective measures can be taken on the final questionnaire.

Patterns to be sought among responses to the pilot testing are missing responses, lack of range in responses, many responses in the "other" category, and extraneous comments. For example, if one used several Likert-scale items and all the respondents answered "strongly agree," this may mean the item was worded so positively that no reasonable person would ever disagree with the statement. Rewording should create an item that is more likely to elicit a range of responses. Assume that the purpose of a survey is to determine clinicians' attitudes toward long-term care of the elderly. An item worded, "Quality long-term care for the elderly is an important component of the health care system in the United States" would be difficult to deny. Rewording the item to read, "Funding for long-term care of the elderly should take priority over funding for public education" requires the respondent to make choices between funding priorities and would likely elicit a greater range of responses.

An item repeatedly left unanswered may indicate that placement of the item on the page is a problem, the item is so sensitive that people do not wish to answer it, or the item is so complicated that it takes too much energy to answer it. A multiple-choice item frequently answered with the response category of "other" may indicate that the choices given were too limited.

Final Revision

Rewording of items, elimination of items, addition of items, or revision of the questionnaire format may all be indicated by the results of the pilot study. If a great many problems were identified in the pilot study, the researcher may wish to retest the questionnaire with a new group of pilot participants before investing the money and time in the final questionnaire.

Motivating Prospects to Respond

After the individuals to whom a questionnaire will be sent are identified, it is the researcher's job to sell them on the idea of completing the questionnaire. The cover letter that accompanies the survey is the major sales tool. It must be attractive, be brief but complete, and provide potential respondents with a good reason to complete the study. Figures 17-2 and 17-3 provide two examples of cover letters annotated with comments on their good and bad points. The inclusion of a stamped envelope addressed to the researcher for return mailing of the questionnaire is a necessary courtesy that will likely increase response. Other methods of motivating participants are the inclusion of incentives in the initial mailing (e.g., inexpensive, lightweight items such as a packet of instant cocoa or a dollar bill), entry into a random drawing for a more valuable incentive when the completed questionnaire is returned, or offering the results of the study when the analysis is complete.

Implementation Details

There are a number of implementation details that need to be planned when conducting a mailed survey: addressing options, envelopes, postage, and follow-up. If the researcher has a choice between printing the address directly on the outer envelope and using mailing labels, the former has the advantage of appearing to be more individualized. If the questionnaire packet that goes to prospective participants fits in a business-sized envelope, the researcher can choose between enclosing a folded business-sized return envelope or using a slightly smaller return envelope designed to fit flat within a business envelope. The latter option provides for a flatter packet and a more professional look. The budget may dictate whether bulk or first-class mailing rates are used to send the questionnaires. Whenever possible, first-class mailing should be done because bulk mail receives lower priority and is often not delivered in a timely fashion. The researcher needs to decide whether to use first-class or business-reply postage for return envelopes. First-class postage must be affixed to each return envelope with the knowledge that a proportion of the investment in return postage will be lost to nonrespondents. Business-reply postage costs more per envelope than first-class postage, but this higher cost is charged only on the returned envelopes. The researcher needs to compare costs between these postage options, assuming various return rates, to make a good decision about which option will be more cost effective.

Plans for follow-up mailings, if needed to achieve the desired return rate, need to be made in advance of the first mailing. To provide for the possibility of following up nonrespondents, the researcher numbers the master list of participants and in the envelope going to each participant places a return envelope or postcard with that participant's number on it. If the numbering is done on the return envelope, the corresponding participant is crossed off when his or her numbered envelope is returned; then the questionnaire and envelope are separated from one another, and the envelope with the identifying information is discarded and never associated with the corresponding questionnaire. This maintains the confidentiality of participant responses but depends on researcher integrity to do so.

A postcard system for follow-up maintains even greater anonymity. A numbered postcard is included with the questionnaire packet, and the participant is instructed to mail the postcard and questionnaire back separately so that the questionnaire and participant number will never be directly linked as they are if the return envelope is coded. However, a postcard system increases mailing and printing costs, and participants may forget to mail the postcard.

If the return rate is lower than desired by 7 to 10 days after the first responses were due, a second mailing to nonrespondents should be done. This follow-up packet should contain a new cover letter and a duplicate copy of the questionnaire. It is often appropriate to differentiate between first and second returns so that one can check to see whether there is a difference of opinions between those who initially responded and those who required a second prodding. This can be done by using a different-colored questionnaire for the follow-up mailing or by making an inconspicuous mark on all the

can hear participants and give them their full attention. If many interviewers are being used, a centralized calling area that enables the researcher to monitor the quality of the calls and answer questions as they arise is helpful. If in-person interviews take place on the participant's "turf," the interviewer needs to be prompt. If the interviews are being conducted at, for example, the interviewer's office, a receptionist should be available to greet arriving participants or take calls from participants who will be late or unable to keep their appointment. The comfort of participants should be taken into account by providing both a comfortable seating area and an appropriate arrangement of interviewer and participant and by making water or soft drinks available during the interview.

The interviewer needs to be prepared with an adequate supply of paper and working pens or pencils. If the interviews are to be recorded, the interviewer needs to be familiar with the recording equipment and ensure that the supply of tapes and batteries is adequate to meet the needs of the day.

When several interviewers are used within a study, the primary researcher needs to provide for their training. An interviewer manual should be developed and ought to include information on interviewing techniques and guidelines, the responsibilities of the interviewers, the rationale for interview questions, and a complete set of forms and procedures. The training process should include demonstration of good interview techniques, practice interviews, and observation and feedback to new interviewers.

SUMMARY

Surveys are systems for collecting self-reported information from participants. In general, the term *survey research* is applied to nonexperimental research with prospective data collection. Self-report instruments can be used to collect facts, determine knowledge, describe behavior, determine opinion, or document personal characteristics. Self-report instruments can include open- and closed-format items. Closed-format items include multiple-choice items, Likert-type scales, semantic differentials, and Q-sorts. Sound survey design requires meticulous attention to the details of sampling, interview, or questionnaire design; interview implementation or questionnaire distribution; and follow-up. The advantages and disadvantages of personal interviews, telephone interviews, mailed questionnaires, or Internet questionnaires must be considered when determining the method of data collection.

REFERENCES

1. Fink A: *The Survey Handbook, The Survey Kit,* Volume 1, 2nd ed, Thousand Oaks, Calif, 2003, Sage.
2. Chevan J, Chevan A: A statistical profile of physical therapists, 1980 and 1990, *Phys Ther* 78:301–312, 1998.
3. Balogun JA, Kaplan MT, Miller TM: The effect of professional education on the knowledge and attitudes of physical therapist and occupational therapist students about acquired immunodeficiency syndrome, *Phys Ther* 78:1073–1082, 1998.
4. Hagberg K, Brånemark R: Consequences of non-vascular trans-femoral amputation: A survey of quality of life, prosthetic use and problems, *Prosthet Orthot Int* 25:186–194, 2001.
5. Nadler SF, Prybicien M, Malanga GA, Sicher D: Complications from therapeutic modalities: Results of a national survey of athletic trainers, *Arch Phys Med Rehabil* 84:849–853, 2003.
6. Wagner AK, Stewart PJB: An internship for college students in physical medicine and rehabilitation: Effects on awareness, career choice, and disability perceptions, *Am J Phys Med Rehabil* 80:459–465, 2001.
7. Tepe ES, Deutsch ES, Sampson Q, et al: A pilot survey of vocal health in young singers, *J Voice* 16:244–250, 2002.
8. Carter RE, Stoecker J: Descriptors of American Physical Therapy Association physical therapist members' reading of professional publications, *Physiother Theory Pract* 23:263–278, 2006.
9. Brown T, Tseng MH, Casey J, et al: Predictors of research utilization among pediatric occupational therapists, *Occup Ther J Res* 30:172–183, 2010.
10. Macht M, Wimbish T, Clark BJ, et al: Diagnosis and treatment of post-extubation dysphagia: Results from a national survey, *J Crit Care* 27:578–586, 2012.
11. Archer KR, MacKenzie EJ, Bosse MJ, et al: Factors associated with surgeon referral for physical therapy in patients with traumatic lower-extremity injury: Results of a national survey of orthopedic trauma surgeons, *Phys Ther* 89:893–905, 2009.
12. Fink A: *How to Ask Survey Questions, The Survey Kit,* Volume 2, 2nd ed, Thousand Oaks, Calif, 2003, Sage.
13. Rozier CK, Raymond MJ, Goldstein MS, Hamilton BL: Gender and physical therapy career success factors, *Phys Ther* 78:690–704, 1998.
14. Osgood CE, Suci GJ, Tannenbaum PH: *The Measurement of Meaning,* Urbana, Ill, 1957, University of Illinois Press.
15. Streed CP, Stoecker JL: Stereotyping between physical therapy students and occupational therapy students, *Phys Ther* 71:16–24, 1991.
16. Stephenson W: *The Study of Behavior: Q Technique and Its Methodology,* Chicago, Ill, 1975, University of Chicago Press.
17. Kovach CR, Krejci JW: Facilitating change in dementia care: Staff perceptions, *J Nurs Admin* 28:17–27, 1998.
18. Dillman DA, Smyth JD, Christian LM: *Internet, Mail, and Mixed-Mode Surveys: The Tailored Design Method,* 3rd ed, Hoboken, NJ, 2009, John Wiley & Sons.
19. Fink A: *How To Conduct Surveys: A Step-By-Step Guide,* 4th ed, Thousand Oaks, Calif, 2009, Sage.

20. Fink A, editor: *The Survey Kit*, 2nd ed, Thousand Oaks, Calif, 2003, Sage.

21. DigitalGov. Lost and Found Mapping Page. Available at: http://www.digitalgov.gov/about/lost-and-found-mapping-page/. Accessed February 12, 2015.

22. Science Buddies. Designing a Survey. Available at: http://www.sciencebuddies.org/science-fair-projects/project_ideas/Soc_survey.shtml. Accessed February 12, 2015.

23. Evans M, Robling M, Maggs Rapport F, et al: It doesn't cost anything to ask, does it? The ethics of questionnaire-based research, *J Med Ethics* 28:41–44, 2002.

24. Sneed RC, May WL, Stencel C, Paul SM: Pediatric physiatry in 2000: A survey of practitioners and training programs, *Arch Phys Med Rehabil* 83:416–422, 2002.

25. Domholdt E, Stewart JC, Barr JO, Melzer BA: Entry-level doctoral degrees in physical therapy: Status as of Spring 2000, *J Phys Ther Educ* 16:60–68, 2002.

26. Sim J, Adams N: Therapeutic approaches to fibromyalgia syndrome in the United Kingdom: A survey of occupational therapists and physical therapists, *Eur J Pain* 7:173–180, 2002.

27. *Survey Research Using Statistical Package for the Social Sciences (SPSS)*, Chicago, Ill, 1998, SPSS, Inc.

28. Fink A: *How to Sample in Surveys, The Survey Kit*, Volume 7, 2nd ed, Thousand Oaks, Calif, 2003, Sage.

29. Borque LB, Fielder EP: *How to Conduct Self-Administered and Mail Surveys, The Survey Kit*, Volume 3, 2nd ed, Thousand Oaks, Calif, 2003, Sage.

30. Spies RA, Carlson JF, Geisinger KF, editors: *The Eighteenth Mental Measurements Yearbook*, Lincoln, Neb, 2010, Buros Institute of Mental Measurements of the University of Nebraska-Lincoln.

31. Murphy LL, Geisinger K, Carlson JF, Spies RA, editors: *Tests in Print VIII*, Lincoln, Neb, 2011, Buros Institute of Mental Measurements of the University of Nebraska-Lincoln.

32. Frank-Stromborg M, Olsen SJ: *Instruments for Clinical Health Care Research*, 3rd ed, Sudbury, Mass, 2004, Jones & Bartlett.

33. Koopman W: Needs assessment of persons with multiple sclerosis and significant others: Using the literature review and focus groups for preliminary survey questionnaire development, *Axon* 24:10–15, 2003.

34. Peterson RA: *Constructing Effective Questionnaires*, Thousand Oaks, Calif, 1999, Sage.

35. Bashi HL, Domholdt E: Use of support personnel for physical therapy treatment, *Phys Ther* 73:421–436, 1993.

36. Goodman CM: The Delphi technique: A critique, *J Adv Nurs* 12:729–734, 1987.

37. Finger ME, Cieza A, Stoll J, et al: Identification of intervention categories for physical therapy, based on the International Classification of Functioning, Disability and Health: A Delphi exercise, *Phys Ther* 86:1203–1220, 2006.

38. Domholdt E, Kerr LR, Mount KA: Entry-level doctoral degrees in physical therapy: Status as of Spring 2003, *J Phys Ther Educ* 20:68–76, 2006.

39. Survey Suite. Available at: http://intercom.virginia.edu/SurveySuite/Guide/Guide.php?index=1. Accessed December 5, 2014.

40. Survey Share. Available at: www.surveyshare.com. Accessed December 5, 2014.

41. Survey Monkey. Available at: www.surveymonkey.com/. Accessed December 5, 2014.

42. Qualtrics. http://qualtrics.com/. Accessed December 5, 2014.

43. Klein J: Issues surrounding the use of the Internet for data collection, *Am J Occup Ther* 56:340–343, 2002.

44. Borque LB, Fielder EP: *How to Conduct Telephone Surveys, The Survey Kit*, Volume 4, Thousand Oaks, Calif, 2003, Sage.

45. Oishi SM: *How to Conduct In-Person Interviews for Surveys, The Survey Kit*, Volume 5, Thousand Oaks, Calif, 2003, Sage.

46. Korner-Bitensky N, Barrett-Bernstein S, Bibasand G, Poulin V: National survey of Canadian occupational therapists' assessment and treatment of cognitive impairment post-stroke, *Aust Occup Ther J* 58:241–250, 2011.

47. Freburger JK, Carey TS, Holmes GM: Physical therapy for chronic low back pain in North Carolina: Overuse, underuse, or misuse? *Phys Ther* 91:484–495, 2011.

CHAPTER 18

Measurement Theory

CHAPTER OUTLINE

Definitions of Measurement
Variable Properties
Scales of Measurement
  Nominal Scales
  Ordinal Scales
  Interval Scales
  Ratio Scales
  Determining the Scale of a
    Measurement
Types of Variables
**Statistical Foundations of
  Measurement Theory**

Frequency Distribution
Mean
Variance
Standard Deviation
Normal Curve
Correlation Coefficient
Standard Error of Measurement
Measurement Frameworks
**Measurement Reliability and
  Validity**
Measurement Reliability
  Two Theories of Reliability

Components of Reliability
Quantification of Reliability
Measurement Validity
  Construct Validity
  Content Validity
  Criterion Validity
Responsiveness to Change
Summary

Rehabilitation professionals use measurements to help them decide what is wrong with patients or clients, how to intervene, and when to discontinue treatment. Health care insurers rely on these measurements when they make decisions about whether to reimburse for rehabilitation services. Researchers use measurements to quantify the characteristics they study. In fact, some investigators focus the majority of their research on the evaluation of rehabilitation measures. Researchers may also use measurements to quantify the amount of the treatment being delivered to their subjects. However, knowledge about the usefulness of measurements is not reserved for these research specialists—clinicians also need to understand the meaning and usefulness of the measures they use.

This chapter presents a framework for understanding and evaluating the measurements used by rehabilitation professionals. The chapter presents several definitions of measurement; discusses properties of variables, scales of measurement, and types of variables; introduces the statistical concepts required to understand measurement theory; and discusses measurement reliability, validity, and responsiveness to change. Chapter 19 builds on this framework by presenting strategies for conducting research about measurements.

DEFINITIONS OF MEASUREMENT

The broadest definition of measurement is that it is "the process by which things are differentiated."[1] A narrower definition is that measurement "consists of rules for assigning symbols so as to (1) represent quantities of attributes numerically (scaling) or (2) define whether the objects fall in the same or different categories with respect to a given attribute (classification)."[2] This text uses the following simpler definition of measurement: Measurement is the systematic process by which things are differentiated. Thus, this definition emphasizes that measurement is not a random process, but one that proceeds according to rules and guidelines.

Differentiation can be accomplished with names, numerals, or numbers. For example, classifying people as underweight, normal weight, or overweight involves the assignment of names to differentiate people according to the characteristic of ideal body composition. If these groups are relabeled as Groups 1, 2, and 3, then each person is assigned a numeral to represent body composition. A *numeral* is a symbol that does not necessarily have quantitative meaning[3(p. 392)]; it is a form of naming. Describing people not by groups but also by their specific percentage of body fat (e.g., 10% or 14%) would involve the assignment of a *number* to represent the quantity of body fat. A number, then, is a numeral that has been assigned quantitative meaning.

VARIABLE PROPERTIES

When we measure changes in a variable, we are measuring some property or attribute of the variable. It is this aspect of the variable that is specified in the operational definition of the dependent variable. Generally, the types of properties that may be measured are at least one of the following:

- *Distance* (e.g., height jumped or distance walked)
- *Duration:* how long a behavior occurs (e.g., time walked)
- *Frequency:* how often a behavior occurs; *rate* is a property used when the frequency of behavior occurrence is in different durations of time
- *Magnitude:* how large a response is (e.g., the size of sound may be measured in decibels, or the amount of pressure measured in some form of weight, such as ounces or pounds)
- *Topography:* position or alignment of body parts in a posture or movement task, but also can be a pattern of movements
- *Latency:* how long after a signal or cue a specific behavioral response occurs
- *Pattern:* a sequence of behaviors

The property that is to be measured must be reflective of the theoretical constructs or concepts of the independent variable (IV). For example, if the scientist-practitioner is using an intervention that theoretically affects the "ease" or "fluidity" of gait, measuring the property of distance walked is inappropriate because distance walked is a measure of endurance. Measuring the amount of time in stance phase for each lower extremity during gait would be a more appropriate measure of "fluidity" of gait.

SCALES OF MEASUREMENT

Four classic scales, or levels, of measurement are presented in the literature. These scales are based on the extent to which a measure has the properties of a real-number system. A real-number system is characterized by order, distance, and origin.[4(p. 12)] *Order* means that higher numbers represent greater amounts of the characteristic being measured. *Distance* means that the magnitude of the differences between successive numbers is equal or logarithmic (i.e., the distance between successive numbers is an equal multiple). *Origin* means that the number 0 (zero) represents an absence of the measured quality.

Nominal Scales

Nominal scales have none of the properties of a real number system. A nominal scale provides classification without placing any value on the categories within the classification. Because there is no order, distance, or origin to the classification, the classification can be identified by name or numeral. However, it is often better to give classifications names instead of numerals so that no quantitative difference among categories is implied. For example, the classification of types of cerebral palsy based on body parts involved (e.g., quadriplegia, diplegia, and hemiplegia) is an example of a nominal measurement. The classification itself is valueless (i.e., does not have quantitative value). It does not rank, for example, the functional impairment of the individual—that depends on level of spasticity, intellectual functioning, and a host of other factors not implied by the classification itself.

Ordinal Scales

Ordinal scales have only one of the three properties of a real number system: order or rank. Thus, an ordinal scale can be used to indicate whether a person or object has more or less of a certain quality. Ordinal scales do not ensure that there are equal intervals between categories or ranks. Because the intervals on an ordinal scale are either not known or are unequal, mathematical manipulations such as addition, subtraction, multiplication, or division of ordinal numbers are not meaningful.

Many instruments that measure functional performance are ordinal. The amount of assistance a patient needs to ambulate is often rated as maximal assistance, moderate assistance, minimal assistance, standby assistance, or independent. Is the interval between maximal assistance and moderate assistance the same as the interval between minimal assistance and standby assistance? Probably not. Sometimes numerals are assigned to points on an ordinal scale, but the validity of this procedure has been questioned because the numerals are often treated as if they were quantitative numbers.[5]

Figure 18-1 illustrates the phenomenon of unequal intervals between points on an ordinal scale of gait independence. Assume that the underlying quantity

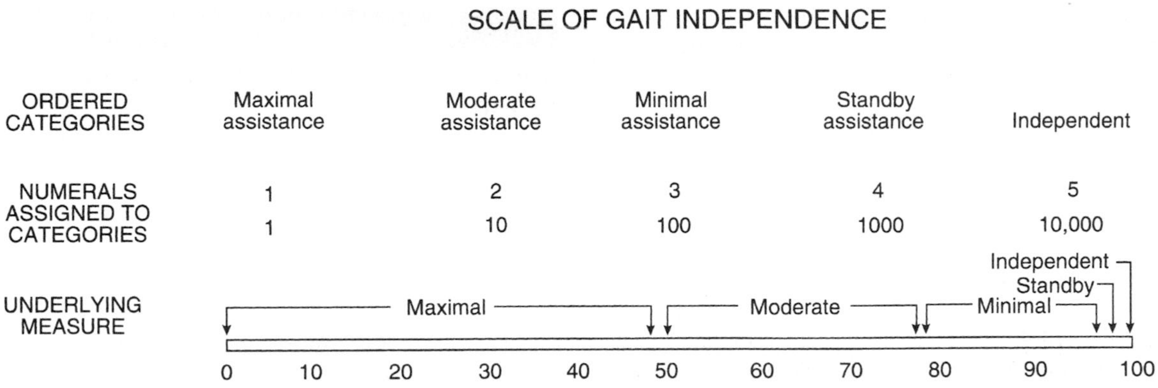

SCALE OF GAIT INDEPENDENCE

ORDERED CATEGORIES	Maximal assistance	Moderate assistance	Minimal assistance	Standby assistance	Independent
NUMERALS ASSIGNED TO CATEGORIES	1	2	3	4	5
	1	10	100	1000	10,000

UNDERLYING MEASURE

Independent — Standby — Minimal — Independent

Maximal — Moderate — Minimal

0   10   20   30   40   50   60   70   80   90   100

Figure 18-1 Level of assistance in gait as an ordinal measurement. The top row shows the assistance categories as used by many clinicians. The bottom row shows a theoretical underlying distribution of the categories based on what percentage of effort is being exerted by the patient. The middle two rows show two vastly different numbering schemes; in both schemes the numbers get larger as the amount of effort exerted by the patient increases.

represented by the assistance categories is the proportion of the total work of ambulation that is exerted by the patient. If the patient and clinician are expending equal energy to get the patient walking, then the patient is exerting 50% of the total work of ambulation. If the patient is independent and the clinician does not need to expend any energy, then the patient is exerting 100% of the total work of ambulation. The top line of Figure 18-1 shows the assistance categories. The middle two lines show numerals that could be assigned to the assistance categories. Either set of numerals would meet the order criterion—higher numerals indicate higher levels of independence. The magnitude of the two sets of numerals varies greatly and shows the danger of thinking of ordinal numbers as real quantities. The bottom scale shows how the assistance categories might fall along a continuum of total work percentage. The categories "minimal," "standby," and "independent," as used by most clinicians, probably fall in the top 20% of the scale. The categories "maximal" and "moderate" probably fall in the bottom 80% of the scale. Thus, the gait independence classification used by clinicians is clearly an ordinal scale: the classification has order but does not represent equal intervals of the underlying construct, "independence," that is being measured.

A second type of ordinal scale is a ranking. During 2003, sisters Serena Williams and Venus Williams were the first- and second-ranked women tennis players in the world, respectively. Although the interval between these two players was slight, the difference between the second- and third-ranked players was much greater. The intervals between ranks are usually unknown and cannot be assumed to be equal.

Interval Scales

Interval scales have the real-number system properties of order and distance, but they lack a meaningful origin. A meaningful zero point represents the absence of the measured quantity. The Celsius and Fahrenheit temperature scales are examples of interval scales. The zero points on the two temperature scales are arbitrary: On the Fahrenheit scale, it is the temperature at which salt water freezes, and on the Celsius scale, it is the temperature at which fresh water freezes. Neither implies the absence of the basic property of heat—the temperature can go lower than 0° on both scales. Both scales, however, have regular (but different) intervals. Because of the equal intervals, addition and subtraction are meaningful with interval scales. A 10° increase in temperature means the same thing whether the increase is from 0° to 10° or from 100° to 110°. However, multiplication and division of Fahrenheit or Celsius temperature readings are not useful because these operations assume knowledge of zero quantities. A Fahrenheit temperature of 100° is not twice as hot as a temperature of 50°; it is merely 50° hotter.

Ratio Scales

Ratio scales exhibit all three components of a real-number system: order, distance, and origin. All the arithmetic functions of addition, subtraction, multiplication, and division can be applied to ratio scales. Length, time, and weight are generally considered ratio scales because their absence is scored as zero, and the intervals between numbers are known to be equal. The Kelvin temperature scale is an example of a ratio scale because the intervals between degrees are equal and the zero point represents the absence of heat.

Determining the Scale of a Measurement

To determine the scale of a measure, the researcher must ascertain whether there is a true zero (origin), whether intervals between numbers are equal (distance), and whether there is an order to the numbers or names that constitute the measure (order). Although this sounds simple enough, a number of twists come into play when determining the scale of a measurement.

For example, does the classification of patients as underweight, normal weight, and overweight represent a nominal or ordinal scale? The numbers are placed into classes, but these classes also have an order, so the scale is ordinal. As another example, do scores on the Sickness Impact Profile (SIP) represent ordinal or interval data? Summed scales—that is, those scored by summing the values of responses on many questions—are often treated as interval scales even though it can be argued that the underlying construct being measured is too abstract to permit the assumption that intervals between scores are equal. When ordinal scales can take many values (e.g., with a summed score that can range from 0 to 100 as opposed to a gait assistance scale with only five values), data may have the mathematical characteristics of an interval scale. Because the scale of measurement determines which mathematical manipulations are meaningful, controversy about measurement scales soon becomes controversy about which statistical tests are appropriate for which types of measures. These statistical controversies are discussed in Chapter 21.

TYPES OF VARIABLES

With respect to measurement, variables can be classified as continuous or discrete (Table 18-1). A discrete variable is one that can assume only distinct values. Levels of variables in a nominal scale are, by definition, discrete: The individuals being classified (e.g., having classifications of cerebral palsy) must fit into a distinct category (e.g., quadriplegic); they cannot be placed between the categories. Discrete variables that can assume only two values are called dichotomous variables. Examples of dichotomous variables are presence or absence of a behavior or disease state. Variables that are counts of behaviors or persons are discrete variables because fractional people or behaviors are not possible, though any behaviors, because they are usually complex, must be rigorously defined. If the measure of interest is the number of times a child names an object correctly in 10 trials, it is not possible to get a score of 7.5 on a single trial. Note, however, that it is possible

Table 18-1

Scales or Levels of Measurement and Types of Variables

Variable Type	Scale or Level	Order	Distance	Origin
Discrete	Nominal	—	—	—
	Ordinal or Rank	X	—	—
Continuous	Interval	X	X	—
	Ratio	X	X	X

to have an average score of 7.5 if the 10-trial sequence is repeated on 4 subsequent days with scores of 8, 6, 9, and 7 (8+6+9+7=30; 30/4=7.5). If discrete variables can assume a fairly large range of values, have the properties of a real-number system, or are averaged across trials, they become similar to continuous variables.

Traditionally, variables that are ordinal have been considered discrete variables. How ordinal variables are treated statistically is open to discussion among some statisticians. The controversy over the treatment of ordinal variables is discussed briefly later.

A continuous variable is one that theoretically can be measured to a finer and finer degree.[4(p. 15)] Clinicians interested in hand function might record the time it takes for someone to transfer 25 objects from one tray to another. Depending on the sophistication of the measurement tools, the clinician might measure time to the nearest second or to the nearest one thousandth of a second. If the smallest increment on a clinician's watch is the second, then measurements cannot be recorded in smaller increments even though the clinician knows that the true time required for completion of a task is not limited to whole seconds. Thus, the limits of technology dictate that continuous variables will always be measured discretely.

Why are we concerned with these scales of measurement and the types of variables? Most notably, different kinds of statistics are employed when particular measurement scales are used. Generally, nominal data are analyzed with nonparametric statistics, whereas interval and ratio data are analyzed using parametric statistics. Traditionally, nonparametric statistics have been used to analyze ordinal data, as well; however, recent reasoning and theory support the use of parametric statistics with ordinal data, arguing that parametric statistics are so robust that they may be used with ordinal data even though the distance between intervals is unknown. This will be discussed in more detail in Chapter 21.

STATISTICAL FOUNDATIONS OF MEASUREMENT THEORY

Seven basic concepts underlie most of measurement theory: frequency distribution, mean, variance, standard deviation, normal curve, correlation coefficient, and standard error of measurement (SEM). These concepts are introduced here and are expanded on in Chapters 20 and 23.

Frequency Distribution

A frequency distribution is nothing more than the number of times each score is represented in the data set. If a therapist measures a patient's knee flexion 10 times during 1 day, the following scores might be obtained: 100, 100, 90, 95, 110, 110, 95, 105, 95, 100. Table 18-2

Table **18-2**

Frequency Distribution of 10 Knee Flexion Measurements

Score	Frequency
90	1
95	3
100	3
105	1
110	2

and Figure 18-2 show two ways of presenting the frequency distribution for these 10 scores.

Mean

The arithmetic mean of a data set is the sum of the observations divided by the number of observations. Mathematical notation for the mean is as follows:

$$\bar{X} = \frac{\sum X}{N}$$

(Formula 18-1)

where $\bar{X}$ is the symbol for the sample mean and is sometimes called "X-bar"; Σ is the uppercase Greek letter sigma and means "the sum of"; X is the symbol for each observation; and N is the symbol for the number of observations. In words, the mean equals the sum of all the observations divided by the number of observations. The mean of the data set presented earlier is calculated as follows:

$$\bar{X} = (90 + 95 + 95 + 95 + 100 + 100 \\ + 100 + 105 + 110 + 110)/10 = 100$$

The population mean, μ, is calculated the same way but is rarely used in practice because researchers do not have access to the entire population.

Variance

The variance is a measure of the variability around the mean within a data set. To calculate the variance, a researcher converts each of the raw scores in a data set

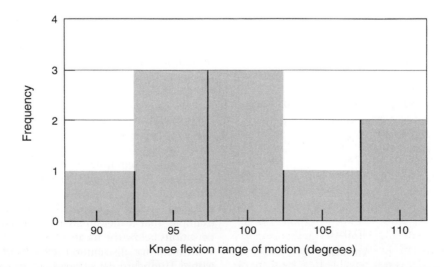

Figure 18-2 Histogram of the frequency distribution of hypothetical knee flexion data.

to a deviation score by subtracting the mean of the data set from each raw score. In mathematical notation,

$$x = X - \bar{X}$$

(Formula 18-2)

The lowercase x is the symbol for a deviation score. The deviation score indicates how high or low a raw score is compared with the mean. The first two columns of Table 18-3 present the raw and deviation scores for the knee flexion data set, followed by their sums and means. Note that both the sum and the mean of the deviation scores are zero. In order to generate a nonzero index of the variability within a data set, the deviation scores must be squared. The variance is then calculated by determining the mean of the squared deviations. In mathematical notation,

$$\sigma^2 = \frac{\sum x^2}{N}$$

(Formula 18-3)

where σ is the lowercase Greek sigma and when squared is the notation for the population variance. The third column in Table 18-3 shows the squared deviations from the group mean, the sum of the squared deviations, and the mean of the squared deviations. The variance is the mean

Table 18-3

Computation of the Variance in the 10 Knee Flexion Measurements

X	x	x^2	z score
90	10	100	1.59
95	5	25	.79
95	5	25	.79
95	5	25	.79
100	0	0	0
100	0	0	0
100	0	0	0
105	5	25	.79
110	10	100	1.59
110	10	100	1.59
Σ 1000	0	400	
μ 100	0	40.0 = σ^2, Variance	

of the squared deviation scores. In practice, there are different symbols and slightly different formulas for the variance, depending on whether the observations represent the entire population of interest or just a sample of the population. This distinction is addressed in Chapter 20.

Although the variance is useful in many statistical procedures, it does not have a great deal of intuitive meaning because it is calculated from squared deviation scores. A measure that does have intuitive meaning is the standard deviation.

Standard Deviation

The standard deviation is the square root of the variance and is expressed in the units of the original measure:

$$\sigma = \sqrt{\sigma^2} = \sqrt{\frac{\sum x^2}{N}}$$

(Formula 18-4)

The mathematical notations for the standard deviation and the variance make their relationship clear: The notation for the variance (σ^2) is simply the square of the notation for standard deviation (σ). The standard deviation of the knee flexion data presented in Table 18-3 is the square root of 40, or 6.3°.

Normal Curve

Groups of measurements frequently approximate a bell-shaped distribution known as the *normal* or *Gaussian curve*. The normal curve is a symmetrical frequency distribution that can be defined in terms of the mean and standard deviation of a set of data. Any raw score within the distribution can be converted into a z score, which indicates how many standard deviations the raw score is above or below the mean. A *z score* is calculated by subtracting the mean from the raw score, creating a deviation score, and then dividing the deviation score by the standard deviation:

$$Z = \frac{x}{\sigma}$$

(Formula 18-5)

The fourth column of Table 18-3 shows each raw score as a *z score*. Raw scores were transformed into *z scores* by dividing each of the deviation scores (x) by the standard deviation of 6.3°. The *z score* tells us, for example, that a measurement of 90° is 1.59 standard deviations below the mean.

In a normal distribution, 68.27% of the scores fall within 1 standard deviation above or below the mean,

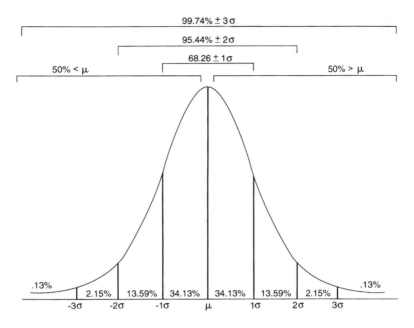

Figure 18-3 Probabilities of the normal curve. μ=mean; σ=standard deviation.

95.44% of the scores fall within 2 standard deviations above or below the mean, and 99.74% of the scores fall within 3 standard deviations above or below the mean. Figure 18-3 shows a diagram of the normal curve, with the percentages of scores that are found within each standard deviation. Figure 18-4A shows the normal curve that corresponds to the knee flexion data set. The mean is 100, and the standard deviation is 6.3. Figure 18-4B shows that if the knee flexion scores are normally distributed, we can expect about 98% of our measurements to exceed the score of 87.4 (the shaded area in the figure). Figure 18-4C shows that we can expect about 68% of our measures to fall between 93.7° and 106.3°. Predicting the probability of obtaining certain ranges of scores is one of the most basic of statistical functions.

Correlation Coefficient

A correlation coefficient is a statistical summary of the degree of relationship that exists between two or more measures. The relationship can be between either different variables (such as bone density and age) or repeated measures of the same variables (such as blood pressures of the same individual taken by three different clinicians). There are many different types of correlation coefficients (Table 18-4); the computational distinctions between them are discussed in Chapter 23. A group of correlations known as *intraclass correlation coefficients* are commonly used to document measurement reliability.

A correlation coefficient of 0.0 means that there is no relationship between the variables; a correlation coefficient of 1.0 indicates that there is a perfect relationship between the variables. Values in between these two extremes indicate intermediate levels of relationship. Some correlation coefficients can also have values from 0.0 to ~1.0. A negative correlation indicates an inverse relationship between variables (i.e., as the values for one variable become larger, the values for the other become smaller). In this text, *r* is used as a general symbol for a correlation coefficient. The specific notation for each type of coefficient is introduced when needed.

Standard Error of Measurement

In addition to knowing the relationship between repeated measurements, the researcher may wish to know how a given score is related to a "true" score for the person, as well as how much a score might vary with repeated measurements of the same individual. To determine the amount of measurement error, a researcher can take many repeated measures of the same participant and calculate the standard deviation of the scores; this standard deviation is known as the standard error of measurement (SEM). In practice, it is difficult to determine the SEM directly. Consider the effect of measuring wrist flexion up to 100 times in someone with limited wrist motion to determine the SEM. The individual's wrist flexion might improve during the course

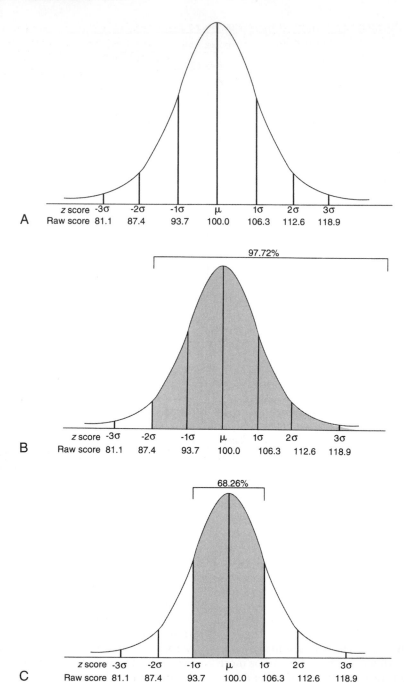

Figure 18-4 Probabilities of the normal curve applied to hypothetical range-of-motion data with a mean of 100 and a standard deviation of 6.3. **A,** The range-of-motion values that correspond to 1, 2, and 3 standard deviations above the mean. **B,** The probability of obtaining a score greater than 87.4° F (the *shaded area*) is 97.72%. **C,** The probability of obtaining a score between 93.7° and 106.3° F (the *shaded area*) is 68.26%. μ=mean; σ=standard deviation.

Table 18-4

Correlation Coefficients

Name of Coefficient	Type of Data Required	No. of Repeated Measures Compared
Pearson product moment correlation	Continuous	Two
Intraclass correlation	Continuous	Two or more
Spearman rank order correlation	Ranked	Two
Kendall's tau	Ranked	Two
Cohen's kappa	Nominal	Usually two; can be modified to accommodate more than two

of testing by virtue of the exercise associated with taking so many measurements. Conversely, the individual's wrist flexion might be reduced as the joint becomes progressively more painful. In any event, taking so many repeated measurements would likely result in a confounding of measurement error with actual treatment effects.

Because of the difficulty in directly determining the SEM, it is often estimated as follows:[6,7(p. 117)]

$$SEM = \sigma\sqrt{1-r}$$

(Formula 18-6)

Assume that a researcher takes two wrist flexion measurements on each of 10 patients. If the standard deviation of the measures is 5 and the intraclass correlation coefficient between the two measures is .80, then the estimated SEM is 2.2.

$$\begin{aligned} SEM &= 5\sqrt{1-.80} \\ &= 5\sqrt{.20} \\ &= 5(.44) \\ &= 2.2 \end{aligned}$$

(Formula 18-7)

The SEM is a standard deviation of measurement errors, and measurement errors are assumed to be normally distributed. Thus, by combining our knowledge of the probabilities of the normal curve with this value for the SEM, we can conclude there is a 68% probability that a person's true wrist flexion would be within 1 SEM or ±2.2° of the original measurement. Approximately 96% of the time, true wrist flexion would be within 2 SEM or ±4.4° of the original measurement.

To determine how much a measure would be expected to vary with repeated measurement, the SEM is multiplied by the square root of the number of measurements and added and subtracted from the original measurement, as above.[6,7(p. 144)]

$$\begin{aligned} SEM_{repeated} &= \sqrt{2}\left(5\sqrt{1-.80}\right) \\ &= 1.414\left(5\sqrt{.20}\right) \\ &= (1.414)(2.2) \\ &= 3.1 \end{aligned}$$

(Formula 18-8)

There is a 68% probability that a repeated measure of wrist flexion would be within ±3.1° of the original measurement. Approximately 96% of the time, a repeated measure of wrist flexion would be within ±6.2° of the original measurement.

MEASUREMENT FRAMEWORKS

There are two basic frameworks in which measurement is conducted and evaluated: norm referenced and criterion referenced. Norm-referenced measures are those used to judge individual performance in relation to group norms. The statistical concepts of the mean and standard deviation are integral to norm-referenced measures. Measurements that use norm-referenced frameworks may use raw scores that are compared with tables of raw-score norms. More commonly, raw scores are standardized in some way to present them in relationship to the mean and standard deviation of the sample on which the norms were established. These standardized scores may be *z scores* (based on a mean of 0 and an SD of 1), T-scores (based on a mean of 50 and an SD of 10, thereby eliminating negative scores), percentile ranks (converting the *z scores* to a percentile ranking based on the normal distribution), or a measure-specific system such as the Scholastic Achievement Test (SAT; based on a mean of 500 and a standard deviation of 100).[8]

Many clinical measurements are norm referenced. Blood pressure and pulse rates are evaluated against a range of normal values, muscle performance can be compared with average performance for age- and sex-matched groups, and developmental status may be compared against norms established with typically developing children. Clinicians who often work with norm-referenced measures may wish to consult a more detailed measurement text to develop a stronger knowledge base in the use of norm-referenced tests.[8]

A criterion-referenced measure is one in which each individual's performance is evaluated with respect to some absolute level of achievement. When a teacher establishes 75% as the minimum passing score in a course, this is a criterion-referenced measurement. If all students exceed the 75% criterion, all pass. If only 25% exceed the criterion, only 25% pass. Clinicians use a criterion-referenced framework when they set specific performance criteria that patients have to meet in order to resume athletic competition, be released from an inpatient setting, or take an assistive device home.

MEASUREMENT RELIABILITY AND VALIDITY

An imperative in rehabilitation practice, as well as research, is that measurements must be trustworthy. The trustworthiness of a measure is evaluated on its reliability and its validity. If we are to make decisions based on data we must believe the data are accurate. Because we can never truly know if a measurement is accurate, we do the next best thing: We reproduce the measurements. Above all else, we must have "trust" that the measurements are consistent, that is, are reproducible. If we can't reproduce the measurement, then we can't be certain the first measurement was accurate. If we can reproduce the measurement, we say we have reliable measures, or the measurement is consistent. When we have a high level of agreement on measurements of the same behavior taken by two or more observers, we have consistency of measurement, and then we consider the measure reliable. In order for there to be consistency of measurement (i.e., agreement) with the same observer, there must be a minimum of two measurements of the same behavior by the same person or two different persons.

In addition to a measure being consistent, another premise of measurement trustworthiness is that the measures must have meaning. That is, the measurement tool must measure what it intends to measure. This aspect of measurement trustworthiness evaluates the theoretical soundness or construct validity of the measure, usually referred to as measurement validity. Measurement tools presume to measure attributes of behaviors that can be explained by some theory. The theory presumes to explain how the patient's behavior occurred according to certain theoretical principles or constructs. Hence, theoretical soundness addresses how well a measurement tool

actually measures what it says it should be measuring. When a measure has theoretical soundness, or validity, we can infer that the results from the study sample of subjects would be similar for a different sample of subjects drawn from the same population.

When we are determining whether a measure is useful, we must first be concerned with the measurement's reliability, that is, how consistent the measurement is. As stated earlier, measurement reliability is usually determined through some form of agreement between observers (often referred to as interrater reliability/agreement or interobserver reliability/agreement) or within an observer (intrarater or intraobserver reliability/agreement). Furthermore, a measure may have reliability, but not have testable validity, and still be a useful tool. For example, a measure that focuses on a single behavior, such as the ability of a client to obtain full elbow extension, is a useful measure if it has very good reliability. If we measure the elbow extension with a goniometer, and we know that the measurement tool (i.e., the goniometer) is reliable, we do not need to know if the measure is valid (i.e., that it has theoretical soundness). We are only concerned with full elbow extension. There's no theory behind elbow extension. It is what it is. In other words, the behavior of elbow extension is not based on any theory: It is an observable, measurable behavior, and that is sufficient in itself. Alternatively, if a measurement tool has items that are based on theoretical principles or constructs, but is not reliable, that instrument is useless. Thus, reliability is a necessary prerequisite for a measurement tool to be useful.

Measurement Reliability

Reliability is the "degree to which test scores are free from errors of measurement."[9(p. 19)] Other terms that are similar to reliability are *accuracy, stability*, and *consistency*. Despite its conceptual simplicity, one pair of writers notes that "it is devilishly difficult to achieve a real understanding of … reliability."[7(p. 126)] Despite this difficulty, this section of the chapter forges ahead and introduces reliability theories, components, and measures.

Two Theories of Reliability

Two basic measurement theories—classical measurement theory and generalizability theory—provide somewhat different views of reliability. Classical measurement theory rests on the assumption that every measurement, or obtained score, consists of a true component and an error component. In addition, each person has a single true score on the measurement of interest. Because we can never know the true score for any measure and, thus, whether a measure is accurate, we try to reproduce the measurement using the relationship between repeated measurements to estimate measurement errors. A measurement is said to be reliable if the error component is small, allowing *consistent* estimation of the true quantity of interest. With classical measurement theory, all variability within a person's score is viewed as measurement error.[10]

Classical theories of reliability have been extended into what is known as *generalizability theory*. Generalizability theory recognizes that there are different sources of variability for any measure. Measurements are studied in ways that permit the researcher to divide the measurement error into sources of variability, or facets, of interest to the researcher.

To understand the differences between these two approaches, consider the measurement of forward head position with a device that provides a measurement in centimeters. Classical measurement theory assumes that every person has a true value for forward head position and that variations in a person's scores are measurement errors about the true score. In contrast, generalizability theory recognizes that differences in scores may be related to any number of different facets. Facets of interest to a given researcher for this example might be the subject's level of relaxation, his or her level of comfort with the particular examiner taking the measurement, the skill of the examiner, and the accuracy of the device used to measure forward head position. The generalizability approach seems to have a great deal of promise for the study of measurements in rehabilitation because it acknowledges and provides a way to quantify the many sources of variability that rehabilitation professionals see in their patients or clients from day to day.

Components of Reliability

Several components of reliability are examined frequently: instrument, intrarater, interrater, and intrasubject reliability. Although it is often difficult to completely separate these components, readers of the literature need to be able to conceptualize the different components so that they can determine which components or combinations of components are being studied.

Instrument Reliability The reliability of the instrument itself may be assessed. There are three broad categories of rehabilitation measurements: biophysiological, self-report, and observational. Different instruments are used to take the different types of measurements, and the appropriate approach for determining an instrument's reliability depends on the type of instrument.

Biophysiological measurements are obtained through the use of mechanical or electrical tools such as the dynamometer, goniometer, spirometer, scale, and electromyograph. Certain devices may require calibration

by an independent service before measurements are taken. In those instances, the device is compared to a particular gold standard. Following calibration, typically, the reliability of these instruments is assessed by taking repeated measurements across the range of values expected to be found in actual use of the device. Assessment of scores on two or more administrations of a test is called test-retest reliability. For example, Stratford and colleagues[11] determined the test-retest reliability of a handheld dynamometer by repeated application of known loads from 10 to 60 kg. If the output of a device is in analogue format (i.e., the tester determines the value by examining a scale on the device), then it is impossible to separate the reliability of the device from the examiner's ability to read the scale accurately. If the device output is in digital format, separation of device reliability from examiner reliability is easier because the digital reading leaves little room for examiner interpretation. Of course this assumes the device has been appropriately calibrated.

Self-report measurements are obtained through the use of instruments that require participants to give their own account of the phenomenon under study. Written surveys, standardized tests, pain scales, and interviews may include self-report items or be all self-report. Forms of reliability for self-report measures, as well as standardized tests, include test-retest reliability, in which subjects take the same test on two or more occasions; parallel-form (sometimes called "alternate-form") reliability, in which similar forms of a test are each administered once; split-half reliability, in which portions of a test are compared with each other; and internal consistency, in which responses to individual items are evaluated. The reader is referred to standard texts on health, educational, or psychological measurement for a fuller description of assessment of the reliability of written tests.[12(pp. 39–46),13,14]

Observational measurements require only a human instrument with systematic knowledge of what to observe. The examiner may be an unobtrusive observer or may play a more active role by requesting that the participant execute a series of actions. The knowledge may be in the examiner's head, as is often the case when a clinician observes gait patterns or other movement strategies, or examiners may use formal checklists to organize their observations. Regardless of format, the observations to be made should be behaviorally defined and operationalized to increase reliability.

Performing manual muscle testing, placing patients into gait or transfer independence categories, determining developmental status, and documenting the accessibility of home or work environments are additional examples of rehabilitation measures that require only a human instrument with the knowledge of what to observe. The reliability of observational scales with multiple items can be examined for internal consistency in much the same manner as written tests. Because the tester is the instrument, determining the reliability of observational measures is linked to determining intrarater and interrater reliability, described next.

Furthermore, instruments in each of these broad categories may be classified as "standardized" or "researcher developed." What differentiates a standardized instrument from a researcher-developed instrument? Standardized instruments have test items that must be strictly administered as described, with no deviation from the description. If the test administrator deviates from the way the test item is to be administered or fails to administer a required item, the psychometrics of the instrument will be compromised. A standardized instrument also has a published manual presenting the psychometrics of the instrument as well as specific instructions for administering the instrument. These instructions may include environment or setting requirements (e.g., ambient noise levels, lighting requirements, room temperature, location within in a house) and specific instructions for delivering a test item to the client or subject (e.g., the test administrator may be required to first demonstrate the task to be tested, such as vertically stacking four 1-inch cubes, one on top of the other, deconstructing the stack, pushing the cubes to the child, and saying to the child, "now you build the tower of cubes"). Alternatively, for our purposes, researcher-developed instruments are developed specifically for use in a study or a series of related studies. Typically, the psychometrics for these instruments is largely limited to measurement reliability. There is little intention of the researchers for the instruments to be widely used. See Chapter 19 for a more thorough discussion of standardization and how it may be applied to measurement or testing instruments.

Both standardized and researcher-developed instruments occur in all three categories of instruments. An example of a standardized biophysiological instrument would be the Bruce Treadmill Test[15] for measuring cardiac function, in which an established and published testing protocol is to be followed for an accurate estimate of cardiac function to be determined. An example of a researcher-developed biophysiological instrument protocol can be obtained from Watkins and colleagues'[16] study of goniometric range-of-motion measurement reliability. The authors examined the goniometric measurement reliability under typical clinical conditions, not training the assessors in a standardized method of obtaining goniometric measures of knee range of motion. Similarly, an example of a standardized self-report measure would be the Western Ontario and McMasters Universities Arthritis Index (WOMAC 3.1),[17]

which is a self-administered assessment of knee and hip osteoarthritis from three aspects—pain, disability, and joint stiffness. An example of a researcher-developed self-report instrument is illustrated in Levangie's study of various factors (e.g., number of vaginal delivery occurrences, age of pregnancies, hours driving in a car, and smoking status) associated with low back pain.[18]

In the observation instrument categories, numerous examples of standardized instruments abound. For example, among the more than 470 standardized tests listed on the American Speech-Language-Hearing Association's Web site,[19] there are Assessment of Language-Related Functional Activities, the Burns Brief Inventory of Communication and Cognition, and the Cognitive Linguistic Quick Test. For physical therapists, the assessments Timed Up and Go,[20] the Test of Infant Motor Performance,[21] and the Six-Minute Walk Test[22] serve as examples of standardized observational instruments. An example of a researcher-developed observational instrument might be a physical therapist counting the percentage of nonheel-strike steps a client takes when walking a specific number of steps, or an occupational therapist measuring the frequency and type of extraneous movements that may occur when a child with cerebral palsy attempts to write her name in cursive.

Intrarater Reliability A strict definition of intrarater reliability is "the consistency with which one rater assigns scores to a single set of responses on two occasions."[23(p. 152)] If a researcher is using a video clip to analyze speech patterns, he or she can watch and listen on two different dates. Because the behavior being assessed both times is identical, any variability in scores is, in fact, related to measurement errors of the researcher. For most of the measurements we take in rehabilitation, however, we do not have the ability to exactly reproduce the movement of interest, as a videotape would. If a clinician wishes to assess intrarater reliability of knee extension performance as measured by a hand-held dynamometer, the patient will have to perform the movement two or more times. In doing so, any variability in the force measurements can be attributed to either the examiner's measurement error or the subject's inconsistent performance. It is often difficult to separate the two.

Interrater Reliability A strict definition of interrater reliability holds that it is the "consistency of performance among different raters or judges in assigning scores to the same objects or responses.... [It] is determined when two or more raters judge the performance of one group of subjects at the same point in time."[23(p. 140)] If two clinicians simultaneously observe and rate an infant's spontaneous movements as part of a developmental assessment, the comparison between their scores will be a pure measure of interrater reliability because they observed the exact same episode of movement. If they observe the child at two different times, however, it will be impossible to separate the variability attributable to differences in the examiners from the variability attributable to actual differences in the child's behavior from time to time. Note, however, that if two or more raters can observe the exact same responses, such as on a videotape, simultaneity of measurement is not essential.

A variation of interrater reliability, triangulation, is used to document the consistency of the results of qualitative research. Triangulation consists of comparing responses across several different sources,[24] which in effect become different raters of the phenomenon of interest. The literature of qualitative research provides additional detail about reliability issues in qualitative research.[24,25]

Intrasubject Reliability The final component of reliability is associated with actual changes in subject performance from time to time. Some measurements in rehabilitation may appear to be unreliable simply because the phenomenon being measured is inherently variable. It may be unreasonable to think, for example, that single measurements of spasticity could be reproducible because spasticity is such a changing phenomenon. Unless one has a perfectly reliable instrument and a perfectly reliable examiner, it is impossible to derive a pure measure of subject variability. Thus, most test-retest reliability calculations reflect some combination of instrument errors, tester errors, and true subject variability. Chapter 19 presents research designs for evaluating the different reliability components or combinations of components.

Quantification of Reliability

Reliability is quantified in two ways: as either relative or absolute reliability. Relative reliability examines the relationship between two or more sets of repeated measures; absolute reliability examines the variability of the scores from measurement to measurement.[10,11]

Relative Reliability Relative reliability is based on the idea that if a measurement is reliable, individual measurements within a group will maintain their position within the group on repeated measurement. For example, people who scored near the top of a distribution on a first measure would be expected to stay near the top of the distribution even if their actual scores changed from

time to time. Relative reliability is measured with some form of a correlation coefficient, which, as mentioned earlier in this chapter, indicates the degree of association between repeated measurements of the variable of interest. Different correlation coefficients are used with different types of data, as shown in Table 18-4.[26–28] The mathematical basis of correlation coefficients and the rationale for choosing a particular coefficient are discussed in greater detail in Chapter 23.

We know that a correlation coefficient of 1.0 indicates a perfect association between repeated measures. How much less than 1.0 can a correlation be if it is to be considered reliable? This question is not easily answered. Currier[29(p. 167)] cites two different sources in which adjectives were used to describe ranges of reliability coefficients (e.g., 0.80–1.00 was described as "very reliable," and 0.69 and below was said to constitute "poor reliability"). Streiner and Norman[7(p. 145)] cite two different authors who recommend minimum reliability coefficients of 0.94 and 0.85—but then imply that such arbitrary judgments are foolish. There are several problems with using adjectives to describe ranges of correlation coefficients or setting minimum acceptable reliability coefficients. First, there are many different formulas for correlation coefficients, and these different formulas may result in vastly different coefficients for the same data.[30] Second, there is no universal agreement about the appropriateness of the different formulas.[31,32] Third, acceptable levels of reliability may differ depending on whether one is using the measurement to make judgments about individual change (as in clinical practice) or group change (as in traditional group research designs), with judgments about individual change requiring higher levels of reliability.[7(p. 145),12(p. 44)]

Fourth, the value of a correlation coefficient is greatly affected by the range of scores used to calculate the coefficient. Correlation coefficients evaluate the consistency of an individual's position within a group; if the group as a whole shows little variability on the measure of interest, there is little mathematical basis for determining relative positions, and the correlation between the repeated measurements will be low. Thus, other things being equal, the interrater reliability correlation coefficient calculated on a group of patients with knee flexion range-of-motion values between 70° and 90° would be lower than one calculated on a group with a broader range of values, say, between 30° and 90°.

Fifth, most of the correlation coefficients are not very good at detecting systematic errors. A systematic error is one that is predictable. For example, assume that on a first measurement of limb girth, a researcher used one tape measure and on a second measurement used a different tape measure that was missing the first centimeter. There would be a systematic measurement error of 1 cm on the second measure. However, if each subject's position within the group were maintained, the correlation coefficients would remain high despite the absolute difference.

Because of these five issues, a rigid criterion for acceptable reliability is inappropriate. In addition, the component of reliability being studied affects the interpretation of the correlation coefficient. For example, one would ordinarily expect there to be less variability in scores recorded on a single day than in scores recorded over a longer period. Similarly, intrarater reliability coefficients are generally higher than interrater reliability coefficients. Finally, if a researcher is deciding which of two measurement tools to use and has found that one has an intrarater reliability of .99 and the other an intrarater reliability of .80, then .80 seems unacceptable. On the other hand, if a highly abstract concept is being measured and a researcher is deciding between two instruments with intertester reliability coefficients of .45 and .60, then .60 may become acceptable. Because of the limitations of determining relative reliability with correlation coefficients, researchers should often supplement relative information with absolute information.

Absolute Reliability   Absolute reliability indicates the extent to which a score varies on repeated measurement. The statistic used to measure absolute reliability is the SEM, described earlier in the chapter. For a clinician or researcher to make meaningful statements about whether a patient's or participant's condition has changed, he or she must know how much variability in the scores could be expected solely because of measurement errors. This is illustrated in Ferriero and colleagues'[33] study of the reliability of a device to measure the surface mobility of surgically scarred skin. The intrarater reliability coefficient (an intraclass correlation coefficient) for repeated measurements of the surface mobility of normal skin was 0.97. The SEM of the surface mobility area measurement was calculated to be 4.59 mm². This indicates that approximately 96% of the time, the true value for surface mobility area would be expected to fall within ±9.18 mm² of the observed measurement (observed score ±2 SEMs), and a repeated measurement would be expected to fall within ±6.49 mm² of the first measurement (first measurement ±2$\left[\sqrt{2}\right]$ [SEM]).

Thus, the correlation coefficient and the SEM provide different types of information about a measure. From the very high correlation coefficient, we learned that the relative reliability of the measure was very

high: Participants in the group must have maintained their relative positions almost perfectly on repeated measurements. From the SEM, we learned how much error, expressed in the units of the measure, we might expect with this measurement. Knowing the SEM of a measurement—and a little bit about the normal curve—enables rehabilitation professionals to evaluate clinical changes in patients in comparison to changes that might be expected solely from measurement error.

Measurement Validity

Measurement validity is the "appropriateness, meaningfulness, and usefulness of the specific inferences made from test scores."[9(p. 9)] Reliability is a necessary, but not sufficient, condition for validity. An unreliable measure is also an invalid measurement because measurements with a great deal of error have little meaning or utility. A reliable measure is valid only if, in addition to being repeatable, it provides meaningful information.

Earlier we defined research validity as the extent to which the conclusions of research are believable and useful (see Chapter 8). Note that although the two types of validity relate to different areas—measurement and research design, respectively—they are similar in that they both relate to the utility of findings and not to the findings themselves. Thus, measurement validity is not a quality associated with a particular instrument or test, but rather is a quality associated with the way in which test results are applied.

For example, the size of a child's spoken vocabulary may provide a valid gross indication of cognitive function in children without communication disorders. The same measure of spoken vocabulary may not be a valid indicator of cognitive function in children who have difficulty producing certain sounds and who may therefore elect to limit the words they choose to speak. Measurement validity is often subdivided into several categories: construct, content, and criterion validity.

Construct Validity

Construct validity is the validity of the abstract theoretical principles or constructs that underlie measures. For example, strength is a construct that is poorly delineated in the rehabilitation literature. When rehabilitation professionals speak of strength, they may mean many different things. Strength may be conceptualized as the ability to move a body part against gravity, the ability to generate speed-specific torque, the ability to lift a certain weight a certain number of times in a certain time period, or the ability to accomplish some functional task. Manual muscle tests, isokinetic tests, work performance tests, and functional tests may all be valid measures of a particular conceptualization of strength or muscle performance.

To maximize construct validity, rehabilitation researchers must first be very clear about the constructs they wish to measure. If strength is an important construct within a study, is it best conceptualized as functional strength, static strength, eccentric strength, or some other aspect of this extremely broad construct? After the underlying construct of interest is clarified, it must be operationalized to make it measurable. An operational definition is a specific description of the way in which a construct is presented or measured within a study. For example, Mathiowetz[34] studied fatigue in persons with multiple sclerosis. He chose his measurement tool based on an operational definition of fatigue found in a clinical practice guideline for multiple sclerosis: "a subjective lack of physical and/or mental energy that is perceived by the individual or caregiver to interfere with usual and desired activities."[35(p. 2)] The Fatigue Impact Scale used within the study appears to be consistent with the construct, in that it includes subscales related to physical, cognitive, and social impact of fatigue. Although developing operational definitions is necessary for construct validity, it does not guarantee construct validity. One might, for example, argue that Mathiowetz did not determine the perceptions of both individuals with multiple sclerosis and their caregivers (for those who were not independent in all activities), thereby failing to include all elements of the operational definition within the measurement design of his study. Supplying readers with the operational definitions used in a study allows them to form their own opinion of the validity of the measurements.

In addition to the intellectual task of determining the match between constructs and their measurement, another way to determine construct validity is to use "known-group" comparisons. In this approach, groups of individuals who are expected to perform differently on a measurement are compared to determine whether the hypothesized differences materialize. For example, in a validation study of the Hong Kong Chinese Version of the Lawton Instrumental Activities of Daily Living (IADL) scale, the authors administered the test to older adults living in a hostel and to those in a care-and-attention home.[36] The construct validity of the scale was demonstrated when the scale successfully differentiated between individuals in the different living situations.

Content Validity

Content validity is the extent to which a measure is a complete representation of the concept of interest. Content validity is more often a concern with self-report or observational tools than with biophysiological ones. When students come away from a test saying, "Can you believe how many questions there were on ...?" they are talking about the content validity of the test because they are questioning whether the emphasis on the examination was an accurate representation of the course content.

Murney and Campbell[37] tested a form of content validity of the Test of Infant Motor Performance (TIMP) when they tested what they referred to as the "ecological relevance" of the test items. They found that 98% of the items in the test corresponded to environmental demands placed on the infant during normal daily activities. In a more traditional way of testing content validity, the test developers also asked a panel of experts to review the items in the test to ensure that a wide range of possible environmental demands was included within the test. When a researcher is designing a questionnaire or a functional scale, he or she should have its content validity evaluated by knowledgeable peers or evaluated in natural settings as part of the pilot testing of the instrument. These evaluation procedures may lead to the addition of items, the deletion of irrelevant or redundant items, or reassessment of the emphasis given to particular topics.

Criterion Validity

Criterion validity is the extent to which one measure is systematically related to other measures or outcomes. Whereas relative reliability compares repeated administrations of the same measurement, criterion validity compares administration of different measures. The mathematical basis for determining the degree of association between two different measures is similar to that for determining the association between repeated administrations of the same measurement. Therefore the correlation coefficients used to determine relative reliability are often used to measure criterion validity as well. The epidemiological concepts of specificity and sensitivity, described in Chapter 15, are also useful for determining criterion validity. Criterion validity can be subdivided into concurrent and predictive validity on the basis of the timing of the different measures.

Concurrent validity is at issue when one is comparing a new tool or procedure with a measurement standard. Clark and colleagues[38] determined the concurrent validity of a new procedure to detect occult ankle fracture (presence of a 15-mm ankle effusion on a plain radiograph) with that of the gold standard of computed tomography (CT). Often, however, a true gold standard against which the new measurement can be compared does not exist. For example, in the study of the measurement of fatigue in individuals with multiple sclerosis, introduced earlier in the chapter, the Fatigue Impact Scale (FIS) was validated by correlating FIS scores with those of another self-reported fatigue scale and with the various subscales of the SF-36 instrument used to document health-related quality of life.[34] None of these comparison tools can be considered gold standards in the way that CT is the definitive tool for diagnosing some conditions.

Predictive validity relates to whether a test done at one point in time is predictive of future status. Flegel and Kolobe[39] studied the predictive validity of the TIMP by comparing scores on the TIMP at up to 4 months of age with scores on the Bruininks-Oseretsky Test of Motor Proficiency (BOTMP) of the same children at 4 to 7 years of age. More than 89% of children were correctly classified by the TIMP. That is, 89% of children were "true positives" (classified as at risk for developmental delay by the TIMP and later classified as developmentally delayed by the BOTMP) or "true negatives" (classified as not at risk for developmental delay by the TIMP and later classified as not developmentally delayed by the BOTMP). Only 11% of children were "false positives" (classified as at risk by the TIMP and not delayed by the BOTMP) or "false negatives" (classified as not at risk by the TIMP but as delayed by the BOTMP). Determining the predictive validity of a screening measure such as the TIMP is an essential but time-consuming process. The premise of many screening tests is that they allow early identification of some phenomenon that is not usually apparent until some later date. The usefulness of such measures cannot be determined unless their predictive validity is known. In clinical application, the scientist-practitioner is concerned with predictive validity of different tests in order to establish a reasonable prognosis for a client.

RESPONSIVENESS TO CHANGE

A third critical issue is the responsiveness to change of a measurement. Practitioners are generally hoping to effect change in their patients or clients, so measures that can reflect such changes in individuals are desirable. Consider two individuals, both of whom have goals related to weight change. One is a man who weighs 250 lb and wishes to reduce to 190 lb. The other is a premature infant who weighs 2500 g and is fighting to get to 4000 g. For the man who is dieting, a bathroom scale with 1-lb increments will be responsive enough to document his weight loss. For the premature infant, a bathroom scale obviously will not be responsive enough to measure the small changes in weight

that are expected to occur; a more precise scale that can measure to the nearest gram is needed. Measurements, then, must be selected with an eye to how responsive to change they will be given the characteristics of the individuals being studied. Also referred to in the literature as "sensitivity to change," in this text the term "responsiveness" is used instead to eliminate any confusion with the epidemiological concept of sensitivity.

Responsiveness to change can be defined as "the extent to which practically or theoretically significant changes in the subject's 'state' are reflected in substantive changes in observed values."[6(p. 33S)] Responsiveness of a measure is related to both the reliability and validity of the measure. If a measure is not very reliable, as indicated by a large SEM, then changes that indicate true change in the status of clinical clients or research participants must be larger still to represent more than measurement error. Conversely, if the measure is very reliable, with a small SEM, then even small changes in the measure will represent true changes in a participant's state, thereby being "responsive" to change.

A measure that is not a good conceptual fit with the construct being measured (i.e., it does not have construct validity) is unlikely to be responsive to change. For example, the Barthel Index of Activities of Daily Living has been used as a generic outcomes tool for individuals with spinal cord injury. However, some have questioned whether its items are specific enough to document the small changes in function that might be expected for some individuals with quadriplegia. In response to these concerns, Gresham and colleagues[40] developed a Quadriplegia Index of Function (QIF) and tested its responsiveness to change compared with the Barthel Index. They found that the average percentage of improvement from admission to discharge for individuals with quadriplegia at a rehabilitation hospital was 46% for the QIF, but only 20% for the Barthel Index, demonstrating better responsiveness to change for the QIF.

Responsiveness to change is also a function of the number of values that a scale can take. If a scale can take only a few values (e.g., the familiar grading scale of A, B, C, D, F), then relatively large changes in performance are needed before a change in grade is registered on the scale. Conversely, if the grading scale includes + and − grades, then relatively small changes in performance may change a grade from B− to B and then to B+.

Ceiling and floor effects also have an impact on the responsiveness of a measure. A floor effect occurs when an individual scores at the bottom of a scale and no further declines in the quantity being measured can be registered even if performance would require it. Ceiling effects occur at the top of a scale so that no further improvement can be registered. Depending on how far "under" the floor (or "over" the ceiling) an individual's true state, substantial change may occur without registering a change on the measurement scale. In Smith and associates'[41] study of the relationship between generic measures of health-related quality of life and ambulatory function, they documented large floor and ceiling effects on some of the SF-36 subscales for their study sample of veterans with peripheral neuropathy. For example, they found that 46% of their sample was at the floor of the role limitation/physical subscale and that 30% were at the ceiling of the social function subscale. Had this been a longitudinal study of physical and social impact of peripheral neuropathy, they would have been unable to detect declines in physical role limitations or improvements in social functioning for substantial numbers of individuals within their study.

Researchers or clinicians who wish to use measures that are responsive to change should look for measures with good reliability and validity for the population they are studying or treating, that can take a number of different values, and that are unlikely to have large floor or ceiling effects for the population of interest. Like reliability and validity, responsiveness to change is not an invariant characteristic of the measure; rather, it varies based on the conditions under which it is applied and the population in which it is used.

Of late, two terms have been used in efforts to afford clinical application of change. These are *minimal detectable difference* (MDD) and *minimal clinically important difference* (MCID) or *minimal important difference* or *change* (MID and MIC, respectively). The former is concerned with the smallest amount of change that can occur that exceeds measurement error, and it is determined mathematically. The latter is considered a measure of the smallest meaningful change to the patient. Of course, this meaningfulness is subjective and dependent on a number of different perspectives. Does the patient consider the change as meaningful? Does the patient's caregiver (e.g., family member or physical therapist) consider the change as meaningful?

SUMMARY

Measurement is a systematic process by which things are differentiated. Measurements can be identified by scale (nominal, ordinal, interval, or ratio), type (discrete or continuous), and framework (norm referenced or criterion referenced). Statistical concepts of importance to measurement theory include the frequency distribution, mean, variance, standard deviation, normal curve, correlation, and standard error of measurement. Reliability is the extent to which a measure is free from error. The components of reliability include instrument, tester, and subject variability. Relative measures of reliability are correlation coefficients; the absolute measure of reliability is the standard error of measurement. Validity is the meaningfulness and utility of an application of a measurement. The components of validity include construct, content, and criterion validity. Responsiveness to change is the extent to which a change in status is reflected in a change in the measured value. Responsiveness to change depends on both the reliability and validity of a measure and is specific to the population being measured.

REFERENCES

1. Hopkins KD, Stanley JC: *Educational and Psychological Measurement and Evaluation*, 6th ed, Englewood Cliffs, NJ, 1981, Prentice-Hall.
2. Nunnally JC: *Psychometric Theory*, 3rd ed, New York, NY, 1994, McGraw-Hill.
3. Kerlinger FN, Lee HB: *Foundations of Behavioral Research*, 4th ed, Fort Worth, Tex, 2000, Harcourt College.
4. Safrit MJ: An overview of measurement. In Safrit MJ, Wood TM, editors: *Measurement Concepts in Physical Education and Exercise Science*, Champaign, Ill, 1989, Human Kinetics.
5. Merbitz C, Morris J, Grip JC: Ordinal scales and foundations of misinference, *Arch Phys Med Rehabil* 70:308–312, 1989.
6. Hyde ML: Reasonable psychometric standards for self-report outcomes measures in audiological rehabilitation, *Ear Hear* 21:24S–36S, 2000.
7. Streiner DL, Norman GR: *Health Measurement Scales: A Practical Guide to Their Development and Use*, 3rd ed, Oxford, UK, 2003, Oxford University Press.
8. Anastasi A, Urbina S: Norms and the meaning of test scores. In Anastasi A, Urbina S, editors: *Psychological Testing*, 7th ed, Upper Saddle River, NJ, 1997, Prentice Hall.
9. American Educational Research Association, American Psychological Association, National Committee on Measurement in Education: *Standards for Educational and Psychological Testing*, Washington, DC, 1999, American Psychological Association.
10. Morrow JR: Generalizability theory. In Safrit MJ, Wood TM, editors: *Measurement Concepts in Physical Education and Exercise Science*, Champaign, Ill, 1989, Human Kinetics.
11. Stratford PW, Norman GR, McIntosh JM: Generalizability of grip strength measurements in patients with tennis elbow, *Phys Ther* 69:276–281, 1989.
12. McDowell I, Newell C: *Measuring Health: A Guide to Rating Scales and Questionnaires*, 3rd ed, New York, NY, 2006, Oxford University Press.
13. Anastasi A, Urbina S: *Reliability: Psychological Testing*, 7th ed, Upper Saddle River, NJ, 1997, Prentice Hall.
14. Litwin MS: *How to Assess and Interpret Survey Psychometrics*, The Survey Kit, Volume 5, Thousand Oaks, Calif, 2003, Sage.
15. Pescatello LS, editor: *ACSM guidelines for exercise testing and prescription*, ed 9, Philadelphia, Pa, 2014, Lippincott Williams & Wilkins.

16. Watkins MA, Riddle DL, Lamb RL, Personius WJ: Reliability of goniometric measurements and visual estimates of knee range of motion obtained in a clinical setting, *Phys Ther* 71:90–97, 1990.

17. WOMAC Osteoarthritis Index: WOMAC 3.1 Index. Available at: http://www.womac.org/womac/index.htm. Accessed June 3, 2015.

18. Levangie PK: Association of low back pain with self-reported risk factors among patients seeking physical therapy services, *Phys Ther* 79:757–766, 1999.

19. American Speech-Language-Hearing Association: *Directory of speech-language pathology assessment instruments.* Available at: http://www.asha.org/assessments.aspx. Accessed June 3, 2015.

20. Centers for Disease Control and Prevention. Available at: http://www.cdc.gov/homeandrecreationalsafety/pdf/steadi-2015.04/TUG_Test-a.pdf. Accessed June 13, 2015.

21. Infant Motor Performance Scales: *The test of infant motor performance and the harris infant neuromotor test.* Available at: http://thetimp.com. Accessed June 3, 2015.

22. American Thoracic Society: *Guidelines for the six-minute walk test.* Available at: https://www.thoracic.org/statements/resources/pfet/sixminute.pdf. Accessed June 3, 2015.

23. Waltz CF, Strickland OL, Lenz ER: *Measurement in Nursing Research,* 4th ed, New York, NY, 2010, Springer.

24. Denzin NK, Lincoln YS: *Handbook of Qualitative Research,* 4th ed, Thousand Oaks, Calif, 2011, Sage.

25. Miles MB, Huberman AM, Saladaña J: *Qualitative Data Analysis: A Methods Sourcebook,* 3rd ed, Thousand Oaks, Calif, 2014, Sage.

26. Cohen J: A coefficient of agreement for nominal scales, *Educ Psychol Meas* 20:37–46, 1960.

27. Haley SM, Osberg JS: Kappa coefficient calculation using multiple ratings per subject: A special communication, *Phys Ther* 69:970–974, 1989.

28. Bartko JJ: The intraclass correlation coefficient as a measure of reliability, *Psychol Rep* 19:3–11, 1966.

29. Currier DP: *Elements of Research in Physical Therapy,* 3rd ed, Baltimore, Md, 1990, Williams & Wilkins.

30. Shrout PE, Fleiss JL: Intraclass correlations: Uses in assessing rater reliability, *Psychol Bull* 86:420–428, 1979.

31. Bartko JJ, Carpenter WT: On the methods and theory of reliability, *J Nerv Ment Dis* 163:307–317, 1976.

32. Hart DL: Invited commentary, *Phys Ther* 69:102–103, 1989.

33. Ferriero G, Vercelli S, Salgovic L, et al: Validation of a new device to measure postsurgical scar adherence, *Phys Ther* 90:776–783, 2010.

34. Mathiowetz V: Test-retest reliability and convergent validity of the Fatigue Impact Scale for persons with multiple sclerosis, *Am J Occup Ther* 57:389–395, 2003.

35. Multiple Sclerosis Council for Clinical Practice Guidelines: *Fatigue and Multiple Sclerosis: Evidence-Based Management Strategies for Fatigue in Multiple Sclerosis,* Washington, DC, 1998, Paralyzed Veterans of America.

36. Tong AYC, Man DWK: The validation of the Hong Kong Chinese Version of the Lawton Instrumental Activities of Daily Living scale for institutionalized elderly persons, *OTJR Occup Particip Health* 22:132–142, 2002.

37. Murney ME, Campbell SK: The ecological relevance of the Test of Infant Motor Performance elicited scale items, *Phys Ther* 78:479–489, 1998.

38. Clark TWI, Janzen DL, Logan PM, et al: Improving the detection of radiographically occult ankle fractures: Positive predictive value of an ankle joint effusion, *Clin Radiol* 51:632–636, 1996.

39. Flegel J, Kolobe THA: Predictive validity of the Test of Infant Motor Performance as measured by the Bruininks-Oseretsky Test of Motor Proficiency at school age, *Phys Ther* 82:762–771, 2002.

40. Gresham GE, Labi ML, Dittmar SS, et al: The Quadriplegia Index of Function (QIF): Sensitivity and reliability in a study of thirty quadriplegic patients, *Paraplegia* 24:38–44, 1986.

41. Smith DG, Domholdt E, Coleman KL, et al: Ambulatory activity in men with diabetes: Relationship between self-reported and real-world performance-based measures, *J Rehabil Res Dev* 41:571–580, 2004.

19

Methodological Research

CHAPTER OUTLINE

Reliability Designs
  Sources of Variability
  Levels of Standardization
    Nonstandardized Approach
    Highly Standardized Approach
    Partially Standardized Approach
  Participant Selection

Range of Scores
Optimization Designs
  Standardization Designs
  Mean Designs
Reliability in Nonmethodological
    Studies
Validity Designs

Construct Validation
Content Validation
Criterion Validation
Responsiveness Designs
Summary

The goals of methodological research are to document and improve the reliability, validity, and responsiveness of clinical and research measurements. Because measurement is an integral part of clinical and research documentation, research that examines measurements is important to all of the rehabilitation professions. In addition to the importance of measurement as a topic in its own right, documentation of the reliability and validity of the measures used within a study is a necessary component of all research. This chapter provides a framework for the design of methodological research. Reliability designs are presented first, followed by validity designs and responsiveness designs.

RELIABILITY DESIGNS

The reliability of a measurement is influenced by many factors, including (1) the sources of variability studied, (2) the participants selected, and (3) the range of scores exhibited by the sample. Each of these factors is illustrated in this chapter by a hypothetical example of measurement of joint range of motion. The hypothetical example is supplemented by relevant examples from the literature. After these three general factors are discussed, two specialized types of reliability studies are considered: reliability optimization and reliability documentation within nonmethodological research.

Sources of Variability

Differences found in repeated measurements of the same characteristic can be attributed to instrument,

intrarater (intratester), interrater (intertester), and intra-subject components. Within each of these four reliability components, there are many additional sources of variability. When designing reliability studies, researchers must clearly delineate which of the reliability components they wish to study and which sources of variability they wish to study within each component. To assist with this task, it is helpful to list the four reliability components and all possible sources of variation for each component. Box 19-1 shows some potential sources of variability in passive range-of-motion scores as measured with a universal goniometer.

After the sources of variability within the measurement are delineated, the researcher must determine which of the components will be the focus of his or her methodological study. As is the case with all research design, the investigator designing methodological research must identify a problem that needs to be studied. Is there a knowledge deficit about the interinstrument reliability of goniometers of different sizes or designs? Is it important to establish the degree of variation that can be expected in a particular measurement made by a single clinician? What is the magnitude of differences that could be expected if several clinicians take measurements of the same person? Is participant or patient performance consistent across days or weeks?

Each of these questions relates to one of the four components of reliability: instrument, intrarater, interrater, and intrasubject. However, in many methodological studies, more than one of the reliability components are examined, or the reliability components are intertwined and cannot be separated clearly.

Box 19-1

Sources of Variability in Passive Range-of-Motion Measurements with a Universal Goniometer

Instrument
Loose axis (slips during measurement)
Tight axis (too difficult to move precisely)
Interinstrument differences

Intrarater
Variations in participant positioning
Inconsistent identification of landmarks
Variable end-range pressure
Inconsistent stabilization
Reading errors

Interrater
Variations in participant positioning
Inconsistent identification of landmarks
Variable end-range pressure
Inconsistent stabilization
Differing ability to gain participants' trust
Different end-digit preference
Reading errors

Intrasubject
Varying levels of pain
Differing tolerance to end-range pressure
Mood changes
Differing activities before measurement
Biological variation

For example, Cataneo and associates[1] examined the test-retest interrater reliability of four balance scales: two that were administered by physical therapists and two that were self-administered by patients, with two measurements of each taken on two different days. When a study examines more than one type of reliability, completely separating one reliability (e.g., test-retest reliability and intrarater reliability) from another may not be possible.

Levels of Standardization

After the sources of variability have been determined, it is necessary to determine the degree of standardization in the measurement protocol. The degree of standardization is the number of sources of variability within a reliability component that are controlled.

Consider three different reasons to study interrater reliability of goniometric measurements. The purpose of one study might be to determine interrater reliability of goniometric measurements as they occur in the clinic, without any standardization of technique between clinicians. The purpose of a second study might be to determine the upper limits of interrater reliability with a highly standardized protocol. The purpose of a third study might be to determine interrater reliability with a level of standardization that would be feasible for most clinics to achieve.

The preceding three purpose statements correspond to three general approaches to reliability that are seen in the literature: nonstandardized, highly standardized, and partially standardized. The three approaches differ in the extent to which the sources of variability are controlled within each of the reliability components under study. For interrater reliability in the measurement of passive motion with a goniometer, Box 19-1 lists seven possible sources of variability: positioning, landmark identification, end-range pressure, stabilization, patient trust in the clinician, end-digit preference (some clinicians always round measurements to the nearest 5°, others round to even numbers only, and others do not round off at all), and reading errors. Let us consider how nonstandardized, highly standardized, and partially standardized studies would be applied to these sources of variability to determine interrater reliability of goniometric measurement.

Nonstandardized Approach

A completely nonstandardized approach would control none of these sources of variability and would establish the lower limit for the reliability component studied. The basic design of a nonstandardized study of interrater reliability would be to have each clinician take measurements privately so as not to influence the technique of the other clinicians within the study.

Watkins and associates[2] studied the reliability of goniometric measures of knee range of motion. Because they wished to study reliability under typical clinical conditions, they did not train their examiners in standardized procedures. In fact, they ensured that the second clinician never saw the first clinician taking measurements, nor did they require standardized positioning of the patient or the goniometer.

Highly Standardized Approach

In contrast to a nonstandardized approach, a highly standardized approach would control many of the possible sources of variability to determine the upper limits of the reliability of the component. Whereas a nonstandardized approach seeks to document the reliability of measurements as they commonly occur, a highly standardized approach seeks to document reliability in an ideal situation. A highly standardized approach to taking measurements may be a useful way of separating measurement error from participant variability.

In a highly standardized study of interrater goniometric reliability, positioning, stabilization, landmarks, end-range pressure, and end-digit preference would all be controlled. Positioning for shoulder internal rotation, for example, could be controlled by having all clinicians take the measurements with the patient supine on the same firm plinth. Stabilization could be controlled by strapping the patient's chest to prevent substitution of scapular or trunk movements. To control inconsistent identification of landmarks, landmarks could be marked on the participants and left in place while all clinicians take their measurements. End-range pressure could be standardized by having an assistant provide a predetermined force as documented by a handheld dynamometer. Finally, end-digit preference could be controlled by instructing clinicians to report the measurement to the nearest degree. The experimental protocol for such a study might be that one clinician positions each patient and three other clinicians each take a measurement in rapid succession. Such a protocol would establish the upper limits of interrater reliability and would eliminate the effects of participant variation because the participant would not be moved between measurements.

Mayerson and Milano[3] used a highly standardized approach to study goniometric measurement reliability. A healthy participant was positioned in 22 consistent extremity joint positions; two clinicians each took two measurements at each position. The protocol eliminated variability resulting from participant positioning, stabilization, end-range pressure, and changes in participant motion. Thus, the protocol provided a test of the reliability of goniometer placement and reading, at least for the two clinicians. They found that both interrater and intrarater differences could confidently be expected to fall within 4° of each other in a highly standardized measurement protocol. This study might have been expanded to include a greater number of clinicians.

Partially Standardized Approach

The third approach to determining the sources of variability to be studied within an investigation of reliability is the partially standardized approach. As indicated by its name, this approach falls between the extremes of the nonstandardized and highly standardized approaches by standardizing a few sources of variability while leaving others nonstandardized. The sources of variability that are standardized often reflect the realities of the clinic. The hypothetical, highly standardized study of internal-rotation range of motion described previously is probably unrealistic for routine clinical use; an assistant is not always available to position the patient, and landmarks are likely to be washed off between treatment sessions. A partially standardized measurement protocol might therefore standardize positioning and stabilization but allow landmark determination and end-range pressure to vary among clinicians. The experimental protocol for a partially standardized study requires educating the examiners in the standardized methods to be used in the study.

Youdas and colleagues[4] used a partially standardized approach to study the reliability of cervical range-of-motion measurements taken by visual estimation, with a universal goniometer, and with a cervical range-of-motion instrument. Clinicians were trained in the use of a standardized protocol for positioning of the participants; placement of the measuring devices and a warm-up protocol for participants were also standardized.

The appropriate level of standardization for reliability studies depends on the research question, and each approach can be useful for specific purposes. Nonstandardized studies describe reliability as it is; highly standardized studies present idealized reliability estimates and examine the impact of limited sources of variability on reliability; and partially standardized studies describe reliability with moderate levels of standardization that could be achievable in clinical settings.

Participant Selection

As is the case with all types of research, participant selection in reliability studies influences the external validity of the study; the study results can be generalized only to the types of participants studied. Therefore, the reliability of an instrument should be determined using the individuals on whom the instrument will be used in practice. If the measure is a clinical one, it is best to determine its reliability on patients who would ordinarily require this measurement as part of their care. In a study of genotype-phenotype correlates of infants and children with metachromatic leukodystrophy (MLD), a disease of inborn metabolism error resulting in the rapid deterioration of motor and cognitive performance ultimately leading to early death, Biffi and colleagues[5] employed the Gross Motor Function Measure (GMFM) to assess motor development of the subjects. The GMFM was developed for use with children with cerebral palsy, a nonprogressive neuromotor disorder, whereas MLD is a degenerative disorder. The authors employed the GMFM without reporting any reliability. Regardless of the level of reliability, the use of a test with patients with a diagnosis differing from a test's intended use, as was done with the children with MLD, may result in unreliable outcomes, lending the collected data unusable. The inappropriate use of normal participants to establish the reliability of some clinical measures has the potential to inflate reliability estimates because normal participants may be easier to measure than affected patients. Pain, obliteration of landmarks because of deformity, or difficulty following directions because of neurological impairment may make it difficult to take measurements in patients.

If a researcher ultimately wishes to determine norms for certain characteristics, it is appropriate to determine the reliability of the measurements using normal participants. If the measurement in question is part of a screening tool, such as a flexibility test that might be administered at a fitness fair, then a broad sampling of the individuals likely to be screened should be used to establish the reliability of the measurement. Use of tests comparing performance of clinical clients to norms from nonclinical populations is quite common in speech-language pathology.

Range of Scores

The reliability of a measure should be determined over the range of scores expected for that measure. There are two reasons for this. First, as discussed in Chapter 18, a restricted range of scores leads to low reliability coefficients, even in the presence of small absolute differences in repeated measurements. The use of normal participants can restrict the range of scores within a study, thereby reducing the reliability coefficients and underestimating the reliability of the measure in clinical use. In contrast, using an extremely heterogeneous group (e.g., a mixed group of patients and nonpatients) would generally overestimate the reliability of the measure for clinical use but might be the ideal mix of individuals for establishing the reliability of the tool for screening purposes. In considering use of norm-referenced procedures, clinicians need to pay attention to the constitution of the "norm" group as well as the rationale for constituting the norm group in a particular way.

Second, reliability may vary at different places in the range of scores because of difficulties unique to taking measurements at particular points in the range. For example, Nussbaum and Downes[1] found that interrater reliability was greatest when testing participants with lower pain thresholds. Researchers need to carefully consider the characteristics of the individuals on whom the test or tool will be used and select a research sample that matches those characteristics.

Optimization Designs

In many instances, researchers have found less than optimal reliability for rehabilitation measures. Such research is useful because it may lead to a healthy skepticism about the measurements we use. In and of itself, however, documenting the reliability of a clinical measure does nothing to improve its reliability. Improving the reliability of rehabilitation measures requires that researchers study ways to optimize reliability. There are two basic designs for optimization research: standardization and mean designs.

Standardization Designs

Standardization designs compare the reliabilities of measurements taken under different sets of conditions. For example, suppose that the result of a nonstandardized reliability study was that the standard error of measurement (SEM) for passive internal-rotation range of motion was 10°. Furthermore, suppose the result of a highly standardized, but clinically unfeasible, study was that the SEM was 1°. A standardization study might be developed with a goal of determining what level of standardization is needed to achieve an SEM of 3°. To do so, a researcher might determine reliability with standardized positioning. If, despite the positioning change, the SEM is still too large, both position and upper chest stabilization might be standardized. The level of standardization would be increased until the reliability goal was met. A reverse sequence could also be implemented by starting with a highly standardized procedure and eliminating standardization procedures that are not feasible in the clinic.

Mean Designs

Mean designs compare the reliabilities of single measurements and also compare the reliabilities of measurements averaged across several trials. This design is particularly appropriate for measures that are difficult to standardize for clinical use or for characteristics that are expected to show a great deal of natural variation.[6] Connelly and colleagues[7] used a mean strategy to study the reliability of walking tests in a frail elderly population. Two raters took three measures of walking on each of 2 days. They then computed reliability coefficients, comparing the means for each day between raters, the best score for each day between raters, and the first measure for each day between raters. They found that the reliability coefficients were highest when they used the mean of three measures, were worst when they used the first measure, and were intermediate when they used the best measure. Such information helps clinicians and researchers make knowledgeable decisions about whether to rely on single measures or whether to average the results of repeated measurements.

Reliability in Nonmethodological Studies

Useful research studies are based on reliable measurements. Measurement reliability in nonmethodological studies should be addressed at two times during the study: during the design phase and during the implementation phase, regardless of the reported reliability from cited methodological studies. In single-subject studies, in which specific behaviors are measured by specific behavioral objectives, reporting of rater reliability training (during each phase of the study) is standard practice.

In the design phase, the researcher must determine which of several possible instruments to choose, which of several possible measurement protocols to follow, and which of several raters to use. Studies of interinstrument, interrater, or intrarater reliability components may be needed to make these decisions.

When conducting a pilot reliability study, the researcher needs to simulate the research conditions as closely as possible. For example, Tsorlakis and colleagues[8] used a test (GMFM) that had high intrarater and interrater reliability, as well as high test-retest reliability in the actual and pilot study. In the pilot reliability study Tsorlakis and colleagues established high interrater reliability, reported as an intraclass correlation coefficient (ICC = 0.994) with an independent assessor, as well as high intrarater reliability level (ICC = 0.997) using subjects similar to the study subjects, before the start of the study. In addition, they established test-retest reliability (ICC = 0.996) by comparing the initial assessment results of the pilot study subjects to a second assessment conducted several days later.

Furthermore, when conducting a pilot reliability study with participants similar to those in the actual study, the pilot study also should have settings, time pressures, and the like similar to those that would occur in the actual study. The results of a pilot reliability study conducted after clinic hours, when researchers and participants have more time and few distractions, may differ from those of the actual study if the actual study takes place during clinic hours, when time is short and distractions abound.

Reliability measures should also be taken during all phases of implementation of a study, as in some instances in which the reliability attained during training phases has been shown to decline during experimental phases.[9,10] In addition, a description of the retraining method of the raters should the raters fail to maintain reliability criteria during the study is desirable.

Researchers can establish reliability during the course of a study by taking repeated measures of all participants, using pretest and posttest scores of a control group as the reliability indicator, or taking repeated measures of selected participants at random. Using a single-subject research design, Embrey and associates[11] reported the interrater reliability of the independent assessor during both baseline phase and randomly selected sessions of the intervention phase.

Which strategy for conducting pilot and actual study reliability is adopted depends on factors such as the expense of the measures, the risks of repeated measurements to participants, and the number of participants in the study.

VALIDITY DESIGNS

As discussed previously, the validity of a measurement is the extent to which a particular use of the measurement is meaningful. Measures are validated through argument about and research into the soundness of the interpretations made from them. To make sound interpretations, a researcher must first be confident that the measurements are reproducible, or reliable. Recall that although reliability is necessary for validity, it does not validate the meaning behind the measure. This section of the chapter presents several designs for research to determine the construct, content, and criterion validity of measurements.

Construct Validation

Constructs are theoretical frameworks that are not directly observable. Strength, function, and pain are constructs used frequently in rehabilitation. Because the constructs themselves are not directly observable, there are no absolute standards against which measurements can be compared to determine whether they are valid indicators of the constructs. Consider, for example, all the different measures that rehabilitation professionals use to represent the construct of strength: manual muscle testing, the number of times that a particular weight can be lifted, handheld dynamometers, and a multitude of isokinetic tests. All are appropriate for some purposes, but none is a definitive measure of strength.

In the absence of a clear-cut standard, persuasive argument becomes one means by which the construct validity of measurements is established.[12] A researcher who wishes to assess strength gains following a particular program of exercise must be prepared to defend the appropriateness of the measurements he or she used for the type of exercise program studied. Such considerations include whether the measure should test concentric or eccentric contractions, whether the test should be isometric or should sample strength throughout the range of motion, and whether the test should be conducted in an open or closed kinetic chain position.

A second way in which construct validity is established is by making predictions about the patterns of test scores that should be seen if the measure is valid.[13(pp. 178–185)] One method is to examine the convergence and divergence of measures thought to represent similar and different constructs, respectively. For example, Mercer and colleagues[14] sought to validate several clinical methods of measuring standing weight bearing (Step Test [ST] and the knee extension component of the Upright Motor Control Test [UMCe]) and weight transfer (Repetitive Reach Test [RR]) to vertical ground reaction forces (GRFs), as measured by force platforms, of patients after stroke as measures of paretic-limb loading. The researchers predicted that each of the clinical measures would correlate with increased GRF during task performances. They found the ST correlated well with peak GRFs, serving as a valid measure of paretic lower-extremity weight bearing in patients after stroke; however, they found only weak correlations of the UMCe to peak GRFs in some of the UMCe tasks, as well as with the RR, thus suggesting the questionable validity of these measures' ability to measure weight bearing and weight transfer onto the paretic limb of patients after stroke.

Construct validity is best supported when the scores on items thought to represent the same construct are highly associated (convergence) and when scores on items that are theoretically different have a low association (divergence).

Another set of predictions often used to establish construct validity relates to the performance of "extreme groups" or "known groups" on the test of interest. A known-groups approach was used by Megens and colleagues[15] to determine the ability of the Harris Infant Neuromotor Test to screen infants at low risk for neuromotor delays from those infants at high risk. In each of four age groups, they were able to distinguish between infants at high risk for neuromotor delays and those at low risk, and in a fifth age group, the detection approached statistical difference.

Content Validation

Content validation involves documenting that a test provides an adequate sampling of the behavior or knowledge that it is measuring. To determine the content validity of a measure, a researcher compares the items in the test against the actual practice of interest.

There are four basic issues a researcher must consider when determining content validity: (1) the sample on whom the measure is validated, (2) the content's completeness, (3) the content's relevance, and (4) the content's emphasis. Chi and Wan[16] determined the content validity of an assessment of activities of daily living (ADL) specific to patients with chronic obstructive pulmonary disease (COPD), noting that patients with COPD have unique health issues that other ADL assessments fail to determine. The authors recruited 12 patients with COPD to review, before discharge, their 25-item Activities of Daily Living Inventory (ADLI). For all but three items, the patient panel indicated 97% agreement that the items were representative of the ADL issues the patients encountered. Further, on panel recommendation, an additional item was added to the ADLI for construct validation, which was also examined in this study.

Criterion Validation

The criterion validation of a measure is determined by comparing it with an accepted standard of measurement. The major considerations in designing a criterion validation study are selecting the criterion, timing the administration of the tests, and selecting a sample for testing.

Three different criteria against which a test is compared are found in the literature. The first criterion is essentially instrumentation accuracy. The accuracy of the measurement provided by an instrument is determined by comparing the reading on the device with a standard measure. Examples in the literature include comparing the angular measurements of a goniometer with known angles[2] and testing a digitizer against known lengths.[17] Complex instruments have specific standardization procedures that allow the investigator to check the instrument against known standards and either make adjustments until the device readings accurately reflect the standard or develop equations that can be used to correct for inaccuracies.[18] For example, clinical audiometers are calibrated according to Standard S3.6–2010 of the American National Standards Institute.[19] Often, practice settings will engage in an analogous activity known as instrument calibration, although the standard to which the clinic instruments are compared may not be as rigorous as would occur in a methodological study.

The second criterion is a concurrent one. A concurrent criterion is applied at the same time the test in question is validated. Hallegraeff and colleagues[20] examined the concurrent validity of the Brief Illness Perception Questionnaire (IPQ-B), comparing it to the mental health component score of the SF-36 (SF-36 MCS) with Dutch patients who had acute nonspecific low back pain. Administering the two scales twice each, 1 week apart, the authors reported adequate concurrent validity between the IPQ-B and the SF-36 MCS.

The third criterion is predictive. A measure has predictive validity if the result of its administration at one point in time is highly associated with future status. There are three difficulties in doing predictive studies: determining the criterion itself, determining the timing of administration of the criterion, and maintaining a good sample of participants measured on both occasions. Flegel and Kolobe[21] studied the predictive validity of the Test of Infant Motor Performance (TIMP) by comparing children's scores on the test when they were younger than 4 months with an assessment of their motor proficiency between the ages of 4 and 7 years.

The importance of timing is also illustrated in the TIMP validity study. By assessing motor proficiency between the ages of 4 and 7 years, Flegel and Kolobe[21] could test a broad range of skills, including fine motor skills needed for handwriting and drawing. If they had tested at only 1 to 2 years of age, they would not have been able to look at these skills. On the other hand, if they had tested children at the age of 12 years, they might have identified more subtle coordination problems as the children began to participate in sports activities.

The third difficulty with predictive validity studies is the sample available for study. Because these studies extend over time, there may be differential loss of participants. For example, in Flegel and Kolobe's[21] study, only 65 children from the initial sample of 137 who were tested with the TIMP could be located for the later testing. If, for example, a disproportionate number of children determined by the TIMP to be at high risk for developmental delay were among the 65 children available for later testing, this might lead to inflated predictive validity estimates. Flegel and Kolobe were able to guard against this possibility by stratifying the 65 children into age and risk groups and then randomly sampling children within each group for their study.

RESPONSIVENESS DESIGNS

Studies of the responsiveness of a measure to changes in status generally involve (1) identification of a group of patients who can be assumed to have made a true change in the underlying construct of interest, (2) use of the measure of interest at pretreatment and posttreatment to calculate various measures of responsiveness, and (3) comparison of the responsiveness of the measure of interest to other related measures to determine the relative responsiveness of the different measurement tools.

For example, Beaton and colleagues[22] conducted a study of the validity, reliability, and responsiveness of the Disabilities of the Arm, Shoulder, and Hand (DASH) outcome measure for different regions of the upper extremity. They first identified a sample of patients who were awaiting treatment for a variety of upper extremity conditions. They assumed that the group as a whole would improve following treatment and that measurements taken before treatment and 12 weeks after treatment would reflect these improvements. However, they recognized that not everyone in the sample might improve, so they created two subgroups of patients about whom the assumption of improvement was more likely to be valid: One subgroup was for those who said their upper-limb condition had improved with treatment, and one subgroup was for those who said their upper-limb function had improved with treatment. In addition, for their question about the responsiveness to change for conditions affecting different parts of the upper extremity, they further subdivided their patients into those with shoulder conditions and those with wrist and hand conditions.

The primary measure of interest was the DASH, and pretreatment and posttreatment measures of the DASH were recorded for all of the participants. The extent to which the DASH changed was represented by three different measures: a change score, an effect size, and a standardized response mean (SRM). A change score is simply the difference between the posttreatment and pretreatment scores. If a study is only examining responsiveness of a single measurement tool, then examining change scores may be sufficient to determine responsiveness. The effect size is the mean change score divided by the standard deviation of the pretreatment score, and the SRM is the mean change score divided by the standard deviation of the change scores. Effect size or SRM is used when comparing the responsiveness of different measurement tools with different measurement scales. By dividing the change score by some measure of variability (either variability at baseline for the effect size or variability of the change scores for SRM), the level of responsiveness is standardized and can be compared across tools with different measurement scales. Beaton and colleagues[22] found that DASH scores were reduced by an average of 13.3 points for all patients and by an average of 19.7 points for the subset of patients who reported that their function was better.

Because they were not just interested in the responsiveness of the DASH by itself, but in the responsiveness of the DASH compared with some more specific tools, Beaton and colleagues[22] also took pretreatment and posttreatment measures using the Shoulder Pain and Disability Index (SPADI) and the Brigham carpal tunnel questionnaire. To compare across these tools, they moved beyond change scores by calculating effect scores and SRM scores. For a subset of shoulder patients who rated their function as better after treatment, the DASH SRM of 1.44 showed more responsiveness to change than the SPADI SRM of 1.13. For a subset of wrist and hand patients who rated their function as better after treatment, the DASH SRM of 0.91 showed marginally more responsiveness to change than the Brigham carpal tunnel questionnaire SRM of 0.87.[22]

Similar methods have been used to compare the responsiveness of the Quadriplegia Index of Function with the Barthel Index[23] and the Western Ontario and McMaster Universities Osteoarthritis Index (WOMAC) with the SF-36,[24,25] and the Knee Society Clinical Rating System.[26]

SUMMARY

Methodological research is conducted to document and improve measuring tools by assessing their reliability, validity, and responsiveness. The major components of reliability are instrument, intrarater, interrater, and intrasubject reliability. Reliability research can be classified according to whether the measurement protocol used is nonstandardized, partially standardized, or highly standardized. Participants should be selected based on whether they would likely be assessed with the tool in clinical situations; in addition, participants who demonstrate a wide range of scores should be selected. Construct validity is determined through logical argument and assessment of the convergence of similar tests and divergence of different tests. Content validity is determined by assessing the completeness, relevancy, and emphasis of the items within a test. Criterion validity is determined by comparing one measure with an accepted standard of measurement. Responsiveness of a measure is determined by examining the change scores, effect scores, or standardized response means for the measure for a group that is assumed to have undergone a true change in the underlying construct of interest.

REFERENCES

1. Cattaneo D, Jonsdottir J, Repetti S: Reliability of four scales on balance disorders in persons with multiple sclerosis, *Disabil Rehabil* 29:1920–1925, 2007.
2. Watkins MA, Riddle DL, Lamb RL, Personius WJ: Reliability of goniometric measurements and visual estimates of knee range of motion obtained in a clinical setting, *Phys Ther* 71:90–97, 1991.
3. Mayerson NH, Milano RA: Goniometric reliability in physical medicine, *Arch Phys Med Rehabil* 65:92–94, 1984.
4. Youdas JW, Carey JR, Garrett TR: Reliability of measurements of cervical spine range of motion-comparison of three methods, *Phys Ther* 71:98–104, 1991.
5. Biffi A, Cesani M, Fumagalli F, et al: Metachromatic leukodystrophy: Mutation analysis provides further evidence of genotype–phenotype correlation, *Clin Genet* 74:349–357, 2008.
6. Stratford PW: Summarizing the results of multiple strength trials: Truth or consequence, *Physiother Can* 44:14–18, 1992.
7. Connelly DM, Stevenson TJ, Vandervoort AA: Between- and within-rater reliability of walking tests in a frail elderly population, *Physiother Can* 48:47–51, 1996.
8. Tsorlakis N, Evaggelinou C, Grouios G, Tsorbazoudi C: Effect of intensive neurodevelopmental treatment in gross motor function of children with cerebral palsy, *Dev Med Child Neurol* 46:740–745, 2004.
9. Mitchell SK: Interobserver agreement, reliability, and generalizability of data collected in observational studies, *Psychol Bull* 86:376–390, 1979.
10. Taplin PS, Reid JB: Effects of instructional set and experiment influence on observer reliability, *Child Dev* 44:547–554, 1973.
11. Embrey DG, Yates L, Mott DH: Effects of neuro-developmental treatment and orthoses on knee flexion during gait: A single-subject design, *Phys Ther* 70:626–637, 1990.
12. Cronbach LJ: *Essentials of Psychological Testing*, New York, NY, 1990, Harper & Row.
13. Streiner DL, Norman GR: *Health Measurement Scales: A Practical Guide to Their Development and Use*, 3rd ed, Oxford, UK, 2003, Oxford University Press.
14. Mercer VS, Freburger K, Chang S-H, Purser JL: Measurement of paretic-lower-extremity loading and weight transfer after stroke, *Phys Ther* 89:653–664, 2009.
15. Megens AM, Harris SR, Backman CL, Hayes VE: Known-groups analysis of the Harris Infant Neuromotor Test, *Phys Ther* 87:164–169, 2007.
16. Chi TS, Wan DWK: Development and validation of Activities of Daily Living Inventory for the rehabilitation of patients with chronic obstructive pulmonary disease, *OTJR Occup Particip Health* 28:149–159, 2008.
17. Norton BJ, Ellison JB: Reliability and concurrent validity of the Metrecom for length measurement on inanimate objects, *Phys Ther* 73:266–274, 1993.
18. Geddes LA, Baker LE: *Principles of Applied Biomedical Instrumentation*, 3rd ed, New York, NY, 1989, John Wiley & Sons.
19. American National Standards Institute (ANSI): *ANSI S3.6–2010 Specification for Audiometers*, Washington, DC, 2010, ANSI.
20. Hallegraeff JM, van der Schans CP, Krijnen WP, de Greef MHG: Measurement of acute nonspecific low back pain perception in primary care physical therapy: Reliability and validity of the brief illness perception questionnaire, *BMC Musculoskel Disord* 14:53–59, 2013.
21. Flegel J, Kolobe THA: Predictive validity of the Test of Infant Motor Performance as measured by the Bruininks-Oseretsky Test of Motor Proficiency at school age, *Phys Ther* 82:762–771, 2002.

22. Beaton DE, Katz JN, Fossel AH, et al: Measuring the whole or the parts? Validity, reliability, and responsiveness of the Disabilities of the Arm, Shoulder, and Hand outcome measure in different regions of the upper extremity, *J Hand Ther* 14:128–146, 2001.

23. Gresham GE, Labi ML, Dittmar SS, et al: The Quadriplegia Index of Function (QIF): Sensitivity and reliability in a study of thirty quadriplegic patients, *Paraplegia* 24:38–44, 1986.

24. Angst F, Aeschlimann A, Steiner W, Stucki G: Responsiveness of the WOMAC osteoarthritis index as compared with the SF-36 in patients with osteoarthritis of the legs undergoing a comprehensive rehabilitation intervention, *Ann Rheum Dis* 60:834–840, 2001.

25. Lingard EA, Katz JN, Wright J, et al: Validity and responsiveness of the Knee Society Clinical Rating System in comparison with the SF-36 and WOMAC, *J Bone Joint Surg Am* 83:1856–1864, 2001.

26. Tong AYC, Man DWK: The validation of the Hong Kong Chinese Version of the Lawton Instrumental Activities of Daily Living scale for institutionalized elderly persons, *OTJR: Occup Particip Health* 22:132–142, 2002.

CHAPTER 20

Statistical Reasoning

CHAPTER OUTLINE

Data Set
Frequency Distribution
Frequency Distribution with
    Percentages
*Grouped Frequency Distribution with
    Percentages*
Frequency Histogram
Stem-and-Leaf Plot
Central Tendency
Mean
Median
Mode
Variability
Range

Variance
Standard Deviation
Normal Distribution
z Score
Percentages of the Normal
    Distribution
Sampling Distribution
Confidence Intervals of the
    Sampling Distribution
Significant Difference
Null Hypothesis
Alpha Level
Probability Determinants
    Between-Groups Difference

Within-Group Variability
Effect Size
Sample Size
Errors
Power
Statistical Conclusion Validity
Low Power
Lack of Clinical Importance
Error Rate Problems
Violated Assumptions
Failure to Use Intention-to-Treat
    Analysis
Summary

Statistics has a bad name. Consider this tongue-in-cheek sampling from the irreverent *Journal of Irreproducible Results*:

> We all know that you can prove anything with statistics. So I recently proved that nobody likes statistics, except for a few professors. If you don't believe that, just ask the person on the street. I did. The first person I saw referred to the subject as "sadistics." The second person, an old gentleman along the Mississippi River, muttered something about "liars, damned liars, and statisticians."[1]

Although quips about statistics may be amusing, the discipline of statistics should not be confused with the conclusions that researchers draw from statistical analyses. Statistics is a discipline in which mathematics and probability are applied in ways that allow researchers to make sense of their data. Although there are many different statistical tests and procedures—too many to include even in textbooks devoted solely to statistics—there are remarkably few central concepts that underlie all of the tests.

In this chapter, the central concepts of statistics are introduced. Readers should be prepared to read this chapter, and Chapters 21 through 24, which cover particular statistical tests, very slowly. Careful reading, examination of the tables and figures, and independent calculation of the examples in this chapter should provide a strong basis for understanding not only the following chapters but also, more important, the data analysis and results portions of research articles in the rehabilitation literature.

The chapter begins by presenting a data set that is used for all of the statistical examples in this and the following four chapters. Next, the concepts of frequency distribution, central tendency, variability, and normal distribution, which were introduced in Chapter 18, are reviewed and expanded. Then the new concepts of sampling distribution, significant difference, and power are explained. Finally, the concepts are integrated by a discussion of statistical conclusion validity.

DATA SET

Achieving a conceptual understanding of statistical reasoning is greatly enhanced by performing simple computational examples. Thus, a small hypothetical data set has been developed for use throughout this and several of the following chapters. Because it would be difficult to develop a small data set relevant to the practice of all of the rehabilitation professions, the data set was developed around a set of hypothetical patients who have undergone the common surgical procedure of total knee arthroplasty. If readers do not have experience treating individuals who have had total knee replacement, surely they have relatives or acquaintances who have undergone this common procedure. Our data set consists of 30 hypothetical patients, 10 at each of three clinics, who have undergone rehabilitation for a total

knee arthroplasty. Eighteen pieces of information are available for each patient:

Case number
Clinic attended
Sex
Age
Three-week knee flexion range of motion (ROM)
Six-week knee flexion ROM
Six-month knee flexion ROM
Six-month knee extensor torque
Six-month knee flexor torque
Six-month gait velocity
Four 6-month activities of daily living (ADL) indexes
Four 6-month deformity indexes

The ADL and deformity indexes were adapted for the purposes of this data set from a knee-rating system that was used at Brigham and Women's Hospital in Boston.[2] Table 20-1 provides an outline of the data set, indicating abbreviations for each variable, the unit of measurement when appropriate, and the meaning of any numerical coding. Table 20-2 presents the actual data set.

Table 20-1

Data Set Specifications for Patients Who Underwent Rehabilitation After Total Knee Arthroplasty

Variable Code	Variable Name	Variable Values
CASE	Case number	01–30
CN	Clinic number	1 = Community Hospital
		2 = Memorial Hospital
		3 = Religious Hospital
SEX	Patient sex	0 = Male
		1 = Female
AGE	Patient age	In years at last birthday
W3R	3-week range of motion (ROM) at each clinic	To nearest degree
W6R	6-week ROM	To nearest degree
M6R	6-month ROM	To nearest degree
E	6-month extension torque	To nearest Newton meter (N•m)
F	6-month flexion torque	To nearest N•m
V	Gait velocity	To nearest cm/s
DFC	Deformity: flexion contracture	$1 = >15°$
		$2 = 6°–15°$
		$3 = 0°–5°$
DVV	Deformity: varus/valgus angulation in stance	$1 = >10°$ valgus
		$2 = >5°$ varus or $6°–10°$ valgus
		$3 = 5°$ varus to $5°$ valgus

Table **20-1—cont'd**

Data Set Specifications for Patients Who Underwent Rehabilitation After Total Knee Arthroplasty

Variable Code	Variable Name	Variable Values
DML	Deformity: mediolateral stability	1 = marked instability 2 = moderate instability 3 = stable
DAP	Deformity: anteroposterior stability with knee at 90-degree flexion	1 = marked instability 2 = moderate instability 3 = stable
ADW	Activities of daily living (ADLs): distance walked	5 = unlimited 4 = 4–6 blocks 3 = 2–3 blocks 2 = indoors only 1 = transfers only
AAD	ADLs: assistive device	5 = none 4 = cane outside 3 = cane full-time 2 = two canes or crutches 1 = walker or unable to walk
ASC	ADLs: stair climbing	5 = reciprocal, no rail 4 = reciprocal, with rail 3 = one at a time, with or without rail 2 = one at a time, with rail and assistive device 1 = unable to climb stairs
ARC	ADLs: rising from a chair	5 = no arm assistance 4 = single-arm assistance 3 = difficult with two-arm assistance 2 = needs assistance of another 1 = unable to rise

FREQUENCY DISTRIBUTION

A frequency distribution is a tally of the number of times each score is represented in a data set. There are four ways of presenting a frequency distribution: frequency distribution with percentages, grouped frequency distribution with percentages, frequency histogram, and stem-and-leaf plot.

Frequency Distribution with Percentages

Table 20-3 shows a frequency distribution with percentages for the variable, "3-week ROM." The first column lists the scores that were obtained. The second column, absolute frequency, lists the number of times that each score was obtained. For example, two patients had 3-week ROM values of 67°. The third

Table **20-2**

Data Set for Patients Who Underwent Rehabilitation After Total Knee Arthroplasty

Case	CN	Sex	Age	W3R	W6R	M6R	E	F	V	DFC	DVV	DML	DAP	ADW	AAD	ASC	ARC
01	1	1	50	95	90	100	170	100	165	2	1	2	1	5	5	5	5
02	1	0	87	32	46	85	100	60	100	2	2	1	1	3	4	4	2
03	1	0	66	67	78	100	130	70	130	1	1	2	2	4	5	5	4
04	1	0	46	92	85	105	175	95	170	2	2	1	2	5	5	5	5
05	1	0	53	87	85	105	157	86	150	1	2	2	2	5	4	5	5
06	1	0	76	58	50	95	88	52	135	2	1	2	2	4	4	4	4
07	1	1	43	92	95	110	120	75	153	1	1	1	1	5	5	5	5
08	1	1	46	88	90	100	130	90	145	2	3	3	2	4	5	5	5
09	1	1	43	84	80	95	132	92	147	1	1	1	2	5	5	5	4
10	1	1	48	81	90	105	156	98	145	2	2	3	2	5	5	4	5
11	2	0	92	34	63	90	87	53	95	3	2	2	2	3	3	3	3
12	2	0	65	56	71	90	160	95	150	2	3	2	2	4	4	5	5
13	2	0	76	45	63	78	92	60	120	1	2	1	2	4	3	3	4
14	2	0	92	27	35	65	85	49	85	3	3	3	3	2	1	1	2
15	2	1	68	76	70	95	170	102	165	2	3	2	2	4	3	5	5
16	2	1	79	49	56	98	81	37	93	2	2	2	1	3	2	3	2
17	2	1	85	47	58	84	87	46	70	3	2	2	2	2	1	2	2
18	2	1	82	50	60	80	93	63	94	1	1	2	2	3	2	2	2
19	2	0	81	40	40	83	96	58	101	2	2	2	2	3	2	1	2
20	2	1	90	67	70	95	103	63	103	1	1	3	2	2	2	2	3
21	3	0	66	32	67	105	180	105	180	1	2	1	1	5	5	5	5
22	3	0	72	50	67	105	150	85	150	2	3	3	2	5	4	4	4
23	3	0	68	60	65	95	154	89	156	2	3	3	2	4	4	4	4
24	3	0	77	84	80	105	141	83	146	2	2	2	1	3	3	4	3
25	3	0	60	81	85	100	168	93	178	3	3	3	2	4	5	5	5
26	3	1	75	81	94	110	146	84	135	2	1	3	3	5	5	5	5
27	3	1	73	84	90	100	120	74	134	2	2	2	3	4	4	4	4
28	3	1	72	81	95	103	110	68	120	2	1	2	3	4	5	3	4
29	3	1	72	82	90	104	116	74	126	3	2	3	1	4	3	4	3
30	3	1	63	91	95	106	137	86	131	2	1	3	3	4	5	5	5

Note: All variables are identified in Table 20-1.

column, relative frequency, lists the percentage of patients who received each score. This is calculated by dividing the number of patients with that score by the total number of patients. From this column we find that the four patients who had scores of 81 represent 13.3% of the sample [4/30×100=13.3%]. The fourth column, cumulative frequency, is formed by adding the relative frequencies of the scores up to and including the score of interest. For example, a researcher might be interested in the percentage of patients who had ROM scores of less than 50° 3 weeks postoperatively. From the cumulative frequency column, one finds that 26.7% of the sample had ROM values of 49° or less.

Table **20-3**

Frequency Distribution of 3-Week Range-of-Motion Values

Score (°)	Absolute Frequency	Relative Frequency (%)	Cumulative Frequency (%)
27	1	3.3	3.3
32	2	6.7	10.0
34	1	3.3	13.3
40	1	3.3	16.7
45	1	3.3	20.0
47	1	3.3	23.3
49	1	3.3	26.7
50	2	6.7	33.4
56	1	3.3	36.7
58	1	3.3	40.0
60	1	3.3	43.3
67	2	6.7	50.0
76	1	3.3	53.3
81	4	13.3	66.6
82	1	3.3	70.0
84	3	10.0	80.0
87	1	3.3	83.3
88	1	3.3	86.6
91	1	3.3	90.0
92	2	6.7	96.7
95	1	3.3	100.0
Total	**30**	**100.0**	

Table **20-4**

Frequency Distribution of 3-Week Range-of-Motion Scores, Modified for Missing Values

Score (°)	Absolute Frequency	Relative Frequency (%)	Adjusted Frequency (%)	Cumulative Frequency (%)
27	1	3.3	3.7	3.7
32	2	6.7	7.4	11.1
34	1	3.3	3.7	14.8
40	1	3.3	3.7	18.5
45	1	3.3	3.7	22.2
47	1	3.3	3.7	25.9
49	1	3.3	3.7	29.6
50	2	6.7	7.4	37.0
56	1	3.3	3.7	40.7
58	1	3.3	3.7	44.4
60	1	3.3	3.7	48.1
67	1	3.3	3.7	51.8
76	1	3.3	3.7	55.5
81	4	13.3	14.8	70.3
82	1	3.3	3.7	74.3
84	3	10.0	11.1	85.1
88	1	3.3	3.7	88.8
91	1	3.3	3.7	92.5
92	1	3.3	3.7	96.2
95	1	3.3	3.7	100.0
Missing	3	10.0	Missing	
Total	**30**	**100.0**	**100.0**	

A variation of this basic display is needed if there are missing values in the sample. Suppose that Patients 3 through 5 missed their 3-week evaluation appointments. Table 20-4 presents a revised frequency distribution that accounts for these three missing pieces of data. Note that another column, adjusted frequency, has been added. The adjusted frequency is calculated by dividing the number of observations for each score by the number of valid scores for each variable, rather than by the number of participants. In this case, there are 27 valid scores. The adjusted frequency of a ROM score of 81° is now 14.8% [4/27×100=14.8%]. The cumulative frequency is the sum of the adjusted frequencies. If many data points are missing, it is often misleading to

present the frequencies as percentages of the total sample; use of adjusted frequencies corrects the problem.

Grouped Frequency Distribution with Percentages

The grouped frequency distribution is another way frequency information is commonly presented. When there are many individual scores in a distribution, the characteristics of the distribution may be grasped more easily if scores are placed into groups. Table 20-5 presents a grouped frequency distribution for the 3-week ROM values. From this grouped distribution, it is readily apparent that the group with the highest frequency is that with scores from 80° to 89°.

Table 20-5

Grouped Frequency Distribution for 3-Week Range-of-Motion Values

Scores (°)	Frequency	Relative Frequency (%)	Cumulative Frequency (%)
20–29	1	3.3	3.3
30–39	3	10.0	13.3
40–49	4	13.3	26.7
50–59	4	13.3	40.0
60–69	3	10.0	50.0
70–79	1	3.3	53.3
80–89	10	33.3	86.7
90–99	4	13.3	100.0
Total	**30**	**100.0**	

A disadvantage of the grouped frequency distribution is that information is lost. Table 20-5 indicates that there are three subjects whose scores range from 30° to 39°; however, this could mean that all three patients had scores of 39, three patients had scores of 30, or the three had a variety of scores within this range.

Frequency Histogram

Another way to present a grouped frequency distribution is a histogram. A histogram presents each grouped frequency as a bar on a graph. The height of each bar represents the frequency of observations in the group. Figure 20-1 shows a histogram of the 3-week ROM data. As with the grouped frequency distribution from which the histogram is generated,

information is lost because one does not know how the scores are distributed within each group.

Stem-and-Leaf Plot

A final way of presenting frequency data is the stem-and-leaf plot. This plot presents data concisely, without losing information in the grouping process. Each individual score is divided into a "stem" and a "leaf," as shown in Table 20-6. In this instance, the stem is the digit representing the multiple of 10 (20, 30, 40, and so on), and the leaf is the digit representing the multiple of 1 (1, 2, 3, 4, and so on). The row with the stem of 5 has leaves of 0, 0, 6, and 8. The stems and leaves together represent the four scores of 50, 50, 56, and 58. The stem-and-leaf plot, like the histogram, provides a good visual picture of the frequency distribution.

Table 20-6

Stem-and-Leaf Plot of 3-Week Range-of-Motion Frequency Distribution

Stem	Leaf	Total
2	7	1
3	2 2 4	3
4	0 5 7 9	4
5	0 0 6 8	4
6	0 7 7	3
7	6	1
8	1 1 1 1 2 4 4 4 7 8	10
9	1 2 2 5	4
Total		**30**

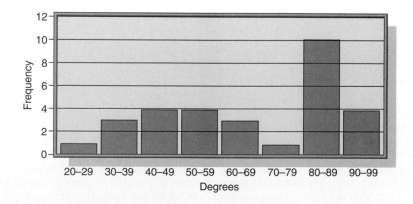

Figure 20-1 Histogram of 3-week range-of-motion scores.

CENTRAL TENDENCY

Researchers often wish to collapse a set of data into a single score that represents the whole set; that is, the researcher is interested in the central tendency of the data. The measures of central tendency, along with the measures of variability that will follow, are known as *descriptive statistics*. The three commonly used measures of central tendency are the *mean*, the *median*, and the *mode*. If a distribution is perfectly symmetrical, then the mean, median, and mode are all identical. If the distribution is asymmetrical, they differ.

Mean

The arithmetic mean of a data set is the sum of the observations divided by the number of observations. Recall from Chapter 18 that mathematical notation for the mean is as follows:

$$\bar{X} = \frac{\sum X}{N}$$

(Formula 20-1)

In words, this equation says the mean is the sum of all the observations divided by the number of observations. For example, the mean of the 3-week ROM scores for Clinic 1 is 77.6° [(95+32+67+92+87+58+92+88+ 84+81)/10=77.6]. The mean is a versatile measure of central tendency because it uses information from all the scores in the distribution. However, extreme values can distort the mean. In this example, 7 of the 10 scores are greater than 80°, but the very low score of 32° pulls the mean down to 77.6°.

Median

The median is the "middle" score of a distribution, or the score above which half of the distribution lies. To calculate the median, a researcher must first rank the scores. When the distribution has an odd number of scores, the middle score is easy to locate: $(N+1)/2$=the middle-ranked score. Thus, in a sample of 987 scores, the 494th ranked score is the median. When the number of scores in a distribution is even, as in our example, the median is calculated by finding the mean of the two middle scores: $[N/2]$ and $[(N/2)+1]$. In a sample with 988 scores, the median is the mean of the 494th and 495th ranked scores. Table 20-7 presents the frequency distribution for the ten 3-week measurements we are considering. The median, as shown, is 85.5°. The median is a useful measure of central tendency when the distribution contains a few extreme values that distort the

Table **20-7**

Median and Mode Calculations for 3-Week Range-of-Motion Values for Clinic 1

Score (°)	Absolute Frequency	Cumulative (%)	Median*	Mode[†]
32	1	10.0		
58	1	20.0		
67	1	30.0		
81	1	40.0		
84	1	50.0		
			85.5	
87	1	60.0		
88	1	70.0		
92	2	90.0		92
95	1	100.0		

*Median is the "middle" score. When there is an even number of scores, the two middle scores are averaged. In this example, the median is (84+87)/2=85.5.
[†]Mode is the score that occurs most frequently.

mean. In addition, the median is often used to describe the central tendency of ordinal measurements, particularly if further statistical analysis of the measures will be done with nonparametric statistics (to be described in more detail in Chapter 21). The disadvantage of the median is that it does not include information from all of the scores in the distribution.

Mode

The mode is the score that occurs most frequently in a distribution. If there are two modes, the distribution is termed bimodal. Our example of 3-week ROM scores has a mode of 92, as shown in Table 20-7. The mode is often used to describe nominal data, which have neither the property of order nor the property of distance and therefore cannot provide a median and mean (see Chapter 18).

VARIABILITY

The variability of a data set is the amount of spread in the data. Two different groups might have the same mean score yet have very different characteristics. For example, a sample of female college athletes might have the same mean weight as a sample of female nonathletes at the school. However, the athletes would be expected to have a relatively narrow range of weights, whereas the nonathletes would be expected to range in weight from the very underweight to the very overweight. The three measures of variability are *range, variance*, and *standard deviation*.

Range

The range is the difference between the highest and lowest values in the distribution. In the group of 10 patients from Clinic 1, the range is 63° (95 – 32 = 63). Although the range is technically a single score, it is often reported by presenting both the high and low scores so that readers will understand not only the range but also the magnitude of the scores in the distribution. The range can be used as a measure of variability with any of the measures of central tendency but is particularly appropriate for use with the median.

Variance

The variance is a measure of variability that, like the mean, requires that every score in the distribution be used in its calculation. Therefore, the variance, along with the closely related standard deviation, is generally reported in concert with the mean. Although the calculation of the variance is presented in Chapter 18, it is reviewed here with our 3-week ROM data from Clinic 1. To calculate the variance, we convert each of the raw scores in the data set to a deviation score by subtracting the mean of the data set from each raw score. In mathematical notation,

$$x = X - \bar{X}$$

(Formula 20-2)

Recall from Chapter 18 that the lowercase, italic x (x) is the symbol for a deviation score. The deviation score indicates how high or low a raw score is compared with the mean. The first two columns of Table 20-8 present the raw and deviation scores for the knee flexion data set and, below them, their sums and means. Note that both the sum and the mean of the deviation scores are zero. To generate a nonzero index of the variability within a data set, we must square the deviation scores. We can then calculate the population variance by determining the mean of the squared deviations. In mathematical notation,

$$\sigma^2 = \frac{\sum x^2}{N}$$

(Formula 20-3)

We know from Chapter 18 that σ is the lowercase Greek sigma and when squared is the notation for the variance. The third column in Table 20-8 shows the squared deviations from the group mean and, below them, their sum and mean. The population variance is used when all of the members of a population are known. In practice this rarely occurs, so the sample variance is used to estimate the population variance. The sample variance is calculated by dividing the sum of the squared deviations by $N-1$, as follows:

$$s^2 = \frac{\sum x^2}{N-1}$$

(Formula 20-4)

The symbol for the sample variance is s^2. In our example, the sample variance is calculated by dividing 3542.40 (the sum of the squared deviations) by 9 ($N-1$), as shown in Table 20-8.

The rationale for dividing the sum of the squared deviations by $N-1$ rests on the concept of degrees of freedom. Although an abstract concept, degrees of freedom can be understood in a general sense through the use of an illustration. In a sample of 10 values with a known mean, 9 of the values are "free" to fluctuate, as long as the investigator has control over the final value. For our sample of 10 observations with a mean of 77.6°, the sum of those 10 observations is 776. If we wanted to generate another sample with a mean of 77.6°, we could select 9 numbers randomly as long as we could manipulate the 10th value. If 9 randomly selected numbers each have a value of 100, they add to a total of 900. The sample can still have a mean value of 77.6° if the 10th value is manipulated to be –124 (900 – 124 = 776/10 = 77.6). This phenomenon is termed *degrees of freedom*, or the number of items that are free to fluctuate. Thus, for the mean, there are always $N-1$ degrees of freedom. Statisticians have found that using the degrees of freedom for the mean as the denominator of the sample variance formula leads to an unbiased estimation of the population variance. The degrees of freedom concept is used in the computation of many different statistical tests.

Standard Deviation

As just defined, the *population variance* is the mean of the squared deviations from the mean, and the *sample variance* is the sum of the squared deviations from the mean, divided by the degrees of freedom for the mean. Although the variance is useful in many statistical procedures, it does not have a great deal of intuitive meaning because it is calculated from squared

Inserting the values of 77.6° ($\bar{X}$) and 6.27° (SEM), we find the following:

$$90\% \text{ CI} = 67.3° \text{ to } 87.9°$$

$$95\% \text{ CI} = 65.3° \text{ to } 89.9°$$

$$99\% \text{ CI} = 61.4° \text{ to } 93.7°$$

We are 90% confident that the true population mean is somewhere between 67.3° and 87.9°; we are 99% confident that it lies somewhere between 61.4° and 93.7°. The computations given here are for the simplest calculation of a CI for the population mean. CIs can also be calculated for population proportions, for the difference between population proportions, and for the difference between population means.[4 (pp. 123–129)]

SIGNIFICANT DIFFERENCE

Researchers often wish to do more than describe their data. They wish to determine whether there are differences between groups who have been exposed to different treatments. The branch of statistics that is used to determine whether, among other things, there are significant differences between groups is known as *inferential statistics*. The theoretical basis of inferential statistics is that population parameters can be inferred from sample statistics. The determination of whether two sample means are significantly different from one another is actually a determination of the likelihood that the two sample means are drawn from populations with the same means. The sampling distribution of the mean is used as the basis for making these inferential statements—it is the link between the observed samples and the theorized population.

When we compare two groups who have received different experimental treatments, we almost always find that there is some difference between the means of the two groups. For example, assume that we wish to determine the effect of continuous passive motion on 3-week ROM in our patients who have had total knee arthroplasty. Assume that the patients at Clinic 1 received continuous passive motion postoperatively and that the patients at Clinic 3 did not. The mean 3-week ROM score for Clinic 1 is 77.6°; for Clinic 3, it is 72.6°. This is a difference of 5.0°. We wonder whether this difference is a true difference between the two groups or chance variation caused by sampling error.

If it is highly likely that the difference was caused by sampling error, we conclude that there is no (statistically) significant difference between the two group means. In other words, if sampling errors are a likely explanation for the difference between the means of the groups, it is

likely that the two groups were drawn from populations with the same means. Conversely, if it is highly unlikely that the difference between the groups was the result of sampling errors, we conclude that there is a significant difference between the groups. If sampling error is not a likely explanation for differences between the groups, it is likely that the two groups come from populations with different means. To determine whether the difference between groups is significant, we test a null hypothesis at a particular alpha level, as described next.

Although the traditional basis for determining statistical differences is presented in the following section, it should be noted that there is a long history of dissatisfaction with this approach to statistical analysis.[5,6] Objections include the need to make all-or-none decisions, the arbitrary nature of conventional levels for determining statistical significance, the sensitivity of results to sample size, and the inability of statistical tests to make value judgments about the clinical importance of statistically significant findings.[6] Despite these objections, significance testing remains the norm for statistical testing, and researchers and readers need to understand the conventions on which it is based.

Null Hypothesis

The seemingly convoluted language needed to describe the meaning of a statistically significant difference derives from the fact that the statistical hypothesis being tested is the hypothesis of "no statistically significant difference." This hypothesis is referred to as the *null hypothesis*, or H_0. The formal null hypothesis for determining whether there are different mean 3-week ROM scores between Clinics 1 and 3 is as follows:

$$H_0 : \mu1 = \mu3$$

Thus, the null hypothesis is that the population mean for Clinic 1 ($\mu1$) is equal to the population mean for Clinic 3 ($\mu3$). For now we will assume that the alternative hypothesis, or H_1, is that the population mean of Clinic 1 is greater than the population mean of Clinic 3:

$$H_1 : \mu1 > \mu3$$

Alternative hypotheses are addressed later with specific statistical tests. In statistical testing, we determine the probability that the null hypothesis is true. If the probability is sufficiently low, we conclude that the null hypothesis is false, accept the alternative hypothesis, and conclude that there are significant differences between the groups. If the probability that the null hypothesis is true is high, we conclude that the null hypothesis is true, accept the null hypothesis, and conclude that there are no significant differences between the groups. The clinical importance of any significant differences that are identified cannot be assumed; researchers and readers need to determine the clinical importance of statistical findings in light of clinical knowledge and experience.

Alpha Level

Before conducting a statistical analysis of differences, researchers must determine how much of a probability of drawing an incorrect conclusion they are willing to tolerate. To use null hypothesis terminology, how low is the "sufficiently low" probability needed to detect a significant difference? The conventional level of chance that is tolerated is 5%, or .05. This is referred to as the alpha (α) level. If a difference in means is significant at the .05 level, this means that 5% of differences of this magnitude would have been the result of chance fluctuations caused by sampling errors. That is, 95% of the time the difference would represent a true difference, and 5% of the time the difference would represent sampling error. Occasionally the more stringent level of .01 is used, as is the more permissive level of .10.

Two twists occur with alpha levels as they are reported in research. The first is the distinction between the alpha level and the obtained probability; the second is inflation and correction of the alpha level during performance of multiple statistical tests.

The distinction between the alpha level and the obtained probability (*p*) level is the distinction between what the researcher is willing to accept as chance and what the actual results are. The alpha level is specified before the data analysis is conducted; the probability level is a product of the data analysis. Researchers may set the alpha level at .05, meaning that they are willing to accept a 5% chance that significant findings may actually be the result of sampling error. In studies in which significant differences are found, the actual probability that a given result will occur by chance may be much less than the alpha level set by the researcher.

Assume that the result of a statistical test comparing two group means is that the probability that the difference will occur by chance is .001. This means that in only 1 of 1000 instances would a difference of this magnitude likely be the result of sampling error. Now that computers are available to calculate statistics, such precise probability levels are often reported. Because the obtained probability level of .001 is less than the preset alpha level of .05, the researcher concludes that there is a statistically significant difference between the groups. Does the reporting of the obtained probability level of .001 somehow indicate that the researcher changed the alpha level during the course of the data analysis? No. The reporting of a specific probability level simply indicates to the reader the extent to which the obtained probability was lower or higher than the alpha set by the researcher.

The second twist given to an alpha level in a study is called *alpha level inflation*. This occurs when researchers conduct many statistical tests within a given study. Using an alpha level of 5%, we know that the probability that differences occurred by chance is 5% for each test. If we conduct many tests, the overall probability of obtaining chance significant differences increases. This increase is alpha level inflation. When researchers conduct multiple tests, they may correct for alpha level inflation by using a more stringent alpha level for each individual test. They may obtain a more stringent alpha by using, for example, the Bonferroni adjustment. This adjustment divides the total alpha level for the experiment, called the experiment-wise alpha level, by the number of statistical tests conducted to determine a test-wise alpha level.[7] For example, a researcher may set the experiment-wise alpha level at .05 and conduct 10 tests, each with a test-wise alpha level of .005 (.05/10=.005). Some researchers consider this adjustment too stringent and compensate by setting a higher experiment-wise alpha level. For example, if a researcher sets the experiment-wise alpha at .15 and conducts seven tests, the adjusted test-wise alpha level would be .0214. Although the Bonferroni adjustment is commonly used, statisticians do not always agree on when to adjust for alpha inflation, nor do they all agree that the Bonferroni adjustment is the best procedure to use when an adjustment is desired.[8,9]

Two articles illustrate somewhat different reasons for using a Bonferroni adjustment. Murray[10] used the adjustment when doing multiple comparisons among four groups of subjects on a variety of spoken language variables. The four groups were those with Huntington's disease (HD), those with Parkinson's disease (PD), and a control group matched to each of the diagnostic groups (CON-HD and CON-PD). This study looked at three comparisons of interest: HD versus CON-HD, PD versus CON-PD, and HD versus PD. Each statistical test of these differences was conducted at an alpha level of .016 (.05/3=.016). Mueller and colleagues[11] used a Bonferroni adjustment because of the large number of dependent variables used in their study of functional status after transmetatarsal amputation. One of the measures, the physical performance test, can have a total score as well as be subdivided into eight subscores. Mueller chose to conduct a statistical test on the total score at an alpha level of .05. Then, he conducted eight more tests on the subscores, each at a divided alpha level of .006 (.05/8=.006).

Statistical analysis requires that the researcher set an alpha level. If the statistical test results in an obtained probability that is less than the predetermined alpha level, the result is deemed statistically significant. Whether a result is statistically significant or not often depends on the way in which the researcher sets the alpha level. Thus, tests of statistical significance do not provide absolute conclusions about the meaning of data. Rather, these tests provide the researcher with information about the probability that the obtained results occurred by chance. The researcher then draws statistical conclusions about whether a statistically significant difference exists. Researchers and readers then need to interpret the statistical conclusions in light of their knowledge of the subject being studied.

Probability Determinants

Three pieces of information are essential to the determination of statistical probabilities: (1) the magnitude of the differences between groups (or between levels of the independent variable when there is only one group), (2) variability within a group, and (3) sample size. In this section, the effect of each of these determinants is illustrated conceptually, without determination of actual probabilities. Actual probabilities are determined in subsequent chapters when specific statistical tests are discussed.

Between-Groups Difference

To illustrate the influence of the size of the difference between two groups, let us compare the differences in mean 3-week ROM scores between Clinics 1, 2, and 3. Clinic 1 has a mean of 77.6°, Clinic 2 a mean of 49.1°, and Clinic 3 a mean of 72.6°. If within-group variability and sample size are held constant, a larger between-groups difference is associated with a smaller probability that the difference occurred by chance. Thus, there is a relatively low probability that the large 28.5° difference in the 3-week ROM means for Clinics 1 and 2 occurred by chance. Conversely, there is a relatively high probability that the smaller 5.0° difference in the 3-week ROM means for Clinics 1 and 3 did occur by chance.

Within-Group Variability

The second piece of information used to determine the probability that a difference is a true difference is the variability within a group. If the between-groups difference and sample size are held constant, the differences between groups with lower within-group variability have a lower probability of occurring by chance than differences between groups with high within-group variability. Assume that we have two groups of 100

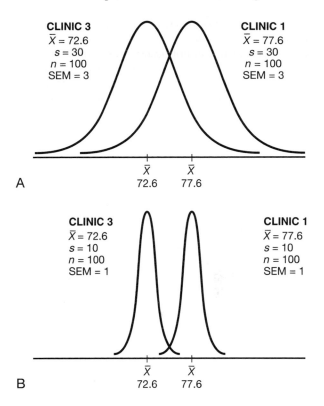

Figure 20-4 Effect of within-group variability on the overlap of sampling distributions. **A,** High variability leads to overlap of sampling distributions. **B,** Low variability leads to minimal overlap of sampling distributions. n = number of subjects; s = standard deviation; SEM = standard error of the mean; $\overline{X}$ = mean.

with means of 72.6° and 77.6°. If the groups have high within-group variability—say, standard deviations of 30.0°—curves representing their sampling distributions would look like those drawn in Figure 20-4A. The sampling distributions, which each have an SEM of 3 $(30/\sqrt{100}=3)$, overlap a great deal.

Because of the overlap in sampling distributions, there is a high probability that the two samples came from populations that have the same mean. Because this probability is high, we conclude that the difference in means occurred by chance; that is, the difference between the means of the two groups is not significant.

Contrast Figure 20-4 parts A and B. Figure 20-4B illustrates the same between-groups difference, 5.0°. However, the within-group variability has been reduced sharply. In this example, each group standard deviation is set at 10.0, meaning that the SEM is 1° $(10/\sqrt{100}=1)$. With an SEM of only 1°, the two curves overlap very little. Because they do not overlap very much, there is a low probability that the samples could have been drawn from populations with the same mean. Because this probability is low, we can conclude that the difference in means did not occur by chance; that is, the difference between the means of the two groups is a significant one. Even small differences between groups can be statistically significant if the within-group variability is sufficiently low.

Effect Size

The two pieces of information listed previously can be combined into a single concept known as *effect size*. The effect size is the between-groups difference divided by a pooled version of the standard deviations of the groups being compared. Large between-groups differences and small within-group variability result in large effect sizes. Small between-groups differences and large within-group variability result in small effect sizes. Computing effect size allows the relative magnitude of experimental effects to be compared across variables with different measurement characteristics. Convention has it that an effect size of 0.20 is considered small, 0.50 is considered medium, and 0.80 is considered large when comparing two group means.[12]

Sample Size

The third piece of information used to determine the probability that a difference is a true difference is the sample size. We already know that the mean of a large sample is more stable than a mean of a small sample. Assume that we have two groups of 100, each with a standard deviation of 10.0°, and a mean difference between the groups of 5.0°. Because of the large sample sizes, we are confident that the mean values are stable indicators of the means of the populations from which the samples are drawn. The estimated SEM for each group's sampling distribution is 1.0° ($10/\sqrt{100}=1$); Figure 20-5A shows the minimal overlap between the two sampling distributions. This minimal overlap leads us to conclude that it is unlikely that the differences between the two groups are due to chance; in other words, there is a significant difference between the groups.

Now assume that we have two groups of 10 participants each. The mean difference between the groups is the same as the previous example (5.0°), as is the standard deviation of each group (10.0°). Because we know that sample sizes of only 10 are sensitive to extreme values, we know that the mean of a sample of 10 is considerably less stable than a mean from a sample of 100. This is reflected in the calculation of the estimated SEM. With a standard deviation of 10° and a sample size of 10, the SEM becomes 3.16° ($10/\sqrt{10}=3.16$). Figure 20-5B shows the curves that correspond to the sampling distributions of our smaller samples. The curves overlap

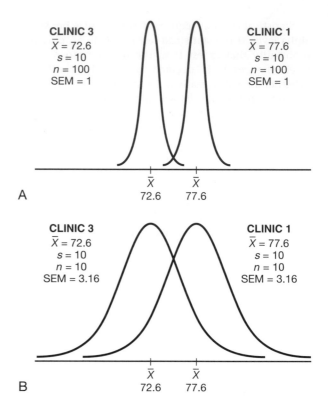

Figure 20-5 Effect of sample size on the overlap of sampling distributions. **A,** Large sample size leads to low overlap. **B,** Small sample size leads to extensive overlap. *n* = number of subjects; *s* = standard deviation; SEM = standard error of the mean; $\bar{X}$ = mean.

considerably, leading us to conclude that the samples might well have been drawn from populations with the same mean; that is, there is no significant difference between the means of the two groups. Thus, if the sample size is large enough, even small between-groups differences may be statistically significant, and conversely, if the sample size is too small, even large between-groups differences may not be statistically significant.

ERRORS

Because researchers determine statistical differences by making probability statements, there is always the possibility that the statistical conclusion has been reached in error. Unfortunately, researchers never know when an error has been made; they only know the probability of making that error. There are two types of statistical errors, labeled simply type I and type II. Figure 20-6 shows the difference between them. The columns represent the two possible states

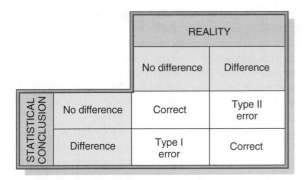

	REALITY	
	No difference	Difference
No difference	Correct	Type II error
Difference	Type I error	Correct

STATISTICAL CONCLUSION (row label)

Figure 20-6 Type I and type II errors reflect the relationship between statistical conclusions and reality.

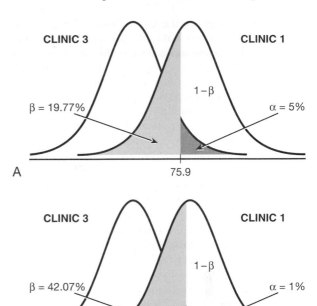

Figure 20-7 Relationship between type I and type II errors. **A,** Alpha (α; probability of making a type I error) is 5%, and beta (β; probability of making a type II error) is 19.77%. **B,** α is 1%, and β is 42.07%.

of reality: There is or is not a difference between groups. The rows represent the two statistical conclusions that can be drawn: There is or is not a difference between groups. The intersection of the columns and rows creates four different combinations of statistical conclusions and reality. If the statistical conclusion is that there is no difference between groups, and if there is in fact no difference, then we have made a correct statistical conclusion. If the statistical conclusion is that there is a difference between groups, and if this is in fact the case, then we have also come to a correct statistical conclusion.

However, if the statistical conclusion is that there is a difference between groups when in fact there is no difference, then we have come to an erroneous statistical conclusion. This error is called a *type I error*. The probability of making a type I error is alpha. Recall that researchers set alpha according to the amount of chance they are willing to tolerate. An alpha level of .05 means that the researcher is willing to accept a 5% chance that significant results occurred by chance. Thus, alpha is the probability that significant results will be found when in fact no significant difference exists. Researchers never know when they have committed a type I error; they only know the probability that one occurred. If researchers wish to decrease the probability of making a type I error, they simply reduce alpha.

A type II error occurs when the statistical conclusion is that there is no difference between the groups when in reality there is a difference. The probability of making a type II error is beta. Beta is related to alpha but is not as easily obtained. Figure 20-7 shows the relationship between alpha and beta.

For this example, we assume samples of 25 with standard deviations of 10°, giving us an SEM of 2.0° (10/√25=2). We also assume that Clinic 3, with a mean of 72.6°, is the standard against which Clinic 1, with a

mean of 77.6°, is being compared. Our null hypothesis is that $\mu_1 = \mu_3$. Our alternative hypothesis is that $\mu_1 > \mu_3$. In words, we wish to determine whether the mean of Clinic 1 is significantly greater than the mean of Clinic 3. Alpha is set at 5% in Figure 20-7A.

To determine beta, we first must determine the point on the Clinic 3 curve above which only 5% of the distribution lies. From the z table we find that .05 corresponds to a z score of 1.645. A z score of 1.645 corresponds in this case to a raw score of 75.9° (through algebraic rearrangement, $\bar{X} + [z][SEM] = X$; 72.6+[1.645][2]=75.9). Thus, if Clinic 1's mean is greater than 75.9° (1.645 SEM above Clinic 3's mean), it would be considered significantly different from Clinic 3's mean of 72.6° at the 5% level. The dark shading at the upper tail of Clinic 3's sampling distribution corresponds to the alpha level of 5% and is the probability of making a type I error. This darkly shaded area is sometimes referred to as the *rejection region* because the null hypothesis of no difference between groups would be rejected if a group mean within this area were obtained. Any group mean less than 75.9° would not be identified as statistically different from the group mean of 72.6°.

The entire part of the curve below the rejection region (including the parts that are lightly shaded) is termed the *acceptance region* because the null hypothesis of no difference between groups would be accepted if a group mean within this area were obtained.

Shift your attention now to the lightly shaded lower tail of the sampling distribution of Clinic 1. Using the z table, we can determine the probability of obtaining sample means less than 75.9°, if the population mean was actually 77.6°. To do so, we convert 75.9° to a z score in relation to 77.6°: $z = (X - \bar{X})$ /SEM; $(75.9 - 77.6)/2 = -.85$. Using the z table, we find that 19.77% of Clinic 1's sampling distribution will fall below a z score of −.85. This percentage is the probability of making a type II error. If Clinic 1, in reality, has a mean that is significantly greater than Clinic 3's mean, we would fail to detect this difference almost 20% of the time because of the overlap in the sampling distributions. Almost 20% of Clinic 1's sampling distribution falls within the acceptance region of Clinic 3's sampling distribution.

There is an inverse relationship between the probability of making type I and II errors. When the probability of one increases, the probability of the other decreases. Figure 20-7B shows that, for this example, when the probability of making a type I error is decreased to 1%, the type II error increases to 43%. Thus, in setting the alpha level for an experiment, the researcher must find a balance between the likelihood of detecting chance differences (type I error: alpha) and the likelihood of ignoring important differences (type II error: beta).

POWER

The power of a test is the likelihood that it will detect a difference when one exists. Recall that beta was the probability of ignoring an important difference when one existed. The probability of detecting a true difference, or power, is therefore $1 - \beta$, as shown in the Clinic 1 curves in Figure 20-7. Recall that the size of the between-groups difference, the size of the sample, and the variability within the sample are the factors that determine whether significant differences between groups are detected. When the sampling distributions of the groups have minimal overlap, the power of a test is high. Factors that contribute to nonoverlapping sampling distributions are large between-groups differences, small within-group differences, and large sample sizes.

Many authors have shown that power is often lacking in the research of their respective disciplines: medicine,[13] nursing,[14] psychology,[15] occupational therapy,[16] and rehabilitation.[17] This is because between-groups differences are often small, sample sizes are often small, and within-group variability is often large. This lack of statistical power in our literature may mean that promising treatment approaches are not pursued because research has failed to show a significant advantage to the approaches. The power of a given statistical test can be determined by consulting published power tables[12,18] or using power software available commercially or online.[19,20]

Researchers may increase a test's statistical power in four ways. First, they can maximize between-groups differences by carefully controlling extraneous variables and making sure they apply experimental techniques consistently. Note, however, that rigid controls may reduce a study's external validity by making the conditions under which it was conducted very different from the clinical situation to which the researcher wishes to generalize the results.

Second, researchers can reduce within-group variability by studying homogeneous groups of subjects or by using subjects as their own controls in repeated measures designs. Note that these strategies may also reduce external validity by narrowing the group of patients to whom the results can be generalized.

Third, researchers can increase sample size. Increasing sample size does not have the negative impact on external validity that the other two solutions have. However, the increased cost of research with more subjects is an obvious disadvantage to this strategy.

Fourth, researchers can select a more liberal alpha level at which to conduct their statistical tests (e.g., $p = .10$ or $p = .15$). The obvious problem here is that, unlike the other solutions, this one flies in the face of statistical convention and is unlikely to be acceptable to the scientific community judging the research. The exception to this is research that is clearly exploratory, pilot work designed to determine whether an approach has promise, rather than to provide definitive evidence about the approach.

Power tables or programs can also be used to determine what sample size is needed to achieve a particular level of power. The variables needed to determine sample size requirements are as follows:

- Desired power (the conventional level recommended is .80 or 80%)
- The alpha level that will be used in the research
- An estimate of the size of the between-groups difference that would be considered clinically meaningful
- An estimate of the within-group variability expected

A researcher can obtain estimates of the between-groups and within-group values from previous research or from a pilot study. For example, to achieve 80% power in their investigation of dosing effects of therapeutic massage on neck pain, Sherman and colleagues[21] employed a 35% to 70% improvement of the intervention groups and a 7% of the control groups and assumed a 10% loss of subjects to arrive at a group size of 38 subjects. When there is no previous information on which to base these estimates, researchers typically substitute effect sizes, determining whether they wish to have enough power to detect small, medium, or large effects, as previously defined. In their investigation of breathing retraining for persons with asthma Grammatopoulou and associates[22] employed an effect size (1.01) obtained from a pilot study of another intervention with persons with asthma, in their *a priori* power analysis. As a result they determined they needed a total of 26 subjects for their study in order to achieve a power of .80.

STATISTICAL CONCLUSION VALIDITY

Readers have previously been introduced to the research design concepts of internal, external, and construct validity (see Chapter 8). The final type of design validity that a researcher must consider when evaluating a research report is statistical conclusion validity. Four threats to statistical conclusion validity, modified from Cook and Campbell,[23] are presented in this section, along with a fifth threat commonly cited in reviews of randomized controlled trials.

Low Power

When statistically insignificant results are reported, readers must ask whether the nonsignificant result is a true indication of no difference or the result of a type II error. Researchers who give power estimates provide their readers with the probability that their analysis could detect differences and, in doing so, provide information readers need to make a decision about the potential usefulness of further study in the area. The editors of the *Journal of Bone and Joint Surgery*, for example, encourage authors to analyze or discuss power when they report *p* values between .05 and .15.[9]

Whether or not a power analysis is provided, readers should examine nonsignificant results to determine whether any of the nonsignificant changes were in the desired direction or of a clinically important magnitude. If the nonsignificant differences seem clinically useful and the probability of making a type II error seems high (the sample size was small, the within-group variability was large, or an analysis showed less than 80% power), then readers should be cautious about dismissing the results altogether. Studies with promising nonsignificant results should be replicated with more powerful designs.

An example of a study with low power is Palmer and associates'[24] report of the effects of two different types of exercise programs in patients with Parkinson's disease. Seven patients participated in each exercise program. No significant changes were found in measures of rigidity, although some showed nonsignificant changes in the desired direction. A power analysis of this study reveals that it had, at most, a 50% power level.[17] Because the probability of making a type II error was so high, the nonsignificant findings should not necessarily be taken to mean that exercise was not useful for these patients. A logical next step in investigating the effects of exercise for patients with Parkinson's disease is to replicate this study with a more powerful design.

Lack of Clinical Importance

If the power of a test is sufficiently great, it may detect differences that are so small that they are not clinically meaningful. This occurs when samples are large and groups are homogeneous. Just as readers need to examine the between-groups differences of statistically insignificant results to determine whether there is promise in the results, they must also use their clinical reasoning skills to examine statistically significant between-groups differences to determine whether they are clinically meaningful.

Two measures have increasingly been reported in rehabilitation research—minimal detectable difference (MDD) and minimal clinically important difference (MCID or MID)—as efforts to increase the clinical importance of research. MDD refers to the amount of change in a score that is necessary to reflect that a true difference has occurred. The MDD considers the amount of measurement error that must be overcome before the scientist-practitioner can consider that a performance change has occurred. The MDD is usually reported in conjunction with the reliability of the dependent variable measure. The more accurate a measure is, the smaller is the MDD. Huijbregts and colleagues[25] examined the ability of the 16-item, 112-point maximum Continuing Care Activity Measure (CCAM) to measure changes of physical function of persons who resided in long-term care (LTC) facilities. The study sample was a heterogeneous population, although there were several homogeneous subgroups within the sample. The subgroups were residents of nursing homes, residents of complex continuing care facilities (CCCs), and residents who had low tolerance for activity but were receiving long-duration care (LTLD). Using the standard error of difference, Huijbregts and colleagues[25] reported that the overall MDD score was 8.63 points, suggesting that a resident required a total CCAM change score of nearly 9 points on a 16-point measure from one administration to the next to have any kind of detectable change. When the MDD for the different subgroups was examined, the authors noted that the MDD for the nursing home group and that for the LTLD group were much less (3.3 and 5.1, respectively).

MCID typically has been reported as the minimum amount of change in a score that is meaningful in the care of the patient. The perspectives of meaningfulness have included those of the patients, their caretakers, and their rehabilitation therapists. Several different ways of determining this meaningfulness include expert consensus,[26] SEM,[27] and receiver operating characteristics (ROC).[28] Palombaro and associates[28] used both expert consensus and ROC to determine the MCID of change in gait speed for patients who had a successful fixation or hip replacement for fractured hip. For expert opinion MCID, the authors had a group of five experts, who frequently studied and published on gait with populations of frail elderly people, determine the MCID. For ROC-determined MCID, the authors took a subsample of patients for whom the Timed Up and Go (TUG) was measured. The MDD on the TUG was calculated for this subsample, and the gait speed sensitivity and specificity were then plotted from the TUG data. The authors reported the median MCID estimate of the five experts and the ROC MCID as equivalent.

Error Rate Problems

Inflation of alpha when multiple tests are conducted within a study is referred to as an *error rate problem* because the probability of making a type I error rises with each additional test. As discussed earlier, some researchers compensate for multiple tests by dividing an experiment-wise alpha among the tests to be conducted. Although division of alpha controls the experiment-wise alpha, it also dramatically reduces the power of each test. Readers must determine whether they believe that researchers who have conducted multiple tests have struck a reasonable balance between controlling alpha and limiting the power of their statistical analyses.

A study of balance function in elderly people illustrates alpha level inflation.[29] In this study, three groups were tested: nonfallers, recent fallers, and remote fallers. Five different measures of balance function were obtained on each of two types of supporting surfaces for each of two types of displacement stimuli. The combination of all these factors produced 20 measures for each subject. In the data analysis, nonfallers were compared with recent fallers, recent fallers were compared with remote fallers, and nonfallers were compared with remote fallers on each of the 20 measures. This yielded a total of 60 different tests of statistical significance. With this many tests, the overall probability that a type I error was committed was far higher than the .05 level set for each analysis. Statistical techniques that would have permitted comparison of more than two groups or more than one dependent variable simultaneously could have been used to prevent this alpha level inflation; these techniques are presented in Chapters 21 and 22.

Violated Assumptions

Each of the statistical tests that are presented in Chapters 21 through 24 is based on certain assumptions that should be met for the test to be valid. These assumptions include whether the observations were made independently of one another, whether participants were randomly sampled, whether the data were normally distributed, and whether the variance of the data was approximately equal across groups. These assumptions, and the consequences of violating them, are discussed in detail in Chapters 21 through 24.

Failure to Use Intention-to-Treat Analysis

Contemporary critics of the quality of randomized controlled trials call for an approach to statistical analysis that is referred to as "intention-to-treat" analysis.[30] The historically more common analysis approach can be referred to as "completer" analysis because only those participants who completed the entire study were included in the data analysis.[6] The problem with the completer approach to statistical analysis is that treatment effects can be greatly overestimated if large numbers of unsuccessful participants drop out of the study. For example, consider a weight loss research study that begins with 200 participants randomized to participate in either a year-long supervised diet and exercise program or a year-long trial of an over-the-counter weight-loss supplement. Twenty participants complete the diet and exercise program with an average weight loss of 20 lb. Seventy participants complete the supplement program with an average weight loss of 5 lb. In a traditional completer analysis, the statistical analysis would be run on only those participants who completed the study, and the likely conclusion would be that the diet and exercise program resulted in significantly more weight loss than the supplement program.

In an intention-to-treat analysis, everyone who was entered into the study is included in the final data analysis according to the treatment they were intended to have, whether or not they completed the study.

For those individuals who did not complete the study, typically the last data point they provided is used in lieu of an actual ending point.[6,31] In the hypothetical weight loss study, if some individuals came to the first session and never showed up again, their baseline weight would be entered as their final weight. If some individuals participated for 11 of the 12 months, their last weigh-in values would be entered as their final weight. Another approach to determining the missing final data is to follow up with dropouts to obtain the best data possible—perhaps some of the individuals who dropped out of the weight loss study would be willing to come in for a 12-month weigh-in even if they did not participate throughout the year-long program. If we assume that all of the dropouts in the hypothetical weight loss study maintained their baseline weight, an intention-to-treat analysis would show an average weight loss of 4 lb for the diet and exercise group (400 total lb lost by the 20 completers + 0 lb lost by the 80 dropouts = 4 lb per participant) and an average weight loss of 3.5 lb for the supplement group (350 total lb lost by the 70 completers + 0 lb lost by the 30 dropouts = 3.5 lb per participant). Compared with the completer analysis, the intention-to-treat approach shows a very different picture of the relative effectiveness of the two approaches to weight loss.

In an environment that emphasizes research on the effectiveness of clinical treatments, delivered in the context of actual clinical care, intention-to-treat analysis is an important part of capturing the overall effectiveness of treatment for broad groups of patients. In the hypothetical weight loss study, the intention-to-treat analysis tells us that over the course of a year, neither the diet and exercise program nor the supplement program resulted in impressive average weight reductions. However, the completer analysis tells us that the diet and exercise program led to substantial average weight reductions for the small subgroup of individuals who persisted with the program. Therefore, despite the contemporary emphasis on intention-to-treat analysis, supplemental completer analysis may be appropriate to document the impact of treatment for those who actually complete the treatment of interest.

SUMMARY

All statistical analyses are based on a relatively small set of central concepts. Descriptive statistics are based on the concepts of central tendency (mean, median, or mode) and variability (range, variance, and standard deviation) within a data set. The distribution of many variables forms a bell-shaped curve known as the normal distribution. The percentage of scores that fall within a certain range of the normal distribution is known and can be used to predict the likelihood of obtaining certain scores. The sampling distribution is a special normal distribution that consists of a theoretical distribution of sample means.

Inferential statistical tests use sampling distributions to determine the likelihood that different samples came from populations with the same characteristics. A significant difference between groups indicates that the probability that the samples came from populations with the same characteristics is lower than a predetermined level, alpha, that is set by the researcher. There is always a probability that one of two statistical errors will be made: a type I error occurs when a significant difference is found when in fact there is no difference; a type II error occurs when a difference actually exists but is not identified by the test. The power of a test is the probability that it will detect a true difference. The validity of statistical conclusions is threatened by low power, results that are not clinically meaningful, alpha level inflation with multiple tests, violation of statistical assumptions, and failure to use intention-to-treat analysis.

REFERENCES

1. Chottiner S: Statistics: Toward a kinder, gentler subject, *J Irreproducible Results* 35(6):13–15, 1990.
2. Ewald FC, Jacobs MA, Miegel RE, et al: Kinematic total knee replacement, *J Bone Joint Surg Am* 66:1032–1040, 1984.
3. Tickle-Degnen L: Where is the individual in statistics? *Am J Occup Ther* 57:112–115, 2003.
4. Elston RC, Johnson WD: *Essentials of Biostatistics*, Philadelphia, Pa, 1987, FA Davis.
5. Sterne JA, Smith GD: Sifting the evidence—what's wrong with significance tests? *BMJ* 322:226–231, 2001.
6. Kazdin AE: Statistical methods of data evaluation. In Kazdin AE, editor: *Research Design in Clinical Psychology*, 4th edn, Boston, Mass, 2003, Allyn & Bacon, pp 436–470.
7. Shott S: *Statistics for Health Professionals*, Philadelphia, Pa, 1990, WB Saunders.
8. Aickin M, Gensler H: Adjusting for multiple testing when reporting research results: The Bonferroni vs Holm methods, *Am J Public Health* 86:726–727, 1996.
9. Senghas RE: Statistics in the *Journal of Bone and Joint Surgery*: Suggestions for authors, *J Bone Joint Surg Am* 74:319–320, 1992.
10. Murray LL: Spoken language production in Huntington's and Parkinson's diseases, *J Speech Lang Hearing Res* 43:1350–1366, 2000.
11. Mueller MJ, Salsich GB, Strube MJ: Functional limitations in patients with diabetes and transmetatarsal amputations, *Phys Ther* 77:937–943, 1997.
12. Cohen J: *Statistical Power Analysis for the Behavioral Sciences*, Hillsdale, NJ, 1988, Lawrence Erlbaum.

13. Moher D, Dulberg CS, Wells GA: Statistical power, sample size, and their reporting in randomized controlled trials, *JAMA* 272:122–124, 1994.

14. Polit DF, Sherman RE: Statistical power in nursing research, *Nurs Res* 39:365–369, 1990.

15. Kazantzis N: Power to detect homework effects in psychotherapy outcome research, *J Consult Clin Psychol* 68:166–170, 2000.

16. Ottenbacher KJ, Maas F: How to detect effects: Statistical power and evidence-based practice in occupational therapy, *Am J Occup Ther* 5:181–188, 1999.

17. Ottenbacher KJ, Barrett KA: Statistical conclusion validity of rehabilitation research: A quantitative analysis, *Am J Phys Med Rehabil* 69:102–107, 1990.

18. Kraemer HC, Thiemann S: *How Many Subjects? Statistical Power Analysis in Research*, Newbury Park, Calif, 1987, Sage.

19. DuPont WD, Plummer WD Jr. PS: Power and Sample Size Calculation. Available at: http://biostat.mc.vanderbilt.edu/wiki/Main/PowerSampleSize. Accessed February 17, 2015.

20. Statistical Power. Available at: http://www.danielsoper.com/statcalc3/default.aspx. Accessed February 18, 2015.

21. Sherman KJ, Cook AJ, Wellman RD, et al: Five-week outcomes from a dosing trial of therapeutic massage for chronic neck pain, *Ann Fam Med* 12:112–120, 2014.

22. Grammatopoulou EP, Skordilis EK, Stavrou N, et al: The effect of physiotherapy-based breathing retraining on asthma control, *J Asthma* 48:593–601, 2011.

23. Cook T, Campbell D: *Quasi-Experimentation: Design and Analysis Issues for Field Settings*, Chicago, Ill, 1979, Rand McNally.

24. Palmer SS, Mortimer JA, Webster DD, et al: Exercise therapy for Parkinson's disease, *Arch Phys Med Rehabil* 67:741–745, 1986.

25. Huijbregts MPJ, Teare GF, McCullough C, et al: Standardization of the Continuing Care Activity Measure: A multicenter study to assess reliability, validity, and ability to measure change, *Phys Ther* 89:546–555, 2009.

26. Wyrwich KM, Metz SM, Kroenke K, et al: Measuring patient and clinician perspectives to evaluate change in health-related quality of life among patients with chronic obstructive pulmonary disease, *J Gen Int Med* 22:161–170, 2007.

27. Wyrwich KW, Tierney WM, Wolinsky FD: Using the standard error of measurement to identify important changes on the Asthma Quality of Life Questionnaire, *Qual Life Res* 11:1–7, 2002.

28. Palombaro KM, Craik RL, Mangione KK, Tomlinson JD: Determining meaningful changes in gait speed after hip fracture, *Phys Ther* 86:809–816, 2006.

29. Ring C, Nayak US, Isaacs B: Balance function in elderly people who have and who have not fallen, *Arch Phys Med Rehabil* 69:261–264, 1988.

30. Moher D, Schulz KF, Altman D, for the CONSORT Group: The CONSORT statement: Revised recommendations for improving the quality of reports of parallel-group randomized trials, *JAMA* 285:1987–1991, 2001.

31. Mazumdar S, Liu KS, Houck PR, Reynolds CF: Intent-to-treat analysis for longitudinal clinical trials: Coping with the challenge of missing values, *J Psychiatr Res* 33:87–95, 1999.

21

Statistical Analysis of Differences: The Basics

CHAPTER OUTLINE

Distributions for Analysis of Differences
t Distribution
F Distribution
Chi-Square Distribution
Assumptions of Tests of Differences
Random Selection from a Normally Distributed Population
Homogeneity of Variance
Level of Measurement
Independence or Dependence of Samples

Steps in the Statistical Testing of Differences
Statistical Analysis of Differences
Differences Between Two Independent Groups
Independent t *Test*
Mann-Whitney or Wilcoxon Rank Sum Test
Chi-Square Test of Association
Differences Between Two or More Independent Groups
One-Way ANOVA

Kruskal-Wallis Test
Chi-Square Test of Association
Differences Between Two Dependent Samples
*Paired-*t *Test*
Wilcoxon Signed Rank Test
McNemar Test
Differences Between Two or More Dependent Samples
Repeated Measures ANOVA
Friedman's ANOVA
Summary

Researchers use statistical tests when they wish to determine whether a statistically significant difference exists between two or more sets of numbers. In this chapter, the general statistical concepts presented in Chapter 20 are applied to specific statistical tests of differences commonly reported in the rehabilitation literature. The distributions most commonly used in statistical testing are presented first, followed by the general assumptions that underlie statistical tests of differences. The sequence of steps common to all statistical tests of differences is then outlined. Finally, specific tests of differences are presented. In this chapter, basic tests using one independent variable are presented. Each is illustrated with an example from the hypothetical knee arthroplasty data set presented in Chapter 20. In Chapter 22, more advanced tests using two independent variables are presented, as are a variety of specialized techniques for analyzing differences. In Chapters 23 and 24, statistical tests of relationships among variables are presented.

DISTRIBUTIONS FOR ANALYSIS OF DIFFERENCES

In Chapter 20, the rationale behind statistical testing was developed in terms of the standard normal distribution and its *z* scores. Use of this distribution assumes that the population standard deviation is known. Because the population standard deviation is usually not known, we cannot ordinarily use the standard normal distribution and its *z* scores to draw statistical conclusions from samples. Therefore, researchers conduct most statistical tests using distributions that resemble the normal distribution but are altered somewhat to account for the errors that are made when population parameters are estimated. The three most common distributions used for statistical tests are the *t*, *F*, and chi-square (χ^2) distributions, as shown in Figure 21-1. Just as we determined the probability of obtaining certain *z* scores based on the standard normal distribution, we can determine the probability of obtaining certain *t*, *F*, and chi-square

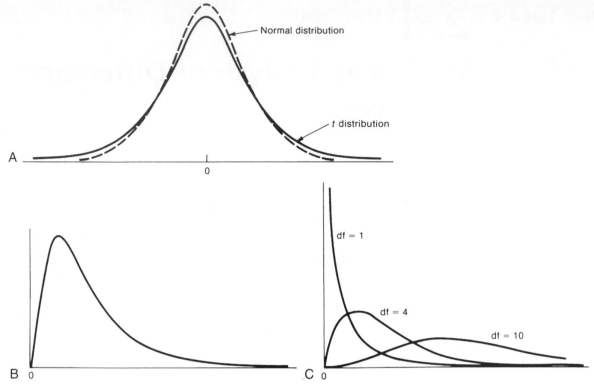

Figure 21-1 Distribution of test statistics. **A,** The solid *t* distribution with 5 degrees of freedom (df) compared with the dashed normal distribution. **B,** *F* distribution with 6 and 12 degrees of freedom. **C,** Chi-square distribution with 1, 4, and 10 degrees of freedom. (From Shott S: *Statistics for Health Professionals,* Philadelphia, Pa, 1990, WB Saunders, pp 75, 148, 208.)

statistics based on their respective distributions. The exact shapes of the distributions vary with the degrees of freedom associated with the test statistic. The degrees of freedom are calculated in different ways for the different distributions, but in general are related to the number of participants within the study or the number of levels of the independent variable, or both. When test statistics are reported within the literature, they often include a subscript that indicates the degrees of freedom.

t Distribution

The *t* distribution is a symmetrical distribution that is essentially a "flattened" *z* distribution (see Fig. 21-1A). Compared with the *z* distribution, a greater proportion of the *t* distribution is located in the tails and a lesser proportion in the center of the distribution. The *z* distribution is spread to form the *t* distribution to account for the errors that are introduced when population parameters are estimated from sample statistics. The shape of a *t* distribution varies with its degrees of

freedom, which is based on sample size. Because estimation of population parameters is more accurate with larger samples, *t* distributions become more and more similar to *z* distributions as sample size and degrees of freedom increase.

F Distribution

The *F* distribution is a distribution of squared *t* statistics (see Fig. 21-1B). It is asymmetrical and, because it is generated from squared scores, consists only of positive values. The actual shape of a particular *F* distribution depends on two different degrees of freedom: one associated with the number of groups being compared and one associated with the sample size.

Chi-Square Distribution

The chi-square distribution is a distribution of squared *z* scores (see Fig. 21-1C). As is the case with the *t* and *F* distributions, the shape of the chi-square distribution varies with its degrees of freedom.

ASSUMPTIONS OF TESTS OF DIFFERENCES

Statistical tests of differences are either parametric or nonparametric. *Parametric tests* are based on specific assumptions about the distribution of populations. They use sample statistics such as the mean, standard deviation, and variance to estimate differences between population parameters. The two major classes of parametric tests are *t* tests and analyses of variance (ANOVAs).

Nonparametric tests are not based on specific assumptions about the distribution of populations. They use rank or frequency information to draw conclusions about differences between populations.[1] Parametric tests are usually assumed to be more powerful than nonparametric tests and are often preferred to nonparametric tests, although this has not always proved to be the case with closer scrutiny.[2] However, parametric tests cannot always be used because the assumptions on which they are based are more stringent than the assumptions for nonparametric tests. Two parametric assumptions are commonly accepted: random selection and homogeneity of variance. A third assumption is controversial and relates to the measurement level of the data. Gravetter and Wallnau[3] offer four instances when nonparametric tests are commonly used: when it is simpler to obtain category data versus actual score data; when original scores violate basic assumptions of *t* tests and ANOVA, such as normal distribution; when original scores have extremely high variance; and when an original score is infinite or cannot be determined.[(pp. 522–523)] Generally, though, "Nonparametric tests are most useful when data cannot in any manner be construed as interval level, when the distribution is markedly non-normal, or when the sample size is very small."[4(p. 411)]

Random Selection from a Normally Distributed Population

The first basic assumption of parametric testing is that the participants are randomly selected from normally distributed populations. However, researchers may violate this assumption as long as the data sets used in the analysis are relatively normally distributed. Even when the data sets are not normally distributed, statistical researchers have shown that the various statistical tests are robust, meaning that they usually still provide an appropriate level of rejection of the null hypothesis. The extent to which a data set is normally distributed may be tested; however, the details are beyond the scope of this text.

When data are extremely nonnormal, one data analysis strategy is to convert, or transform, the data mathematically so that they become normally distributed. Squaring, taking the square root of, and calculating a logarithm of raw data are common transformations. Parametric tests can then be conducted on the transformed scores. A second strategy for dealing with nonnormality is to use nonparametric tests, which do not require normally distributed data.

Homogeneity of Variance

The second basic assumption of parametric testing is that the population variances of the groups being tested are equal, or homogeneous. Homogeneity of variance may be tested statistically. If homogeneity of variance is tested and the variances of the groups are found to differ significantly, nonparametric tests must be used. When the sample sizes of the groups being compared are the same, differences in the variances of the groups become less of a concern.[5] Therefore, researchers generally design their studies to maximize the chance of having equal, or nearly equal, sample sizes across groups.

Level of Measurement

The third, and most controversial, assumption for parametric testing concerns the measurement level of the data. As noted earlier, one distinction between parametric and nonparametric tests is that the two types of tests are used with different types of data. Nonparametric tests require rankings or frequencies; nominal and ranked ordinal data meet this need, and interval and ratio data can be converted into ranks or grouped into categories to meet this need. Parametric tests require data from which means and variances can be calculated; interval and ratio data clearly meet this need, whereas nominal data clearly do not. The controversy, then, surrounds the use of parametric statistics with ordinal measurements.

The traditional belief that parametric tests can be conducted only with interval or ratio data is no longer considered valid.[6,7] Although ordinal-scaled variables do not have the property of equal intervals between numerals, the distribution of ordinal data is often approximately normal. As long as the data themselves meet the parametric assumptions, regardless of the origin of the numbers, parametric tests can be conducted. As is the case with all statistical tests of differences, the researcher must interpret parametric statistical conclusions that are based on ordinal data in light of their clinical or practical implications.

For example, a common type of ordinal measurement used by rehabilitation professionals is a scale of the amount of assistance a patient needs to accomplish various functional tasks. The categories maximal, moderate, minimal, standby, and no assistance could be coded numerically from 1 to 5, with 5 representing no assistance. Assume that four different groups have mean scores of 1.0, 2.0, 4.0, and 5.0 and that these group means have been found to be significantly different from one another. If the researchers believe that the "real" interval between maximal and moderate assistance is greater than the interval between standby and no assistance, they may interpret the difference between the groups with means of 1.0 and 2.0 to be more clinically important than the difference between the groups with means of 4.0 and 5.0. It is reasonable to conduct parametric tests with ordinal data as long as interpretation of the tests accounts for the nature of the ordinal scale.

INDEPENDENCE OR DEPENDENCE OF SAMPLES

Another important consideration for either parametric or nonparametric testing concerns whether the different sets of numbers being compared are "independent" or "dependent." Two scores, for example, are independent "if the occurrence of the first event has no effect on the probability of the second event."[3(p. 223)] When two or more groups consist of different, unrelated individuals, the observations made about the samples are independent. For example, the 3-week range-of-motion (ROM) scores for patients in Clinics 1 through 3 in our hypothetical knee arthroplasty study (see Chapter 20) are independent of one another. Knowing the 3-week ROM values for patients at Clinic 1 provides us with no information about 3-week ROM values of the different patients being seen at Clinic 2 or Clinic 3. Ideally, the samples should be randomly assigned,[8] but this is not always the case.

When the sets of numbers consist of repeated measures on the same individuals, they are said to be dependent. The 3-week, 6-week, and 6-month ROM scores for patients across the three clinics are dependent measures. A patient's 6-week score is expected to be related to the 3-week score. Repeated measures taken on the same individual are not the only type of dependent measures, however. If we compare male and female characteristics by using brother-sister pairs, we have dependent samples. If we study pairs or trios of individuals matched for factors such as income, education, age, height, and weight, then we also have dependent samples.

Different statistical tests are used with independent versus dependent samples, and the assumption of either independence or dependence must not be violated. The researcher must select the correct test according to whether the samples are independent or dependent.

STEPS IN THE STATISTICAL TESTING OF DIFFERENCES

The statistical testing of differences can be summarized in 10 basic steps, regardless of the particular test used. A general assumption of these steps is that researchers plan to perform parametric tests and resort to the use of nonparametric tests only if the assumptions for parametric testing are not met. The steps are as follows:

1. State the null and alternative hypotheses in parametric terms.
2. Decide on an alpha level for the test.
3. Determine whether the samples are independent or dependent.
4. Determine whether parametric assumptions are met. If they are not met, revise hypotheses for nonparametric testing.
5. Determine the appropriate statistical test, given the aforementioned information.
6. Calculate the test statistic.
7. Determine the degrees of freedom for the test statistic.
8. Determine the probability of obtaining the calculated test statistic, taking into account the degrees of freedom. Computer statistical packages generate the precise probability of obtaining a given test statistic for the given degrees of freedom.
9. Compare the probability obtained in step 8 with the alpha level established in step 2. If the obtained probability is less than the alpha level, the test has identified a statistically significant difference; that is, the null hypothesis is rejected. If the obtained probability is equal to or greater than the alpha level, the test has failed to identify a statistically significant difference; that is, the null hypothesis is not rejected.
10. Evaluate the statistical conclusions in light of clinical knowledge. If the result is statistically significant but the differences between groups do not seem to be important from a clinical perspective, this discrepancy should be discussed. If the result is statistically insignificant but the differences between groups appear clinically important, a power analysis should be conducted and discussed in light of the discrepancy between the statistical and clinical conclusions.

Table 21-1 lists these steps. The first column shows how the steps are implemented when a computer program is

Table **21-1**		
Ten Steps in the Statistical Testing of Differences		
	COMPUTATION METHOD	
Step	**Computer Package**	**Calculator and Tables**
1	State hypotheses.	
2	Determine alpha level.	
3	Determine whether samples are independent or dependent.	
4	Run frequency and descriptive programs to determine whether parametric assumptions are met.	Plot frequencies and calculate descriptive statistics to determine whether parametric assumptions are met.
5	Determine appropriate test.	
6	Use appropriate programs to calculate test statistic.	Use appropriate formulas to calculate test statistic.
7	Program calculates the degrees of freedom.	Calculate the degrees of freedom.
8	Program calculates the probability of obtaining the test statistic given the degrees of freedom.	Determine the critical value of the test statistic given the degrees of freedom and predetermined alpha level.
9	Compare the obtained probability with the alpha level to draw statistical conclusion. When the obtained probability is less than alpha, a statistically significant difference has been identified.	Compare the obtained test statistic with the critical value of the test statistic to draw statistical conclusion. When the obtained test statistic is greater than the critical value, a statistically significant difference has been identified.
10	Evaluate the statistical conclusions in light of clinical knowledge.	

used for the statistical analysis; the second column shows how the steps are implemented in the increasingly rare instances when calculators and tables are used to perform the statistical analysis. Steps that are common to both computation methods cross the two columns. The remainder of this chapter illustrates how these 10 steps are implemented for several different statistical tests of differences.

STATISTICAL ANALYSIS OF DIFFERENCES

The hypothetical total knee arthroplasty data set presented in Chapter 20 is used in the rest of this chapter to illustrate different statistical tests of differences. All the analyses were conducted with SPSS, a statistical package originally known as the Statistical Package for the Social Sciences.[9] Formulas and computations are included with the first few examples to illustrate how the test statistics are calculated. However, the purpose of this chapter is to enable readers to understand the results of tests, not to perform statistical analyses. Researchers

who wish to analyze small data sets by hand can refer to any number of good biostatistical references for the formulas and tables needed to do so.[3,5,10-12]

The tests presented in this chapter are organized by the type of difference being analyzed, rather than by statistical technique. For each type of difference being analyzed, both a parametric test and a nonparametric test are given. Although the number of tests may seem daunting, there are actually only a few basic tests that are varied according to the number of groups being compared, whether the samples are independent or dependent, the nature of the data, and whether parametric assumptions are met. Table 21-2 presents an overview of the tests presented in this chapter.

Differences Between Two Independent Groups

Assume that Clinics 1 and 2 have different postoperative activity protocols for their patients who have had total knee arthroplasty. We wonder whether there are

Table **21-2**

Basic Statistical Tests for Analyzing Differences

Design	INDEPENDENT LEVELS OF THE INDEPENDENT VARIABLE		DEPENDENT LEVELS OF THE INDEPENDENT VARIABLE	
	Parametric	**Nonparametric**	**Parametric**	**Nonparametric**
One independent variable with two levels; dependent variables analyzed one at a time	Independent *t* test	Mann-Whitney (ranks) Wilcoxon rank sum (ranks) Chi-square (frequencies)	Paired-*t* test	Wilcoxon signed rank (ranks) McNemar (frequencies)
One independent variable with two or more levels; dependent variables analyzed one at a time	One-way analysis of variance (ANOVA)	Kruskal-Wallis (ranks) Chi-square (frequencies)	Repeated measures ANOVA	Friedman's ANOVA (ranks)

Table **21-3**

Independent *t* Test

Clinic		1		2	
Data	3	2	2	7	
	5	8	3	4	
	6	7	4	0579	
	8	1478	5	06	
	9	225	6	7	
			7	6	
Mean		$\bar{X}_1 = 77.6$	$\bar{X}_2 = 49.1$		
Variance		$s_1^2 = 393.62$	$s_2^2 = 212.58$		
Standard deviation		$s1 = 19.84$	$s2 = 14.58$		

$$t = \frac{\bar{X}_1 - \bar{X}_2}{\left[\sqrt{\frac{(n_1 - 1)s_1^2 + (n_2 - 1)s_2^2}{n_1 + n_2 - 2}}\right]\left[\sqrt{\frac{1}{n_1} + \frac{1}{n_2}}\right]} = \frac{28.5}{(17.4)(.447)} = 3.66$$

differences in 3-week ROM results between patients at Clinic 1 and Clinic 2. The null and alternative hypotheses that we intend to test are as follows:

$$H_0 : \mu1 = \mu2$$
$$H_1 : \mu1 \neq \mu2$$

We set alpha at 5% and determine that we have independent samples because different, unrelated patients make up the samples from the two clinics. Now we have to determine whether our data meet the assumptions for parametric testing. Table 21-3 shows the descriptive statistics and stem-and-leaf plots for the 3-week ROM data for the two groups. The variances, although not identical, are at least of similar magnitude. The ratio of the larger variance to the smaller variance is 1.85, which is less than the 2.0 maximum recommended for meeting the homogeneity-of-variance assumption for the independent *t* test.[13(p. 117)] Typically, only large differences in variance are of concern, and if unsure, investigators may use more sophisticated procedures such as Bartlett's, Levene's, or Brown-Forsythe.[14] Returning to our example, we see the plot for Clinic 1 is positively skewed; that is, it has a long tail of higher numbers. The plot for Clinic 2 looks fairly symmetrical (see Table 20-2 for raw data). Under these conditions, some researchers would proceed with a parametric test, and others would use a nonparametric test because of the nonnormal shape of the Clinic 1 data. The parametric test of differences between two independent sample means is the independent *t* test; the nonparametric test is either the Mann-Whitney test or the Wilcoxon rank sum test.

Independent t Test

Like most test statistics, the test statistic for the independent *t* test is the ratio of the differences between the groups to the differences within the groups. Conceptually, the difference between the groups, or the numerator, is "explained" by the independent variable (i.e., clinic). The variance within the groups, or the denominator, is "unexplained" because we do not know what leads to individual differences between subjects. Therefore, the test statistic formula "partitions" the variability in the data set into explained and unexplained variability. When the variability explained by the independent variable is sufficiently large compared with the unexplained variability, the test statistic is large, and a statistically significant difference is identified.

The pooled formula for the independent *t* is presented at the bottom of Table 21-3. The numerator is simply the difference between the two sample means. The denominator is a form of a standard error of the mean created by pooling the standard deviations of the samples and dividing by the square root of the pooled sample sizes. When the *t* formula is solved by inserting the values from our example, a value of 3.66 is obtained. A separate variance formula can be used if the difference between the two group variances is too great to permit pooling.[10] The computer-generated two-tailed probability of obtaining a *t* statistic of 3.66 with 18 degrees of freedom (n_1+n_2-2) is .002. Because .002 is less than the predetermined alpha level of .05, we reject the null hypothesis. We conclude that the mean 3-week ROM scores of the populations from which the Clinic 1 and Clinic 2 patients are drawn are significantly different from one another. The difference between the means of the two groups is 28.5°. Because this difference seems clinically important, our statistical and clinical conclusions concur.

In determining our statistical conclusions in the paragraph above, a two-tailed probability was used. The *t* test is one of only a few statistical tests that require the researcher to differentiate between directional and nondirectional hypotheses before conducting the test. The alternative hypothesis given at the beginning of this section, $\mu_1 \neq \mu_2$, is nondirectional, meaning that we

are open to the possibility that Clinic 1's mean ROM is either greater than or less than Clinic 2's mean ROM. If Clinic 1's mean is greater than Clinic 2's mean, as in our example, the *t* statistic will be positive. If, however, Clinic 2's mean is greater than Clinic 1's mean, the value of *t* will be negative. Because our research hypothesis allows for either a positive or a negative *t*, the probability that *t* will be greater than +3.66 and the probability that *t* will be less than −3.66 must both be accounted for. The two-tailed probability of .002 is the sum of the probability that *t* will exceed +3.66 and the probability that *t* will be less than −3.66.

A directional hypothesis is used occasionally as the alternative to the null hypothesis. A directional hypothesis specifies which of the means is expected to be greater than the other. Use of a directional hypothesis is justified only if there is existing evidence of the direction of the effect or when only one outcome is of interest to the researcher. Researchers who use a directional hypothesis are interested in only one tail of the *t* distribution. Because the two-tailed probability is the sum of the probabilities in the upper and lower tails of the distribution, the one-tailed probability is determined by dividing the two-tailed probability in half. Thus, for our example, the two-tailed probability of .002 becomes a one-tailed probability of .001.

In this example, both the one- and two-tailed probabilities are so low that both lead to the same statistical conclusion. Imagine, however, if the two-tailed probability for a test was .06. If we set alpha at .05 and conduct a two-tailed test, there is no significant difference between groups. However, if we conduct a one-tailed test, we divide the two-tailed probability in half to get a one-tailed probability of .03. This is less than our alpha level of .05; thus, with the one-tailed test, we conclude that there is a significant difference between groups. As can be seen, the one-tailed test is more powerful than the two-tailed test. Researchers should not be tempted to abuse this power by conducting one-tailed tests unless they have an appropriate rationale for doing so.

Independent *t* tests are often used to analyze pretest-posttest designs when there are only two groups and two measurements on each participant. One strategy is to perform an independent *t* test on the pretest data; if there is no significant difference between groups at pretest, then an independent *t* test is run on the posttest data to determine whether there was a significant treatment effect. A second strategy is to create gain scores by subtracting the pretest value from the posttest value for each participant. An independent *t* test is then run on the gain scores to determine whether one group had a significantly greater change than the other. Egger and Miller[15] provide a useful description of different options for analyzing pretest–posttest designs, along with guidelines for making decisions among the options.

Mann-Whitney or Wilcoxon Rank Sum Test

The Mann-Whitney and Wilcoxon rank sum tests are two equivalent tests that are the nonparametric alternatives to the independent *t* test. If the assumptions for the independent *t* test are violated, researchers may choose to analyze their data with one of these tests. When nonparametric tests are used, the hypotheses need to be stated in more general terms than the hypotheses for parametric tests. Hypotheses in nonparametric research are classified as *null* or *alternate* (also called the research hypothesis). Alternate hypotheses may be directional, or one-tailed, which predicts a significant change in a particular direction; they may also be nondirectional.[1(p. 4)] Following are examples of null and (directional) corresponding alternate hypotheses:

H_0: The populations from which Clinic 1 and Clinic 2 samples are drawn are identical.

H_1: One population tends to produce larger observations than the other population.

To perform the Mann-Whitney test, a researcher ranks the scores from the two groups, regardless of original group membership. Table 21-4 shows the ranking of 3-week ROM scores for Clinics 1 and 2. When a number occurs more than once, its ranking is the mean of the multiple ranks it occupies. For example, the two 67s are the 11th and 12th ranked scores in this distribution, so each receives a rank of 11.5. The next-ranked number, 76, receives the rank of 13.

Table **21-4**

Mann-Whitney or Wilcoxon Rank Sum Test

	Clinic 1 Score (Rank)	Clinic 2 Score (Rank)
	32 (2)	27 (1)
	58 (10)	34 (3)
	67 (11.5)	40 (4)
	81 (14)	45 (5)
	84 (15)	47 (6)
	87 (16)	49 (7)
	88 (17)	50 (8)
	92 (18.5)	56 (9)
	92 (18.5)	67 (11.5)
	95 (20)	76 (13)
Rank sum	**(142.5)**	**(67.5)**

The sum of the Clinic 1 ranks is 142.5; the sum of the Clinic 2 ranks is 67.5.

To understand the logic behind the Mann-Whitney, imagine that our two clinics have vastly different scores that do not overlap at all. The Clinic 2 ranks would be 1 through 10, which add up to 55; the Clinic 1 ranks would be 11 through 20, which add up to 155. Now suppose the opposite case, in which the scores are very similar. The Clinic 2 scores might get all the odd ranks, which add up to 100; the Clinic 1 scores might get all the even ranks, which add up to 110. When the two samples are similar, their rank sums will be similar. When the samples differ greatly, the rank sums will be very different. The rank sums (67.5 and 142.5) of our two samples of patients with total knee arthroplasty fall between the two extremes of (a) 55 and 155 and (b) 100 and 110. To come to a statistical conclusion, we need to determine the probability of obtaining the rank sums of 67.5 and 142.5 if in fact the populations from which the samples are drawn are identical. To do so, we transform the higher rank sum into a *z* score and calculate the probability of obtaining that *z* score.

An alternative form of the Mann-Whitney test uses a *U* statistic, which is converted into a *z* score. In this example, the computer-generated *z* score is 2.84, and the associated two-tailed probability is .0046. We conclude from this that there is a significant difference between the scores from Clinic 1 and the scores from Clinic 2. Given the 28.5° difference in the means and the 37.5° difference in the medians between the clinics, this difference seems clinically important. Once again, our statistical and clinical conclusions concur.

Chi-Square Test of Association

Assume that we still wish to determine whether there are differences in the 3-week ROM scores of Clinics 1 and 2. However, let us further assume that previous research has shown that the ultimate functional outcome after total knee arthroplasty depends on having regained at least 90° of knee flexion by 3 weeks after surgery. If such evidence existed, we might no longer be interested in the absolute 3-week ROM scores at our clinics. We might instead be interested in the proportion of patients who achieve 90° of knee flexion 3 weeks postoperatively. In this case, we would convert the raw ROM scores into categories: "less than 90°" and "greater than or equal to 90°." Then we would use a chi-square test of association to determine whether the two clinics had similar proportions of patients with and without 90° of knee flexion at 3 weeks postoperatively. A complete chi-square example is presented in the next section on analysis of differences among two or more independent groups.

..

Differences Between Two or More Independent Groups

If Clinics 1 through 3 all have different postoperative protocols for their patients who have undergone total knee arthroplasty, we might wonder whether there are significant differences in mean 3-week ROM scores among the three clinics. To test this question statistically, we develop the following hypotheses:

H_0: $\mu_1 = \mu_2 = \mu_3$

H_1: At least one of the population means is different from another population mean.

We set alpha at .05 for the analysis. The samples are independent because they consist of different, unrelated participants. The descriptive measures and stem-and-leaf plots for all three clinics are presented in Table 21-5. The scores for both Clinics 1 and 3 appear to be nonnormal; however, the variances are similar. If we believe that the parametric assumptions have been met, we test the differences with a one-way ANOVA. If we do not believe that the parametric assumptions have been met, the comparable nonparametric test is the Kruskal-Wallis test. A chi-square test of association can be used to test differences between groups when the dependent variable consists of nominal-level data.

One-Way ANOVA

ANOVA techniques partition the variability in a sample into between-groups and within-group variability. Conceptually, this is the same as the partitioning described for the independent t test, although the F statistic generated within an ANOVA is a squared version of the t statistic. This F ratio is created with between-groups variability as the numerator and within-group variability as the denominator and is distributed as shown in Figure 21-1B, discussed earlier. Because the F distribution is a squared t distribution, F cannot be negative. This means that all the extreme values for F are in the upper tail of the distribution, eliminating the need to differentiate between one- and two-tailed tests. The ANOVA is a versatile statistical technique, and there are many variations.[16] All of the ANOVA techniques are based on partitioning variability to create an F ratio that is evaluated against the probabilities of the F distribution.

The ANOVA required in our example is known as a *one-way ANOVA*. "One-way" refers to the fact that only one independent variable is examined. In this case, the independent variable is clinic, and it has three levels: Clinic 1, Clinic 2, and Clinic 3. Table 21-6 shows the calculations needed to determine the F statistic. Although time consuming, the calculations presented here are not difficult. To compute the F statistic, we must first know the individual group means as well as the grand mean. The *grand mean* is the mean of all of the scores across the groups; for our three samples, the grand mean is 66.4°.

The total variability within the data set is determined by calculating the sum of the squared deviations of each individual score from the grand mean. This is called the *total sum of squares* (SST). The SST calculation is shown at the bottom of the fourth column of Table 21-6. The second column shows the raw scores; the third column, the deviation of each raw score from the grand mean; and the fourth column, the squared deviations. The sum of these squared deviations across all 30 subjects is the SST.

The within-group variability is determined by calculating the sum of the squared deviations of the individual scores from the group mean. This is known as the *within-group sum of squares* (SSW). The second column of Table 21-6 shows the raw scores; the fifth column, the deviations of each raw score from its group mean; and the final column, the squared deviations. The sum of all of the 30 squared deviation scores at the bottom of the sixth column is the SSW.

The between-groups variability is determined by calculating the sum of the squared deviations of the group means from the grand mean, with each deviation weighted according to sample size. This is known as the *between-groups sum of squares* (SSB) and is shown at the bottom of Table 21-6.

Table **21-5**

Frequencies and Descriptive Statistics for 3-Week Range of Motion at Clinics 1 Through 3

Clinic	1		2		3	
Data			2	7		
	3	2	3	4	3	2
	4		4	0579	4	
	5	8	5	06	5	0
	6	7	6	7	6	0
	7		7	6	7	
	8	1478			8	111244
	9	225			9	1
$\bar{X}$		77.6		49.1		72.6
s^2		393.62		212.58		357.38
s		19.84		14.58		18.90

Table 21-6

One-Way Analysis of Variance Calculations of Sum of Squares Total (SST), Within Group (SSW), and Between Groups (SSB)

Clinic No.	Raw Score	Deviation from Grand Mean	Deviation^2	Deviation from Group Mean	Deviation^2
1	32	−34.4	1183.36	−45.6	2079.36
1	58	−8.4	70.56	−19.6	384.16
1	67	.6	.36	−10.6	112.36
1	81	14.6	213.16	3.4	11.56
1	84	17.6	309.76	6.4	40.96
1	87	20.6	424.36	9.4	88.36
1	88	21.6	466.56	10.4	108.16
1	92	25.6	655.36	14.4	207.36
1	92	25.6	655.36	14.4	207.36
1	95	28.6	817.96	17.4	302.76
2	27	−39.4	1552.36	−22.1	488.41
2	34	−32.4	1049.76	−15.1	228.01
2	40	−26.4	696.96	−9.1	82.81
2	45	−21.4	457.96	−4.1	16.81
2	47	−19.4	376.36	−2.1	4.41
2	49	−17.4	302.76	−.1	.01
2	50	−16.4	268.96	.9	.81
2	56	−10.4	108.16	6.9	47.61
2	67	.6	.36	17.9	320.41
2	76	9.6	92.16	26.9	723.61
3	32	−34.4	1183.36	−40.6	1648.36
3	50	−16.4	268.96	−22.6	510.76
3	60	−6.4	40.96	−12.6	158.76
3	81	14.6	213.16	8.4	70.56
3	81	14.6	213.16	8.4	70.56
3	81	14.6	213.16	8.4	70.56
3	82	15.6	243.36	9.4	88.36
3	84	17.6	309.76	11.4	129.96
3	84	17.6	309.76	11.4	129.96
3	91	24.6	605.16	18.4	338.56
Σ			13,303.40 (SST)		8671.70 (SSW)

$$SSB = (77.6 - 66.4)^2(10) + (49.1 - 66.4)^2(10) + (72.6 - 66.4)^2(10) = 4631.7$$

Note: Grand mean = 66.4°, Clinic 1 mean = 77.6°, Clinic 2 mean = 49.1°, and Clinic 3 mean = 72.6°.

The SST is the sum of the SSB and the SSW. Conceptually, then, the total variability in the sample is partitioned into variability attributable to differences between the groups and variability attributable to differences within each group.

The next step in calculating the *F* statistic is to divide the SSB and SSW by appropriate degrees of freedom to obtain the mean square between groups (MSB) and the mean square within each group (MSW), respectively. The degrees of freedom for the SSB is the number of groups minus 1; the degrees of freedom for the SSW is the total number of participants minus the number of groups. The *F* statistic is the MSB divided by the MSW. Thus, for our example, the MSB is 2315.85:

$$MSB = \frac{SSB}{(groups-1)} = \frac{4631.7}{2} = 2315.85$$

The MSW is 321.17:

$$MSW = \frac{SSW}{(N-groups)} = \frac{8671.7}{27} = 321.17$$

The *F* statistic is 7.21:

$$F = \frac{MSB}{MSW} = \frac{2315.85}{321.17} = 7.21$$

Large *F* values indicate that differences between the groups are large compared with the differences within groups. Small *F* values indicate that the differences between groups are small compared with the differences within groups. The computer-generated probability for our *F* of 7.21 with 2 and 27 degrees of freedom is .0031. Because this is less than our predetermined alpha level of .05, we can conclude that there is at least one significant difference among the three means that were compared.

If a one-way ANOVA does not identify a significant difference among means, then the statistical analysis is complete. If, as in our example, a significant difference is identified, the researcher must complete one more step. Our overall, or omnibus, *F* test tells us that there is a difference among the means. It does not tell us whether Clinic 1 is different from Clinic 2, whether Clinic 2 is different from Clinic 3, or whether Clinic 1 is different from Clinic 3. To determine the sources of the differences identified by the omnibus *F*, we must make multiple comparisons between pairs of means.

Conceptually, conducting multiple-comparison tests is similar to conducting *t* tests between each pair of means, but with a correction to prevent inflation of the alpha level. A comparison of two means is called a *contrast*.

Common multiple-comparison procedures, in order of decreasing power (i.e., continually more cautious or conservative, with continually smaller risks of type I error), are as follows:
- Planned orthogonal contrasts
- Newman-Keuls test
- Tukey HSD (honestly significant difference) test
- Bonferroni test
- Scheffé test[17(p. 386)]

The more powerful tests identify smaller differences between means as significant. Various assumptions must be met for the different multiple-comparison procedures to be valid.

A Newman-Keuls procedure used on our example indicates that the mean ROM scores for Clinic 1 (77.6°) and Clinic 3 (72.6°) were not found to be significantly different, and the mean ROM score for Clinic 2 (49.1°) was found to differ significantly from the mean ROM scores for both Clinics 1 and 3. From a clinical viewpoint, it seems reasonable to conclude that the 5° difference between Clinics 1 and 3 is not important, but the difference of more than 20° between Clinic 2 and Clinics 1 and 3 is.

There are two additional twists to the multiple-comparison procedure: (1) whether the contrasts are planned or post hoc and (2) whether the multiple-comparison results are consistent with the omnibus test.

In planned contrasts, the researcher specifies which contrasts are of interest before the statistical test is conducted. If, for some reason, the researcher is not interested in differences between Clinics 2 and 3, then only two comparisons need to be made: Clinic 1 versus Clinic 3, and Clinic 1 versus Clinic 2.

If planned contrasts are not specified in advance, all possible multiple comparisons should be conducted as post hoc tests. As more multiple comparisons are conducted, each contrast becomes more conservative to control for alpha inflation.

Occasionally, the omnibus *F* test identifies a significant difference among the means, but the multiple-comparison procedure fails to locate any significant contrasts. One response to these conflicting results is to believe the multiple-comparison results and conclude that despite the significant *F*, there is no significant difference among the means. Another response is to believe the *F*-test results and use progressively less conservative multiple-comparison procedures until the significant difference between means is located.

Kruskal-Wallis Test

The Kruskal-Wallis test is the nonparametric equivalent of the one-way ANOVA. If the assumptions of the parametric test are not met, the nonparametric test should be performed. Following our guidelines for nonparametric tests, we may state null and alternative hypotheses as follows:

H_0: The three samples come from populations that are identical.

H_1: At least one of the populations tends to produce larger observations than another population.

To conduct the Kruskal-Wallis test, a researcher ranks the scores, regardless of group membership. The ranks for each group are then summed and plugged into a formula to generate a Kruskal-Wallis (KW) statistic. The distribution of the KW statistic approximates a chi-square distribution. The computer-generated value of the KW statistic for our example is 11.10; the respective probability is .0039. Because .0039 is less than the alpha level of .05 that we set before conducting the test, we conclude that there is a significant difference somewhere among the groups.

An appropriate multiple-comparison procedure to use when a Kruskal-Wallis test is significant is the Mann-Whitney test with a Bonferroni adjustment of alpha. We have three comparisons to make, and each is tested at an alpha of .017 (the original alpha of .05 divided by three for the three comparisons). The probabilities associated with the three Mann-Whitney tests are as follows: For Clinic 1 compared with Clinic 2, $p=.0046$; for Clinic 1 compared with Clinic 3, $p=.2237$; and for Clinic 2 compared with Clinic 3, $p=.0072$. Thus, the multiple comparisons tell us that there is no significant difference between Clinics 1 and 3 and that Clinic 2 is significantly different from both Clinics 1 and 3. In this example, the nonparametric conclusions are the same as the parametric conclusions.

Chi-Square Test of Association

Assume that we still wish to determine whether there are differences in the 3-week ROM scores of the three clinics. However, let us assume, as we did when the chi-square test was introduced earlier, that previous research has shown that the ultimate functional outcome after total knee arthroplasty depends on having regained at least 90° of knee flexion by 3 weeks postsurgery. In light of such evidence, we might no longer be interested in the absolute 3-week ROM scores at our three clinics. Our interest, instead, would be in the relative proportions of patients with at least 90° of motion across the three clinics. Our hypotheses would be as follows:

H_0: There is no association between the clinic and ROM category proportions.

H_1: There is an association between the clinic and ROM category proportions.

Table 21-7 presents the data in the contingency table format needed to calculate chi-square. A contingency

---

Table 21-7

Chi-Square (χ^2) Test of Association

Clinic No.	THREE-WEEK KNEE FLEXION RANGE-OF-MOTION CATEGORY	
	<90°	≥90°
1	7 (8.67)	3 (1.33)
2	10 (8.67)	0 (1.33)
3	9 (8.67)	1 (1.33)
Total	26	4

$$\chi^2 = \sum \frac{(O-E)^2}{E} = (.32)+(.20)+(.01)+(2.10) \\ +(.01)+(.08)=4.04*$$

Note: Values are actual frequencies. Expected frequencies are in parentheses.
*$p=.1327$.

---

table is simply an array of data organized into a column variable and a row variable. In this table, clinic is the row variable and consists of three levels. ROM category is the column variable and consists of two levels. Calculation of the chi-square statistic is based on differences between observed frequencies and frequencies that would be expected if the null hypothesis were true.

To determine the observed frequencies, we need to examine the raw data and place each participant in the appropriate ROM category. To determine the expected frequencies, we need to determine the distribution of scores if the proportion in each ROM category were equal across the clinics. In our example, 26 of the 30 participants overall have ROM scores less than 90°. If these patients were equally distributed among the clinics, each clinic would be expected to have 8.7 (26/3=8.7) patients with ROM less than 90°. There are four participants with ROM greater than or equal to 90°. If these four participants were equally distributed among clinics, each clinic would be expected to have 1.3 (4/3=1.3) participants with ROM greater than or equal to 90°. In this example, the expected frequencies are easy to calculate because there is an equal number of patients in each group. If there are unequal numbers, the expected frequencies are proportionate to the numbers in each group.

An alternative test, the chi-square test of goodness of fit, compares the observed frequencies with hypothesized expected frequencies. For example, if we knew of previous research results that indicated that 80% of patients with total knee arthroplasty achieved 90° of motion by 3 weeks postoperatively, then we might test each of our clinic proportions against this hypothesized proportion.

To compute the chi-square statistic, the squared deviation of each expected cell frequency from the observed frequency is divided by the expected frequency for that cell; this is done for every cell, and the values are added together, as shown at the bottom of Table 21-7.

Table 21-7 shows the chi-square calculation for our example. The chi-square of 4.04, with 2 degrees of freedom (the number of columns − 1 × number of rows − 1), is associated with a probability of .1327. Because this probability is higher than the .05 we set as our alpha level, we conclude that there is no significant difference in the proportions of patients in the two ROM categories across the three clinics.

Note that the statistical conclusions of the chi-square analysis differ from those of the ANOVA and Kruskal-Wallis test. The ANOVA, which used all the original values of the data for the analysis, detected a difference among groups. The Kruskal-Wallis test, based on a ranking of the original data, also detected a difference. However, the chi-square test of association—using only nominal data, which eliminated much of the information in the original data set—failed to detect a difference among the groups. But, if the 90° benchmark is really our measure of interest, then, clinically, the chi-square test is the more salient result.

In general, if ratio or interval data exist, it is not wise to convert them to a lower measurement level unless there is a strong theoretical rationale for doing so. Given the hypothetical rationale that was used to set up this chi-square example, we would conclude that patients at all three clinics are likely to have equally poor functional outcomes because of the low proportion of patients at any of the clinics who achieved 90° of motion by 3 weeks postoperatively.

Differences Between Two Dependent Samples

Suppose that we are interested in whether there is a change in ROM from 3 weeks postoperatively to 6 weeks postoperatively for patients across all three of our clinics. The hypotheses we test are as follows:

H_0: $\mu_{\text{3-week ROM}} = \mu_{\text{6-week ROM}}$

H_1: $\mu_{\text{3-week ROM}} \neq \mu_{\text{6-week ROM}}$

We set the alpha level at .05. In this example, the two levels of the independent variable of interest are dependent—they are repeated measures taken on the same individuals. When determining whether the data are suitable for parametric testing, remember that the relevant data are the differences between the pairs, rather than the raw data. Table 21-8 presents the distributions of the differences for the entire sample. The differences were calculated by subtracting the 3-week

ROM values from the 6-week ROM values given in Table 20-2. A positive difference therefore indicates an improvement in ROM over the 3-week time span. The distribution of difference scores is asymmetrical, with a greater proportion of scores in the lower end of the range. The parametric test of differences for two dependent samples is the paired-*t* test. The corresponding nonparametric test is the Wilcoxon signed rank test. The test of differences between two dependent samples for nominal data is the McNemar test.

Paired-t Test

To calculate the paired-*t* test, we first determine the difference between each pair of measurements. The mean difference and standard deviation of the differences are calculated, and then the mean is compared with a mean difference of zero. The mean of our example differences is 7.0; the standard deviation of the differences is 10.03. We calculate the *t* statistic for paired samples by dividing the mean difference by the standard error of the mean differences, as shown at the bottom of Table 21-8. The probability associated with the *t* statistic of 3.82 with 29 degrees of freedom (number of pairs − 1) is .001. Because .001 is less than the alpha level of .05, we conclude that there is a significant difference between 3-week and 6-week ROM scores. Clinically, an average 7.0 difference in motion over 3 weeks seems modest for this population, particularly considering that few patients are even close to achieving the maximal mechanical ROM of their new knee joints. Therefore, the statistical conclusion must be tempered with a statement about the relatively small size of the difference.

Table **21-8**

Difference Between 6-Week and 3-Week Range-of-Motion Scores Across Clinics

0	8 7 6 5 4 4 2
0	0 2 3 3 4 4 5 6 7 8 8 9
1	0 1 1 3 4 4 5 7 8
2	9
3	5

Mean of the differences: 7.0°

Standard deviation of the differences: 10.03°

$$t = \frac{\bar{X}_d}{\dfrac{S_d}{\sqrt{n}}} = \frac{7.0}{\dfrac{10.03}{\sqrt{30}}} = 3.82$$

Wilcoxon Signed Rank Test

The Wilcoxon signed rank test is the nonparametric version of the paired-*t* test. The nonparametric hypotheses relate to the median:

H_0: The difference between the population medians is equal to zero.

H_1: The difference between the population medians is not equal to zero.

To conduct the Wilcoxon signed rank test, we calculate the difference between each pair of numbers. We rank the nonzero differences according to their absolute value and then separate them into the ranks associated with positive and negative differences. If there is no difference from one time to the next, then the sum of the positive ranks should be approximately equal to the sum of the negative ranks. Table 21-9 shows the sums of the positive and negative ranks for this example. As is the case with the Mann-Whitney procedures for analyzing differences between independent samples, the ranked information is transformed into a *z* score. The computer-generated *z* score and probability for this example are 3.298 and .001, respectively. This probability being less than our alpha of .05, we conclude that there is a significant difference between 3-week and 6-week ROM.

To determine the clinical importance of the difference, we examine the median of the difference between the two samples. The median difference for this example is 6.5°. This seems a fairly modest gain for a 3-week period. Once again, we should temper our statistical conclusion with a statement about the relatively small size of the median difference.

McNemar Test

The McNemar test is the nominal-data analogue to the paired-*t* test and the Wilcoxon signed rank test. It can also be viewed as the dependent samples version of the chi-square test. In fact, a review of rehabilitation research showed that chi-square tests were often used inappropriately for dependent samples when the McNemar test would have been more appropriate.[18] The McNemar test can only be used to analyze 2×2 contingency tables, and thus its usefulness is limited. Suppose we want to determine whether there is a predictable change in ROM from 3 weeks to 6 weeks and are interested not in absolute range scores, but only in whether patients have greater than or less than 90° of motion. Our hypotheses are as follows:

H_0: The proportion of patients with less than 90° of motion at 3 weeks postoperatively is identical to the proportion of patients with less than 90° of motion at 6 weeks postoperatively.

H_1: The population proportions are not equal at the two time intervals.

Table 21-9

Wilcoxon Signed Rank Test

Difference	Rank by Absolute Value	Positive Difference Rank	Negative Difference Rank
0			
−2	1.5		1.5
2	1.5	1.5	
3	3.5	3.5	
3	3.5	3.5	
−4	6.5		6.5
−4	6.5		6.5
4	6.5	6.5	
4	6.5	6.5	
−5	9.5		9.5
5	9.5	9.5	
−6	11.5		11.5
6	11.5	11.5	
7	13.5	13.5	
−7	13.5		13.5
−8	16		16
8	16	16	
8	16	16	
9	18	18	
10	19	19	
11	20.5	20.5	
11	20.5	20.5	
13	22	22	
14	23.5	23.5	
14	23.5	23.5	
15	25	25	
17	26	26	
18	27	27	
29	28	28	
35	29	29	
Σ signed ranks		370	65

To perform the McNemar test, we generate a 2×2 table of frequencies, as shown in Table 21-10. Each participant is represented only once in the table. For example, a participant who had less than 90° of motion at 3 weeks and still had less than 90° of motion at 6 weeks

Table 21-10

McNemar Test

Three-Week Range of Motion	SIX-WEEK RANGE OF MOTION	
	Limited Progress Motion (<90°)	**Normal Progress (≥90°)**
Limited progress (<90°)	20	6
Normal progress (≥90°)	1	3

Table 21-11

Stem-and-Leaf Displays of Range-of-Motion Data at Three Times

Stem	Week 3	Week 6	Month 6
2	7		
3	224		
4	0579	06	
5	0068	0568	
6	077	033577	5
7	6	0018	8
8	1111244478	00555	0345
9	1225	000004555	00555558
10			00000345555556
11			00

is one of the 20 individuals indicated in the upper left corner of the table. If the proportion of patients in each category stays the same from 3 weeks to 6 weeks, we would expect that (1) some patients will not change categories (upper left and lower right cells) and (2) the number of patients who change categories will be distributed evenly between those moving from less than to greater than 90° and those moving from greater than to less than 90° (lower left and upper right cells). Table 21-10 shows that 23 patients did not change ROM categories, 6 improved from less than to greater than 90°, and only 1 had a decline in motion from greater than to less than 90°.

The probability of such an occurrence, if in fact there is no difference in proportions, is .1250, as generated by the computer program. Being greater than .05, we conclude that the change in proportions from 3 weeks to 6 weeks is not significant. Clinically, a change of categories in only 7 of 30 patients seems to indicate minimal effectiveness of the intervention over the 3-week time span. Thus, the statistical conclusion of an insignificant difference in proportions concurs with our clinical impression.

Differences Between Two or More Dependent Samples

We now wish to determine whether patients show a pattern of ROM improvement from 3 weeks postoperatively, to 6 weeks postoperatively, to 6 months postoperatively. Our hypotheses for such a question are as follows:

H_0: $\mu_{\text{3-week ROM}} = \mu_{\text{6-week ROM}} = \mu_{\text{6-month ROM}}$

H_1: At least one population mean does not equal another population mean.

We set alpha at .05. The samples are dependent because each participant is measured three times. Table 21-11 shows the stem-and-leaf displays for the

ROM scores at all three time periods; none is symmetrical. Additional assumptions about the variances and covariances of the measures must be met, but a full discussion of these is beyond the scope of this text. The parametric test of differences between more than two dependent means is the repeated measures ANOVA. The corresponding nonparametric test is Friedman's ANOVA.

Repeated Measures ANOVA

Just as the one-way ANOVA is the extension of the independent *t* test from two groups to more than two groups, the repeated measures ANOVA is the extension of the paired-*t* test to more than two dependent samples. There are three different approaches to a repeated measures ANOVA: multivariate, univariate, and adjusted univariate. The assumptions for the univariate approach are more stringent than those for the multivariate approach; statistical packages provide a test (Mauchly test of sphericity) of the assumptions to guide researchers in deciding which approach to use.[13(p. 169)] The univariate approach is similar to the one-way ANOVA and is discussed here.

Recall the procedure used for the paired-*t* test. We started with a group of subjects with ROM scores ranging from 32 to 95 (see Table 21-4). To determine the test statistic, we calculated the difference between the 3-week and 6-week measures. Taking the difference of the paired scores effectively eliminated the widespread variability between participants in the sample and allowed us to focus on the changes within participants with time. Like the paired-*t* test, the repeated measures ANOVA mathematically eliminates between-subjects variability to focus the analysis on within-subject variability.

Recall that the one-way ANOVA partitioned the variability in the data set into between-groups and within-group categories. The univariate repeated measures ANOVA first partitions the variability in the data set into between-subjects and within-subject categories. The within-subject variability is then subdivided into between-treatments and error (or residual) components (Table 21-12). Two F ratios can be generated from a repeated measures ANOVA: One is the ratio of between-subjects to within-subject variability; the other is the ratio of between-treatments to residual variability. The first ratio is sometimes reported but is not relevant to the research question we are addressing here. A significant between-subjects F ratio would merely tell us that there is substantial variability between individual participants, and a nonsignificant between-subjects F ratio would tell us that participants are fairly homogeneous. Neither result is relevant to the question of whether there are differences between treatments. Thus, the between-treatments F ratio is the one that is relevant to our research question. It is the ratio of the between-treatments variability to the variability that is left after the variability caused by differences between participants is removed. Thus, the variability that makes up the denominator of the F ratio is called the *residual*. It is also referred to as *error* because this represents random differences in participants caused by sampling errors.

If a repeated measures ANOVA identifies a significant difference among the means, the next step is to make multiple comparisons between pairs of means to determine which time frames are significantly different from one another. The multiple-comparison procedures for repeated measures must be based on assumptions of dependence between the pairs being compared. Maxwell[19] recommends the use of paired-t

tests with a Bonferroni adjustment of alpha. However, both Gravetter and Wallnau[3(p. 427)] and Kiess and Green[20(p. 351)] indicate that, with a slight modification of formula,[3(p. 427)] post-hoc analysis for repeated measures ANOVA proceeds in the same manner as for between-subjects ANOVA, and they recommend either the Tukey HSD test or Scheffé test.

In our example, a significant difference between treatments was identified: $F_{2,58}=94.06$, $p=.0001$. Three paired-t tests are used as the multiple comparisons to determine where the differences lie. Because three comparisons are needed, the overall alpha level of .05 becomes .017 ($.05/3=.017$). The results of the paired-t tests are as follows: For 3-week versus 6-week scores, $t_{29}=3.83$, $p=.001$; for 3-week versus 6-month scores, $t_{29}=10.38$, $p=.000$; and for 6-week versus 6-month scores, $t_{29}=11.51$, $p=.000$. (Note that the probability is never actually zero, but in this case it is low enough that it can be rounded off to zero.)

To determine the clinical relevance of these differences, we need to examine the means for the different time periods: 3 weeks—66.4, 6 weeks—73.4, and 6 months—96.4. As noted previously, the average 7.0 difference between weeks 3 and 6 seems small, but the 23.0 difference between week 6 and month 6 seems highly important.

Friedman's ANOVA

Friedman's ANOVA is the nonparametric equivalent of the repeated measures ANOVA. Hypotheses are as follows:

H_0: All possible rankings of the observations for any subject are equally likely.

H_1: At least one population tends to produce larger observations than another population.

Calculation is based on rankings of the repeated measures for each participant. Two different formulas can be used to calculate either a Friedman's F or a

---

Table 21-12

Summary of a Repeated Measures Analysis of Variance

Source	Sum of Squares	Degrees of Freedom	Mean Square	F	p
Between subjects	20,710.46	29	714.15	2.23	.0047
Within subject	19,244.66	60	320.74		
Between treatments	14,709.42	2	7354.71	94.06	.0001
Residual	4535.24	58	78.19		
Total	**39,955.12**	**89**			

Friedman's chi-square. The computer-generated chi-square for the differences in ROM at 3 weeks, 6 weeks, and 6 months postoperatively is 48.75, and the associated probability is .0000. Because .0000 is less than our preset alpha of .05, we conclude that at least one time frame is different from another. An appropriate nonparametric multiple-comparison procedure is the Wilcoxon signed rank test with a Bonferroni adjustment of the alpha level for each test. All three multiple comparisons show significant differences: For 3-week ROM versus 6-week ROM, $p = .001$; for 3-week ROM versus 6-month ROM, $p = .000$; and for 6-week ROM versus 6-month ROM, $p = .000$. Thus, for this example, the nonparametric and parametric results agree.

SUMMARY

Statistical testing of differences between samples is based on 10 steps: (1) stating the hypotheses, (2) deciding on the alpha level, (3) examining the frequency distribution and descriptive statistics to determine whether the assumptions for parametric testing are met, (4) determining whether samples are independent or dependent, (5) determining the appropriate test, (6) using the appropriate software or formulas to determine the value of a test statistic, (7) determining the degrees of freedom, (8) determining the probability of obtaining the test statistic for the given degrees of freedom if the null hypothesis is true, (9) evaluating the obtained probability against the alpha level to draw a statistical conclusion, and (10) evaluating the statistical conclusions in light of clinical knowledge.

The independent *t*, Mann-Whitney or Wilcoxon rank sum, and chi-square tests are used to evaluate differences between two independent samples; the one-way ANOVA, Kruskal-Wallis, and chi-square tests can be used for two or more independent samples. The paired-*t*, Wilcoxon signed rank, and McNemar tests are used to evaluate differences between two dependent samples; the repeated measures ANOVA and Friedman's ANOVA can be used for two or more dependent samples.

REFERENCES

1. Corder GW, Foreman DI: *Nonparametric Statistics for Non-statisticians*, Hoboken, NJ, 2009, John Wiley & Sons.
2. Fitzgerald S, Dimitrov D, Rumrill P: The basics of nonparametric statistics, *Work* 16:287–292, 2001.
3. Gravetter FJ, Wallnau LB: *Essentials of Statistics for the Behavioral Sciences*, 7th ed, Belmont, Calif, 2011, Wadsworth.
4. Polit DF, Beck CT: *Nursing Research: Generating and Assessing Evidence for Nursing Practice*, 9th ed, Philadelphia, Pa, 2012, Lippincott Williams & Wilkins.
5. Dawson-Saunders B, Trapp RG: *Basic and Clinical Biostatistics*, 4th ed, New York, NY, 2004, Lange Medical/McGraw-Hill.
6. Gaito J: Measurement scales and statistics: Resurgence of an old misconception, *Psychol Bull* 87:564–567, 1980.
7. Nunnally JC, Bernstein IH: *Psychometric Theory*, 3rd ed, New York, NY, 1994, McGraw-Hill.
8. IBM. Independent Samples *t*-Test. Available at: http://pic.dhe.ibm.com/infocenter/spssstat/v20r0m0/index.jsp?topic=%2Fcom.ibm.spss.statistics.help%2Fidh_ttin.htm. Accessed December 9, 2014.
9. IBM. SPSS Software. Available at: http://www-01.ibm.com/software/analytics/spss/. Accessed December 9, 2014.
10. Plichta SB, Kelvin EA, Munro BH: *Munro's Statistical Methods for Health Care Research*, 6th ed, Philadelphia, Pa, 2013, Wolters Kluwer Health/Lippincott Williams & Wilkins.
11. Polit DF: *Statistics and Data Analysis for Nursing Research*, Boston, Mass, 2010, Pearson.
12. Elston RC, Johnson WD: *Essentials of Biostatistics*, Philadelphia, Pa, 1994, FA Davis.
13. Shott S: *Statistics for Health Professionals*, Philadelphia, Pa, 1990, Saunders.
14. Tests for Homogeneity of Variance. Available at: http://www.math.montana.edu/~jobo/st541/sec2e.pdf. Accessed December 9, 2014.
15. Egger MJ, Miller JR: Testing for experimental effects in the pretest-posttest design, *Nurs Res* 33:306–312, 1984.
16. Fitzgerald SM, Rumrill P, Hart RC: Using analysis of variance (ANOVA) in rehabilitation research investigations, *Work* 15:61–65, 2000.
17. Glass GV, Hopkins KD: *Statistical Methods in Education and Psychology*, 2nd ed, Englewood Cliffs, NJ, 1984, Prentice-Hall.
18. Ottenbacher KJ: The chi-square test: Its use in rehabilitation research, *Arch Phys Med Rehabil* 76:678–681, 1995.
19. Maxwell SE: Pairwise multiple comparisons in repeated measures designs, *J Educ Stat* 5:269–287, 1980.
20. Kiess HO, Green BA: *Statistical Concepts for the Behavioral Sciences*, 4th ed, Upper Saddle River, NJ, 2010, Pearson.

22

Statistical Analysis of Differences: Advanced

CHAPTER OUTLINE

Advanced ANOVA Techniques
Differences Between More Than
One Independent Variable
Between-Subjects Two-Way ANOVA
Mixed-Design Two-Way ANOVA
Differences Across Several
Dependent Variables
Effect of Removing an
Intervening Variable
Analysis of Single-Subject Designs
Celeration Line Analysis

Level, Trend, Slope, and Variability
Analysis
Two Standard Deviation Band
Analysis
C Statistic
Survival Analysis
Survival Curves
Differences Between Survival Curves
**Hypothesis Testing with Confidence
Intervals**

Review of Traditional Hypothesis
Testing
Foundations for Confidence Interval
Testing
Interpretation and Examples
Power Analysis
Power Analysis—Design Phase
Power Analysis—Analysis Phase
Summary

The analyses presented in Chapter 21 provide broad coverage of the most commonly reported statistical tests of differences. Readers will, however, find articles of interest that include a variety of advanced or special data analysis techniques. It seems likely that the use of these advanced techniques will increase because the widespread availability of sophisticated statistical analysis software eliminates the computational burden of these techniques. This chapter provides an overview of these more advanced or specialized techniques. First, the following advanced analysis of variance (ANOVA) techniques are covered: factorial ANOVA and the important concept of interaction (including between-subjects and mixed-design models), multivariate analysis of variance (MANOVA), and analysis of covariance (ANCOVA). Second, four specialized techniques for analyzing single-subject data are presented: celeration lines; analysis of level, trend, and slope; the two standard deviation band approach; and the C statistic. Third, the concepts of survival analysis and determining differences between survival curves are introduced. Fourth, the use of confidence intervals for hypothesis testing is discussed. Finally, the related concepts of power analysis and effect size are presented.

ADVANCED ANOVA TECHNIQUES

From Chapter 21, we know that ANOVA is a powerful statistical technique that can be used to evaluate differences among two or more independent or dependent groups by partitioning the variance in the data set in different ways. The same general process can be extended to analyze differences between more than one independent variable at a time, to analyze the differences between more than one dependent variable simultaneously, and when it is desirable, to mathematically remove the impact of an intervening variable.

Differences Between More Than One Independent Variable

There are several instances in which researchers wish to determine the impact of more than one independent variable on a dependent variable. Different forms of advanced ANOVA techniques are used for such analysis, depending on the nature of the independent variables selected for analysis. Using the data set presented in Chapter 20, we might wish to know whether there are differences in 3-week range-of-motion (ROM) values between clinics and between the sexes. This particular question involves two between-subjects factors, meaning that neither factor consists of repeated measures on the same participants. A different research question is whether ROM differences between clinics (a between-subjects factor) are consistent across time (a repeated, within-subject factor). The first research question is analyzed with a two-factor ANOVA for two between-subjects factors; the second is analyzed with a two-factor ANOVA for one between-subjects and one within-subject factor. The second analysis is sometimes referred to as a mixed-design ANOVA.

Whenever we examine the influence of more than one independent variable on a dependent variable, we must also examine whether there is an interaction between the independent variables. In the between-subjects example, the interaction question is whether the responses of men and women to treatment depend on the clinic at which they are treated. In the mixed design, the interaction question is whether changes across time are consistent across the clinics. Each of these two variations on two-factor ANOVA is discussed subsequently.

Between-Subjects Two-Way ANOVA

The statistical hypotheses for the between-subjects two-way ANOVA are as follows:

H_0: There is no interaction between clinic and sex.

H_1: There is an interaction between clinic and sex.

H_0: $\mu C_1 = \mu C_2 = \mu C_3$

H_C: At least one clinic population mean is different from another clinic population mean.

H_0: $\mu W = \mu M$

H_S: The population mean for women is different from the population mean for men.

There are null and alternative hypotheses for the interaction between clinic and sex, for the main effect of clinic, and for the main effect of sex. The overall alpha level is set at .05. This particular test is known as a two-way or two-factor ANOVA because two independent variables are examined. It can also be described as a 3×2 ANOVA, describing the number of levels of each of the factors. Three- and four-way ANOVAs are also possible. Table 22-1 shows the data, and Table 22-2 summarizes the ANOVA for this example.

Because interpretation of two-way ANOVAs depends on the interaction result, let us examine the interaction first. The F ratio for interaction (the Clinic×Sex row in Table 22-2) is only .070, and the probability is .932. Because the probability exceeds the .05 alpha level we set before the analysis, we conclude that there is no interaction between sex and clinic. This means that men and women respond the same across the clinics. Interactions can be interpreted best if the cell means are graphed as shown in Figure 22-1.

Note that although the means for men and women are different, the pattern of response is the same across clinics: Both men and women do best at Clinic 1, slightly worse at Clinic 3, and the worst at Clinic 2. The

Table 22-1

Three-Week Range-of-Motion Data for Two-Factor Between-Subjects Analysis of Variance

Clinic	SEX	
	Men	**Women**
1	32, 67, 92, 87, 58 $\bar{X}_{1M} = 67.2$	95, 92, 88, 84, 81 $\bar{X}_{1W} = 88.0$
2	34, 56, 45, 27, 40 $\bar{X}_{2M} = 40.4$	76, 49, 47, 50, 67 $\bar{X}_{2W} = 57.8$
3	32, 50, 60, 84, 81 $\bar{X}_{3M} = 61.4$	81, 84, 81, 82, 91 $\bar{X}_{3W} = 83.8$

Table 22-2

Summary of a Two-Factor Between-Subjects Analysis of Variance

Source	Sum of Squares	Degrees of Freedom	Mean Square	F	p
Clinic	4631.66	2	2315.83	9.963	.001
Sex	3060.30	1	3060.30	13.165	.001
Clinic×Sex	32.60	2	16.30	.070	.932
Residual	5578.80	24	232.45		
Total	13,303.36	29			

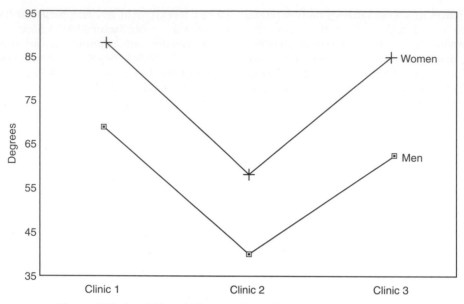

Figure 22-1 Parallel lines indicate no interaction between clinic and sex.

nearly parallel lines between the means of the men and women across clinics provide a visual picture of what is meant by no interaction.

Because no interaction has been identified, we now examine the main effects for clinic and sex. The main effect for clinic is determined by comparing the means of all subjects at each clinic, regardless of whether they are men or women. The main effect for sex is calculated by determining the sum of squares for men and women, regardless of the clinic at which they are treated. Analysis of the main effects depends on the assumption that the factors do not interact and that therefore each factor can be examined independently, without concern for the other factors. In this example, the main effects for both clinic and sex are significant: $F_{2,24}=9.96$, $p=.001$, and $F_{1,24}=13.16$, $p=.001$, respectively (see Table 22-2). Because the sex variable has only two levels, we do not need to conduct post hoc testing to locate the difference. Because the clinic variable has three levels, multiple comparisons are needed, as described in the one-way ANOVA example in Chapter 21.

When an interaction is present, the data analysis generally proceeds differently. To illustrate this, the data presented previously have been altered to create a significant interaction between clinic and sex. Table 22-3 shows the new data, Table 22-4 summarizes the ANOVA, and Figure 22-2 shows the modified graph of the cell means. The lines in Figure 22-2 are not parallel, indicating an interaction. Although women do better than men at Clinics 2 and 3, men do better than women at Clinic 1.

Table 22-3

Three-Week Range-of-Motion Data for Two-Factor Analysis of Variance Revealing an Interaction

	SEX	
Clinic	**Men**	**Women**
1	95, 92, 87, 92, 88	32, 67, 58, 84, 81
	$\bar{X}_{1M} = 90.8$	$\bar{X}_{1W} = 64.4$
2	34, 56, 45, 27, 40	76, 49, 47, 50, 67
	$\bar{X}_{2M} = 40.4$	$\bar{X}_{2W} = 57.8$
3	32, 50, 60, 84, 81	81, 84, 81, 82, 91
	$\bar{X}_{3M} = 61.4$	$\bar{X}_{3W} = 83.8$

When a significant interaction is present, the main effects for the individual variables are often difficult to interpret. For example, although Table 22-4 indicates that the main effect for clinic is significant, it would be erroneous for us to make any general statements about differences between clinics because these differences are not uniform across men and women. Likewise, the main effect for sex would lead us to conclude that there are no differences between men and women. However, it is clear that there are differences between the sexes at each clinic—the opposite directions of these differences

Table 22-4

Summary of a Two-Factor Analysis of Variance Revealing an Interaction with Simple Main Effects for Clinic Within Sex

Source	Sum of Squares	Degrees of Freedom	Mean Square	F	p
Clinic	4631.66	2	2315.83	11.301	.000
Sex	149.63	1	149.63	.730	.401
Clinic × Sex	3604.06	2	1802.03	8.794	.001
Clinic within sex (women)	1826.53	2	913.27	4.457	.023
Clinic within sex (men)	6409.20	2	3204.60	15.639	.000
Residual	4918.00	24	204.91		
Total	13,303.36	29			

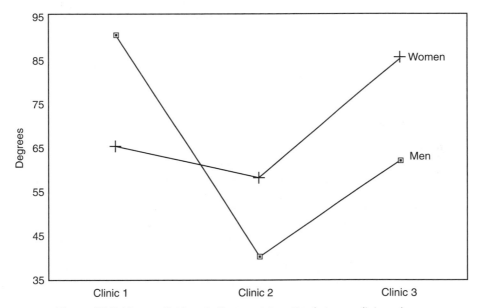

Figure 22-2 Nonparallel lines indicate an interaction between clinic and sex.

cancel out any main effect and erroneously make it appear that there are no differences between the sexes.

When a significant interaction is identified, the researcher typically analyzes simple main effects, rather than overall main effects. A simple main effect is one in which the differences among the levels of one factor are assessed separately for each level of the other factor. In this example, there are significant differences between clinics for the men and for the women (see Table 22-4). These results might be summarized in a journal article as follows:

DATA ANALYSIS: A two-way analysis of variance was used to determine whether there were significant differences between clinics and sexes for 3-week range of motion and whether there was a significant interaction between clinic and sex. Identification of a significant interaction led to further analysis of a simple main effect for clinic and post hoc analysis of significant simple main effects with the Newman-Keuls procedure. Alpha was set at .05 for each analysis.

RESULTS: As illustrated in Figure 22-2, there was a significant interaction between clinic and sex ($F_{2,24}=8.794$, $p=.001$). For both the men and the women, the simple main effect of clinic was significant, as shown in Table 22-4. Post hoc analysis revealed that all clinics were significantly different for the men, whereas only Clinics 2 and 3 were significantly different for the women.

An example of a two-factor ANOVA can be found in Magalhaes and colleagues'[1] study of differences in bilateral motor coordination on three different tasks based on age and sex. The age variable had five levels: 5, 6, 7, 8, and 9 years old. The sex variable had two levels: boys and girls. In this study, no interactions were found, so the main effects were interpreted for each of the analyses.

Mixed-Design Two-Way ANOVA

We are now interested in determining whether there are differences in ROM across the three clinics and across the three times that measurements are taken: 3 weeks, 6 weeks, and 6 months. Clinic is a between-subjects factor because different participants are measured at each clinic. Time is a within-participant factor because ROM measures are repeated on each of the participants across the time intervals in the study. The hypotheses for our test are as follows:

H_0: There is no interaction between clinic and time.

H_1: There is an interaction between clinic and time.

H_0: $\mu_{C1}=\mu_{C2}=\mu_{C3}$

H_C: At least one clinic population mean is different from another clinic population mean.

H_0: $\mu_{\text{3-week ROM}}=\mu_{\text{6-week ROM}}=\mu_{\text{6-month ROM}}$

H_T: At least one time population mean is different from another time population mean.

Interpretation of a mixed-design ANOVA follows the same sequence of analysis as the two-factor, between-subjects ANOVA. Table 22-5 presents the

Table 22-5

Mean Range of Motion over Time at Clinics 1 Through 3

Clinic	Three Weeks	Six Weeks	Six Months
1	77.6°	78.9°	100.0°
2	49.1°	58.6°	85.8°
3	72.6°	82.8°	103.3°

means for our example, and Table 22-6 presents the F ratios and p levels associated with each comparison. As shown in Figure 22-3, there is no interaction between clinic and time. This indicates that all the clinics had the same pattern of change across time. Because there is no interaction, the main effects for clinic and time are examined, and there is a significant effect for each. Post hoc analysis shows that all three clinics are significantly different from one another and that all three time periods are significantly different from one another.

The mixed-design ANOVA is frequently used to analyze pretest–posttest control group designs. In the simplest design, there is a treatment factor with two levels (treatment group and control group) and a time factor with two levels (pretest and posttest). The ideal results for such a study would be for the two groups to be essentially the same at the pretest, the control group to remain unchanged at posttest, and the treatment group to be improved considerably at posttest. Figure 22-4 shows a graph of these ideal results. A significant interaction is illustrated: The treatment group responded differently over time than did the control group. Thus, when a mixed-design two-factor ANOVA is used to analyze a pretest–posttest design, the research question is answered by examining the interaction between the

Table 22-6

Summary of Two-Factor Mixed-Design Analysis of Variance

Source	Sum of Squares	Degrees of Freedom	Mean Square	F	p
Clinic	9138.76	2	4569.38	10.66	.000
Error	11,571.70	27	428.58		
Time	10,709.42	2	7354.71	100.89	.000
Clinic × Time	598.64	4	149.66	2.05	.100
Error	3936.60	54	72.90		

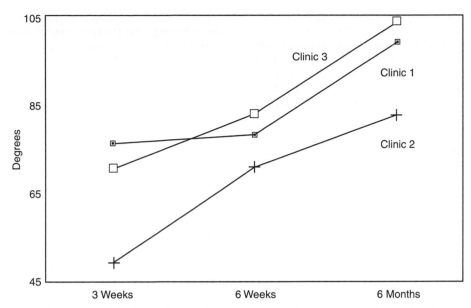

Figure 22-3 Nearly parallel lines indicate no interaction between clinic and time.

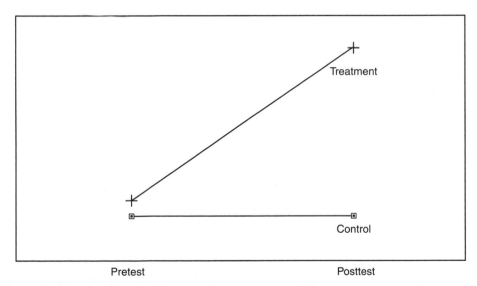

Figure 22-4 Ideal pretest–posttest results. The two groups are almost equal at pretest, the control group does not change at posttest, and the treatment group shows significant improvement at posttest. The nonparallel lines indicate a significant interaction between group and time.

group factor and the time factor. These results might be summarized in a journal article as follows:

DATA ANALYSIS: A 3×3 analysis of variance with one between-subjects factor (clinic) and one within-subject factor (time) was used to analyze differences between range-of-motion (ROM) means at an alpha level of .05. Post hoc comparisons were made for the clinic factor, with Newman-Keuls tests at alpha=.05, and for the time factor, with paired-*t* tests at alpha=.017.

RESULTS: The mean ROM for each group at each point in time is presented in Table 22-5. There was no significant interaction between clinic and time ($F_{4,54}=2.05$, $p=.100$). There were significant main effects for both clinic ($F_{2,27}=10.66$, $p=.000$) and time ($F_{2,54}=100.89$, $p=.000$). Overall means for Clinic 1 (85.5) and Clinic 3 (86.2) were not significantly different; Clinic 2's mean (64.5) was significantly different from those of Clinics 1 and 3. Means for all three time periods were significantly different from one another (3-week mean=66.4, 6-week mean=73.4, and 6-month mean=96.4).

A mixed-design two-factor ANOVA was used by Nobusako and associates[2] in their examination of the effectiveness of a gaze direction recognition task (GDR) on neck pain over 12 sessions. They had two levels of group, the intervention group that received the GDR and the control group, while the session variable had 12 levels. The researchers found simple main effects for group and for session and an interaction effect of session and group.

Differences Across Several Dependent Variables

Researchers are often interested in the effects of their treatments on several different dependent variables. In our sample data set, we are now interested in whether several 6-month outcomes are different between clinics: ROM, knee extensor strength, knee flexor strength, and gait velocity. One analysis approach is to run a one-way ANOVA for each dependent variable. There are two potential problems with this approach. The first is the alpha level inflation that results from conducting multiple tests. The second is the possibility that although no single variable exhibits significant differences across clinics, small, consistent differences across several dependent variables are present. Because an ANOVA can handle only one dependent variable at a time, a cumulative effect over several dependent variables would be undetected.

Multivariate procedures solve these problems by analyzing several dependent variables simultaneously. Multivariate analyses should not be confused with multifactor analyses: The former analyze several dependent variables simultaneously; the latter analyze several independent variables simultaneously. Although the mathematical basis for multivariate testing of differences is beyond the scope of this text, the interpretation of multivariate results is simply an extension of what has already been learned about ANOVA procedures.

A multivariate analysis of variance (MANOVA) uses an omnibus test to determine whether there are significant differences on the factor of interest (in our case, clinic) when the dependent variables of interest are combined mathematically. The multivariate test statistic used most frequently is Wilks' lambda, although several others are often reported by computer statistical packages. Wilks' lambda is usually converted to an estimated F statistic, and the probability of this estimated F is determined to test the null hypothesis.[3]

If the omnibus F level is significant, then a univariate ANOVA is conducted for each dependent variable to determine where among the dependent variables the differences lie. After the dependent variables that are significantly different are identified, multiple-comparison procedures can be conducted to determine which levels of the independent variable are different on the dependent variables for which significant differences have been identified. However, just as an ANOVA can produce inconsistent findings between the omnibus and multiple comparison procedures, so too can a MANOVA yield inconsistent findings between the omnibus multivariate test and the univariate tests on each dependent variable.

In the total knee arthroplasty example, the omnibus F is 3.53 and is significant at the .003 level. Table 22-7 presents univariate and post hoc results for each of the dependent variables. This analysis might be reported in a journal article as follows:

DATA ANALYSIS: Differences in 6-month status across clinics were examined with a multivariate analysis of variance (MANOVA) for the following dependent variables: 6-month range of motion, extension torque, flexion torque, and gait velocity. Univariate F tests with Newman-Keuls post hoc analyses were conducted to determine the sources of any difference identified by the MANOVA.

RESULTS: The multivariate F of 3.53 was significant at the .003 level. Table 22-7 shows the mean for each dependent variable for each clinic, the F and p values for the test for differences across clinics for each dependent variable, and an indication of which multiple comparisons showed significant differences between clinics. All four dependent variables were significantly different across clinics. In addition, all four dependent variables showed the same pattern of pairwise differences among clinics: None of the dependent variable means was significantly different between Clinics 1 and 3; all were significantly different between Clinics 1 and 2 and between Clinics 2 and 3.

Grammatopoulou and associates[4] employed a 2×4 MANOVA to analyze one of the health outcomes of a physiotherapy breathing retraining program for persons with controlled asthma. The MANOVA was employed to determine differences of the two groups of participants on the physical component (PC) and the mental component (MC) of the SF-36 at four different measurement times (0, 1, 3, and 6 months). They reported a significant interaction between the intervention and the four measurement times concerning the two SF-36 factors. After employing a univariate analysis with a Bonferroni

Table 22-7

Multivariate Analysis of Variance for Four Dependent Variables

Dependent Variable	INDEPENDENT VARIABLE			STATISTIC		MULTIPLE COMPARISONS		
	Clinic 1	Clinic 2	Clinic 3	F	p	1/2	1/3	2/3
Six-month range of motion (°)	100.0	85.8	103.3	15.63	.000	*		*
Extension torque (N•m)	135.8	105.4	142.2	4.90	.015	*		*
Flexion torque (N•m)	81.8	62.6	84.1	5.12	.013	*		*
Gait velocity (cm/s)	144.0	107.6	145.6	8.25	.002	*		*

Note: Asterisk indicates a significant difference between the means of the indicated pair of clinics.

adjustment, the researchers reported a significant inter-action between intervention and time for the PC, but not for the MC of the SF-36.

Effect of Removing an Intervening Variable

In our examples thus far, we have identified signifi-cant differences between clinics. However, scrutiny of patient characteristics at the three clinics shows that Clinic 2 has a patient population that is much older ($\bar{X}$ = 81.0 years) than the patients at Clinic 1 ($\bar{X}$ = 55.8 years) and Clinic 3 ($\bar{X}$ = 69.8 years). If younger

patients tend to gain ROM faster than older patients, perhaps the age difference between the clinics, rather than differences in the quality of care, explains the dif-ference in early ROM results.

The ANCOVA procedure uses the overall relationship between a dependent variable and an intervening vari-able, or covariate, to adjust the dependent variable scores in light of the covariate scores. For example, let us reex-amine the differences between clinics on the 3-week ROM variable by using age as a covariate. In our example, there is a strong negative correlation between age and 3-week ROM; that is, younger patients tend to have higher scores, and older patients tend to have lower scores (Fig. 22-5).

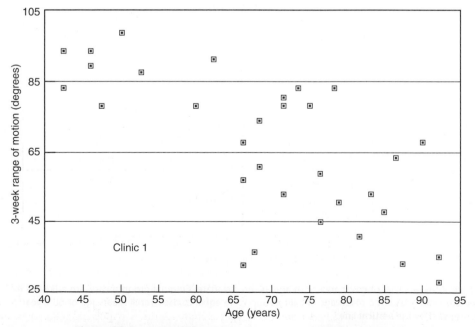

Figure 22-5 Relationship between age and 3-week range of motion.

An ANCOVA essentially takes each participant's 3-week ROM score and adjusts it to a predicted value as if the participant's age was the same as the mean age of the sample. In our total sample of 30 patients, the mean age is 68.8 years. Thus, the 3-week ROM scores of participants who are younger than 68.8 years are reduced and those of participants who are older than 68.8 years are increased. After this mathematical adjustment has taken place, an ANCOVA is run on the adjusted data. Figure 22-6 shows this adjustment graphically. The ANCOVA is summarized in Table 22-8. After age is accounted for, the differences between the groups disappear—the F value of 1.88 is not significant ($p = .173$).

The preceding example used a patient characteristic (age) as the covariate. Another typical use of an ANCOVA is to test for differences between posttest scores using pretest scores as covariates. If pretest scores between groups are significantly different, as is common in clinical research when random assignment to groups has not been possible, then posttest scores can be adjusted to mathematically eliminate the pretest differences.[5,6] However, it is preferable to have equivalent groups at the start of the study because there are any number of assumptions that must be met before an ANCOVA can be used legitimately. The ANCOVA results in the total knee

Table 22-8

Analysis of Covariance of 3-Week Range of Motion (ROM)

Clinic	Mean Age (yr)	Actual 3-Week ROM	Adjusted 3-Week ROM*
1	55.8	77.6°	64.54°
2	81.0	49.1°	61.22°
3	69.8	72.6°	73.53°

*No significant differences among clinics; $F_{2,26} = 1.88$, $p = .173$.

arthroplasty example might be reported in a journal article as follows:

DATA ANALYSIS: An analysis of covariance was used to determine whether there were significant differences between clinics after the effect of participant age was removed. Alpha was set at .05.

RESULTS: Table 22-8 shows the mean values for age, actual 3-week range of motion (ROM), and adjusted 3-week ROM across the three clinics. The difference among the adjusted means was not statistically significant.

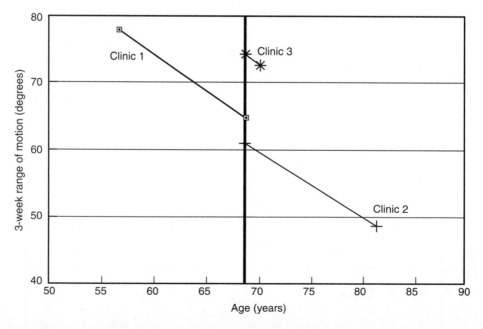

Figure 22-6 Analysis of covariance with age as the covariate. Original group means are adjusted to predicted values as if the mean age of each group were equal to the overall mean age of 68.8 years, represented by the vertical line.

The first ANCOVA example from the literature shows the use of extraneous variables as covariates. Employing an analysis of covariance (ANCOVA), with milk type as a covariant, Vignochi and colleagues[7] investigated the effects of 5 days per week of physical therapy for 4 weeks on the bone density of premature infants. The authors compared two randomly assigned groups of infants born prematurely, matched for gestational age and birth weight, reporting significantly greater gains in bone mass content and bone mass density for the group receiving physical therapy.

A second ANCOVA example illustrates the use of a pretest score as the covariate. Flynn and associates[8] used this kind of ANCOVA in their study of whether an audible pop is necessary for a manipulation to be successful. Dependent variables were a pain rating scale, lumbopelvic range of motion, and scores on the Oswestry Disability Questionnaire, all measured before manipulation and at a follow-up visit 2 to 4 days after the manipulation. Because it was impossible to randomize which patients would experience an audible pop while receiving the manipulation, the chance that the two groups (those with and those without an audible pop during manipulation) would be different at baseline was a real possibility. Therefore, ANCOVA was used to adjust each participant's posttest values in light of his or her pretest values.

ANALYSIS OF SINGLE-SUBJECT DESIGNS

Thus far, most of our analyses have examined group differences by making inferences to the populations from which the groups were drawn.

Although group differences may have statistical significance, they may not have clinical impact. This approach is not satisfactory for single-subject designs, in which our interest is in whether an individual has changed over time. Typically, in single-subject designs, the analysis emphasis is on specific observable behaviors that have clinical significance to the subject. Thus, visual analysis of "significant" change in the graphed dependent variable data, indicative of clinical impact, is preferred to statistical analysis. Assume that a patient has extremely limited ROM 10 weeks after total knee arthroplasty. After treating the patient for 10 weeks with manual stretching and exercise, the therapist decides that more drastic measures are needed and implements a new treatment for 10 weeks, which has the results shown in Figure 22-7. It appears that the new treatment results in an improvement over the baseline, but is there any way to express this more quantitatively? In fact, many different techniques can be used to analyze single-subject data.[9] [15] These references provide specific calculation details and discuss when to use which of the analyses. In this chapter, four

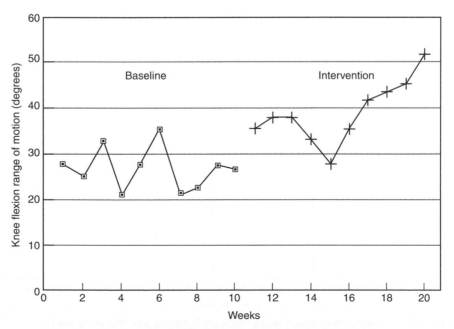

Figure 22-7 Single-subject data.

of the more commonly used techniques are summarized: celeration line analysis; analysis of level, trend, and slope; the two standard deviation band analysis approach; and the C statistic.

Celeration Line Analysis

In celeration line analysis, a researcher compares data in different phases by generating a line or lines based on the median of subsets of data in each phase (Fig. 22-8). To determine the celeration line through the baseline data, the researcher splits the data in half and splits each half in half again. The median of each of the halves is plotted on vertical lines (the points in Fig. 22-8 represent these two medians). A line is drawn through these two points and is extended into the intervention area. The number of data points in the intervention phase and the number exceeding the celeration line are counted. The probability of having a certain proportion of scores above the celeration line can be generated from a table based on the binomial distribution.[12(p. 184)] The table indicates that in a one-tailed test at an alpha level of .05, 9 or 10 intervention-phase numbers must be above the celeration line for a significant difference to have occurred. Because all 10 intervention-phase points are above the celeration line, we can conclude that significant improvement occurred during the treatment phase.

A basic assumption of the celeration line approach is that the baseline data do not exhibit serial dependency, a phenomenon associated with the ability to predict the next point from the previous point.[12(p. 170)]

A sample analysis with celeration lines is presented in the next section. In the literature, Vaz and colleagues[16] used extended celeration lines and two standard deviation band widths to analyze the effects of treadmill training three times a week in 20-minute sessions for 10 weeks on a number of gait measures, including gait speed, cadence, and quality, as well as standing balance of two persons who had ataxia due to head trauma.

Level, Trend, Slope, and Variability Analysis

In addition to the results related to the extended celeration line, observation or quantification of changes in graphed data levels, trends, slopes, and variability may facilitate the description of the patterns seen across time (Fig. 22-9). Remember from Chapter 21, when analyzing single-subject data, only adjacent phases are to be compared. To evaluate these changes, a researcher may calculate a celeration line for each phase of the study or may use these concepts to guide their visual analysis of the data.

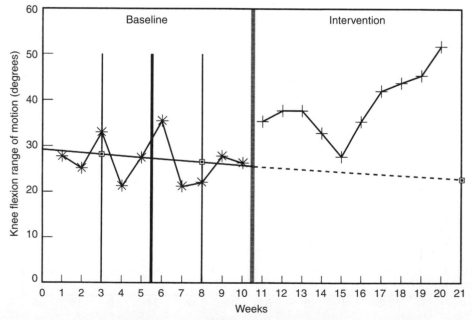

Figure 22-8 Celeration line approach to analysis of single-subject data. The celeration line determined for the baseline phase *(solid line)* is extrapolated into the intervention phase *(dotted line)*.

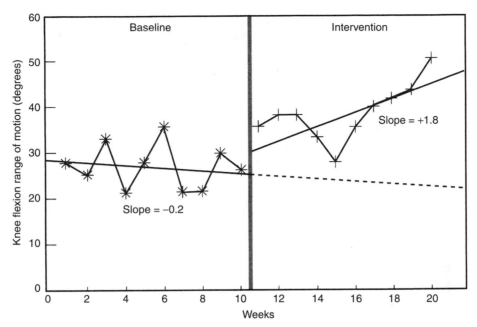

Figure 22-9 Level, trend, and slope analysis of single-subject data. Celeration lines are calculated for each phase. There is a four-level change, indicated by the intersections of the celeration lines in each phase with the vertical line separating the phases. There is a change in trend from downward to upward and a change in slope from −0.2 to +1.8.

Level is the difference between the numerical value of observations in one phase and the numerical value of observations in a subsequent phase. A change in level is quantified by calculating the difference between the end of one celeration line and the beginning of the celeration line in the subsequent phase. There is a difference of +4° in level between the baseline and intervention phases of our example.

Trend is the direction of change in the pattern of results. In our example there has been a reversal of the trend: It was downward in the baseline phase and is upward in the intervention phase. Trend can be quantified by calculating the slopes of the lines. Slope is the amount that the Y value changes for each unit change in X. To calculate slope, we select two data points on the celeration line. The slope is the difference between the two Y values divided by the difference between the X values. In our example, the data points used to generate the baseline celeration line are (3,28) and (8,27). The slope is calculated as follows: $(27 - 28)/(8 - 3) = -1/5 = -0.2$. This means that, on average, the patient loses 0.2° of motion each week during the baseline phase. The slope of the intervention-phase celeration line is calculated similarly and is +1.8. On average, the patient gained 1.8° of motion each week in the intervention phase. Thus, not only does the

trend reversal indicate a positive treatment effect, but the difference in the magnitude of the slopes also indicates that treatment led to a fairly rapid improvement in ROM in the intervention phase compared with the baseline phase.

Variability in single-subject data is a change in the range of scores in one phase compared with the range of scores in an adjacent phase. To more accurately determine this change, several have advocated adding a "best fit" line to the phase data, such as that provided by a celeration line. Variability will be the sum of the differences or "distances" between the individual data points and the corresponding celeration line values in one phase compared with the summed differences of the data points and corresponding celeration line values in an adjacent phase.[12,17] Typically, the "distances" are summed disregarding the negative and positive value signs. For example, in Figure 22-10, we have a celeration line in both the baseline and intervention phases. If we add the difference values (without minus or plus values) between each data point and the corresponding point on the celeration line for each phase, we have a summed distance from the baseline celeration line of 115 for all baseline data points, whereas the summed distance from data points to the celeration line in the intervention phase is 30. This is also presented in Table 22-9.

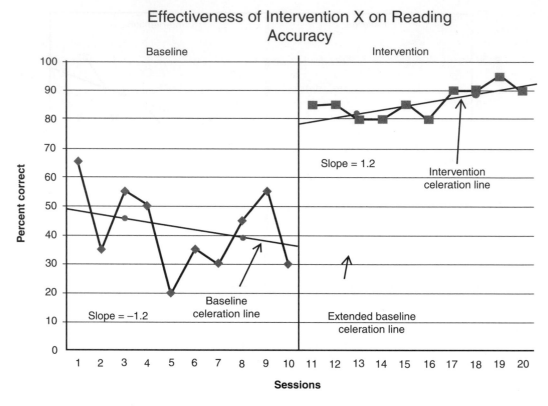

Figure 22-10 A celeration line in both the baseline and intervention phases.

Table	**22-9**

Effectiveness of Intervention X on Reading Fluency

Data Point Values	Baseline Celeration Line Values	Difference	Data Point Values	Intervention Celeration Line Values	Difference
65	48	17	85	80	5
35	46	11	85	82	3
55	45	10	80	83	3
50	44	6	80	84	4
20	43	23	85	85	0
35	42	7	80	86	6
30	41	11	90	88	2
45	39	6	90	89	1
55	38	17	95	90	5
30	37	7	90	91	1
		Total 115			**Total 30**

The results of this example analysis might be reported in a journal article as follows:

DATA ANALYSIS: Celeration lines for the baseline and intervention phases were developed using the split-middle approach. In addition, differences between phases were described through calculation of trend, slope, level, and variability changes from phase to phase. To determine whether the difference between the baseline and intervention phase was statistically significant, we extended the celeration line for the baseline phase into the intervention phase and evaluated the distribution of scores above and below the line in the intervention phase against a tabled value based on binomial probabilities. Alpha was set at .05.

RESULTS: Figure 22-9 shows the data and celeration lines for each phase of the study. The baseline trend was downward and the intervention trend upward, as indicated by the direction of the slopes, −1.2 and +1.2, respectively. The change in level, or the extent of discontinuity between the celeration lines where they intersect the vertical line separating the two phases, was +43%. Data became more stable as indicated by the summed difference of data point values from corresponding "best fit" celeration line values for the baseline phase (115) compared with the summed difference of data point values from corresponding "best fit" celeration line values for the intervention phase (30) (see Table 22-9). All 10 data points in the intervention phase fall above the extended baseline celeration line; this indicates a statistically significant treatment effect at $p = .05$.

Visual analysis of trend and slope was part of the data analysis strategy of Cadenhead and colleagues[18] as they examined the effect of passive ROM exercises on lower-extremity ROM of adults with cerebral palsy.

Two Standard Deviation Band Analysis

A third way to analyze single-subject data is to calculate the mean and standard deviation of the baseline points. Using this information, a horizontal line representing the mean is drawn across the baseline and intervention phases that are being compared. Two other horizontal lines are drawn in at two standard deviations above and below the mean. The area between the two new lines is the "two standard deviation (2-SD)" band. This band represents the "likely" scores for the patient if there is no change as a result of the treatment. If there is a

change, one would expect that several scores during the intervention phase would fall outside the 2-SD band. In fact, Ottenbacher,[12(p. 188)] citing earlier authors, indicates that a general rule of thumb is that when two successive points fall outside of the 2-SD band, a statistically significant (at an alpha of .05) difference has been detected between the baseline and intervention points. Figure 22-11 shows that the 2-SD band method of analysis leads to the conclusion that a significant difference does exist between the baseline and intervention scores. The results of this example analysis might be reported in a journal article as follows:

DATA ANALYSIS: The two standard deviation (2-SD) band analysis technique was used to determine whether there was a significant difference between baseline and intervention scores. The mean and standard deviation of the baseline data were calculated, and a 2-SD band around the baseline data was plotted across both the baseline and intervention phases (see Fig. 22-11). Our statistical decision rule was that a significant difference between baseline and intervention phases would be identified if two successive intervention points fell outside the 2-SD band.[11(p. 188)]

RESULTS: Figure 22-11 shows that more than two successive intervention points fell outside the 2-SD band, indicating a statistically significant difference between the baseline and intervention phases.

Earlier we noted that Vaz and colleagues[16] employed a 2-SD band as well as a celeration line to analyze their outcomes. Miller[19] also used the 2-SD band method to analyze her study of outcomes following body-weight–supported treadmill and overground walking training in a patient after cerebrovascular accident. Significant differences were found between phases for several variables, including the Berg Balance Scale and the 6-minute walk.

C Statistic

The C statistic is a data analysis method thought to be particularly appropriate for small data sets and for data sets with serial dependency.[10] The logic of the C statistic is similar to that of ANOVA: The sum of squared deviation scores related to the treatment effect is divided by the sum of squared deviation scores related to the baseline. Nourbakhsh and Ottenbacher[10] provided instructions for calculating the C statistic, which can be interpreted with a normal probability table such as the one in Appendix B. The C statistic was used as part of

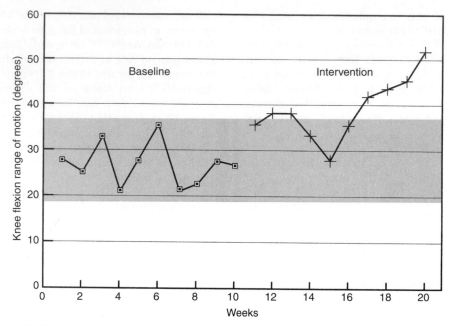

Figure 22-11 Two standard deviation (SD) band method of analyzing single-subject data. The shaded band shows 2 SDs above and below the mean of the baseline data.

the data analysis strategy of Cadenhead and colleagues[18] as they examined the effect of passive ROM exercises on lower-extremity ROM of adults with cerebral palsy.

SURVIVAL ANALYSIS

Survival analysis, as its name implies, is a mathematical tool that was initially used to analyze the changing proportion of survivors over time after some naturally occurring initial event (e.g., survival after stroke) or after some manipulation (e.g., survival after heart transplant surgery). Just as the outcomes movement in health care research, discussed in Chapter 16, has led to widespread use of dependent variables other than mortality, there is now expanded use of survival analysis for outcomes other than death.

Survival Curves

The basic elements needed for survival analysis are two defined events that form the basis for a survival curve: the event that qualifies a patient for inclusion in the analysis and the event that removes the patient from the analysis. In classic survival analysis, for example, a patient would enter the analysis when he or she received a heart transplant and exit the analysis when he or she died. With contemporary survival analysis, the exit event might be one of many outcomes other than death: failure of a prosthetic joint replacement,

resumption of independent ambulation after surgery, admission to an extended care facility, return to a health care practitioner for further consultation for a condition presumed to be resolved, return to sport following injury, or loss of a job following successful placement after completion of a work conditioning program. The exit event may be negative or positive as long as it separates the proportion of individuals who have not yet experienced the event from those who have.

Determining the proportions of patients who have and have not experienced the exit event across time is easier to conceptualize than it is to actually calculate. First, the calculations depend on whether a new proportion is calculated at specified time intervals (actuarial or life table analysis) or each time a patient changes status (Kaplan-Meier analysis).[20(pp. 188–209)] Second, the calculations depend on the handling of subjects who are lost to follow-up or who must leave the study because of an event other than the specified exit event. For example, assume that the exit event is admission to an extended care facility after returning home following an intensive poststroke rehabilitation program. Researchers need to know how to account for patients who die shortly after completing the rehabilitation program but who remained independent in their homes until their death. Computation details and information about the use of statistical analysis programs for survival analysis are beyond the scope of this text but can be found in other resources.[20(pp. 188–209)]

Differences Between Survival Curves

Although researchers may be interested in a single survival curve for participants who have experienced a single event or procedure, they are often more interested in whether there is a significant difference in survival curves for participants who have experienced different events or procedures. Hoenig and associates[21] made such a comparison when they sought to determine whether there were differences in the timing of ambulation after surgical repair of a hip fracture, based on the timing of the surgical repair (early, defined as within 2 days of hospital admission, versus late) and the frequency of physical and occupational therapy (high frequency, defined as more than five sessions per week, versus low frequency). Readers can refer to Chapter 16 and Figure 16-2 for a more complete presentation of their findings.

There are several statistical methods, each using different mathematical principles, that can be used to compare survival curves.[20(pp. 196–203)] The Wilcoxon rank sum test, introduced in Chapter 21, can be used to determine differences in the survival time ranking between two groups. The log-rank test, sometimes referred to with the addition of either or both the Cox and Mantel names, uses chi-square test principles, also introduced in Chapter 21, to compare the observed survivors in each group with the expected survivors based on the combined groups. The Mantel-Haenszel test uses odds ratios, introduced in Chapter 21, to compare the odds of survival for both groups. A final type of test for differences in survival is known as a proportional hazards, or Cox regression, model.[20(p. 221)] This model is based on regression analysis techniques, which are presented in Chapters 23 and 24. Clearly, additional details about these methods are beyond the scope of this text. However, readers should take from this brief discussion two central ideas. First, the array of tests and the varied naming conventions make it difficult for even sophisticated readers to make judgments about the appropriateness of the test chosen. Second, despite the wide variety of tests of differences between survival curves, all of the tests rest on the basic statistical foundations presented elsewhere in this text.

HYPOTHESIS TESTING WITH CONFIDENCE INTERVALS

Up to this point, the process of testing differences between groups or levels has been presented in terms of comparisons between an obtained probability level (*p*) and a predetermined probability of error set by the researcher, the alpha (α) level. Recall that the determinants of the *p* value in any statistical test of differences are (1) the size of the difference in the dependent variable between levels of the independent variable, (2) the amount of variability on the dependent variable within levels of the independent variable, and (3) the sample size. In traditional hypothesis testing, these factors are used within a specific formula for a statistic such as *t* or *F*. The *t* or *F* value is calculated, and computerized statistical analysis programs are used to determine the probability associated with the calculated value of *t* or *F*. If this *p* value is less than the preset alpha level, then a statistically significant finding has been identified.

Critics of this traditional approach note that the emphasis on *p* and alpha levels leads to "lazy thinking"[22(p. 746)] because each decision about the meaningfulness of data is reduced to a dichotomy of "significant" versus "nonsignificant." Put into terms of the steps of statistical analysis that were presented in Chapter 21, these critics believe that an emphasis on *p* values leads many researchers to stop the analysis process with step 9 (comparing the obtained probability with the alpha level to draw a statistical conclusion) instead of proceeding to the final step 10 (evaluating the statistical conclusions in light of clinical knowledge). These critics believe that presentation of statistical results in the form of confidence intervals rather than *p* values facilitates the higher level of evaluation that they believe is important to the proper interpretation of research results.

Review of Traditional Hypothesis Testing

Understanding the basis of the argument for using confidence intervals for hypothesis testing requires revisiting some of the statistical principles originally introduced in Chapter 20. Readers who have difficulty following the greatly abbreviated discussion of these principles should review the appropriate sections of Chapters 20 and 21.

Recall that the mean is a sample statistic. Furthermore, sample statistics are not precise values in and of themselves; rather, they are estimates of population parameters. As estimates, sample means contain a certain amount of error. The magnitude of this error depends on the variability within the data and the size of the sample. Specifically, this error is known as the standard error of the mean (SEM) and can be calculated for each group by dividing the group's standard deviation by the square root of the size of the group. Confidence intervals (CIs) around the mean can be computed by adding and subtracting standard errors to and from the mean. The error that the researcher is willing to tolerate is based on the number of standard deviations above and below the mean that are included in the confidence interval. With large groups of normally distributed data, adding and subtracting 1.645 SEMs yields a 90% CI; 1.96 SEMs yields a 95% CI; and 2.576 SEMs yields a 99% CI.

Earlier, an independent *t* test was used to compare the 3-week ROM values between Clinic 1 ($\bar{X}$ = 77.6°, s = 19.84) and Clinic 2 ($\bar{X}$ = 49.1°, s = 14.58). The independent *t* formula, presented in Table 21-3, is the difference between the means divided by the standard error of the difference between the means ($t = 28.5/7.78 = 3.66$). The computer-generated probability of obtaining this *t* value was .002, which was less than the preset alpha of .05, so a statistically significant difference was identified.

Foundations for Confidence Interval Testing

As noted in the previous section, in traditional hypothesis testing we compute a probability and reach our statistical conclusion when we compare the obtained *p* to a preset alpha level. In hypothesis testing with confidence intervals, we calculate a confidence interval for the difference of interest and reach our statistical conclusion by determining whether the confidence interval includes the value that corresponds to the null hypothesis. For most purposes this value is zero ("0") because the null hypothesis proposes that there will be "no difference" between groups. If the confidence interval contains "0," then we conclude that there is no statistically significant difference between groups. If the confidence interval does not contain "0," then we conclude that there is a statistically significant difference between groups. When using confidence intervals to determine the significance of odds ratios and relative risk ratios, a significant difference is identified when the interval does not contain the number "1". This is because a ratio of 1 means that the risks for the groups being compared are equal.

Using confidence intervals for hypothesis testing means that the concept of confidence intervals for each group must be extended to the concept of a confidence interval for the difference between groups. Doing so involves rearranging the mathematical concepts of the *t* test.[22(p. 749)] The general confidence interval formula for the difference between two independent group means is as follows:

$$CI = (\text{difference between the means})$$
$$\pm (\text{appropriate multiplier})$$
$$\times (\text{standard error of the difference})$$

For this example, the computations given in Chapter 21 (see Table 21-3) give two of the three values needed for computing the confidence interval:

$$CI = 28.5 \pm (\text{appropriate multiplier})(7.78)$$

The third value cannot be determined directly from the information in this text because it depends on access to a complete *t* table, commonly found in texts solely devoted to statistics. However, the conceptual basis for this value can be identified easily. Recall that when determining the confidence interval for a single, normally distributed group, the appropriate multiplier for a 95% confidence interval, based on the normal *z* distribution, was 1.96. Furthermore, recall that the *t* distribution is a slightly flattened *z* distribution. The appropriate multiplier for a 95% confidence interval for the difference between two means is based on the *t* distribution rather than the *z* distribution and is slightly further toward the tail of the distribution at 2.101. Inserting 2.101 into our formula, we find that the 95% confidence interval for the difference between these two means is 12.15° to 44.85°:

$$95\% \text{ CI} = 28.5 \pm (2.101)(7.78)$$
$$95\% \text{ CI} = 28.5 \pm 16.35$$
$$95\% \text{ CI} = 12.15 \text{ to } 44.85$$

Because this confidence interval does not contain "0," we conclude that there is a significant difference between the means of Clinics 1 and 2. This statistical conclusion matches the conclusion we reached with the independent *t* test in Chapter 21. This is not surprising in that the two methods depend on algebraic rearrangement of the same formula. Sim and Reid[23] recommend that confidence intervals be used (1) when sample statistics are used as estimates of population parameters, (2) in addition to or instead of the results of hypothesis testing, (3) as a means to assess the clinical importance of research results, (4) with adjusted confidence levels when multiple intervals are calculated (the equivalent to controlling for alpha inflation), and (5) when reporting the results of individual studies that are included within meta-analyses.

Interpretation and Examples

With the traditional method, the reader is tempted to believe that in our hypothetical example, the "true" difference between the means is 28.5° and that the difference between the means is "really" significant because the *p* value of .002 is so much less than the alpha of .05. With the confidence interval presentation, the reader is reminded that 28.5° is only an estimate of a difference between the means. The confidence interval tells us that there is a 95% chance that the population difference in mean 3-week ROM values is between approximately 12° and approximately 45°. With this information, the researcher or reader has a sound basis on which to judge the clinical importance of the finding.

Van der Windt and colleagues[24] used confidence intervals to supplement their traditional hypothesis testing in a study of the effectiveness of corticosteroid injections versus physical therapy for treatment of painful stiff shoulders. For example, they found a difference of 31% in success rates between groups: 77% of patients treated with the corticosteroid injections were "successes" at 7 weeks compared with only 46% of those treated with physical therapy. The confidence interval for this difference in percentage was 14% to 48%. Because this interval does not contain "0," it corresponds to a statistically significant difference in percentage of treatment successes between groups after 7 weeks of treatment. Prencipe and coworkers[25] used confidence intervals to test the significance of the odds ratio for dementia in elderly, community-dwelling individuals with and without stroke. The odds ratio for dementia was 5.8 with a 95% confidence interval from 3.1 to 10.8. Since this interval does not contain "1," the authors concluded that there was a significant increase in the odds of dementia for individuals who have had stroke compared with those without stroke. Furthermore, there is a 95% chance that the population of individuals with stroke is 3.1 to 10.8 times more likely to have dementia compared with the population of individuals without stroke.

POWER ANALYSIS

Power is the ability of a statistical test to detect a difference when it exists, as discussed in Chapter 20. Maximizing power within a research design involves (1) maximizing the size of the difference in the dependent variable between levels of the independent variable, (2) minimizing the amount of variability on the dependent variable within levels of the independent variable, and (3) maximizing the sample size. In addition, the alpha level selected by the researcher influences power, with higher power associated with larger alpha levels. Power analysis is used at two very different points in the research process: in the design phase and after the analysis phase. Texts[26,27] and computer software[28] can be used to conduct a power analysis at either time.

Power Analysis—Design Phase

During the design phase of a research project, power analysis is used to help the researcher design a study that has "enough" power, typically 80%, to detect differences that exist. To do so, the researchers could estimate the size of the between-group difference that they would consider to be important, the variability they would expect to see within the groups being studied, and the sample size that is reasonable given the constraints of the research setting. From this information, a "dry run" statistical analysis can be done, and the power of the analysis can be calculated. If the power is less than 80%, the researchers need to reconsider some of the elements of the design. Could treatment be extended to maximize the chance of a large between-groups difference? Could a more homogeneous group of subjects be studied to minimize the within-group variability? Could another clinic be involved to increase the sample size?

In the preceding paragraph, the between-groups difference, within-group variability, and sample size were given and the power was calculated based on those givens. When power analysis is used in the design phase of a study, however, it is usually run in "reverse." Rather than solving for "power," researchers usually specify power at 80% and solve for one of the other factors that they can control. Because the nature of the treatment and the characteristics of the subjects are often dictated by the research question, sample size is generally seen to be the most controllable factor related to power. Therefore, power analysis in the design phase is most often used to help estimate the sample size for the study.

When power analysis is used to estimate sample size, researchers must specify their desired power level, as well as the anticipated between-groups differences and within-group variability. In practice, estimating these two factors may be difficult, particularly in topic areas for which little previous research exists. When this is the case, researchers may use the concept of effect size to help them plan their sample sizes. The effect size is a ratio of the difference between the means of the pooled standard deviation of the groups being compared. For a comparison of two group means, an effect size of .20 is considered small, .50 is considered medium, and .80 is considered large.[26] Using these conventions, researchers who do not have reliable estimates of the between-groups differences and within-group variability can determine what sample sizes would be required to detect effect sizes that would be considered small, medium, and large.

Without going into computational details, for power of 80% and an alpha level of .05, the sample size requirements for a two-sample independent *t* test can be shown to be 25 per group to detect a large effect of .80, 63 per group to detect a medium effect of .50, and 392 per group to detect a small effect of .20.[26] This means that a total of 50, 126, or 784 participants would be required to detect large, medium, and small effects, respectively. Of 100 rehabilitation studies reviewed by Ottenbacher and Barrett,[29] the maximum number of participants in a study was 126. In addition, 76 of the 100 studies had fewer than 50 participants. If we assume that all 100 studies were two-group studies, this means that none of the 100 studies had enough participants to detect a small effect, only 1 could detect a medium effect, and only 23 studies could detect a large effect. Clearly, rehabilitation researchers who use group designs should work to design more powerful studies.

Power Analysis—Analysis Phase

The second use of power analysis is to compute the power of a statistical test after it has failed to identify a statistically significant difference. When a difference is not identified, the researcher and the reader wonder whether a correct conclusion has been reached or whether a type II error has been committed. A correct conclusion is ensured when the finding of no difference between the samples corresponds with the reality of no difference between the populations from which the samples were drawn. A type II error is committed when the finding of no difference between the samples is at odds with a true difference between the populations. Because the entire populations are generally not available for study, researchers never know whether they are correct or whether they have committed a type II error. The probability of making a type II error is known as beta, or β (power is $1-\beta$). Because of this relationship between power and type II errors, low probabilities of type II errors are associated with high power values. Power may be expressed as a percentage by moving the decimal two places to the right. By convention, 80% power is desirable. As noted earlier, rehabilitation research often lacks power. Thus, lack of power, or a type II error, is often a likely explanation for a nonsignificant result in rehabilitation research. Many journals require authors to follow the guidelines of the CONSORT statement, which requires that researchers present power analyses.[30] Murray[31] used power analysis in the analysis phase of her study of spoken language production in Huntington's and Parkinson's diseases, noting that the study had 75% power to detect large effect sizes, but only 30% power to detect medium effect sizes.

SUMMARY

Basic ANOVA techniques can be extended to factorial ANOVA (analyzing more than one independent variable simultaneously, including between-subjects and mixed-design models), multivariate ANOVA, or MANOVA (analyzing more than one dependent variable simultaneously) and to analysis of covariance, or ANCOVA (removing the effect of an intervening variable). Four specialized techniques for analyzing single-subject data are presented. Celeration line analysis extrapolates a baseline celeration line into the treatment phase and determines whether the distribution of data points in the treatment phase reflects a significant difference. Level, trend, slope, and variability analysis compares the characteristics of the celeration lines from different phases of the study. Two standard deviation band analysis compares actual values in the treatment phase with values that would be expected if there was no difference between treatment and baseline phases. The C statistic uses logic similar to ANOVA to compare baseline and treatment phases. Actuarial and Kaplan-Meier survival analysis methods are used to determine the proportion of patients who have and have not experienced a defined event at different points in time. Differences in survival curves can be determined by Wilcoxon rank sum, log rank, Mantel-Haenszel, and proportional hazards methods. Some researchers prefer to present their statistical findings in terms of confidence intervals rather than *p* values. Doing so involves algebraic rearrangements of traditional hypothesis-testing formulas. Power analysis can be used in the design phase of a study to determine the sample size needed to detect different effect sizes or can be used in the analysis phase to look for possible explanations of nonsignificant findings.

REFERENCES

1. Magalhaes LC, Koomar JA, Cermak SA: Bilateral motor coordination in 5- to 9-year-old children: A pilot study, *Am J Occup Ther* 43:437–443, 1989.
2. Nobusako S, Matsuo A, Morioka S: Effectiveness of the gaze direction recognition task for chronic neck pain and cervical range of motion: a randomized controlled pilot study. *Rehab Res Pract* 2012:1–13, 2012.
3. Tabachnick BG, Fidell LS: *Using Multivariate Statistics*, 6th ed, Boston, Mass, 2013, Pearson.
4. Grammatopoulou EP, Skordilis EK, Stavrou N, et al: The effect of physiotherapy-based breathing retraining on asthma control, *J Asthma* 48:593–601, 2011.
5. Egger MJ, Miller JR: Testing for experimental effects in the pretest-posttest design, *Nurs Res* 33:306–312, 1984.
6. Dimitrov DM, Rumrill PD: Pretest-posttest designs and measurement of change, *Work* 20:159–165, 2003.

Table 23-3

Characteristics of Different Correlation Coefficients

Coefficient	Characteristics
Pearson product moment correlation	Two continuous variables
Spearman's rho (ρ)	Two ranked variables; shortcut calculation of Pearson
Point biserial	One continuous variable, one dichotomous variable
Kendall's tau (τ)	Two ranked variables
Phi (φ)	Two dichotomous variables; shortcut calculation of Pearson
Cramer's V	Two categorical variables
Kappa (K)	Two or more nominal variables with two or more categories; a reliability coefficient
Intraclass correlation	Two or more continuous variables; a reliability coefficient
Partial correlation	Two variables, with effects of a third held constant
Multiple correlation	More than two variables
Canonical correlation	Two sets of variables

of relationship between two interval or ratio variables. Several are listed in Chapter 18, where correlation is introduced as a concept related to measurement theory, and Table 23-3 lists the characteristics of several additional correlation measures.

Spearman's rho (ρ) and Kendall's tau (τ) correlations are designed for use when both variables are ranked or ordinal. The point-biserial correlation is used with one continuous and one dichotomous variable. The Spearman's rho and point-biserial formulas are simply shortcut versions of the Pearson r.[5(pp. 237–238)] Correlation coefficients for use with nominal data are the phi (φ), Cramer's V, and kappa (κ) coefficients. Phi is another shortcut version of the Pearson r, applicable when both variables are dichotomous, such as in determining the relationship between sex and the answer to a yes-or-no question.[5(p. 237)] Cramer's V is used when there are two

categorical variables. Kappa, discussed in more detail in Chapter 24, is a reliability coefficient that can be used when nominal variables consist of more than two categories.

Correlation coefficients for more than two variables are also available. The intraclass correlation coefficients (ICCs), discussed more fully in Chapter 24, are a family of reliability coefficients that can be used when two or more repeated measures have been collected. Kappa can also be used with more than two nominal repeated measures. Partial correlation is used to assess the relationship between two variables with the effect of a third variable eliminated. Multiple correlation is used to assess the variability shared by three or more variables. Canonical correlation is a technique for assessing the relationships between two sets of variables.

Assumptions of the Correlation Coefficients

Calculation of the Pearson product moment and related correlation coefficients depends on three major assumptions. First, the relationships between variables are assumed to be linear. Analysis of a scatterplot of the data must show that the relationship forms a straight line. Curvilinear relationships (those that do not follow a straight line) may be analyzed, but this requires more advanced techniques than are discussed in this text. Figure 23-2 shows the scatterplot of our hypothetical total knee arthroplasty data showing the relationship between age and a new variable: length of acute care hospital stay postoperatively. There is an obvious relationship between variables, but it is not linear. Both young and very old patients have short lengths of stay, possibly because younger adults reach their ROM goals quickly and older adults are transferred to a skilled nursing facility for continued rehabilitation. Those of intermediate age stay in the hospital somewhat longer, presumably to achieve their ROM goals in the acute care hospital, without transfer to a skilled nursing facility. The Pearson r for this relationship is .3502, indicating a minimal degree of linear relationship between these two variables. If researchers rely solely on Pearson r values to guide their conclusions, they may mistakenly conclude that no relationship exists when in fact a strong nonlinear relationship exists.

The second assumption is homoscedasticity. As shown in Figure 23-3A, homoscedasticity means that for each value of one variable, the other variable has equal variability. Nonhomoscedasticity is illustrated

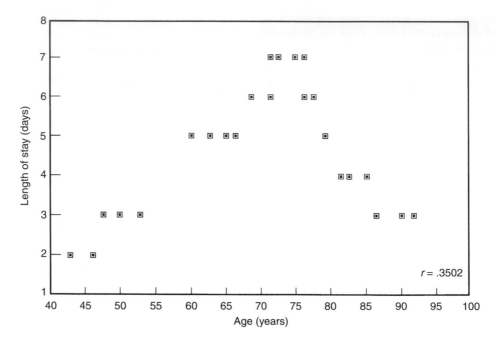

Figure 23-2 Relationship between age and length of stay. There is a strong nonlinear relationship between the two variables. The low *r* value is deceptive because it is designed to detect linear relationships only.

in Figure 23-3B. Because the calculation of Pearson *r* is based on *z* scores, whose calculation in turn depends on standard deviations for each variable, widely varying variances at different levels will distort the calculated value of *r*.

The third assumption is that both variables have enough variability to demonstrate a relationship. If either or both variables have a restricted range, the correlation coefficient will be artificially low and uninterpretable. Figure 23-4A shows the scatterplot of Clinic 3's data for 6-month ROM and gait velocity. There appears to be little relationship between the two because the data cluster in the top right corner of the graph and the Pearson *r* is −.2673. However, the range of ROM values is very restricted, with all participants showing close to full ROM of their prosthetic knees.

Figure 23-4B shows the scatterplot of 6-month ROM and gait velocity for the entire sample of 30 patients. In this example, each variable takes a fairly wide range of values, and the relationship between 6-month ROM and gait velocity is obvious. The Pearson *r* for this set of data is .6399. Thus, the restricted-range data yielded a correlation coefficient that was different in both mag-

nitude and direction from the coefficient calculated on data with a greater range of values. Restricted range issues may be present in just about any study in which relationships among variables are examined within a highly selected group of individuals such as elite athletes, students enrolled in health professions programs, or children who are identified as having marked developmental delays.

Interpretation of Correlation Coefficients

Correlation coefficients are interpreted in four major ways: (1) the strength of the coefficient itself; (2) the variance shared by the two variables, as calculated by the coefficient of determination; (3) the statistical significance of the correlation coefficient; and (4) the confidence intervals about the correlation coefficient. Regardless of which method is chosen, the interpretation should not be extrapolated beyond the range of the data used to generate the correlation coefficient.

Strength of the Coefficient

The first way to interpret the coefficient is to examine the strength of the relationship, which is independent of the

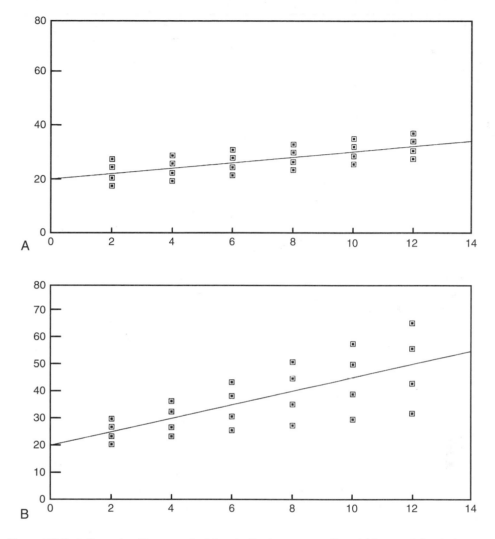

Figure 23-3 A, Example of homoscedasticity; the Y values are equally variable at each level of X. **B,** Example of nonhomoscedasticity; the Y values are not equally variable at each level of X.

direction (direct or inverse) of the relationship. This method of interpretation is exemplified by Munro's[5] descriptive terms for the strength of correlation coefficients:

.00–.25: Little, if any correlation
.26–.49: Low correlation
.50–.69: Moderate correlation
.70–.89: High correlation
.90–1.00: Very high correlation

Such a system of descriptors assumes that the meaningfulness of a correlation is the same regardless of the context in which it is used. This assumption is not necessarily valid. For example, if one is determining the reliability of a strength measure from one day to the next, an *r* of .70 may be considered

unacceptably low for the purpose of documenting day-to-day changes in status. However, if one is determining the relationship between abstract constructs such as self-esteem and motivation that are difficult to measure, then a correlation of .50 may be considered very strong.

Variance Shared by the Two Variables

The second way to evaluate the importance of the correlation coefficient is to calculate what is called the *coefficient of determination*. The coefficient of determination, r^2, is the square of the correlation coefficient, *r*. The coefficient of determination is an indication of the percentage of variance that is shared by the two

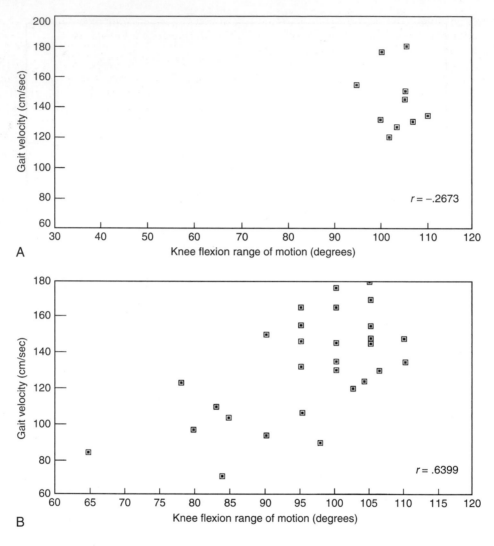

Figure 23-4 A, Restricted range of the X variable results in a low correlation coefficient. **B,** The addition of a broader range of X values reveals a pattern that was not apparent in **A.**

variables. For the relationship between 6-month ROM and gait velocity at Clinic 1 (see Table 23-1), the coefficient of determination is approximately .58 ($.76^2 = .5776$). This means that 58% of the variability within one variable can be accounted for by the other variable. The remaining 42% of the variability is due to variables not yet considered—perhaps height, leg length, pain, age, or sex. Using the coefficient of determination, we find, for example, that a "high" correlation coefficient of .70 accounts for only 49% of the variance among the variables, and a "low" correlation of .30 accounts for an even lower 9% of the variance between the variables.

Statistical Significance of the Coefficient

The third method of interpreting correlation coefficients is to statistically determine whether the coefficient calculated is significantly different from zero. In other words, we determine the probability that the calculated correlation coefficient would have occurred by chance if in fact there was no relationship between the variables. A special form of a *t* test is used to determine this probability. The problem with this approach is that very weak correlations may be statistically different from zero even though they are not very meaningful. This is particularly likely to occur with large samples. For example, Alexander and associates[6] studied the relationship between different components of stroke rehabilitation and health outcomes in 152 individuals and found a statistically significant correlation of .174 between the number of sessions of speech and language therapy and general health 3 months after stroke. Although statistically significant, a correlation of this magnitude probably does not describe a clinically meaningful relationship.

Confidence Intervals Around the Coefficient

The fourth way to determine the meaningfulness of a correlation coefficient is to calculate a confidence interval about the correlation coefficient. To do so, a researcher converts the r values into z scores, calculates confidence intervals with the z scores, and transforms the z score intervals back into a range of r scores. Using steps outlined by Munro,[5(pp. 236–237)] the 95% confidence interval for an r of .76 for 6-month ROM and gait velocity at Clinic 1 is .17 to .94. The confidence interval is very large because the sample is small ($n = 10$) and does not permit accurate estimation. Using the same procedures, the 95% confidence interval for the same r calculated for a sample of 100 participants is approximately .65 to .83, a far smaller interval. As is the case for the confidence intervals calculated in the analysis of differences, larger samples permit more accurate estimation of true population values.

Limits of Interpretation

A consideration common to all four interpretation methods is that the interpretation of correlation coefficients should not extend beyond the range of the original data. For example, Figure 23-5 shows the fairly strong relationship between the 6-month ROM and gait velocity data *(asterisks)*. The line showing the trend of the data is extrapolated to a ROM of 0°. At this ROM, the trend line indicates that the gait velocity would be estimated to be approximately negative 38 cm/s—an impossible figure! Rather than being a linear relationship throughout the ROM, it is likely that the relationship becomes curvilinear as ROM becomes closer to 0°, with gait velocity bottoming out at some low level *(crosses)*. Knowing that the relationship between ROM and gait velocity is strong and linear in the top half of the usual values does not permit us to extrapolate these conclusions to values outside the ranges encountered in the original data collection.

Literature Examples

Alexander and colleagues[6] studied the relationships between different components of stroke rehabilitation

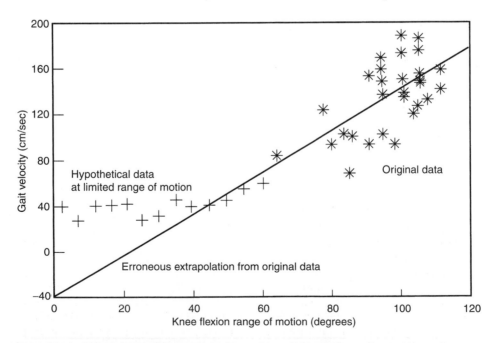

Figure 23-5 Extending interpretation of regression beyond the original data results in invalid conclusions. Original data *(asterisks)* extrapolated past the X and Y values predict that patients with no flexion range of motion will have a negative gait velocity. Crosses indicate the more likely relationship between the two variables in their lower ranges.

and health outcomes. They chose to present an extensive correlation matrix showing the relationships between six measures of rehabilitation inputs (number of sessions of physical therapy, occupational therapy, speech and language therapy, dietetics, podiatry, and community nursing) and 27 measures of outcomes (nine measures, each taken at 1 month, 3 months, and 6 months after stroke). The importance of the various correlations in the study was evaluated by determining the statistical significance of the correlations and by discussing the pattern of significance seen across the variables.

Wert and colleagues[7] investigated the relationship of age, gait biomechanics (hip extension, trunk flexion, and foot-floor angle at heel-strike), and gait characteristics (step width, stance time, and cadence) to energy costs of walking in 50 community-dwelling older adults who ambulated without an assistive device. They determined Pearson or Spearman correlation coefficients for each of the variables, reporting that three of the six gait parameters' relationships (0.373 to 0.523) were important to the energy costs of walking. They calculated 36 correlations and evaluated each for statistical significance.

The alternate correlation coefficient, Cramer's V, was used by Harter and associates[8] to document the relationship between instrumented and manual Lachman ligament laxity testing. They interpreted the V coefficient of .27 with significance testing, finding that the

relationship between the two types of laxity testing was not significant.

LINEAR REGRESSION

Correlational techniques, as discussed earlier, are used to describe the relationships among two or more variables. When the researcher's purpose extends beyond description of relationships to include prediction of future characteristics from previously collected data, the statistical analysis extends from correlation to regression techniques.

Suppose we wish to predict a patient's eventual gait velocity on the basis of an early postoperative indicator such as 3-week ROM. The Pearson product moment correlation between these two variables is .5545, indicating a moderate degree of correlation in which 31% of the variability in gait velocity ($r^2 = .3075$) can be accounted for by variability in 3-week ROM. Unlike correlation techniques, regression techniques require that variables be defined as independent (or a level of an independent variable) or dependent. In this example, the independent variable is 3-week ROM and is used to predict the dependent variable, gait velocity.

Figure 23-6 shows a scatterplot of 3-week ROM and gait velocity scores, with a line showing the best fit between these two variables. This line is generated

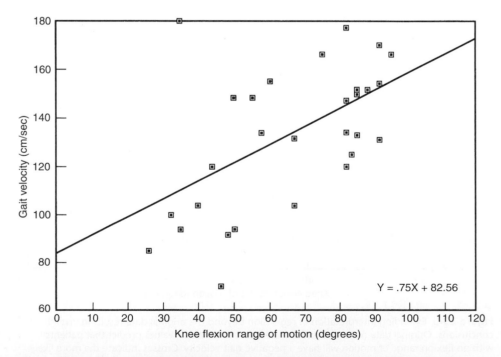

Figure 23-6 Regression of gait velocity on 3-week knee flexion range of motion.

by using the data to solve the general equation for a straight line:

$$Y = bX + a$$

where *b* is the slope of the line and *a* is the intercept (i.e., the Y value at the point at which the line intersects the Y-axis). The slope, *b*, is found by multiplying the Pearson *r* value by the ratio of the standard deviation of Y to the standard deviation of X: [$b=r(sy/sx)$]. The intercept, *a,* is found by subtracting the product of the slope and the mean of X from the mean of Y: ($a=Y\simeq X-b$). As with most statistical analyses today, computer programs can generate regression equations quickly and easily without the need for hand calculations. The formula for the regression line of gait velocity on 3-week ROM is Y=0.75X+82.56. Although this equation defines the best-fitting line through the data, most of the points do not fall precisely on the line. The vertical distance from each point to the line is known as the *residual*, and the mean of the residuals is zero. The standard deviation of the residuals is known as the *standard error of the estimate* (SEE).

After the regression equation is generated, it can be used to predict the gait velocity of future patients by solving for Y (gait velocity) on the basis of the patient's X (3-week ROM) score. For example, suppose that a patient has 70° of ROM 3 weeks postoperatively. The predicted gait velocity for this patient is 135.06 cm/s [0.75(70)+82.56=135.06]. Because we know that this prediction is unlikely to be precise, we can provide additional useful information by generating a confidence interval around the predicted value. The confidence interval around the predicted value is created by using the SEE. A 95% confidence interval, for example, is created by adding and subtracting 1.96 SEEs from the regression line, as shown graphically in Figure 23-7. In this example, the SEE generated by the computer is 24.54 cm/s, and the 95% confidence interval would be found by adding and subtracting 48.09 cm/s to and from the predicted Y value. For patients with 3-week ROM of 70°, we therefore are 95% certain that their gait velocity at 6 months will be between 86.96 and 183.16 cm/s. Ideally, the dependent variable is highly correlated with the independent variable, resulting in small residuals, a small SEE, and a more precise prediction.

The statistical significance of a regression equation is usually determined with an *F* test to evaluate whether r^2, the amount of variance in Y predicted by X, is significantly different from zero. As is the case with statistical testing of the correlation coefficient using a *t* test, r^2 may be statistically different from zero without being terribly meaningful. In our example, the r^2 of .3075 is significantly different from zero at p=.0015. Despite this statistical significance, we know that the 95%

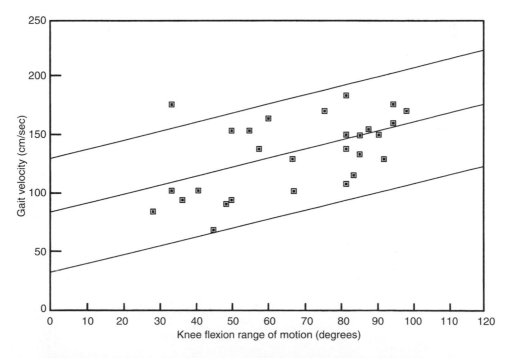

Figure 23-7 Ninety-five percent confidence intervals around the predicted gait velocity.

confidence interval for predicting a single score is quite large and may not allow for clinically useful prediction. For instance, the gait velocity needed to cross most streets safely is approximately 130 cm/s.[9] The range of the confidence interval is great enough that for most patients, we could not predict whether their eventual velocity would enable them to be community ambulators. This reflects the fact that there is only a moderate correlation between the two variables in question.

In practice, then, this regression equation would not likely be perceived to be very useful, and the researchers would search for additional independent variables that would allow for more precise prediction of the dependent variable. When more than one variable is used to predict another variable, the simple linear regression technique is extended to multiple regression, as discussed in Chapter 24.

SUMMARY

Relationship analysis studies are generally nonexperimental, with the researcher observing different phenomena rather than manipulating groups of participants. The magnitude and direction of relationships between variables are expressed mathematically as Pearson product moment correlations or a variety of alternative correlation coefficients. Assumptions for use of the correlation coefficients include linearity, homoscedasticity, and an adequate range of values for each variable. Correlation coefficients are interpreted in several ways: by the strength of the coefficient itself, by the coefficient of determination, by the statistical significance of the correlation coefficient, and by confidence intervals about the correlation coefficient. When the researcher's purpose extends beyond description of relationships to include prediction, the statistical analysis extends from correlation to regression techniques.

REFERENCES

1. Katz-Leuer M, Rotemh H, Lewitus H, et al: Relationship between balance abilities and gait characteristics in children with post-traumatic brain injury, *Brain Inj* 22(2):153–159, 2008.
2. Beaton DE, Katz JN, Fossel AH, et al: Measuring the whole or the parts? Validity, reliability, and responsiveness of the Disabilities of the Arm, Shoulder, and Hand outcome measure in different regions of the upper extremity, *J Hand Ther* 14:128–146, 2001.
3. Godi M, Franchignoni F, Caligari M, et al: Comparison of reliability, validity, and responsiveness of the Mini-BESTest and Berg Balance Scale in patients with balance disorders, *Phys Ther* 93:158–167, 2013.
4. Swartz HM, Flood AB: The corntinental theory of flat and depressed areas: On the relationship between corn and topography, *J Irreproducible Results* 35(5):16–17, 1990.
5. Plichta Kellar S, Kelvin E: *Munro's Statistical Methods for Health Care Research*, 6th ed, Philadelphia, Pa, 2013, Lippincott Williams & Wilkins.
6. Alexander H, Bugge C, Hagen S: What is the association between the different components of stroke rehabilitation and health outcomes? *Clin Rehabil* 15:207–215, 2001.
7. Wert DM, Brach J, Perera S, VanSwearingen JM: Gait biomechanics, spatial and temporal characteristics, and the energy cost of walking in older adults with impaired mobility, *Phys Ther* 90:977–985, 2010.
8. Harter RD, Osternig LA, Singer KM, Cord SA: A comparison of instrumented and manual Lachman test results in anterior cruciate ligament-reconstructed knees, *Athl Train* 25:330–334, 1990.
9. Lerner-Frankiel MB, Vargas S, Brown M, et al: Functional community ambulation: What are your criteria? *Clin Manag Phys Ther* 6(2):12–15, 1986.

CHAPTER 24

Statistical Analysis of Relationships: Advanced

CHAPTER OUTLINE

Reliability Analysis
  Pearson Product Moment
    Correlation with Extensions
  Intraclass Correlation Coefficients
  Kappa
Multiple Regression
  Variable Entry in Multiple
    Regression

Interpretation of the Multiple
    Regression Equation
  Literature Examples
Logistic Regression
  Rationale for Logistic
    Regression
  Literature Examples
Discriminant Analysis

Factor Analysis
  Factor Analysis Steps
  Literature Examples
Summary

Chapter 23 introduced basic correlation and regression techniques by emphasizing bivariate procedures—that is, those in which just two variables are involved. In addition, the techniques presented in Chapter 23 were used to analyze relationships between distinctly different variables such as age and gait velocity. In this chapter, which covers more advanced correlation and regression techniques, these basic concepts are extended in two ways. First, specialized reliability correlation coefficients, in which repeated measures of the same variable are analyzed, are examined. Second, procedures that examine the complex interrelationships among many variables are introduced. These procedures include multiple regression, logistic regression, discriminant analysis, and factor analysis.

RELIABILITY ANALYSIS

A specialized type of relationship analysis is used to assess the reliability of a measure. As discussed in Chapter 18, there are two major classes of reliability measures: those that document relative reliability and those that document absolute reliability. It is the measures of relative reliability that depend on correlational techniques. In some instances, the correlational technique does not provide all of the desired reliability information, and regression or difference analysis techniques are used to supplement the correlational technique. Three techniques used for reliability analysis are

presented here: the Pearson product moment correlation with regression and difference analysis extensions, the intraclass correlation coefficients, and the kappa correlations.

Pearson Product Moment Correlation with Extensions

The discussion of reliability coefficients begins with the Pearson product moment correlation coefficient not because it is an ideal reliability coefficient (it is not), but because it is familiar. The fact that extensions to the Pearson correlation coefficient are needed to make it an acceptable reliability coefficient suggests that researchers might do better with correlations that are specifically designed to quantify reliability.[1] The central problem with the Pearson product moment correlation as a reliability coefficient is that it is only a measure of relative reliability: A high, positive Pearson value indicates that high scores on one measure are associated with high scores on another measure and that low scores on one measure are associated with low scores on another measure. When we compare two different variables, such as 3-week range-of-motion (ROM) and gait velocity, the strength of the relationship is the only information we desire, so the Pearson correlation is ideal.

When comparing paired measurements for the purpose of determining their reliability, however, we are concerned with both the relationship between the two measures and the magnitude of the differences between the two measures. These two forms of reliability are called *relative reliability* and *absolute reliability* (also *association* and *concordance*), respectively. Alone, the Pearson product moment correlation (introduced in Chapter 23) is not a complete tool for documenting reliability because it assesses association and not concordance.

There are three strategies used by researchers to supplement the information gained from the Pearson correlation coefficient: paired-*t* test, slope and intercept documentation, and determination of the standard error of measurement (SEM). They are all demonstrated in this section using a data sample representing repeated measures of 3-week ROM made by Therapists A and B at Clinic 3, as shown in Table 24-1. Therapist B consistently rates participants higher than Therapist A—in fact, an average of 10.8° higher. The participant who scores highest for Therapist A also scores highest for Therapist B, even though the actual ROM scores differ based on which therapist took the measure. Thus, the relative reliability is high, with a Pearson *r* of .977. However, to assume that the scores are interchangeable would clearly be incorrect given the average 10.8° difference between therapist measures.

The first way to extend the reliability analysis beyond the Pearson measure of relative reliability is to conduct a paired-*t* test on the data. For our data, *t* is 8.11, with an associated probability of .000. This means

that there is a very small chance that the difference between therapists' scores occurred by chance, so we conclude that there is a significant difference between the scores of Therapist A and Therapist B. The scores from the two therapists are highly associated but lack concordance.

The second way to extend the reliability analysis beyond the Pearson measure is to generate a regression equation for the data and document the slope and intercept. If a measure is absolutely reliable, the slope will be close to 1.0, and the intercept will be close to 0.0.[2] In Figure 24-1, the dotted line represents perfect concordance between the two repeated measures, with a slope of 1.0 and an intercept of zero. The solid line represents a proportionate bias on the part of Rater 2. The intercept is still zero, but the slope exceeds 1.0. In Figure 24-2, the dotted line again represents perfect concordance between the two repeated measures, with a slope of 1.0 and an intercept of zero. The solid line represents an additive bias on the part of Rater 2, with scores consistently 5 points higher than those of Rater 1. The slope of this regression line is still 1.0, but the intercept is now 5.0. For the Therapist A and B data, the slope is 1.0156, and the intercept is 9.666, as shown in Figure 24-3. This indicates the presence of a largely additive bias on the part of one of the therapists.

The third way to add to the usefulness of the Pearson product moment correlation for documenting reliability is to report the SEM for the paired data. Using the formula presented in Chapter 18, ($SEM = \sigma\sqrt{1-r}$), we find that the SEM for these data is 2.96, meaning that a 95% confidence interval for two repeated measurements would be ±8.2 ($\sqrt{2} \times 2.96 \times 1.96$), permitting us to be 95% confident that repeated measures would fall within 8.2 of one another. The results of an extended Pearson reliability analysis might be written up as follows:

DATA ANALYSIS: To assess the association between the two therapists' scores, the Pearson product moment correlation was calculated. The concordance of the scores was assessed by calculation of the slope and intercept of the regression equation of one therapist's scores on the other, determination of the SEM, and calculation of a paired-*t* test.

RESULTS: The Pearson *r* was found to be .977, indicating a high degree of association between the scores of the two therapists. However, the slope was 1.02, and the intercept was 9.67. The 95% confidence interval for the SEM was 8.2. The paired-*t* test revealed that the 10.8 mean difference between therapist scores was statistically significant at the .000 level.

Table 24-1

Reliability Data for 3-Week Range-of-Motion Measurements by Therapists A and B

Subject	Therapist A	Therapist B	Difference (B ≅ A)
1	32	38	6
2	50	64	14
3	60	73	13
4	84	90	6
5	81	87	6
6	81	93	12
7	84	94	10
8	81	98	17
9	82	98	16
10	91	99	8
Σ	726.0	834.0	108.0
$\bar{X}$	72.6	83.4	10.8

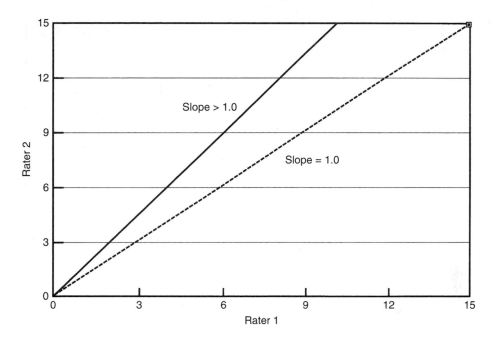

Figure 24-1 Proportionate bias between raters is revealed by a slope greater than 1.0. The *dotted line* represents perfect agreement with a slope of 1.0 and an intercept of 0.0.

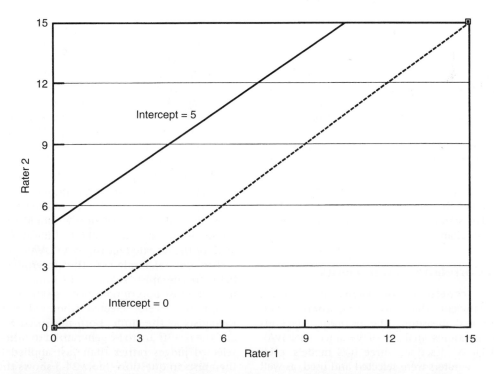

Figure 24-2 Additive bias between raters is revealed by an intercept equal to 5.0. The *dotted line* represents perfect agreement with a slope of 1.0 and an intercept of 0.0.

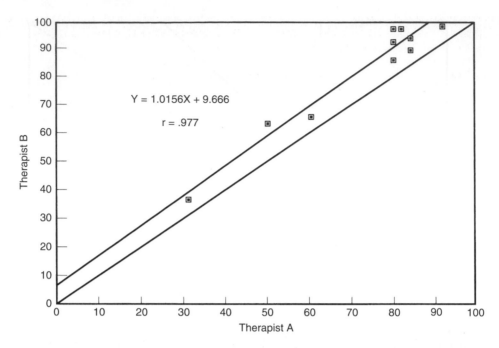

Figure 24-3 Bias between Therapist A and Therapist B. There is almost no proportionate bias (slope=1.0156), but there is a large additive bias (intercept=9.666°).

DISCUSSION: Despite the high degree of association between the measures taken by Therapist A and Therapist B, the absolute difference between scores means that the absolute interrater reliability is too low for the measures of the two therapists to be considered interchangeable.

Readers should recognize that researchers would probably not use all three extensions in a single study. Any one of these extensions in this case would be sufficient to cast doubt on the absolute reliability of the measures. This example also illustrates that the Pearson correlation alone is not an acceptable way to measure reliability, a point that is reinforced in Hyde's[3] analysis of psychometric standards for outcomes measures used in audiological rehabilitation.

Intraclass Correlation Coefficients

The intraclass correlation coefficients (ICCs) are a family of coefficients that allow comparison of two or more repeated measures. The technique depends on repeated measures analysis of variance (ANOVA). Shrout and Fleiss[4] described three ICC models, each differing on how raters were selected and used, as well as to which subjects the raters were assigned. There are also three different forms, which indicate the number

of measurements on which the ICC is calculated. There are at least six different ICC formulas, and the issue of which one to use in a particular calculation has generated considerable confusion.[5] When an ICC is reported, the model and form are to be indicated in parentheses immediately after the coefficient [e.g., ICC=0.84, (2,1)]. Table 24-2 provides two of the formulas and indications for their use, based on the work of Shrout and Fleiss.[4] In addition to being able to handle more than two repeated measures, the ICC is thought to be a better measure than the Pearson *r* because it accounts for absolute as well as relative reliability. However, because they take into account "level" differences, but are not true measures of concordance,[2] researchers who report reliability on the basis of an ICC should still report the results of an absolute reliability indicator such as the SEM[1] or the repeated measures ANOVA.

For our example of the interrater reliability between Therapists A and B at Clinic 3, the ICC (2,1) may be most appropriate because the two therapists in question were selected from a larger group of therapists at the clinic; both measured each patient, and the results are to be generalized to other randomly selected judges rather than just applied to the two therapists in question. Table 24-3 shows the ICC (2,1) calculation to be .854. This is less than the .977 that was calculated with the Pearson product moment

Table 24-2

Calculations of Intraclass Correlation Coefficients (ICCs)

Source of Variation	Degrees of Freedom	Mean Square (MS)
Between subjects	$N* - 1$	Between subjects (BMS)
Within subject	$N(K^\dagger - 1)$	Within subject (WMS)
Between judges	$K - 1$	Between judges (JMS)
Error	$(N-1)(K-1)$	Error (EMS)

Formula	Appropriate Use
$$ICC(1,1) = \frac{BMS - WMS}{BMS + (K-1)WMS}$$	Each subject is rated by different randomly selected judges.
$$ICC(2,1) = \frac{BMS - EMS}{BMS + (K-1)EMS + \dfrac{K(JMS - EMS)}{N}}$$	Each subject is rated by the same randomly selected judges.

*Subjects.
†Judges.

Table 24-3

ICC (2,1) Calculation for 3-Week Range of Motion for Therapists A and B

Source of Variation	Degrees of Freedom	Mean Square (MS)	F	p
Between subjects	9	734.78 (BMS)		
Within subject	10	66.30 (WMS)		
Between judges	1	583.20 (JMS)	65.7	.000
Error	9	8.87 (EMS)		

$$ICC(2,1) = \frac{BMS - EMS}{BMS + (K-1)EMS + \dfrac{K*(JMS - EMS)}{N^\dagger}}$$

$$ICC(2,1) = \frac{734.78 - 8.87}{734.78 + (2-1)8.87 + \dfrac{(2)(583.20 - 8.87)}{10}} = .854$$

*Judges.
†Subjects.

correlation, but it still generally would be interpreted to be a fairly high level of correlation. Thus, it is useful to examine the results of a repeated measures ANOVA, which shows that there is a significant difference between the measures of the two therapists, $F_{1,9} = 65.7$, $p = .000$. Using the repeated measures ANOVA results with an ICC is analogous to using a paired-t test to extend the results of a Pearson product moment correlation reliability analysis.

Although this example of an ICC used only two raters to compare the results with those found with the Pearson product moment correlation analysis in the previous section, the ICC, like the ANOVA it is based on, extends easily to accommodate more than two raters. When only two raters are present, the researcher has a choice between the Pearson and an ICC; when three or more raters measure each participant, an ICC must be used.

Katz-Leuer and colleagues[6] employed an ICC (1,1) to examine within-session reliability of the Modified Functional Reach Test (MFRT) and the Timed Up and Go (TUG) with children with traumatic brain injury (TBI), as well as typically developing (TD) children. They reported that the within-session reliability for the MFRT for both groups of children was excellent (≥0.94) and good for the TUG for both groups (≥0.85). Because the researchers were interested only in the error between the first and second assessments of each test, the ICC (1,1) was appropriate for this study.

Wong[7] examined the interrater reliability of the Berg Balance Scale (BBS), comparing the scores of 16 testers who rated the videotaped performances of five persons, poststroke, on the BBS. Additionally, Wong studied the intrarater reliability of the BBS by comparing the scores of two testers who rated independently, in vivo, the five persons who were poststroke, to the same two testers' scores obtained from the videotaped assessments. In both instances, the two-way random ICC (2,k) was employed. Intrarater reliability and interrater reliability were excellent, with both having ICC of 0.99.

Kappa

Kappa is a reliability coefficient designed for use with nominal data. Suppose that we wanted to determine whether Therapists A and B at Clinic 3 agreed with each other on the stair-climbing ability of their patients. Table 24-4 shows the cross-tabulation of the data of Therapists A and B. For 6 of the 10 patients, the therapists gave identical scores. For 4 of the 10 patients, the therapists differed by one category. The simplest way to express the degree of concordance between the therapists' observations is to calculate the percentage of patients on whose ability the two therapists agreed completely. For this example, the agreement is 60%. However, because there are only a few nominal categories, there is a high probability that some of the agreements occurred by chance. The kappa correlation coefficient adjusts the agreement percentage to account for chance agreements, as shown in the formula at the bottom of Table 24-4.[8] The kappa for this example is .3939.

Kappa can also be weighted to account for the seriousness of the discrepancy.[9] Consider one disagreement in which one rater scores the patient as a 5 in stair climbing (reciprocal, no railing) and the other scores the patient as a 4 (reciprocal, with rail). Contrast this with a disagreement between a 4 and a 3 (one at a time, with or without rail). Some might believe that disagreement on the use of a rail is a less serious reliability problem than disagreement

Table 24-4

Kappa Correlation Calculation

| Therapist B | THERAPIST A | | | | |
	5	4	3	2	Total
5	2 (.20) [.12]	1			3 (.30)
4	2	3 (.30) [.20]			5 (.50)
3			1 (.10) [.02]		1 (.10)
2				1	1 (.10)
Total	4 (.40)	4 (.40)	2 (.20)		10 (1.0)

$$\kappa = \frac{p_0 - p_c}{1 - p_c} = \frac{.60 - .34}{1 - .34} = .3939$$

Note: Numbers are the number of observations in the cell. Numbers in parentheses are the proportion of observations in the cell. Numbers in brackets are the proportion of observations expected by chance in the cell. The proportion expected by chance is calculated by multiplying the marginal proportion (total row or column) for the corresponding row and column.

p_0, sum of the observed probabilities in perfect agreement = .60.
p_c, sum of the chance probabilities for perfect agreement = .34.

about whether the patient can maneuver the stairs reciprocally. A weighted kappa allows the researcher to establish different weights for different disagreements. In addition to occurring in weighted and nonweighted forms, kappa can be extended to more than two raters.[10]

Van Dillen and colleagues[11] studied the reliability of physical examination items used for classification of patients with low back pain. Many of the items required patients to report whether their symptoms were the same, decreased, or increased in response to a particular movement. Other items described alignment and movement, scoring the items as "yes" or "no" based on whether a patient exhibited the various alignment or movement patterns. Because these scoring systems are nominal, the authors used kappa to determine reliability. For the symptom behavior items, the agreement percentage ranged from 98% to 100%, and the corresponding kappas ranged from .87 to 1.00. For the alignment and movement variables, the agreement percentage ranged from 55% to 100%, and the corresponding kappas ranged from .00 to .78. Landis and Koch[12] described the strength of agreement of kappa to be slight for kappas between .00 and .20, fair between .21 and .40, moderate between .41 and .60, substantial between .61 and .80, and almost perfect for .81 to 1.00. According to these descriptors, Van Dillen and colleagues[11] found almost perfect correlations for the symptom behavior items but wide variation in the strengths of agreement (from slight to substantial) for the alignment and movement variables.

MULTIPLE REGRESSION

Multiple regression techniques are designed to analyze complex relationships among many different variables. Traditional multiple regression uses numerical independent variables to predict a numerical dependent variable.[13(pp. 213–222)] With the development of large databases containing many cases and many different variables, multiple regression strategies are more feasible than ever, but no less difficult to implement effectively.[14] In the small data set used throughout this text, gait velocity is a continuous numerical variable that is appropriate for analysis with multiple regression. Many of the independent variables we might use to generate a multiple regression equation would also be numerical variables such as age, height, leg length, and weight. In addition to these variables, however, we might also wish to include some nominal independent variables such as gender (male, female) or postoperative complications (yes, no). Even though multiple regression techniques were designed for use with numerical variables, they can accommodate nominal independent variables if a different number is assigned to each of the nominal levels. For example, the presence of a postoperative complication might be entered as a "1," whereas the absence of a complication would be entered as a "0." This process of assigning arbitrary numbers to nominal independent variables is called *dummy coding*.

In Chapter 23, simple linear regression was used to predict 6-month gait velocity (the dependent variable) from 3-week ROM of patients after total knee arthroplasty. A regression equation was calculated, but it was not very precise, with 3-week ROM accounting for only 31% of the variability in gait velocity. Clearly, there are factors other than 3-week ROM that must account for the gait velocity of these patients.

Because the prediction of gait velocity from 3-week ROM is not precise enough to be useful clinically, the next logical step is to add an additional variable or variables to the equation to determine whether the prediction can be made more precise. For example, suppose we add patients' age to the equation. The general prediction equation for multiple regression is as follows:

$$Y = b_1X_1 + b_2X_2 + b_iX_i + a$$

For each independent variable, there is a corresponding slope, which is referred to in multiple regression as a b-weight. For the entire equation there is one intercept, which is referred to as the constant. The computer-generated regression equation for 3-week ROM and age as predictors of gait velocity is as follows:

$$(\text{velocity}) = -.04(3-\text{week ROM}) - 1.41(\text{age}) + 227.04$$

A 65-year-old patient with 70° of motion 3 weeks postoperatively would be predicted to have a gait velocity of 138.19 cm/s 6 months postoperatively:

$$.04(70) - 1.41(65) + 227.04 = 138.19$$

The raw regression coefficient for age can be interpreted as follows: If ROM is held constant, for each 1-year increase in age, the velocity prediction decreases by 1.41 cm/s. If age is held constant, for each 1° increase in ROM, the velocity prediction increases by only .04 cm/s.

The correlation between all the independent variables and the dependent variable in a multiple regression equation is represented by R, to distinguish it from r, the correlation between the two variables in a simple linear regression equation. For this equation, the multiple correlation, R, is .77483, and the R^2 is .55477. This means that the combination of 3-week ROM and age accounts for 55% of the variability in gait velocity. Recall that 3-week ROM alone accounted for only 31% of the variability in gait velocity. The addition of age to the equation has greatly improved its predictability.

Variable Entry in Multiple Regression

When performing a multiple regression, researchers often specify various decision rules to guide the computer in generating the regression equation. The rules are generally constructed so that the method of variable entry maximizes the accuracy of predictions while minimizing the number of variables in the equation. Variables are retained in the equation if they improve the R^2 by a specified amount or if they are associated with a probability of some specified amount.

In a forward regression strategy, a researcher adds one variable at a time and stops when additional variables do not contribute the preset amount. In a backward regression strategy, the researcher begins with all the possible variables of interest in the equation and deletes them one at a time if their presence does not contribute the preset amount. A stepwise regression strategy combines forward and backward procedures to generate the equation. If any of these strategies were used in our example, the age variable would be entered first, and the 3-week ROM variable would not be entered because it contributes so little beyond that of age. For example, the R^2 associated with age alone is .55432; for age and 3-week ROM combined, it is only .55497, an increase of only .00045. This means that the addition of 3-week ROM to the equation adds only .045% of additional predictability for gait velocity. Clinically, this means that, if our interest is primarily in predicting gait velocity, we can eliminate the possibly inconvenient and expensive measurement of 3-week ROM and substitute the inexpensive, easily obtained age value.

Interpretation of the Multiple Regression Equation

The meaningfulness of the multiple regression equation can be assessed in several ways. First, an F test of R^2 can be conducted to determine whether it is significantly different from zero. For our example, the computer-generated significance of the F test is .0000, indicating that there is a very low probability that the R^2 of .55477 was obtained by chance.

The second way to assess the meaningfulness of a multiple regression equation is to generate a confidence interval. The computer-generated standard error of the estimate (SEE) for the multiple regression equation is 20.03 cm/s, and a 95% confidence interval would add and subtract 39.27 cm/s to the predicted Y value [±1.96 (SEE)]. Thus, we could be 95% certain that our 65-year-old patient with 70° of knee flexion 3 weeks postoperatively would have a 6-month gait velocity of 98.92 to 177.46 cm/s. Recall that the 95% confidence interval for the simple regression of gait velocity on ROM was 86.96 to 183.16 cm/s, as presented in Chapter 23. Because a greater proportion of the variability in gait velocity is accounted for by the multiple regression compared with the simple regression, this multiple regression interval is somewhat narrower than the simple regression interval.

A third way to evaluate the regression equation is to determine the relative contribution of each of the variables to the equation. This can be done by either conducting a t test of the contribution of each variable or dividing the R^2 into the components attributable to each variable. This division is done through beta (β)-weights, which are standardized versions of b-weights. The beta-weight for each variable is multiplied by the correlation coefficient between that variable and the dependent variable. For our example, the mathematical notation is:

$$R^2 = \left(\beta_{3\text{-week ROM}}\right)\left(r_{3\text{-week ROM, velocity}}\right) + \left(\beta_{age}\right)\left(r_{age, velocity}\right)$$

Using computer-generated beta-weights and correlation coefficients, we find the following:

$$.5547 = (.0305)(.5545) + (-.7224)(-.7445)$$
$$= .0169 + .5378$$

This means that of the 55% of the variability in gait velocity predicted by the equation, almost 54% is due to the relationship between age and gait velocity and less than 2% is due to the relationship between 3-week ROM and velocity. The t tests of the contribution of variables yield significance levels of .8711 for 3-week ROM and .0006 for age. Both the division of R^2 and the t tests indicate that age is a much more important predictor of gait velocity than is 3-week ROM.

Recall that in the simple linear regression of gait velocity on 3-week ROM, the ROM variable accounted for approximately 31% of the variability in gait scores. How is it that it now accounts for only 2% of that variability? The answer can be found in an examination of the interrelationships among all three variables. The Venn diagrams in Figure 24-4 illustrate this principle. Independently, 3-week ROM accounts for about 31% of the variability in gait velocity, as shown in Figure 24-4A. Independently, age accounts for about 55% of the variability in gait velocity, as shown in Figure 24-4B. In addition, age and 3-week ROM are highly related, with one variable accounting for approximately 53% ($r_{age, 3\text{-week ROM}} = -.7253$) of the variability in the other, as shown in Figure 24-4C. When all three are examined together, almost all of the variability in velocity that is accounted for by 3-week ROM is also accounted for by the relationship between age and velocity. Thus, in the regression of gait velocity on both age and 3-week ROM, the latter assumes much less importance than when it is the sole variable used to predict gait velocity.

With the availability of computer-based statistical packages, it is deceptively easy to run multiple regression analyses. However, factors that influence the validity of multiple regression procedures include the extent of multicollinearity (high levels of correlation among the predictor variables, which is undesirable), cross-validation of the regression equation with a second sample of participants or with random subsets of the original sample, adequate sample size, and how outlying data points are handled.[15]

The results of this multiple regression analysis might be written up in a journal article as follows:

DATA ANALYSIS: Simple linear regression of gait velocity on 3-week range of motion (ROM) was used initially to test whether early ROM status could be used to predict eventual function as

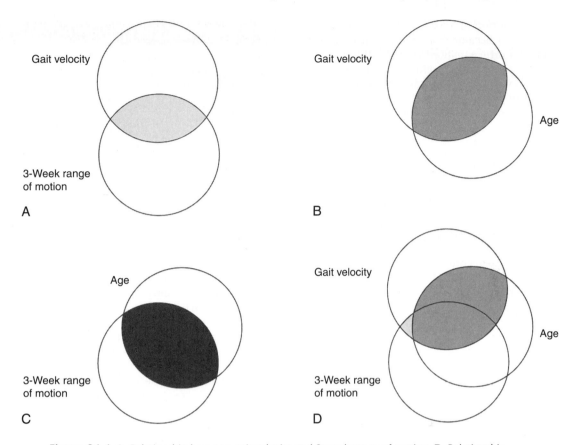

Figure 24-4 A, Relationship between gait velocity and 3-week range of motion. **B,** Relationship between gait velocity and age. **C,** Relationship between 3-week range of motion and age. **D,** Relationship of both age and 3-week range of motion to gait velocity. Most of the variability in gait velocity accounted for by 3-week range of motion is also accounted for by age.

measured by gait velocity. Multiple regression was used to add the variable of age to the prediction equation when 3-week ROM proved to be an inadequate independent predictor. The significance of each variable was determined with a *t* test, the significance of R^2 was determined with an *F* test, and alpha was set at .05. In addition, confidence intervals around the predicted Y value were generated.

RESULTS: For the simple regression of gait velocity on 3-week ROM, *r* was only .5545. Although significantly different from zero (*p*=.0015), this means that only 30.75% of the variance in gait velocity was accounted for by 3-week ROM. The 95% confidence interval around the predicted gait velocity score for a given individual would require that 48.09 cm/s be added to and subtracted from the predicted score.

To enhance predictability, a multiple regression equation was developed to predict gait velocity

from both 3-week ROM and age. The equation developed from the two predictor variables was: velocity=.04(3-week ROM)−1.41(age)+227.04. The R^2 for this equation was .5547 and was significant at *p*=.0000. The contribution of age was .5378 and was significant at *p*=.0006; the contribution of 3-week ROM was only .0169 and was not significant at *p*=.8711. For this equation, the 95% confidence interval around the predicted gait velocity score for a given individual would require that 39.27 cm/s be added to and subtracted from the predicted score.

DISCUSSION: The simple regression of gait velocity on 3-week ROM did not confirm the clinical observation that early ROM status is a good predictor of eventual gait outcome. When age was added to the equation, prediction of gait velocity improved. However, the very strong relationship between age and gait velocity meant that the contribution of 3-week ROM to prediction of gait velocity became insignificant when age was included in the equation. Thus, for this group of patients, eventual gait velocity can be predicted almost as well by age alone as by the combination of age and 3-week ROM.

Literature Examples

Brown and colleagues[16] used multiple regression to study the amount of variance in functional skills that was predicted by cognitive and perceptual abilities of persons who, following a stroke, received intensive rehabilitation. Of the 10 subscales of cognitive performance and 6 subscales of perceptual performance, the investigators reported that 4 and 3 subscales, respectively, were significantly correlated with the measure of functional skill (Barthel Index). The regression analysis found the cognitive variables predicted 64% of the functional performance on the Barthel Index, of which two were found to make significant contributions, whereas 27% of the functional performance was predicted by the perceptual variables, of which only one was found to make a significant contribution to predicting performance on the Barthel Index at discharge.

Goverover and Hinojosa[17] used multiple regression to predict instrumental activities of daily living (IADL) performance based on categorization and deductive reasoning abilities for adults with brain injury. They developed several different regression models to determine how well different combinations of age, education, categorization, and deductive reasoning variables predicted performance on IADLs.

LOGISTIC REGRESSION

Multiple regression procedures, as described previously, can provide useful information for predicting numerical dependent variables. However, therapists are often interested in predicting dichotomous outcomes, such as whether or not a patient achieves independence or whether or not a patient returns home following rehabilitation. For example, we might be interested in determining what factors predict the need for an assistive device 6 months after total knee arthroplasty.

Rationale for Logistic Regression

Using the data set originally presented in Chapter 20, we find that almost 100% of patients in their 40s and 50s, 57% in their 60s, 22% in their 70s, and 0% in their 80s and 90s are independent in gait without an assistive device. Figure 24-5 illustrates these data conceptually with a smoothed line representing the approximate relationship between age and use of gait devices 6 months after total knee arthroplasty. It is obvious that the relationship between these two factors is not linear. Rather, it remains at a high level in the younger age ranges, drops off rapidly for the intermediate ages, and then bottoms out at a low level for the older age ranges.

This S-shaped curve is typical of the relationship between a dichotomous variable and a continuous variable. Because the relationship is nonlinear, standard linear correlation and regression techniques are not appropriate, and techniques that use logarithmic and exponential transformations of the data are used instead.[18(p. 255)] The general technique that is used to predict dichotomous outcomes from numerical independent variables is called logistic regression.

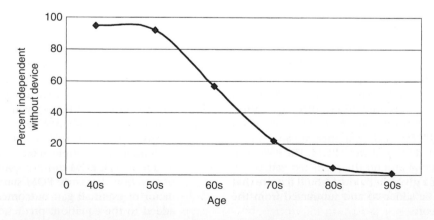

Figure 24-5 Graph illustrates the nonlinear, S-shaped curve that describes the relationship between a continuous variable (age) and a dichotomous variable (independence without an assistive device).

Literature Examples

In the rehabilitation literature, logistic regression has been used to examine the factors that predict falls among the elderly. Because of the complex mathematical transformations involved in logistic regression, the presentation of results can be confusing, and a full discussion is beyond the scope of this text. However, readers should know that there are two common ways of presenting the results of logistic regression: with odds ratios for the variables within the logistic regression equation or by presenting the equation itself.

For example, Resnik and Borgia[19] used logistic regression to identify factors that affected rehabilitation services received by persons in the Veterans Affairs system, as well as the impact of specific lower limb amputation rehabilitation guidelines on various factors. The study reported changes in odds ratios associated with several variables, including geographic area. The authors reported that those residing in the Midwest and West regions were 1.25 to 1.47 times more likely to receive rehabilitation services preoperatively than those residing in the South, whereas those residing in the Northeast were 0.63 to 0.69 times less likely to receive preoperative rehabilitation services than those residing in the South. Further, they reported that after the guidelines were implemented regional differences continued, with those residing in the Midwest being 1.69 times as likely to receive rehabilitation services than those residing in the South, and those living in the Northeast having 0.36 times the odds of receiving rehabilitation services than those residing in the South.

Shumway-Cook and colleagues[20] also used logistic regression to analyze the relationships among falls and a variety of other factors. Rather than presenting their results as odds ratios, they chose to provide readers with the actual logistic regression equation and with some sample predictions from the equations. By doing so, they help readers get past the complex equation that results from any logistic regression to see the implications of the equation. They showed that solving the equation for an individual without a history of imbalance and a Berg Balance Scale score of 54 would result in a prediction of a 5% probability of falling. They also solved their equation for an individual with a history of imbalance and a Berg Balance Scale score of 42 to show a predicted 91% probability of falling.

DISCRIMINANT ANALYSIS

Discriminant analysis is a procedure in which multiple predictor variables are used to place individuals into groups. Essentially, it is a backward multivariate analysis of variance (MANOVA) procedure. Recall that MANOVA uses a grouping factor to examine differences on multiple dependent variables at the same time. For example, MANOVA might be used to determine whether boys and girls differ on the combined communication variables of vocabulary, mean length of utterance, grammatically complete utterances, and complex sentences. In contrast, discriminant analysis uses the set of combined communication variables from each participant to predict whether each is a boy or a girl. Knowing which participants are, in fact, boys and girls allows the researchers to document the proportion of participants who were classified correctly by the discriminant analysis. A data set that produces a MANOVA identifying significant differences between boys and girls on the combined communication variables would produce a discriminant analysis with a high proportion of correct classifications.

In an effort to discriminate persons with chronic fatigue syndrome (CFS) from persons who were sedentary without CFS, Snell and colleagues[21] collected peak oxygen consumption, oxygen consumption at the ventilator threshold (VT), peak workload, and workload at VT data at two times, separated by 24 hours. They reported that 48% of the variance on the tests accounted for the CFS diagnosis, with workload at VT apparently demonstrating the largest decrement in performance.

In another study, Rogers and Case-Smith[22] used handwriting speed and legibility to predict whether students would be fast or slow keyboarders. If handwriting difficulties predict slow keyboarding, then using keyboarding as an alternative way for students with handwriting difficulties to complete school assignments might not be as effective as hoped. The handwriting variables correctly categorized students as fast or slow keyboarders in 71.1% of cases. However, for those not correctly classified, some with handwriting difficulties were actually fast keyboarders (rather than slow keyboarders as predicted). This suggests that at least some students with handwriting difficulties can develop keyboarding skills that may facilitate written work in school.

FACTOR ANALYSIS

Factor analysis is a tool whereby correlational techniques are used to discover which of many variables cluster together as a related unit, separate from other, unrelated clusters. It is a data reduction technique in which many variables are grouped into a smaller number of related groups.

Factor analysis is generally done for one of three reasons: test development, theory development, or theory testing. In test development, factor analysis is often used to help reduce a great number of items into a smaller number. Factor analysis groups items that are related to one another, and the test developer can then select certain questions from each factor for inclusion in the final version of the test. In theory development, factor analysis is used to examine the underlying structure of a set of variables about which the researcher has not developed a conceptual framework. The factors that emerge are then examined and named by the researcher, who then develops hypotheses about interrelationships among the factors. In theory testing, items thought to be representative of certain constructs are factor analyzed to determine whether the items load as hypothesized.

In our sample data set, 12 different pieces of data are recorded for each patient at 6 months postoperatively:
One ROM measure
Two muscle strength measures
Four deformity measures
Four activities of daily living (ADL) measures
One gait velocity measure

A theoretical grouping of these variables might be according to changes in body structure and function and disability, as defined in the World Health Organization's International Classification of Functioning, Disability, and Health.[23] The bodily change variables relate to abnormal structures and would include the ROM measure, the strength measures, and the deformity measures. The disability variables relate to abnormal performance of activities and, in this example, would include the ADL measures and gait velocity. Researchers might hypothesize that if bodily changes and disability are truly different constructs, then a factor analysis of the 12 variables would yield one factor that consists of the bodily change variables and one factor that consists of the disability variables.

Factor Analysis Steps

The result of a factor analysis of these 12 variables is presented here. The mathematical basis of factor analysis has been presented well by others and is therefore omitted so that emphasis may be placed on interpretation rather than calculation.[24] In brief, the steps in a factor analysis are as follows:

1. A group of variables is analyzed for interrelationships.
2. The number of important underlying factors is determined by reviewing eigenvalues associated with each factor.
3. Factors are extracted.
4. The factor solution is rotated to maximize differences between the factors.
5. Rotated factor loadings are examined to determine a simple structure.
6. The resulting factors are interpreted.

Let us examine these steps in sequence for the 12 6-month variables. First, a correlation matrix is developed, as shown in Table 24-5. In this example,

Table **24-5**

Correlation Matrix for 12-Variable Factor Analysis

	F	E	DFC	DVV	DML	DAP	V	ADW	AAD	ASC	ARC
M6R	.56	.59	−.17	−.23	.11	−.15	.63	.68	.70	.71	.65
F		.95	−.19	.19	.04	−.05	.89	.72	.69	.75	.81
E			−.13	.24	.03	−.09	.90	.70	.65	.75	.79
DFC				.46	.45	.14	−.22	−.34	−.26	−.21	−.24
DVV					.27	−.01	.17	−.10	−.19	−.01	.02
DML						.45	−.07	−.16	−.10	−.12	.02
DAP							−.17	−.06	.02	−.17	.12
V								.80	.75	.82	.85
ADW									.83	.78	.81
AAD										.83	.81
ASC											.82

M6R, 6-month range of motion; F, flexion torque; E, extension torque; DFC, deformity-flexion contracture; DVV, deformity-varus/valgus angulation; DML, deformity-mediolateral instability; DAP, deformity-anteroposterior in ability; V, gait velocity; ADW, activities of daily living (ADL)-distance walked; AAD, ADL-assistive device; ASC, ADL-stair climbing; ARC, ADL-rising from chair.

the matrix has been set up so that the theorized bodily change and disability variables are close to one another. If we examine the last five columns of the matrix, which consists of the theorized disability variables, we find that they are all fairly highly correlated with the ROM and strength variables (rows 1 through 3) and with the other disability variables (rows 8 through 11). They are minimally correlated with the deformity variables (rows 4 through 7). Although we can visually detect some patterns within the relationships among variables, the matrix is far too complex for simple visual analysis; hence, there is need for a mathematical tool like factor analysis.

The second step of a factor analysis is to determine the number of factors in the solution. Initially, the variables in the factor analysis problem are used to create the same number of factors. Each factor has an associated eigenvalue, which is related to the percentage of variability within the data set that can be accounted for by the factor. Some factors will account for very little variance and are therefore eliminated from the analysis. One convention for determining the number of factors in the solution is that only factors with eigenvalues of greater than 1.0 are retained. Another method is the scree method, which examines the pattern of eigenvalues graphically.[24(p. 635)] When a researcher is testing a theory, the number of factors he or she retains may simply be the number of theorized factors.

The factor analysis of our 12 variables shows that three factors had eigenvalues greater than 1.0; the scree method would retain either two or three factors, and our theoretical model predicted two factors. For the purpose of this example, then, two factors are selected for extraction, the third step in factor analysis. Terms that describe different extraction techniques are *principal components extraction, image factoring,* and *alpha factoring,* among others.

The fourth step in factor analysis is to rotate the factors. In essence, rotation can be thought of as resetting the zero point within the factor analysis. Doing so maximizes the appearance of differences between factors. Terms that describe different types of rotation techniques are orthogonal, oblique, varimax, and quartimax, among others. After rotation has occurred, one speaks in terms of "factor loadings" rather than "correlation." A factor loading is essentially the correlation between each variable within a factor and the entire factor. Table 24-6 shows the rotated factor loadings determined by the factor analysis.

The fifth step in factor analysis is to determine, if possible, a simple structure for the factors. A simple structure is developed when each variable is associated with only one factor. To determine a simple structure,

Table 24-6

Rotated Factor Loadings

Variable	Factor I	Factor II
V	.94	.10
ARC	.92	.12
ASC	.91	−.03
ADW	.89	−.12
F	.89	.20
E	.88	.24
AAD	.88	−.09
M6R	.76	−.05
DML	−.07	.77
DFC	−.30	.71
DVV	−.00	.71
DAP	−.10	.44
% of variance accounted for	53.7	16.6

V, gait velocity; ARC, activities of daily living (ADL)-rising from chair; ASC, ADL-stair climbing; ADW, ADL-distance walked; F, flexion torque; E, extension torque; AAD, ADL-assistive device; M6R, 6-month range of motion; DML, deformity-mediolateral instability; DFC, deformity-flexion contracture; DVV, deformity-varus/valgus angulation; DAP, deformity-anteroposterior instability.

the researcher decides to retain in each factor only those variables that loaded above some arbitrary point, often .30. In our example, if factor loadings above .30 are retained, the flexion contracture variable remains in both factors because its loading on Factor I is −.305 and its loading on Factor II is .71. Thus, to obtain a simple structure for this analysis, we need to adopt a more restrictive criterion for variable retention. If we adopt a criterion of .35, a simple structure is created.

The final step in factor analysis is to name and interpret the factors. This is done according to the variables that were retained in each factor and is highly subjective. Researchers often name the factors in a manner consistent with the theoretical underpinnings of the study. Factor II in our solution consists of the four deformity variables and could be named "Changes in Body Structure." This name lets the reader know that Factor II consists of a subgroup of the hypothesized construct of bodily change. Factor I is more difficult to name because it consists of a combination of functional, strength, and ROM variables. A name consistent with the theoretical underpinnings would be "Changes in

Table 24-7

Rotated Factor Loadings

Variable	FACTOR	
	Changes in Body Function and Disability	Changes in Body Structure
Gait velocity	.94	
ADL-rising from chair	.92	
ADL-stair climbing	.91	
ADL-distance walked	.89	
Flexion torque	.89	
Extension torque	.88	
ADL-assistive device	.88	
Six-month range of motion	.76	
Deformity-mediolateral instability		.77
Deformity-flexion contracture		.71
Deformity-varus/valgus angulation		.71
Deformity-anteroposterior instability		.44

ADL, activities of daily living.

Body Function and Disability." Table 24-7, a modified version of Table 24-6, illustrates how a simple structure with named factors might be presented. After the factors are named, the implications of the factors are discussed by the researcher. The following is the interpretation of this factor analysis as it might be written in a journal article:

DATA ANALYSIS: Factor analysis with principal components extraction and orthogonal varimax rotation was used to test whether variables loaded as predicted on two theorized factors described in the International Classification of Functioning, Disability, and Health (ICF). A simple structure was developed by including in each factor only those variables with rotated factor loadings higher than .35.

RESULTS: Table 24-7 shows the rotated factor loadings for the two-factor solution. The first factor included all the activities of daily living (ADL) variables, as well as the gait velocity, range of motion (ROM), and torque variables. The second factor included all the deformity variables. Factor I was labeled "Changes in Body Function and Disability" and accounted for 53.7% of the variance; Factor II was labeled "Changes in Body Structure" and accounted for 16.6% of the variance.

DISCUSSION: Our results do not fully support the hypothesized distinction between body changes and disability because some of the body change variables loaded with the disability variables. However, the body change variables did split among the two factors according to the structure and function dimensions described in the ICF. The structural—that is, anatomical—body change variables (the four measures of deformity) all loaded together and were separate from the other eight variables. This indicates that the actual anatomical alignment of the knees was not highly associated with eventual functional recovery. The variables that are more representative of physiological function than anatomical structure (flexion and extension torque and flexion ROM) loaded with the disability variables of ADL status and gait velocity. These results suggest that the constructs of body changes and disability, as defined within the ICF, are not completely valid for patients who have had total knee arthroplasty. However, the fact that body function and body structure variables loaded within different factors supports the notion that these two types of body changes represent distinct different underlying constructs.

Literature Examples

Myers and colleagues[25] surveyed physical therapists (PTs) on factors that affected their involvement in preschool transitions from early intervention programs. The survey had two scales, one addressing factors that affected PTs "involvement" in transition planning, the other scale addressing factors that examined activities that PTs viewed as "facilitative" or supportive of their involvement in transition planning. A factor analysis was conducted on each scale. From the "involvement" subscale, five factors were identified (collaboration with early intervention, family support, evaluation, teaming in preschool programs, and working with preschool teachers) as important to the involvement of PTs in transition planning, whereas two factors were identified from the "facilitative" subscale (perceived value and expertise and external supports) as important to PT involvement.

A different example is Mulligan's[26] use of factor analysis to test a theoretical model of sensory integration dysfunction. The hypothesized model predicted that the different subtests of the Sensory Integration and Praxis Tests (SIPT) would cluster into five separate latent variables. A complex analysis that tested various factor analytic models led the author to conclude that a model with one generalized variable and four latent variables fit the data better than the originally hypothesized model.

SUMMARY

Advanced and special relationship analysis techniques are used to analyze more than two variables simultaneously or to analyze repeated measures of the same variable. Specialized reliability correlation coefficients, in which repeated measures of the same variable are analyzed, include the Pearson product moment correlation with extensions to evaluate the slope and intercept of an associated regression line; intraclass correlation coefficients based on analysis of variance techniques; and kappa, which is used with nominal data. Multiple regression is used to predict a numerical dependent variable from many different independent variables. Logistic regression is used to predict a nominal dependent variable from many different independent variables. Discriminant analysis uses a set of predictor variables to place individuals into groups. Factor analysis is a correlational technique that is used to determine which of many variables cluster together as a related unit separate from other, unrelated clusters.

REFERENCES

1. Rankin G, Stokes M: Reliability of assessment tools in rehabilitation: An illustration of appropriate statistical analysis, *Clin Rehabil* 12:187–199, 1998.
2. Delitto A, Strube MJ: Reliability in the clinical setting, *Res Sect Newsl* 24(1):2–8, 1991.
3. Hyde ML: Reasonable psychometric standards for self-report outcomes measures in audiological rehabilitation, *Ear Hear* 21:S24–S36, 2000.
4. Shrout PE, Fleiss JL: Intraclass correlations: Uses in assessing rater reliability, *Psychol Bull* 86:420–428, 1979.
5. Müller R, Büttner P: A critical discussion of intraclass correlation coefficients, *Stat Med* 13:2465–2476, 1994.
6. Katz-Leurer M, Rotem H, Lewitus H, et al: Functional balance tests for children with traumatic brain injury: Within-session reliability, *Pediatr Phys Ther* 20:254–258, 2008.
7. Wong CK: Interrater reliability of the Berg Balance Scale when used by clinicians of various experience levels to assess people with lower limb amputations, *Phys Ther* 94:371–378, 2014.
8. Cohen J: A coefficient of agreement for nominal scales, *Educ Psychol Measur* 20:37–46, 1960.
9. Cohen J: Weighted kappa: Nominal scale agreement with provision for scaled disagreement or partial credit, *Psychol Bull* 70:213–220, 1968.
10. Fleiss JL: Measuring nominal scale agreement among many raters, *Psychol Bull* 76:378–382, 1971.
11. Van Dillen LR, Sahrmann SA, Norton BJ, et al: Reliability of physical examination items used for classification of patients with low back pain, *Phys Ther* 78:979–988, 1998.
12. Landis JR, Koch GG: The measurement of observer agreement for categorical data, *Biometrics* 33:159–174, 1977.
13. Dawson-Saunders B, Trapp RG: *Basic and Clinical Biostatistics*, 3rd ed, Norwalk, Conn, 2000, Appleton & Lange.
14. Nick TG, Hardin JM: Quantitative research series. Regression modeling strategies: An illustrative case study from medical rehabilitation outcomes research, *Am J Occup Ther* 53:459–470, 1999.
15. Dimitrov D, Fitzgerald S, Rumrill P: Multiple regression in rehabilitation research, *Work* 15:209–215, 2000.
16. Brown T, Mapleston J, Nair A, Molloy A: Relationship of cognitive and perceptual abilities to functional independence in adults who have had a stroke, *Occup Ther Int* 20:11–22, 2013.
17. Goverover Y, Hinojosa J: Categorization and deductive reasoning: Predictors of instrumental activities of daily living performance in adults with brain injury, *Am J Occup Ther* 56:509–516, 2002.
18. Elston RC, Johnson WD: *Essentials of Biostatistics*, Philadelphia, Pa, 1994, FA Davis.
19. Resnik L, Borgia ML: Factors associated with utilization of preoperative and postoperative rehabilitation services by patients with amputation in the VA system: An observational study, *Phys Ther* 93:1197–1210, 2013.
20. Shumway-Cook A, Baldwin M, Polissar NL, Gruber W: Predicting the probability of falls in community-dwelling older adults, *Phys Ther* 77:812–819, 1997.
21. Snell CR, Stevens SR, Davenport TE, Van Ness JM: Discriminative validity of metabolic and workload measurements for identifying people with chronic fatigue syndrome, *Phys Ther* 93:1484–1492, 2013.
22. Rogers J, Case-Smith J: Relationships between handwriting and keyboarding performance of sixth-grade students, *Am J Occup Ther* 56:34–39, 2002.
23. World Health Organization. International Classification of Functioning, Disability, and Health. Available at: www.who.int/classification/icf. Accessed December 14, 2014.
24. Tabachnick BG, Fidell LS: *Using Multivariate Statistics*, 4th ed, New York, NY, 2000, Harper & Row.
25. Myers CT, Effgen SK, Blanchard E, et al: Factors influencing physical therapists' involvement in preschool transitions, *Phys Ther* 91:656–664, 2011.
26. Mulligan S: Patterns of sensory integration dysfunction, *Am J Occup Ther* 52:819–828, 1998.

CHAPTER 25

Evaluating Evidence One Article at a Time

CHAPTER OUTLINE

Elements of a Research Article
Guidelines for Discussing Published
    Research
Generic Evaluation of Original
    Research Studies
    Step 1: Classify the Research and
        Variables
    Step 2: Compare Purposes and
        Conclusions
    Step 3: Describe Design and
        Control Elements
    Step 4: Identify Threats to Research
        Validity

Step 5: Place the Study in the
    Context of Other Research
Step 6: Evaluate the Personal Utility
    of the Study
Generic Evaluation of Review
    Articles
    Step 1: Assess the Clarity of the
        Review Question
    Step 2: Evaluate the Article
        Identification and Selection
        Strategies
    Step 3: Determine How the Authors
        Assess Validity of the Studies

Step 4: Evaluate the Results Against
    the Strength of the Evidence
Step 5: Evaluate the Personal Utility
    of the Review
Structured Evaluation by Clinical
    Research Issues
Evaluation of Levels of Evidence
Evaluation of Randomized
    Controlled Trials
Summary

Evidence-based practice is a major force in health care practice in the 21st century. Influenced by the same forces that advanced the emergence of the outcomes movement (see Chapter 16) in the 1990s, evidence-based practice requires that clinicians use the literature of their professions to guide practice. A common definition of evidence-based medicine (EBM) is that it is "the integration of best research evidence with clinical expertise and patient values."[1(p. 1)] Thus, evidence-based practice does not demand that practitioners be ruled by research evidence; rather, it requires that they integrate research evidence with their own clinical experiences and the values of their patients or clients. To effectively integrate research evidence, practitioners must evaluate research reports critically before applying the results to practice. Such evaluation requires that practitioners apply the principles from the first 23 chapters of this text to the articles they are reading. This chapter provides a number of frameworks for doing so. First, the elements of a research article and a few general "rules of thumb" for discussing published research are listed. Then, generic frameworks for the evaluation of original research articles and review articles are outlined. Next, a more structured approach to evaluation of research according to the clinical issue at hand is presented. Approaches that evaluate levels of evidence are also outlined. Finally, some scoring systems specific to the evaluation of randomized controlled trials are presented.

ELEMENTS OF A RESEARCH ARTICLE

Table 25-1 lists and describes the elements of a research article. The components encountered first are the journal article title and abstract. Following these is the body

345

Table 25-1

Elements of a Research Article

Element	Characteristics
Title	Is concise, yet descriptive. Identifies major variables studied. Provides clues about whether the purpose of the research is description, relationship analysis, or difference analysis through use of phrases such as "characteristics of," "relationship between," or "effects of," respectively.
Abstract	Briefly summarizes research purpose, methods, and results. Depending on journal, is usually 150 to 300 words. Does not include summary of related literature or significant discussion of the limitations and implications of the research.
Introduction	Sets the stage for the presentation of the research. Usually does not have a heading; sometimes is subdivided into Problem, Purpose, or Literature Review sections. Whether subdivided or not, defines the broad problem that underlies the study, states the specific purposes of the study, and places the problem and purposes into the theoretical context of previous work. Often presents research hypotheses. Occasionally contains tables or figures.
Method	Describes the conduct of the study. Usually is subdivided into Subjects, Instruments, Procedures, and Data Analysis sections. Often refers to methods or procedures used by others as the basis for the present study. Often contains figures showing equipment used.
Results	Presents the results without comment on their meaning. Often is subdivided into sections corresponding to the variables studied. Is often brief because much of the information is contained in tables and figures.
Discussion	Presents the authors' interpretation of their results, along with their assessment of study limitations and directions for future research. Often refers to previous work that is related to the findings of the study. May be subdivided into Limitations, Clinical Relevance, and Future Research sections.
Conclusions	Concisely restates the important findings of the research. Presents a conclusion for each purpose outlined in the introduction.
References	Lists references cited in the text of the article. Is followed occasionally by a bibliography that lists relevant work not cited in the article.
Appendix	If included, follows the references. Typically includes survey instruments or detailed treatment protocols.

of the article, which typically consists of introduction, methods, results, discussion, conclusions, and reference sections. Generally, the introduction section argues why the study should be done. Often the argument is delivered by a short review of the literature to illustrate the gap in the research that the proposed study will address. Sometimes the literature review will emphasize the failure of previous research methods to address the problem, or indicate that a specific population has not been studied, or explain that a different method of measuring outcomes has not been tried. The introduction section establishes the theoretical constructs on which the study is based. Additionally, the introduction section

may present data illustrating the magnitude of the problem, such as the incidence or prevalence of a disorder or disability. Importantly, the introduction presents the hypotheses, purposes, or objectives of the study, usually as the last paragraph of this section. Within the typical method section there are several subsections detailing different aspects of the study. For example, there will be a subsection that describes the people who participated in the study, noting how they were selected for the study (e.g., randomly selected or a sample of convenience), the criteria for including and excluding participants in a study, how they were assigned to the different groups, and significant features of the participants (e.g., mean age, mean weight, sex). Other subsections often found in the methods section are: settings or environment, dependent variables, instruments or equipment, procedures or interventions, design, and data analysis. The purpose of this detail is twofold: (1) to provide sufficient information so that the reader may replicate the study, and (2) to justify the different actions taken in each of the subsections by the researchers. Several sections may contain tables, which consist of rows and columns of numbers or words; figures may also be included, which might include photographs, diagrams, graphs, or other visual displays that illustrate important concepts or results within the study. The discussion section is where the authors can compare their study to previous research in the field, emphasizing how the study outcomes have changed the study's theoretical constructs, presenting limitations of the study and how those limitations may have affected the outcomes, and offering suggestions for future studies. Generally, the discussion section begins with a very brief repeat of the results specific to the study's purpose or objectives. Subsequently, the authors will present how the outcomes data compared to studies that were similar in purpose to the authors' study. Often this argument will emphasize design, measurement, or procedural differences, as well as theoretical constructs, thus serving as a foreshadowing of a discussion on the study limitations, followed by the authors' recommendations for future studies. Following the discussion section, often research manuscripts will have a conclusion section. This section will briefly restate the purpose of the study, provide the results of the study, and include a sentence as to the impact of the study. If the study's discussion section was quite large and comprehensive, the conclusion may have a sentence or two indicating how the study fit in the research literature. The reference section follows the conclusion. The reference section will present all of the sources of information the study cited in the preceding sections, including journal articles, texts, and Internet addresses. Sometimes the reference section may include a citation to a personal communication the authors had with someone. The format of the reference section is dictated by the writing style manual that the journal embraces. For example, the flagship journal of the American Physical Therapy Association, and all of its specialty section journals, employs the American Medical Association style manual, whereas the flagship journals of the American Speech-Language-Hearing Association and the American Occupational Therapy Association adhere to the American Psychological Association style manual. Occasionally an article contains an appendix of information that may be useful to readers but is too detailed for inclusion in the body of the report. The appendix will follow the reference section.

GUIDELINES FOR DISCUSSING PUBLISHED RESEARCH

Readers who discuss their reviews in writing or through oral presentation to others should follow four basic style guidelines:
1. Discuss the study in the past tense.
2. Clearly distinguish between their own opinions and those of the authors.
3. Qualify generalizations so that they are not erroneously attributed.
4. Justify each position with evidence from the study, particularly in the discussion section.

Table 25-2 presents examples of inappropriate and appropriate wording in the context of some actual articles[2,3] to illustrate each of the four stylistic guidelines.

GENERIC EVALUATION OF ORIGINAL RESEARCH STUDIES

Single reports of original research should be evaluated from two major perspectives: trustworthiness and utility. Trustworthiness relates to whether sources of invalidity have been controlled as well as is practical, whether authors openly acknowledge the limitations of the study, and whether the conclusions drawn are defensible in light of the methods used in the study. In Chapters 8 and 20, more than 20 sources of invalidity within research studies are identified. Armed with a list of these potential problems, readers of the research literature can easily become overly critical and conclude that all studies are hopelessly flawed and offer nothing of value to the practitioner. However, as we have seen in Chapters 8 and 20, there are no perfect studies because of the reciprocal nature of many of the threats to validity. In many instances, when a researcher controls one source of invalidity, another one rears its ugly head. Thus, there is no absolute standard of trustworthiness to which every study can be held. However, because trustworthiness focuses on the design and interpretation of studies themselves, different readers can be expected to identify common areas of concern related to the trustworthiness of a study.

In contrast, the utility of a study relates to the usefulness of its results to a particular practitioner. Unlike the assessment of trustworthiness, the assessment of utility may vary widely among readers. The results of a well-controlled study of a narrowly defined patient population may be highly trustworthy but of low utility to a practitioner who sees a different patient population. Conversely, a first study of a given phenomenon may be very useful to a particular practitioner even if it suffers from several methodological flaws.

Table 25-2	

Style Guidelines for Writing About Published Research

Inappropriate Wording	Appropriate Wording
Chiarello and colleagues[2] state that there is no difference in outcome between patients who receive short-duration CPM versus long-duration CPM. (This wording implies that the authors still hold this belief.)	Chiarello and colleagues[2] found no differences in outcome between patients who received short-duration CPM versus long-duration CPM. (This wording makes it clear that the authors' statements relate to the particular study under discussion.)
Use of CPM after total knee arthroplasty decreases the need for postoperative manipulation under anesthesia. (This wording does not make it clear whether this is the conclusion of the review author or the author of the study.)	Based on their research, Ververeli and colleagues[3] concluded that CPM after total knee arthroplasty decreased the need for postoperative manipulation under anesthesia. (This wording clearly attributes the statement to the study authors.)
Patients with greater knee range of motion have better functional outcomes after surgery. (This wording implies that this relationship between range of motion and functional outcome is well established.)	Therapists and surgeons often assume that patients with greater knee range of motion have better functional outcomes after surgery. (This wording makes it clear that the relationship between range of motion and functional outcome is an unsubstantiated assumption.)
A number of different dependent variable measures were used in this study (e.g., specific test of quality of life, impairment, and disability).	The authors failed to present any reliability or validity information on the dependent variable measures they used in this study.

When evaluating the literature, readers must balance legitimate criticisms with a realistic sense of the compromises that all researchers must make in designing and implementing a study. Several authors have presented guidelines for evaluating the research literature.[4–8] In fact, many different scales and checklists have been developed to aid readers in evaluating the literature,[9,10] and some are presented later in the chapter. In addition, examples of research evaluations by experienced consumers of the literature can be found as commentaries to published reports in several journals.[11] Although different evaluators of the literature structure their commentaries differently, they all assess the same basic aspects of research articles.

In this section, a six-step generic sequence for evaluating the literature is presented to help novice evaluators structure their critiques. The first steps emphasize classification and description of the research in order to place it in the larger context of research as a vast and varied enterprise. The middle steps emphasize identification of threats to the validity of the research. The final steps involve assessing the place the research has in both the existing literature and one's own practice. Appendix C and Table 3-2 provide two formats of question sets to help readers structure their critiques. Table 3-2 is a matrix that presents where in a manuscript the questions are likely to be addressed and to which subtypes of research validity the questions are relevant. Because of the great variety of research designs and analyses that appear in the published literature, readers should recognize that the questions need to be applied thoughtfully and selectively because they are neither exhaustive nor universally applicable.

In addition, readers need to move from merely answering the questions to evaluating, justifying, and interpreting the implications of the answers in the context of each study they review. For example, one of the questions in Appendix C is "Was the independent variable implemented in a laboratory-like or clinic-like setting?" In one study, a tightly controlled, laboratory-like setting might be exactly what is needed to establish the effectiveness of a particular technique under ideal conditions. In another study of a phenomenon for which effectiveness is already well established, looser, clinic-like control might be exactly what is needed to establish whether the technique still works when the vagaries of actual clinical practice apply. Thus, merely answering the question of "laboratory-like" versus "clinic-like" control of the independent variable does not tell the reader whether the control was appropriate. Rather, the reader, having determined the level of control, then needs to evaluate whether that level of control was appropriate for the study at hand.

To further assist readers embarking on a review of a study, a written critique of Gose's[12] investigation of continuous passive motion (CPM) for patients after total knee arthroplasty (TKA) is provided as an example. The example is developed step by step as each of the six critique steps is presented. Despite the older publication date (1987), this article was selected for review because its design provides many opportunities to illustrate the various control and validity issues addressed in this text. The abstract of Gose's report reads:

The purpose of this study was to evaluate the effects of adding three 1-hour sessions of continuous passive motion (CPM) each day to the entire postoperative program of patients who received a total knee replacement (TKR). A retrospective chart review was completed for 55 patients (8 with bilateral involvement, totalling 63 knees) who received a TKR between 1981 and 1984. The data analysis compared the following variables for 32 patients who received CPM and 23 patients who received no CPM: the length of hospital stay (LOS), the number of postoperative days (PODs) before discharge, the frequency of postoperative complications, and the knee range of motion at discharge. The CPM groups showed significant decreases in the frequency of complication ($p<.05$), the LOS ($p<.01$), and in the number of PODs ($p<.001$). No difference was demonstrated in the ROM of the two groups. These results support the use of postoperative applications of CPM, but not as strongly as those reported from studies that used longer periods of CPM. Further research is indicated to delineate the minimum dosage of CPM needed to obtain the maximum beneficial effects.[12(p. 39)]

Step 1: Classify the Research and Variables

Classification of the research and variables provides an immediate sense of where the individual piece of research belongs in the literature. The information needed to classify the research is found in the abstract, introduction, and methods sections of a journal article. If the reviewer determines that the research is experimental, it should come as no surprise if the authors make causal statements about their results; if the reviewer determines that the research is nonexperimental, the reader's expectations about causal statements should change. If the dependent variables of interest are range-of-motion (ROM) measures, the reviewer should

expect clean, easily understood results; if the dependent measures relate to patterns of interaction between therapists and patients, the reviewer should expect complexity and depth. We might summarize this first evaluative step for Gose's CPM study as follows:

> Gose's study of the effects of continuous passive motion (CPM) on rehabilitation after total knee arthroplasty is an example of a retrospective analysis of differences between groups. The study had one independent variable, treatment, with two levels: usual postoperative therapy and postoperative therapy supplemented with CPM. The type of treatment received by each participant was not actively manipulated, but rather was apparently determined by physician prescription.
>
> There were five dependent variables: total length of stay in the acute care hospital, number of postoperative days in the acute care hospital, frequency of postoperative complications, knee flexion range of motion (ROM) at discharge, and knee extension ROM at discharge. All data were gathered through retrospective chart review.

Step 2: Compare Purposes and Conclusions

Any piece of research needs to be assessed in light of the contribution it was designed to make to the profession. It is not fair to fault a study for not accomplishing a purpose that it was never designed to meet. Before reading the methods, results, and discussion sections of an article, it is often useful to compare the purposes, which may be found in the introduction, and the conclusions. This comparison serves two purposes. First, it indicates whether or not the study is internally consistent. Purposes without conclusions, or conclusions without purposes, should alert the reader to look for the points at which the study strays from its original intent.

The comparison also provides guidance for the critique of the methods, results, and discussion. If the conclusions indicate that statistically significant relationships or differences were identified, then the reader knows to evaluate the remainder of the article with an eye to how well the researcher controlled for alternative explanations for the results and whether the statistical results are clinically important. If the conclusions do not indicate any statistically significant results, then the reader knows to evaluate the study with respect to power and the clinical importance of the results. With regard to Gose's study, we might write up this second step of our critique as follows:

The purpose of this study was clearly stated at the end of the introduction section of the paper: to compare the effects of adding three 1-hour daily sessions of CPM to a postoperative total knee arthroplasty rehabilitation program. The effects measured related to both the physical status of the patient (flexion and extension ROM and frequency of complications) and the cost effectiveness of care (total length of stay and length of postoperative stay).

The conclusions were consistent with the purpose. There were significant differences between the CPM and non-CPM groups for three of the five dependent measures: length of stay, number of days of postoperative hospitalization, and frequency of postoperative complications. There were no significant differences between groups on the two ROM variables: knee flexion and extension.

Step 3: Describe Design and Control Elements

In the third step of the evaluation process, the reviewer completes the description of the study elements and begins to make judgments about the adequacy of the research design. The design of the study is identified so that the sequence of measurement and manipulation (if present) is clear to the reader of the review. This identification can be done in any of the three ways introduced earlier in Chapters 10, 11, 12, and 14:

- Making a diagram of the design
- Using symbols such as Campbell and Stanley's Os and Xs
- Using descriptive terms

The research design alone does not indicate the trustworthiness of the study. For example, a "strong" design such as a pretest–posttest control group design may not yield trustworthy information if the independent variable is not implemented consistently for participants in the treatment group. Thus, a critical reader of the literature needs to determine both the design of the study and the level of control the researchers exerted over implementation of the independent variable, selection and assignment of participants, extraneous variables related to the setting or participants, measurement, and information. The third step in our review of Gose's CPM study can be written as follows:

As noted previously, data for this study were collected retrospectively, with group membership determined by the postoperative rehabilitation program each patient happened to have undergone. This study was therefore of a nonexperimental, ex post facto nature with nonequivalent treatment and control groups. Because all dependent variables were collected at the completion of either rehabilitation program, the study followed a posttest-only design.

The nonexperimental, retrospective nature of data collection means that many design control elements were absent. The implementation of the independent variable took place in the hospital setting and would be expected to vary accordingly. The author did not indicate the proportion of patients who received all of the intended CPM sessions. Because he later discussed how the intended dosage of CPM in this study differs from that reported in other studies, it seems important to know whether the actual dosage received by the patients was equal to, greater than, or less than the intended dosage.

The selection and assignment of participants to groups were accomplished through chart review to determine, first, whether participants met general inclusion criteria and, second, whether they had undergone traditional or CPM-added rehabilitation. The basic inclusion criteria were having undergone a total knee arthroplasty between 1981 and 1984 at one hospital, having had ROM values recorded at admission and discharge, and having accomplished certain rehabilitation tasks by postoperative days (PODs) 2 and 7. These criteria mean that patients with complications severe enough to impede the rehabilitation process were excluded from the study. Thus, the frequency of postoperative complications indicated in this study was likely less than the number of actual complications that occur after total knee arthroplasty.

Assignment of participants to a group was accomplished simply by identification of which type of rehabilitation they had undergone. The author did not indicate what factors might have led one patient to receive CPM-added rehabilitation and another patient to receive traditional rehabilitation. If, for example, certain surgeons prescribed CPM-added rehabilitation and others prescribed traditional rehabilitation, the effects of the type of rehabilitation would be confounded by the surgeon.

If the traditional rehabilitation group had their surgery and rehabilitation in 1981 and 1982 and the CPM-added group received care in 1983 and 1984, then the effects of type of rehabilitation would be confounded with any general changes in surgical technique, knee prosthesis design, hospital staffing patterns, and the like that may have differed between the two time periods.

Because of the retrospective design, extraneous variables such as disease severity and medication received postoperatively were not controlled. In addition, there was no control over ROM measurements taken, such as written procedures for taking ROM measurements or citing studies that reported on knee joint ROM reliability, and no indication of how many different therapists recorded ROM values in the study.

Step 4: Identify Threats to Research Validity

After the type of research has been defined, the purposes and conclusions reviewed, and the design and control elements outlined, the reviewer is able to examine the threats to the validity of the study. This step involves not only assessing the threats to validity but also evaluating the extent to which the authors identify the study's limitations themselves.

As described in Chapter 8, the threats to research validity can be divided into validity subtypes, specifically construct, internal, statistical conclusion, and external validity. Any study should be assessed for construct and external validity, asking, "Do the ideas that undergird the study make sense?" and "To whom and under what conditions can the results of the study be applied?" Studies that use statistical tools should be assessed for statistical conclusion validity, asking, "Were statistical tools used appropriately within this study?" and "Were measurement instruments reliable and valid for the studied population?" Studies that have one or more independent variables and analyze differences between or within groups should be assessed for internal validity, asking "Is the independent variable the most plausible explanation for differences between or within groups?" (In Table 3-2 and Appendix C we have presented where many of the different questions addressing the different validity subtypes may be found in an intervention research manuscript.) Our analysis of all four types of validity for Gose's CPM study might be written as follows:

CONSTRUCT VALIDITY CONCERNS: The major construct validity concerns in Gose's study are construct underrepresentation and interaction of different treatments. The variables studied were a combination of cost-effectiveness variables related to length of stay and patient-oriented variables such as frequency of complications and knee ROM. These variables did not, however, represent a full range of outcomes for patients after total knee arthroplasty. It would have been nice if functional measures such as ambulation or stair-climbing ability had been measured. Presumably, this information would have been as available from the medical record as the ROM data were. In addition to underrepresentation of the dependent variables, the author acknowledged that the independent variable was also underrepresented: The dosage of CPM in this study was low compared with the dosage in other studies. A more complete, prospective study would assess several different dosages of CPM to determine the minimum level needed to obtain desired results.

The interaction of different treatments is always a concern with a retrospective study such as this one. We have no way of knowing, for example, whether the CPM treatments, which were administered by nursing staff, consisted of mechanical application of the unit with minimal interpersonal contact between nurse and patient or took the form of relaxed interchanges that provided an opportunity for education and discussion. If the latter was the case, then this study may have actually been assessing the effects of a combined program of CPM, education, and attention, rather than the isolated addition of CPM to the treatment regimen. The author acknowledged the possibility that differences between groups may be related to factors other than the use of CPM.

INTERNAL VALIDITY CONCERNS: The major internal validity concerns in this study are assignment, mortality, diffusion of treatment, compensatory equalization of treatments, and compensatory rivalry or resentful demoralization of participants. Very little information was given about why a particular patient received either the CPM-added rehabilitation or the non-CPM regimen. As noted earlier, if group membership was confounded with surgeon or time frame, it would be difficult to conclude that differences between groups were related solely to the differences in their rehabilitation regimens.

Regarding the threat of mortality to internal validity, we have no way of knowing how many potential participants in each group were not included in the study because they developed serious complications that prevented them from meeting the inclusion criteria of supervised ambulation on POD 2 and progressive ambulation by POD 7.

A third threat to internal validity comes from having patients from both groups be treated at the same time. It is plausible that members of each group were hospital roommates, and if the roommate in the CPM group extolled the virtues of this new device, perhaps the roommate in the non-CPM group compensated by moving her knee more frequently. If the therapists believed that CPM was beneficial, they could have become upset when some physicians did not prescribe it and compensated by increasing the number of ROM repetitions they included for their patients who were not receiving CPM. Because the author did not clearly indicate whether the two regimens were in effect given simultaneously or sequentially, we cannot speculate about the likelihood that these internal validity threats actually occurred.

STATISTICAL CONCLUSION VALIDITY CONCERNS: No concerns about statistical conclusion validity seem warranted. The sample sizes were reasonable (32 and 23); there was only one statistical test performed per dependent variable; the homogeneity of variance assumptions seem to have been met; the statistically significant results seem clinically important (e.g., the CPM group had an average postoperative length of stay approximately 3.5 days shorter than the non-CPM group); and the statistically insignificant results seem clinically unimportant (the difference in the mean ROM values between groups was only 1.0° for both knee flexion and extension). No dependent variable measurement psychometrics or description of the reliability of the ROM measures was reported owing to the retrospective form of the study.

EXTERNAL VALIDITY CONCERNS: The external validity of the study is strong in some areas and weak in others. The participants seem representative of typical patients who received total knee arthroplasties in the 1980s: elderly women with osteoarthritis. However, the average age of patients receiving total knee arthroplasty continues to move downward, and today it is not uncommon to have individuals in their 40s and 50s undergo the procedure. If individuals who choose total knee arthroplasty at younger ages are both healthier and more active than older adults who received the procedure in the past and more highly committed to returning to active lifestyles, they may have similarly short lengths of stay and low levels of complications regardless of whether CPM is used.

External validity is strengthened, ironically, by the relatively low dosage of CPM provided in this study. At the time the study was done, typical CPM protocols called for many hours per day—often up to 20 hours per day—of CPM. Although 3 hours of CPM per day seemed like a very low dosage at the time of the study, lower daily doses or fewer numbers of days of CPM are more common in contemporary reports. Therefore, compared with other studies of CPM administered in the early 1980s, this study has a dosage per day that more closely matches protocols in use today.

External validity is limited, however, by the dramatic changes in length of stay for almost all diagnoses and surgical procedures during the last 20 years. Although the CPM group's length of stay was significantly less in this study than the non-CPM group's, both lengths of stay (mean of 16.4 and 20.0 days, respectively) were much longer than is typical today, irrespective of the nature of the rehabilitation regimen. This means that although the daily dosage of CPM may match contemporary protocols, the total dosage of CPM given across the hospital stay may be greater than typical in today's short-stay environment.

Step 5: Place the Study in the Context of Other Research

In the fifth and sixth steps of evaluation, the reviewer assesses the utility of the research. First, the reviewer determines how much new information the study adds to what is already known about a topic. Even though only a single study is being critiqued, the question of utility cannot be answered in isolation. For example, if a treatment has consistently been shown to be effective in tightly controlled settings with high internal validity, another well-controlled study may not add much to our knowledge about that treatment. In such a case, what is needed is a study conducted in a realistic clinical setting, where control is difficult. Similarly, a small one-group study of a previously unstudied area might be an important addition to the rehabilitation therapy literature, whereas the same design applied to a well-studied topic may add little.

The best assessments of context are made by reviewers who have extensive knowledge of the literature on the topic. Knowledgeable reviewers can assess whether the authors of a research report have adequately reviewed and interpreted the literature they cite. Reviewers without this knowledge must rely on the authors' descriptions of the literature. Our review of the place Gose's CPM study has in the literature might be written as follows:

Despite the previously noted limitations of Gose's study, this work played an important role in the evolution of CPM from a 20-hour-per-day treatment modality to a modality that is used in varying dosages. The author indicated that previous studies of 20-hour-per-day CPM protocols found shorter lengths of stay, lower frequencies of postoperative complications, and greater early knee ROM in CPM groups compared with non-CPM groups. This study provided preliminary evidence that a low dosage of CPM could reduce the length of stay and frequency of complications in a typical group of older osteoarthritic patients receiving total knee replacement. Interestingly, there is still no consensus on appropriate dosage, as noted by the authors of a meta-analysis of 14 randomized controlled trials of CPM after total knee arthroplasty.[13]

Step 6: Evaluate the Personal Utility of the Study

As the final step in any research critique, the reviewer determines whether the study has meaning for his or her own practice. Whereas the determination of the trustworthiness of a research article will be somewhat consistent across reviewers, the question of personal utility will be answered differently by different reviewers. Hypothetically, we might write our assessment of the personal utility of Gose's CPM study as follows:

The results of this study have some potential application for the setting in which we work. In our setting, we follow an 8- to 10-hour-a-day regimen of CPM with excellent early ROM and relatively short stays. However, for those patients who cannot sleep well with the CPM unit on, this means that they are in the CPM unit during many of their waking hours. We believe that these patients stay in bed too much and are unable to give adequate attention to the development of effective quadriceps femoris muscle power and the development of more functional skills such as walking at a relatively normal velocity and for longer distances.

Although this study provides only partial support for the effectiveness of a low dosage of CPM, its findings are consistent with a more recent report that found no difference between a low-dosage protocol and a high-dosage protocol.[2] On the basis of the results of these studies, as well as our own dissatisfaction with some aspects of high dosages of CPM, we plan to implement and assess a trial of medium to low dosages of CPM in our patients who have had total knee arthroplasty.

The evaluation of personal utility is a very concrete way to conclude a review of a single research study. This ending is a reminder that the first five evaluative steps are not mere intellectual exercises, but rather are the means by which each reader decides whether and how to use the results of a study within his or her own practice.

GENERIC EVALUATION OF REVIEW ARTICLES

Review articles provide practitioners with a time-efficient way of remaining up to date in areas of importance to their practice. In fact, the authors of the "Users' Guide to the Medical Literature," a series of articles appearing in the *Journal of the American Medical Association (JAMA)* beginning in 1993, and now compiled into a book,[14,15] recognize the importance of review articles and go so far as to recommend that "resolving a clinical problem begins with a search for a valid overview or practice guideline as the most efficient method of deciding on the best patient care."[16(p. 2097)] Having made this statement, however, they then indicate that clinicians need help in differentiating good reviews from poor reviews. This section of the chapter provides guidelines to help rehabilitation practitioners make such judgments about review articles. Although there are mathematical ways to synthesize the results of several related studies (see Chapters 12 and 26 for additional information on meta-analysis), the focus in this section is on the conceptual synthesis that is presented in many review articles. The series of points to consider has been compiled from several different resources.[8,17–19]

Step 1: Assess the Clarity of the Review Question

Readers should assess the clarity of the question being posed within the review. Well-formulated questions that can help direct practice should generally address (1) the type of exposure (to a risk factor, an intervention, or a diagnostic test), (2) the outcome of interest, (3) the type of person being studied, and (4) the comparison against which the exposure is being compared.[18] An example that illustrates these four areas is found in van der Heijden and colleagues'[20] systematic review of randomized controlled trials (RCTs) of physiotherapy for patients with soft tissue shoulder disorders. Within the body of the article, the type of exposure (different forms of physiotherapy), the outcomes of interest (success rates, pain reduction, functional status, mobility, and need for drugs or surgery), the type of person being studied (those with soft tissue shoulder disorders; studies reporting on individuals after mastectomy or fracture were excluded, as were studies reporting on shoulder pain with hemiplegia or rheumatoid arthritis), and the comparison groups (some compared various forms of physiotherapy, some compared physiotherapy with placebo treatment, and some compared physiotherapy with other interventions such as drug or injection therapies) were presented.

Step 2: Evaluate the Article Identification and Selection Strategies

The reader should determine whether the method used to identify articles was comprehensive and whether the criteria used to select articles for review were appropriate. The process of identifying articles should be as comprehensive as possible, using the strategies identified in Chapter 4 or by other authors[18,21] and proceeding until new strategies yield only redundant studies. The search strategy should be documented clearly so that the reader has a clear sense of the time span of the review, the search terms used, and the databases that were accessed. After a pool of articles is identified, the reviewers must cull those articles that include the information needed to answer the question posed by the review. In the study of physiotherapy for soft tissue shoulder disorders, the authors of the review reported that their search strategy yielded 47 articles that met five initial criteria: patients had shoulder pain; treatments were randomly allocated; at least one treatment included physiotherapy; outcomes included success rate, pain, mobility, or functional status; and results were published before January 1996. Of these 47 articles, 24 were excluded from the review because the shoulder pain was not related to soft tissue and 3 were excluded because they represented multiple reports of the same data. Thus, 20 papers were ultimately included in the review.[20] Because the authors carefully reported their identification and selection process, readers are in a position to judge the completeness and appropriateness of the articles selected for review. Without this information, readers are left to wonder about the criteria used by the review author in selecting articles on which to report.

Step 3: Determine How the Authors Assess Validity of the Studies

The reader should determine whether and how the review authors assessed the validity of each of the studies within the review. In the study of soft tissue shoulder disorders, the authors compared each trial against eight validity criteria: selection criteria, assignment procedures, similarity of groups at baseline, withdrawals from treatment, missing values, presence of additional interventions, masked application of the intervention, and masked assessment of the outcome.[20] Readers can have a higher level of confidence in reviews in which two or more individuals have reviewed each study independently, with a process for resolving disagreements between reviewers.[8]

Step 4: Evaluate the Results Against the Strength of the Evidence

Readers should determine whether the results of the individual studies are evaluated against the strength of the evidence in those studies as well as in closely related studies. This generally means that the articles are not discussed in an article-by-article fashion (i.e., the reviews do not read as follows: Brown found x, Smith found y, Johnson found z). Rather, the articles are discussed topic by topic, and any single article may be referred to in several different sections of the review. For example, in van der Heijden and associates'[20] systematic review of physiotherapy for soft tissue shoulder disorders, the findings were grouped first by the type of intervention and then by the findings of those studies that were thought to have sufficiently high levels of validity. For example, they first identified six studies that evaluated the effect of ultrasound against various alternatives and judged that four of the six studies had acceptable validity. They then summarized the findings from those four studies, one of which compared ultrasound to cold therapy. Later, they evaluated the effect of cold therapy against various alternatives—one of which was obviously ultrasound. Thus, the one study comparing ultrasound and cold therapy was cited at least twice—once during the discussion of the effectiveness of ultrasound, and once with the discussion of the effectiveness of cold therapy.

Step 5: Evaluate the Personal Utility of the Review

Readers should evaluate the discussion and conclusions sections of the review to determine whether this information is consistent with the findings in the review and whether it has applications to their own practice. As was the case with the evaluation of a single study, readers must place the results of the review within the context of their own practices to determine the usefulness of the information.

STRUCTURED EVALUATION BY CLINICAL RESEARCH ISSUES

Recognizing the wide variety of types of research, some authors have developed more structured evaluation and application systems for different types of articles. As described earlier in Chapter 3, one of the most widely used frameworks is the one for the practice of EBM developed by Sackett and colleagues.[22] In this framework, studies are first classified according to the clinical issue being addressed: diagnosis and screening, prognosis, therapy, and harm. After classification by clinical issue, the study is evaluated for its level of evidence, based largely on types of research design. For this step, the EBM model has a hierarchy of five levels of evidence. Table 25-3 presents a modified version of their levels of evidence. Four different types of research

Table 25-3

Level of Evidence

Level	Characteristics
1a	Systematic review of randomized controlled trials, with homogeneity*
1b	Individual randomized controlled trial with narrow confidence intervals (representing large sample sizes or low variability of participants within groups)
2a	Systematic review of cohort studies, with homogeneity*
2b	Individual cohort study or low-quality randomized controlled trial
3a	Systematic review of case-control studies, with homogeneity*
3b	Individual case-control study
4	Case series and poor-quality cohort and case-control studies
5	Expert opinion without critical appraisal or based on physiology or bench research

*Homogeneity refers to the extent to which confidence intervals from individual studies overlap in a meta-analysis; see Chapter 26 for a more detailed discussion of homogeneity in meta-analysis.
Modified from Sackett DL, Straus SE, Richardson WS, et al: Guidelines. In: *Evidence-Based Medicine: How to Practice and Teach EBM,* 2nd ed, 2000, Edinburgh, UK, Churchill Livingstone, pp 169–182.

designs involving patients are represented, in the following order from the highest to lowest level: RCTs, cohort designs, case-control designs, and case series. Information about these different types of research can be found in Chapters 10 to 17. Each of these levels is divided into an "a" and "b" sublevel, with the "a" sublevel representing a systematic review of several studies at that level and the "b" sublevel representing a report of an individual study at that level or a poor-quality report of a study with a higher level design. A fifth, and lowest, level is reserved for expert opinion without critical appraisal or reports of basic science research that is not applied to patients in a clinical context. The study is then evaluated by working through a series of questions specific to the clinical issue at hand. In Sackett and colleagues'[22] EBM, 11 criteria are used to evaluate studies, with greater emphasis on the first 4 criteria (i.e., subjects were randomly assigned to groups; subject assignment to groups was concealed or "blinded"; study length and study methods were sufficient and complete, respectively, to realize results; and subjects were analyzed by the group to which they were assigned).

Using the more traditional method of evaluating studies for their research validity as advocated by Shadish and colleagues,[23] scientist-practitioners are first asked to determine whether the study results are valid (i.e., how well the study addressed the four subtypes of research validity). If the results are considered valid, readers are then asked to consider the importance or impact of the results. The impact of results is largely considered as the size of the treatment effect.[1] If the results are found to be both valid and important, readers are asked to consider whether they can be applied to the patient at hand.

In an effort to simplify and standardize written critical analyses of research literature, the Centre for Evidence-Based Medicine has developed a format known as critically appraised topics (CATs) and has provided online access to this format as well as other tools to assist the scientist-practitioner in analyzing research studies (see below).[24]

Box 25-1 presents a simplified version of Sackett and colleagues'[22] questions for studies related to therapy, meaning any health care intervention. These questions should seem familiar because they generally relate to concepts of design, control, and validity that have been presented in detail in early chapters of this text.

Box 25-2 presents a simplified version of Sackett and colleagues'[22] questions related to diagnosis, screening, prognosis, and harm. Background information about this kind of research is discussed in Chapter 15. Readers of this literature are encouraged to go to Sackett and colleagues' texts for more detail[25–27] or to any number of

Box 25-1

Structured Questions for Articles About Therapy

Are the results of this individual study valid?

Was the assignment of patients to treatment randomized?

Was follow-up sufficiently long and complete?

Were all patients analyzed in the groups to which they were randomized?

Were patients and clinicians masked to the treatment?

Were groups treated equally, apart from the therapy?

Were groups similar at the start of the study?

Are the results important?

What is the magnitude of the treatment effect?

How precise is the estimate of the treatment effect?

Are the results applicable to our patient?

Is our patient so different from those in the study for which the results do not apply?

Is the treatment feasible in our setting?

What are our patient's potential benefits and harms from the treatment?

Modified from Sackett DL, Straus SE, Richardson WS, et al: Therapy. In: *Evidence-Based Medicine: How to Practice and Teach EBM,* 2nd ed, 2000, Edinburgh, UK, Churchill Livingstone, pp 105–153.

excellent general or discipline specific evidence-based Web sites that feature similar information:

- Centre for Health Evidence (Canada): http://www.cche.net
- Occupational Therapy Evidence-Based Practice Research Group (McMaster University, Canada): http://www.srs-mcmaster.ca
- Centre for Evidence-Based Medicine (University of Toronto, Canada): http://cebm.utoronto.ca
- Evidence Based Medicine Toolkit (University of Alberta): http://www.ebm.med.ualberta.ca/Ebm.html

Web searches of "evidence-based practice," or "evidence-based practice" and "rehabilitation" (or a specific rehabilitation discipline), will yield many useful resources.

EVALUATION OF LEVELS OF EVIDENCE

As noted earlier, the work of Sackett and colleagues[27] is a common framework used in level-of-evidence approaches to evaluating research. Although Sackett and colleagues' framework for levels of evidence is cited frequently, readers should be aware that other,

similar frameworks exist.[28] For example, the American Academy of Cerebral Palsy and Developmental Medicine has modified Sackett's framework with some departures. Significant among those departures is the creation of separate levels of evidence for single-subject research studies, as well as modifications to the EBM levels, such as placing systematic reviews of RCTs and larger RCTs with sample size above 100 and narrow confidence intervals in the first level, while placing smaller RCTs, those with sample size below 100, systematic reviews of cohort studies, and very large "outcomes" studies in the second level.[24,29]

One of the criticisms of taking a level-of-evidence approach to the literature is that readers may simply identify the designs of studies without looking further to determine the quality of the research within the level, as noted by Ciccone: "Some people treat levels of evidence like a poker game in which an RCT beats two cohort studies. That is not always true in evidence-based practice. Studies from lower levels may be better for your purposes or they may be better in terms of the quality of the study."[30(p. 48)]

Another criticism of the level-of-evidence approach is that it places RCTs at the top of the hierarchy, without critically addressing the limitations imposed by the controlled manipulation that is required within an RCT. As discussed in Chapter 16, the outcomes movement developed in part because of the sense that RCTs were limited because they could not often capture the complexity of the clinical environment. A quote from Kane is repeated here:

If the practice of medicine (including rehabilitation) is to become more empiric, it will have to rely on epidemiological methods. Although some may urge the primacy of randomized clinical trials as the only path to true enlightenment, such a position is untenable for several reasons. First, the exclusivity of most trials is so great that the results are difficult to extrapolate to practice. Such trials may be the source of clinically important truths, but these findings will have to be bent and shaped to fit most clinical situations. Second, researchers do not have the time or resources to conduct enough trials to guide all practice. Instead, we need a more balanced strategy that combines targeted trials with well-organized analysis of carefully recorded clinical practice.[31(p. JS22)]

One approach to levels of evidence that bridges the RCT-versus-outcomes research debate is that of the Medical Research Council (London) (MRC), which presents a continuum-of-evidence model

Box 25-2

Structured Questions for Articles About Diagnosis, Screening, Prognosis, and Harm

Diagnosis

Is evidence about a diagnostic test valid?
Was there an independent, masked comparison with a reference standard?
Was the diagnostic test evaluated in an appropriate spectrum of patients?
Was the reference standard applied uniformly?
Was the test validated in a second group of patients?
Does the test accurately distinguish patients who do and do not have the disorder?
What are the sensitivity, specificity, and likelihood ratios?
Are multilevel likelihood ratios used?
Can I apply this test to a specific patient?
Is the test available, affordable, accurate, and precise in our setting?
Can we generate a sensible pretest probability for the patient?
Will resulting posttest probabilities affect the management of our patient?

Screening

Does early diagnosis lead to improved survival or quality of life?
Are patients diagnosed early willing to participate in treatment?
Are the time and energy it will take to confirm the diagnosis and provide care well spent?
Do the frequency and severity of the condition warrant the effort and expenditure of screening?

Prognosis

Is the evidence about prognosis valid?
Was a representative sample of patients assembled at a common point early in the course of the disease?
Was patient follow-up sufficiently long and complete?
Were objective outcome criteria applied in a masked fashion?
If done, was subgroup analysis adjusted and validated appropriately?
Is the evidence about prognosis important?
How likely are the outcomes over time?
How precise are the prognostic estimates?
Can we apply this prognostic evidence to our patients?
Are study patients similar to our own?
Will this evidence have an impact on our conclusions about what to tell our patients?

Harm

Are the results of this harm study valid?
Were groups similar in ways other than exposure to the potentially harmful agent?
Were exposures and outcomes measured in the same way in both groups?
Was the follow-up sufficiently long for the outcome to have occurred?
Is there strong evidence of causation from the exposure?
What is the magnitude of the association between exposure and outcome?
Can this evidence of harm be applied to our patient?
Is our patient so different from those in the study that the results do not apply?
How are risks and benefits balanced for this patient?
What are our patient's preferences, concerns, and expectations from this treatment?
What alternative treatments are available?

Modified from Sackett DL, Straus SE, Richardson WS, et al: *Evidence-Based Medicine: How to Practice and Teach EBM,* 2nd ed, 2000, Edinburgh, UK, Churchill Livingstone.

for studying complex interventions to improve health, including rehabilitation interventions that may involve substantial biopsychosocial elements, training of family members, and behavior modification.[32] The initial model was a linear five-phase continuum of evidence framework with increasing internal validity to investigative studies. The middle three phases of the framework paralleled the EBM hierarchy of evidence, with case studies, level 4 of the EBM model, as phase 2 of the MRC continuum, and RCTs, EBM level 1b, as phase 4 of the MRC continuum. Phase 5 was evaluation of a broader clinical application of the RCTs, accommodating the design to the unique demands of a clinical health setting or policy. More recently, the MRC has revised the model so that the phase continuum linearity is more flexible, while maintaining the ultimate final phase as an evaluation of a broader clinical application of previous research to the unique demands of the clinical health setting or policy.[33]

The beauty of this approach is that it captures the dynamic nature of the research endeavor, differentiates among research designs in a way that highlights the importance of RCTs, and acknowledges the role that pragmatic outcomes research should play once definitive RCTs have been completed.

The levels-of-evidence approach to evaluation of research studies is attractive, in part because of its apparent simplicity. On the surface, assigning a level of evidence requires only a cursory examination of each article to determine the study design. However, a more careful reading of the work on levels of evidence shows that determining the appropriate level of evidence represented by a given piece of research requires both assessment of the quality of the work and identification of the research design. The tools identified in the next section of this chapter can help readers make such quality distinctions.

EVALUATION OF RANDOMIZED CONTROLLED TRIALS

A final approach to the evaluation of original research involves assigning a quality score to the study. Typically, this is done for RCTs and reflects an important step beyond merely identifying the level of evidence of a study. Although many scoring systems exist,[9,10] two scoring systems for RCTs are described here: the Jadad 5-point scale[34] and the PEDro/OTseeker 10-point scale.[35] The Jadad scale has been evaluated for reliability by several authors with conflicting results.[36-39] The single published report of

the reliability of the PEDro scale concluded that the reliability of consensus judgments of the total PEDro scale is acceptable.[40]

Table 25-4 shows the criteria and scoring for both the PEDro and Jadad scales. This table shows that the information that contributes to each score is similar, with both scales including scored criteria related to random allocation, masking of participants and researchers, and retention of participants within the study. In addition, the PEDro scale allocates points for proper use of statistical tools. Operational definitions for each PEDro criterion can be found at the PEDro Web site (http://www.pedro.org.au) or in an appendix to Maher and associates'[40] report on PEDro scale reliability.

Maher and associates[40] also reported on the base rate at which the various PEDro scale items were found in the trials they reviewed. Random allocation was present in about 96% of trials, groups were similar at baseline in about 63%, but in only 19% was the allocation concealed from the person determining participant eligibility for the trial. Assessors were masked in about 42% of trials, but the participant was masked in only about 6% and the clinician in only about 4% of trials. The low levels of participant and clinician masking is to be expected given the interactive, participative nature of many rehabilitation interventions. About 66% of trials had less than 15% of participants drop out of the study, but only about 15% of trials used an intention-to-treat analysis to manage the dropouts. About 93% of trials made between-groups statistical comparisons, and about 88% provided both point measures and variability data. Table 25-5 shows the use of the PEDro score to rate the quality of a sample of RCTs in rehabilitation.

SUMMARY

The major elements of a research article are the title; abstract; introduction, methods, results, discussion, conclusions, and references sections; and, sometimes, an appendix. When discussing previously published work, reviewers should use the past tense and should make clear whether statements are their own or the opinions of the authors whose study they are reviewing. Reviewers of single studies should classify the research and its variables, compare the purposes and conclusions, outline the design and control elements, determine the threats to the validity of the study, place the study in the context of previous work, and assess the study's utility for their personal practice. Evaluators of review articles should

Table 25-4

Scales for Scoring the Quality of Randomized Controlled Trials

Research Concept	PEDro Scale*	Jadad Scale†
Eligibility	1. Eligibility criteria were specified. Not scored.	
Random Allocation and Its Impact on Baseline Characteristics	2. Subjects were randomly allocated to groups (in a crossover study, subjects were randomly allocated to an order in which treatments were received). No=0, Yes=1. 3. Allocation was concealed. No=0, Yes=1. 4. The groups were similar at baseline regarding the most important prognostic indicators. No=0, Yes=1.	1. Was the study described as randomized? No=0, Yes=1. Give 1 additional point if method of randomization was appropriate. Deduct 1 point if method of randomization was inappropriate.
Masking of Participants, Clinicians, and Researchers	5. There was blinding of all subjects. No=0, Yes=1. 6. There was blinding of all therapists who administered the therapy. No=0, Yes=1. 7. There was blinding of all assessors who measured at least one key outcome. No=0, Yes=1.	2. Was the study described as double blind? No=0, Yes=1. Give 1 additional point if method of blinding was appropriate. Deduct 1 point if method of blinding was inappropriate.
Retention of Participants	8. Measures of at least one key outcome were obtained from more than 85% of the subjects initially allocated to groups. No=0, Yes=1. 9. All subjects for whom outcome measures were available received the treatment or control condition as allocated or, when this was not the case, data for at least one key outcome was analyzed by "intention to treat." No=0, Yes=1.	3. Was there a description of withdrawals and dropouts? No=0, Yes=1
Use of Statistical Tools	10. The results of between-groups statistical comparisons were reported for at least one key outcome. No=0, Yes=1. 11. The study provided both point measures and measures of variability for at least one key outcome. No=0, Yes=1.	
Total possible	**10 points**	**5 points**

*PEDro scale. Adapted from PEDro scale download. Available at: http://www.pedro.org.au/english/downloads/pedro-scale/. Accessed February 20, 2015.
†Jadad AR, Enkin MW: Assessing the quality of RCTs: why, what, how, and by whom? In: *Randomized Controlled Trials: Questions, Answers and Musings*, 2nd ed, Malden, MA, 2007, Blackwell Publishing, Inc.

assess the clarity of the review question, evaluate the article identification and selection strategies, determine how the authors assess the validity of the studies, evaluate the results against the strength of the evidence, and evaluate the personal utility of the review. Other methods of evaluating research articles include using structured evaluation checklists for different types of research, evaluating the level of evidence generated by a study, and using scoring systems developed for RCTs.

Table 25-5

PEDro Scoring of Selected Randomized Controlled Trials in Rehabilitation

Primary Author/Study Characteristics	Chin et al, 2001[41*]	Clark et al, 1997[42†]	Kraemer et al, 2001[43]	Mancini et al,[44]	Nilsson et al, 2001[45*]	Perry et al, 1999[46†]	Purdy[47†]
Participant characteristics or diagnosis	Independent living in frail older adults	Independent living in older adults	Healthy women exposed to maximal eccentric exercise	Older adults with Parkinson's disease and drooling	Older adults with hemiparesis after stroke	Adults with bipolar disorder	Children with Down syndrome
Intervention	Exercise and/or enriched foods	Occupational therapy	Compression therapy	Botulinum toxin	Body-weight–supported treadmill training	Patient education	Oral-motor treatment or behavioral modification
PEDro scale scores							
Random allocation	Y	Y	Y	Y	Y	Y	Y
Concealed allocation	Y	N	N	N	Y	Y	N
Baseline similarity	Y	N	Y	Y	Y	Y	N
Participant masking	N	N	N	Y	N	N	N
Clinician masking	N	N	N	Y	N	N	N
Assessor masking	N	Y	N	Y	Y	Y	Y
High retention	N	N	Y	Y	Y	Y	N
Intention to treat	N	Y	Y	Y	N	Y	N
Between-groups comparisons	Y	Y	Y	Y	Y	Y	N
Point and variability	Y	Y	Y	N	Y	Y	Y
Total	**5**	**5**	**6**	**8**	**7**	**8**	**3**

*Rating from PEDro.
†Rating from OTseeker.

REFERENCES

1. Sackett DL, Straus SE, Richardson WS, et al: *Evidence-Based Medicine: How to Practice and Teach EBM*, 2nd ed, Edinburgh, UK, 2000, Churchill Livingstone.
2. Chiarello CM, Gundersen L, O'Halloran T: The effect of continuous passive motion duration and increment on range of motion in total knee arthroplasty patients, *J Orthop Sports Phys Ther* 25:119–127, 1997.
3. Ververeli PA, Sutton DC, Hearn SL, et al. Continuous passive motion after total knee arthroplasty: Analysis of costs and benefits, *Clin Orthop* 321:208–215, 1995.
4. Riegelman RK: *Studying a Study and Testing a Test: Reading Evidence-Based Health Research*, 6th ed, Philadelphia, Pa, 2012, Wolters Kluwer/Lippincott Williams & Wilkins.
5. Chalmers TC, Smith H, Blackburn B, et al: A method for assessing the quality of a randomized control trial, *Control Clin Trials* 2:31–49, 1981.
6. Guyatt GH, Sackett DL, Cook DJ, for the Evidence-Based Medicine Working Group: Users' guides to the medical literature. II: How to use an article about therapy or prevention. A: Are the results of the study valid? *JAMA* 270:2598–2601, 1993.
7. Guyatt GH, Sackett DL, Cook DJ, for the Evidence-Based Medicine Working Group: Users' guides to the medical literature. II: How to use an article about therapy or prevention. B: What were the results and will they help me in caring for my patients? *JAMA* 271:59–63, 1994.
8. Meade MO, Richardson WS: Selecting and appraising studies for a systematic review, *Ann Intern Med* 127:531–537, 1997.
9. Moher D, Jadad AR, Nichol G, et al: Assessing the quality of randomized controlled trials: An annotated bibliography of scales and checklists, *Control Clin Trials* 16:62–73, 1995.
10. Verhagen AP, de Vet HCW, de Bie RA, et al: The art of quality assessment of RCTs included in systematic reviews, *J Clin Epidemiol* 54:651–654, 2001.
11. Rothstein JM: Commenting on commentaries [editor's note], *Phys Ther* 71:431–432, 1991.
12. Gose JC: Continuous passive motion in the postoperative treatment of patients with total knee replacement: A retrospective study, *Phys Ther* 67:39–42, 1987.
13. Milne S, Brosseau L, Robinson V, et al: Continuous passive motion following total knee arthroplasty, *Cochrane Database Syst Rev*, 2:CD004260, 2003.
14. Guyatt G, Rennie D, Meade MO, Cook DJ, editors: *Users' Guides to the Medical Literature: Essentials of Evidence-Based Clinical Practice*, 2nd ed, Chicago, Ill, 2009, American Medical Association.
15. Guyatt GH, Rennie D, editors: *Users' Guides to the Medical Literature: Essentials of Evidence-Based Clinical Practice*, Chicago, Ill, 2002, American Medical Association.
16. Guyatt GH, Rennie D: Users' guides to the medical literature [editorial], *JAMA* 270:2096–2097, 1993.
17. Oxman AD, Sackett DL, Guyatt GH: Users' guides to the medical literature: I. How to get started, *JAMA* 270:2093–2095, 1993.
18. Counsell C: Formulating questions and locating primary studies for inclusion in systematic reviews, *Ann Intern Med* 127:380–387, 1997.
19. Shaughnessy AF, Slawson DC: Getting the most from review articles: A guide for readers and writers, *Am Fam Physician* 55:2155–2160, 1997.
20. van der Heijden GJMG, van der Windt DAWM, de Winter AF: Physiotherapy for patients with soft tissue shoulder disorders: A systematic review of randomised clinical trials, *BMJ* 315:25–30, 1997.
21. Dickersin K, Scherer R, Lefebvre C: Identifying relevant studies for systematic reviews, *BMJ* 309:1286–1291, 1994.
22. Sackett DL, Straus SE, Richardson WS, et al: Guidelines. In: *Evidence-Based Medicine: How to Practice and Teach EBM*, 2nd ed, Edinburgh, UK, 2000, Churchill Livingstone, pp 169–182.
23. Shadish WR, Cook TD, Campbell DT: *Experimental and Quasi-Experimental Designs for Generalized Causal Inference*, Boston, Mass, 2002, Houghton-Mifflin.
24. Centre for Evidence-Based Medicine. Catmaker. Availabe at: http://www.cebm.net/catmaker-ebm-calculators/. Accessed February 20, 2015.
25. Sackett DL, Straus SE, Richardson WS, et al: Diagnosis and screening. In: *Evidence-Based Medicine: How to Practice and Teach EBM*, 2nd ed, Edinburgh, UK, 2000, Churchill Livingstone, pp 67–93.
26. Sackett DL, Straus SE, Richardson WS, et al: Prognosis. In: *Evidence-Based Medicine: How to Practice and Teach EBM*, 2nd ed, Edinburgh, UK, 2000, Churchill Livingstone, pp 95–103.
27. Sackett DL, Straus SE, Richardson WS, et al: Harm. In: *Evidence-Based Medicine: How to Practice and Teach EBM*, 2nd ed, Edinburgh, UK, 2000, Churchill Livingstone, pp 155–168.
28. Law M, Philip I: Evaluating the evidence. In Law M, editor: *Evidence-Based Rehabilitation: A Guide to Practice*, Thorofare, NJ, 2008, Slack, pp 121–142.
29. Darrah J, Hickman R, O'Donnell M, et al. AACPDM Methodology to Develop Systematic Reviews of Treatment Interventions, rev 1.2. 2008. Available at: https://www.aacpdm.org/resources/outcomes/systematicReviewsMethodology.pdf. Accessed May 13, 2014.
30. Glaros S: Evidence is not created equal: A discussion of levels of evidence, *PT Magazine* 11(10):42–49, 52, 2003.
31. Kane RL: Improving outcomes in rehabilitation: A call to arms (and legs), *Med Care* 35(Suppl):JS21–JS27, 1997.
32. Medical Research Council. A Framework for Development and Evaluation of RCTs for Complex Interventions to Improve Health. Available at: http://webarchive.nationalarchives.gov.uk/20140102215327/ http://www.mrc.ac.uk/Utilities/Documentrecord/index.htm?d=MRC003372. Accessed February 20, 2015
33. Medical Research Council. Developing and Evaluating Complex Interventions: New Guidance. Available at: http://webarchive.nationalarchives.gov.uk/20140102215327/ http://mrc.ac.uk/utilities/documentrecord/index.htm?d=mrc004871. Accessed February 20, 2015.
34. Jadad AR, Enkin MW: *Randomized Controlled Trials: Questions, Answers and Musings*, 2nd ed, Malden, MA, 2007, Blackwell Publishing, Inc.

35. PEDro scale. Available at: www.pedro.org.au. Accessed December 15, 2014.

36. Bhandari M, Richards RR, Sprague S, Schemitsch EH: Quality in the reporting of randomized trials in surgery: Is the Jadad scale reliable? *Control Clin Trials* 22:687–688, 2001.

37. Clark HD, Wells GA, Huet C, et al: Assessing the quality of randomized trials: Reliability of the Jadad scale, *Control Clin Trials* 20:448–452, 1999.

38. Oremus M, Wolfson C, Perrault A, et al: Interrater reliability of the modified Jadad quality scale for systematic reviews of Alzheimer's disease drug trials, *Dement Geriatr Cogn Disord* 12:232–236, 2001.

39. Jadad AR, Moore RA, Carroll D, et al: Assessing the quality of reports on randomized clinical trials: Is blinding necessary? *Control Clin Trials* 17:1–12, 1996.

40. Maher CG, Sherrington C, Herbert RD, et al: Reliability of the PEDro scale for rating the quality of randomized controlled trials, *Phys Ther* 83:713–721, 2003.

41. Chin A, Paw MJM, de Jong N, Schouten EG, et al: Physical exercise and/or enriched foods for functional improvement in frail, independently living elderly: A randomized controlled trial, *Arch Phys Med Rehabil* 82:811–817, 2001.

42. Clark F, Azen SP, Zemke R, et al: Occupational therapy for independent-living older adults: A randomized controlled trial, *JAMA* 278:1321–1326, 1997.

43. Kraemer WJ, Bush JA, Wickham RB, et al: Influence of compression therapy on symptoms following soft tissue injury from maximal eccentric exercise, *J Orthop Sports Phys Ther* 31:282–290, 2001.

44. Mancini F, Zangaglia R, Cristina S, et al: Double-blind, placebo-controlled study to evaluate the efficacy and safety of botulinum toxin type A in the treatment of drooling in parkinsonism, *Mov Disord* 18:685–688, 2003.

45. Nilsson L, Carsson J, Danielsson A, et al: Walking training of patients with hemiparesis at an early stage after stroke: A comparison of walking training on a treadmill with body weight support and walking training on the ground, *Clin Rehabil* 15:515–527, 2001.

46. Perry A, Tarrier N, Morriss R, et al: Randomised controlled trial of efficacy of teaching patients with bipolar disorder to identify early symptoms of relapse and obtain treatment, *BMJ* 318:149–153, 1999.

47. Purdy AH, Deitz JC, Harris SR: Efficacy of two treatment approaches to reduce tongue protrusion of children with Down syndrome, *Dev Med Child Neurol* 29:469–476, 1987.

CHAPTER OUTLINE

Reasons to Synthesize the Literature
Ways to Synthesize the Literature
Narrative Reviews
Systematic Reviews Without Meta-Analysis
Systematic Reviews with Meta-Analysis
Preparing for a Systematic Review
Determine the Rationale and Purpose of the Review

Identify the Literature
Select Studies for Inclusion
Synthesizing the Literature
Identify Important Characteristics of Individual Studies
Determine the Quality of the Individual Studies
Identify Important Constructs Across Studies
Make Descriptive Comparisons Across Studies

Pool Statistical Data Across Studies
Specify Problems That Need Further Study
Reporting on Systematic Reviews
Describing Review Methods
Presenting Review Results
Summary

Learning to evaluate research evidence one study at a time is a necessary, but not sufficient, skill for evidence-based practitioners. Because single studies, by themselves, rarely provide definitive answers to guide practice, clinicians must base their work on the aggregate evidence available about a given issue. Sometimes the aggregate evidence needed to answer a clinical question may be available in published reviews completed by other clinicians or researchers or in published guidelines promulgated by various private or government agencies committed to improving the use of evidence in health care.[1,2] Other times the evidence needed to answer a clinical question may not have been aggregated by others, and clinicians need to synthesize the literature themselves. This chapter outlines reasons for synthesizing the literature, defines three approaches to synthesizing the literature, and provides guidance for conducting a systematic review of the literature, including preparation for the review, review methods, and ways of reporting on systematic reviews.

REASONS TO SYNTHESIZE THE LITERATURE

Aggregating evidence to guide practice is one of the most important reasons for synthesizing the literature, but it is not the only reason to do so. Fink,[3] in her text on conducting research literature reviews, outlines five additional reasons for synthesizing the literature: (1)

developing research proposals required for academic degrees, (2) developing proposals required to apply for external research funding, (3) identifying research methods, (4) identifying experts in a given topic area, and (5) identifying funding sources in a given area.

For all these reasons, the ability to synthesize the literature is an essential skill for rehabilitation professionals. Looking across a rehabilitation career, the same professional may need to synthesize the literature to fulfill academic requirements as a student, to guide practice as a clinician, to identify possible consultants for a new program as a service administrator, and to obtain funding for research as an academician.

WAYS TO SYNTHESIZE THE LITERATURE

There are three general approaches to synthesizing research results across several different studies: narrative reviews, systematic reviews without meta-analysis, and systematic reviews with meta-analysis.[4–6] Definitions and characteristics of each approach are presented, with examples from the rehabilitation literature.

Narrative Reviews

Narrative reviews of the literature are often characterized by their limitations, as noted in this humorous quote presented earlier in Chapter 12:

A common method of integrating several studies with inconsistent findings is to carp on the design or analysis deficiencies of all but a few studies—those remaining frequently being one's own work or that of one's students and friends—and then advance the one or two "acceptable" studies as the truth of the matter.[7(p. 7)]

In the past, narrative reviews were the norm, and guidelines for conducting literature searches focused on developing a conceptual understanding of the topic of interest.[8] Narrative reviews rarely provide detailed methods about how the review was conducted, typically do not have independent evaluation of articles by more than one rater, and do not generally include formal evaluation or scoring of the studies. In format, they often read more like book chapters than research articles. Narrative reviews often summarize the reviewed studies in series—Jones found this, Brown found that, Smith found something else altogether—rather than integrating information across the studies.

Although largely replaced by systematic reviews as a means of aggregating evidence to apply to practice, there are still valid reasons to undertake narrative reviews of the literature. Take, for example, Hesse and colleagues'[9] narrative review about treadmill training with partial body-weight support after stroke. The purpose of this review appeared to be to provide practitioners with a broad base of information about a particular therapy regimen, in this case body-weight–supported treadmill training (BWSTT). Thus, their review provided an overview of the motor learning theory and physiological basis for BWSTT, a description of current and emerging technical aspects of BWSTT, and a narrative summary of the clinical literature about BWSTT. So providing thorough information about a particular therapeutic approach is one valid reason to conduct a narrative review.

Another time to conduct a narrative review is when the literature in an area is sparse, yet diverse. For example, Geertzen and colleagues[10] undertook a review of the literature on rehabilitation after lower-limb amputation. They identified 24 articles for inclusion in the review, but these articles covered so many different themes (from functional outcomes to phantom pain and skin problems) and appeared to represent such a wide array of research designs that it would be difficult to apply the more uniform criteria typical of systematic reviews.

Sometimes a narrative review can serve the purpose of examining approaches to treatment over time. Sommers and colleagues[11] undertook a review and critical analysis of treatment research related to articulation and phonological disorders. Their interest was in evaluating research methods across two decades rather than in aggregating evidence about the effectiveness of treatment for articulation and phonological disorders. Indeed, if they had tried to conduct a systematic review of treatment effectiveness, they would have had difficulty given the wide variety of designs they identified and the limited information they found about participant characteristics and extent and duration of treatment.

Narrative write-ups of reviews are also the norm in research and grant proposals and in the introductory sections of research papers. Space is often limited in these formats, so the written literature review highlights only the information needed to "build a case"—that is, justifying the need to investigate a specific intervention, use of a specific measurement tool, or use of a specific design—for the study at hand, even when the researchers have been more systematic in gathering and evaluating evidence on the topic.

Systematic Reviews Without Meta-Analysis

Systematic reviews, which require documented search strategies and explicit inclusion and exclusion criteria for studies used in the review, reduce the sorts of biases noted in the quote in the previous section. Although some systematic reviews include statistical pooling of results across studies (meta-analysis, discussed in the next section), many do not. In some cases, review authors simply do not have the statistical expertise needed to conduct a meta-analysis; in other instances, the body of literature consists of such varied designs and diverse types of data presentation and analysis that statistical pooling of data is not feasible.

Bilney and colleagues[12] conducted a systematic review of literature to determine the effectiveness of physiotherapy, occupational therapy, and speech-language therapy for people with Huntington's disease. Their work exhibits the characteristics typical of a systematic review without meta-analysis: research article format, a documented search strategy, explicit rules for including and excluding studies from the review, independent data extraction by two reviewers, formal ratings of study quality, and results that are presented in tables that summarize important information from each study.

Systematic Reviews with Meta-Analysis

Systematic reviews with meta-analysis are differentiated from other reviews by their meta-analytic component. Meta-analysis is the analysis of analyses (in the same way that meta-theory, introduced in Chapter 2, is theorizing about theory). The basic concept behind meta-analysis is that the size of the differences between treatment groups (the effect size) is mathematically standardized so that it can be pooled across studies with different, but conceptually related, dependent variables. Recent examples in the rehabilitation literature include meta-analyses that synthesized the evidence about the effectiveness of constraint-induced movement therapy (CIMT) for adults poststroke,[13] the effectiveness of physical therapy in treating persons with Parkinson's disease,[14] and the effectiveness of the Picture Exchange Communication System (PECS) as a communication system with children with autism spectrum disorder.[15] McCallum and colleagues[16] conducted a systematic review with a qualitative meta-analysis of quality in physical therapy clinical education. Because this study included both quantitative and qualitative design studies, data pooling was inappropriate. Instead, McCallum and colleagues[16] employed a qualitative content analysis, analyzing the data by clinical education themes.

Having outlined the three general ways of synthesizing the literature, the remainder of this chapter provides more detail on how to conduct a systematic review of the literature, with or without meta-analysis. The methodology of systematic reviews is designed to produce a review that is systematic, explicit, and reproducible.[3] Three important resources provided most of the methodological details for this section. First, the PRISMA Statement Web site[17] includes a checklist of recommendations to consider in preparing a systematic review for publication, divided into categories such as Methods, Results, and Discussion. Each section has several statements to guide authors. For example, the Methods section includes, "State the process for selecting studies (i.e., screening, eligibility, included in systematic review, and, if applicable, included in the meta-analysis)." Also serving as guides in this section are Fink's[3] book on conducting research literature reviews and Law and Philip's[18] chapter on systematically reviewing the evidence. Brief examples based on several studies of continuous passive motion (CPM) use after total knee arthroplasty (TKA) are given to illustrate some of the steps.[19–25] Figure 26-1 reproduces Fink's[3(p. 190)] overview of the steps in conducting a systematic review of the literature.

PREPARING FOR A SYSTEMATIC REVIEW

Three preparatory steps need to be completed before a systematic review can be undertaken: (1) determining the rationale and purpose of the review, (2) identifying literature for potential inclusion in the review, and (3) selecting studies for inclusion.

Determine the Rationale and Purpose of the Review

Just as any research that involves the collection of new data should have a clearly developed rationale and stated purpose, so should a systematic review of the literature. The rationale should identify a problem the systematic review is to address or establish the need for the systematic review. For example, English and associates identified as a problem the amount and pattern of physical activity and sedentary behaviors of persons poststroke and a need for identifying ways of changing behaviors.[26] A systematic review should have a well-developed purpose statement that follows the PICO elements. That is, the purpose statement should specify participant characteristics and diagnoses (P), intervention characteristics (I), the comparative intervention(s) (C), and dependent variables or outcomes of interest (O). The specificity of the purpose statement should match the body of literature that is expected to be identified for the review. For example, the purpose statement for Bilney and colleagues' review of therapy effectiveness in Huntington's disease is relatively broad:

> To assist physiotherapists, occupational therapists, speech-language pathologists, and rehabilitation physicians to effectively treat people with Huntington's disease by providing a review and critical evaluation of the evidence on therapy outcomes.[12(p. 12)]

Contrast this general objective with the far more specific objective of Milne and colleagues' meta-analysis on CPM following TKA:

> The aim of this meta-analysis is to determine the effectiveness of CPM following knee arthroplasty. We will compare CPM to standard physiotherapy treatments done on patients after a total knee arthroplasty. Standard physiotherapy treatment consisted of any combination of the following interventions: range-of-motion (ROM) exercises, muscle strengthening exercises (isometric, dynamic), functional exercises, gait training, immobilization, and ice. The outcome measures of interest for the meta-analysis were active and passive knee ROM, length of hospital stay, pain, knee swelling, fixed flexion deformity and quadriceps strength at end of treatment and during follow-up.[27(p. 2)]

The following objectives and purpose statement of English and associates' systematic review are even more

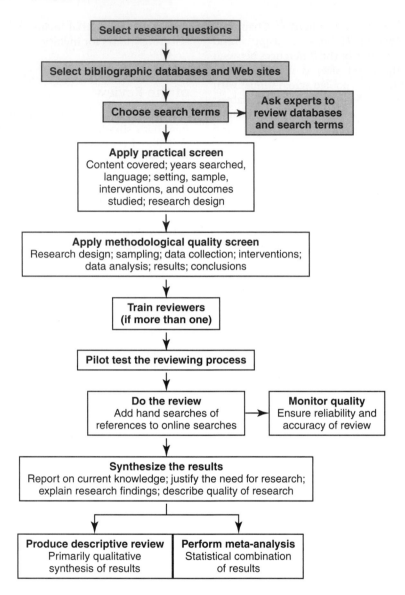

Figure 26-1 An overview of the systematic literature review process. (Modified from Fink A: *Conducting Research Literature Reviews: From the Internet to Paper*, 4th ed, Los Angeles, Calif: 2014, Sage.)

specific, likely reflecting the guidelines of the PRISMA statement:

> The over arching aim of this systematic review is to answer the question: How active are people living in the community with a stroke-related disability? Specifically
>
> 1. How much per day do people with stroke spend sedentary (i.e., sitting or lying down)?
> 2. How much time per day do people with stroke spend engaged in physical activity when they are

active, what is the intensity level (light, moderate, vigorous) of this activity?
> 3. What is the pattern of accumulation of sedentary time and physical activity? And
> 4. What factors influence physical activity levels in people with stroke?[26(p. 186)]

Although Figure 26-1 implies that determining the research question occurs as the first step of the process, in our experience the initial statement of the research question is merely a draft question that is revised and refined as the literature search is undertaken and studies are selected for inclusion in the review. Imagine that Bilney and colleagues[12] started their review hoping to determine the effect of rehabilitation therapies on quality of life in individuals with Huntington's disease. After they searched the literature, they would have discovered that few studies used quality-of-life measures—and they would need to either abandon the review or revise their purpose to include a broader range of dependent variables. Likewise, imagine that Milne and colleagues[27] had not specified their interest in comparing CPM to standard care. On review of the literature, they would discover a large number of studies of CPM following TKA, some of which compared different CPM protocols to one another—requiring that they either examine several different comparisons or limit their purpose to comparing CPM to standard care.

Identify the Literature

Using the techniques outlined in Chapter 4, the researcher must identify a relatively complete set of articles on the topic for possible inclusion in the review. Typically this begins with a search of one or more electronic bibliographic databases. Because a systematic review needs to be explicit and reproducible, the researchers must carefully document the final search strategy used to identify articles for possible inclusion. Of course, most researchers will "play around" in the electronic databases to see what is yielded from different combinations of terms and different limitations on searches—these exploratory searches need not be documented. However, after a set of search terms, databases, and limits (such as the years included in the review, the language of articles) is set, researchers should re-run their searches to obtain a definitive set of articles for possible inclusion in the review. For example, English and associates reported they used the MEDLINE database as the basis for their search and used four additional databases to expand their search.[26] They also reported examples of different Medical Subject Headings (MeSH) for their search terms and indicated the reader could obtain other limiters and "the full search strategy"[26(p. 186)] from the authors.

Select Studies for Inclusion

After a set of articles for possible inclusion in the review is identified, the researchers need to determine which articles are relevant to the question at hand. Typically this will be a two-step process. First, the identified studies from the search will be reviewed by title and abstract for relevancy. Subsequently, the reviewers should review the articles to ensure the studies meet the inclusion criteria for the review. For example, assume that the electronic database searches yield 100 unique articles for possible inclusion in our hypothetical review that compares standard care plus CPM to standard care following TKA.

The next step is to review the article abstracts to ensure that each article is a report of original research, that the participants have undergone TKA, and that at least one of the comparisons in the article is between standard care plus CPM and standard care. Perhaps 25 articles will be review articles or "how-we-do-it" articles, 16 will compare various CPM protocols to one another, and 4 will be "false hits" with participants who have undergone anterior cruciate ligament reconstruction, leaving 55 articles for possible inclusion in the review. Because this is still a relatively large number of articles of varying quality, perhaps the researchers will decide to eliminate any study that includes fewer than 20 participants per group or that uses nonexperimental, retrospective methods. After reviewing the abstracts of the 55 remaining articles, this might reduce the number of articles for possible inclusion to a manageable 35. The researchers might obtain hard copies or PDF files of those 35 articles, using the various strategies presented in Chapter 4. After the hard copies or PDF files of the selected studies are obtained, they should be reviewed to ensure that they meet the specified criteria; in some instances, the abstract will not have included enough information to make this determination; in others, the abstract will have misrepresented the particulars of the study.

After an article review confirms that an article meets the study criteria, its reference list should be reviewed (sometimes referred to as a citation or bibliographic search) to identify other potential studies that meet the inclusion criteria but were missed by the electronic searches. Some reviewers supplement this strategy with "hand searching" of journals expected to be good sources of articles on the topic and with consultation with experts to determine whether they know of relevant studies, particularly unpublished studies that have been missed. Generally, the use of unpublished studies, and sometimes the use of "gray" literature, is discouraged in reviews because the studies are not accessible by traditional academic/research search processes or have not been reviewed by the traditional peer process. English and associates required that a study meet the following six criteria for it to be included in their review: "1) be a report of new original data, 2) be a peer-reviewed full-text article, 3) include adults who had experienced a stroke, 4) include at least one objective measure of free-living physical activity or exercise, 5) have objective measurements that were taken in a free-living situation and over 2 days, and 6) have its full text available in English."[26(p. 187)]

To enhance the reproducibility of the systematic review, two or more reviewers should independently determine which of the 100 initial articles to eliminate from the review and independently determine whether to add any additional articles through citation checking or hand searching. Discrepancies in eliminated or added articles would be resolved by discussion among the reviewers or by consultation with another reviewer who serves as a referee. Alternatively, reviewers may employ a decision rule that excludes any study if there is any doubt the study meets the inclusion criteria by any of the reviewers. English and associates had one reviewer who screened the titles and abstracts of articles and two reviewers who reviewed the articles to ensure they met the inclusion criteria, using consensus to resolve disagreements.[26] For our hypothetical search, assume that two additional studies are identified through citation checking, leaving a core of 37 articles to use in the next phase of the review.

Systematic reviews are always vulnerable to the criticism that the search strategies were incomplete, that the authors selected the wrong set of studies from those identified, and that publication bias could have had an impact on the review conclusions. To guard against these criticisms, authors should use comprehensive search strategies that extend beyond electronic bibliographic databases, should use more than one researcher to select studies, and should make their inclusion and exclusion criteria explicit. The issue with publication bias is the possibility that a higher proportion of studies favorable to the intervention being studied are published than are those unfavorable to the intervention, either because journal editors prefer to publish positive results or because authors more often submit positive results for publication. At minimum, authors should address the possibility of publication bias in their narrative. In meta-analysis, authors may also address the possibility of publication bias with a variety of analytic techniques.[3]

SYNTHESIZING THE LITERATURE

Having identified the core of 37 articles for the review, the next task is to undertake the intellectual task of identifying, organizing, and synthesizing the results across studies, initially examining the articles for methodological issues, and then focusing on content issues. Six steps can guide this process: (1) identifying important characteristics of individual studies, (2) determining the quality of the individual studies, (3) identifying important constructs across the studies, (4) making descriptive comparisons across studies, (5) pooling statistical information across studies if a meta-analysis is being done, and (6) specifying problems in need of further study.

It is useful to create a database for the review, much as one would do for a study of original research. The rows of the database are the included studies, and the columns are the variables related to each study. Garrard[28] has recommended that a database begin with the author in the first column, followed by the journal reference in the second, and the third column the year of the publication. Additionally, she suggests that the subsequent columns will be largely divided into two major areas: methodological features of studies (e.g., design and dependent variables) and content issues specific to the focus of the literature review.

Identify Important Characteristics of Individual Studies

Typically, the first step of a systematic review is "getting to know" each of the studies within the review. Important characteristics of each study are extracted, including items such as primary author, publication date, total number of participants, design features, independent variables, dependent measures, and summary results. It is important that more than one reviewer extract the data and that the review describe the method for resolving conflicts. For example, English and associates had two reviewers independently critique articles and assess for risk of bias, with a third reviewer resolving any disagreements.[26] Table 26-1 shows the individual characteristics that might be recorded for a subset of articles included for a systematic review of CPM use following TKA.

Determine the Quality of the Individual Studies

Many systematic reviews include a formal evaluation of quality, typically a level-of-evidence approach if the study designs vary widely or a scoring approach if the review is limited to randomized controlled trials. For example, Bilney and colleagues[12] identified the levels of evidence represented by each study in their review of therapy outcomes for Huntington's disease, and de Goede and associates[14] scored the trials in their review of the effects of physical therapy for Parkinson's disease, using a tool similar to those presented in Chapter 25. Alternatively, English and associates adapted an existing instrument that had been developed for critiquing case-control studies, broadening its utility to include other types of study designs.[26] They reported that 80%

Table 26-1

Characteristics of Included Studies

Study	Design	N	Comparison Groups	Dependent Variables	Major Results
Chen et al, 2000[20]	RCT	51	Usual care Usual care+CPM	Knee ROM Edema	No differences between groups
MacDonald et al, 2000[19]	RCT	120	Usual care Usual care+0°–50° CPM Usual care+70°–110° CPM	Knee ROM Functional score Pain Length of stay	No differences between groups
Chiarello et al, 1997[21]	RCT	45	Usual care control group Short-duration, set progression CPM Short-duration, as tolerated progression CPM Long-duration, set progression CPM Long-duration, as tolerated progression CPM	Knee ROM	No differences between groups
Pope et al, 1997[25]	RCT	57	Usual care Usual care+0°–40° CPM Usual care+0°–70° CPM	Knee ROM Functional score Pain Complications	No long-term differences between groups
Yashar et al, 1997[24]	RCT	210	Usual care+0°–30° CPM Usual care+70°–100° CPM	Knee ROM Functional score Pain Length of stay Complications	Few long-term differences between groups
Basso & Knapp, 1987[23]	Successive cohorts	23	Usual care+high-dose CPM Usual care+low-dose CPM	Knee ROM Edema Pain Length of stay	No differences between groups
Gose, 1987[22]	Retrospective chart review	55	Usual care Usual care+low-dose CPM	Knee ROM Length of stay Complications	No ROM differences between groups CPM group had shorter length of stay and fewer complications

CPM, continuous passive motion; RCT, randomized controlled trial; ROM, range of motion.

of the 30 included studies used reliable and valid physical activity measures. They also noted that overall the studies had low risk for bias, employing nine criteria to measure risk of bias. Table 26-2 shows how quality scoring might be presented for the randomized controlled trials included in a review of CPM after TKA. In this example, the quality scores are uniform and the item scores are similar, so there would be little reason to place more or less weight on particular studies based on their methodological rigor. Narrative validity analysis, as presented in Chapter 25, is also important to undertake; even randomized controlled trials with high scores for their design may have implementation flaws that limit their usefulness as a source of evidence. For example, if there were a rigorous randomized controlled trial from 1990 that identified shorter lengths of stay for patients who used CPM after TKA, these results would need to be interpreted in light of the much shorter stays typical of contemporary practice.

Identify Important Constructs Across Studies

In this phase of the review, the constructs and variables that undergird the studies become the focus, rather than the individual studies. By doing so, as in Table 26-3, it becomes clear, for example, that knee ROM is a dependent variable for all of the studies in the review, but that edema is a dependent variable in only two of them. Likewise, it is

clear that there are more data to answer a question about the impact of CPM at discharge (seven studies) than there are at 1 year postoperatively (three studies).

Make Descriptive Comparisons Across Studies

After each study has been examined independently, the reviewer compares results across the studies. In this hypothetical review of CPM after TKA, we see that several investigators have examined the impact of CPM on length of stay. Of the four authors who addressed this issue, Gose[22] found shorter lengths of stay with low-dose CPM added to usual care, and the other three researchers (Basso,[23] Yashar,[24] and MacDonald[19]) found no differences in length of stay between those receiving usual care or various types of CPM in addition to usual care. Having identified an inconsistent finding, the task of the review author is to examine this conflicting evidence carefully to determine whether there are differences among the studies that might explain the contradictory results. In this case, the only significant finding is in one of the older studies and the one with the weakest design (the retrospective chart review). The review conclusion would likely be that there is no contemporary evidence that use of CPM leads to reduced length of stay after TKA. Similar comparisons across studies would be made for each of the factors of interest within the review.

Table **26-2**

Quality Scores (PEDro Scale)* of Randomized Controlled Trials Included in the Review

	PRIMARY AUTHOR				
	Chen et al, 2000[20]	MacDonald et al, 2000[19]	Chiarello et al, 1997[21]	Pope et al, 1997[25]	Yashar et al, 1997[24]
Random allocation	Y	Y	Y	Y	Y
Concealed allocation	N	N	N	N	N
Baseline similarity	Y	Y	Y	Y	Y
Participant masking	N	N	N	N	N
Clinician masking	N	N	N	N	N
Assessor masking	Y	Y	N	N	Y
High retention	N	N	Y	Y	Y
Intention to treat	N	N	N	N	N
Between-groups comparisons	Y	Y	Y	Y	Y
Point and variability	Y	Y	Y	Y	N
Total	**5**	**5**	**5**	**5**	**5**

*From http://www.pedro.org.au.

Table **26-3**

Selected Constructs in Studies in the Review

	Constructs	Study*
Design Elements		
Group assignment	Nonrandom	Gose (1987), Basso (1987)
	Random	Pope (1995), Yashar (1997), Chiarello (1997), Chen (2000), MacDonald (2000)
Group comparisons	Usual care vs usual care+CPM	Gose (1987), Chen (2000)
	Usual care vs usual care+different CPM protocols	Chiarello (1997), Pope (1997), MacDonald (2000)
	Usual care+different CPM protocols	Basso (1997), Yashar (1997)
Implementation of CPM		
Dosage	20+ hours/day	Basso (1987), Pope (1997), Yashar (1997), MacDonald (2000)
	10 hours/day	Chiarello (1997)
	3–6 hours/day	Basso (1987), Gose (1987), Chiarello (1997), Chen (2000)
Initial CPM ROM	Not specified	Basso (1987), Chiarello (1997), Chen (2000)
	0° to 30°–50°	Gose (1987), Pope (1997), Yashar (1997), MacDonald (2000)
	0° to 60°–70°	Pope (1997)
	70° to 100°–110°	Yashar (1997), MacDonald (2000)
Outcomes	Knee ROM	Basso (1987), Gose (1987), Chiarello (1997), Pope (1997), Yashar (1997), Chen (2000), MacDonald (2000)
	Functional score	Pope (1997), Yashar (1997), MacDonald (2000)
	Complications	Gose (1987), Yashar (1997), Pope (1997)
	Pain	Basso (1987), Yashar (1997), Pope (1997), MacDonald (2000)
	Edema	Basso (1987), Chen (2000)
	Length of stay	Basso (1987), Gose (1987), Yashar (1997), MacDonald (2000)
Follow-up	Hospital discharge	Basso (1987), Gose (1987), Chiarello (1997), Yashar (1997), Pope (1997), MacDonald (2000), Chen (2000)
	One-year postoperative	Yashar (1997), Pope (1997), MacDonald (2000)

*References associated with each cited article are as follows: Basso,[23] Chen,[20] Chiarello,[21] Gose,[22] MacDonald,[19] Pope,[25] and Yashar.[24]

CPM, continuous passive motion; ROM, range of motion.

English and associates reported on constructs specific to their objectives, including amount of sedentary time per day, time spent in different levels of physical activity, patterns of activity, and factors influencing free-living activity. Among their results, they noted there were no studies that used measures explicit to measuring sedentary behaviors, but they estimated sedentary time from some of the studies. They also noted that when analyzing the studies for levels of activity, 22 of 30 studies measured steps per day, and one study measured the amount of time participants spent in moderate-intensity activity.[26]

Pool Statistical Data Across Studies

When there are enough studies, with enough comparisons in common, and with enough statistical detail, then statistical synthesis of studies can be accomplished through meta-analysis. The details needed to implement a meta-analysis are beyond the scope of this text, but readers are referred to a number of excellent articles, texts, and Web sites for further information.[7,28–38] Many reviewers who undertake a meta-analysis work with statisticians who have expertise in this specialized branch of statistics.

The central concepts that undergird meta-analysis are (1) the use of confidence intervals for hypothesis testing (see Chapter 22) and (2) the pooling of effects across studies. In traditional hypothesis testing, a probability is computed and a statistical conclusion is reached when the obtained p value is compared with a preset alpha level (see Chapter 20). In hypothesis testing with confidence intervals, a confidence interval is calculated for the difference of interest, and a statistical conclusion is reached by determining whether the confidence interval includes the value that corresponds to the null hypothesis (see Chapter 22). In a meta-analysis, the results of each of the studies are converted to confidence intervals, allowing all of the studies to be evaluated against a common indicator of "no difference," even when the variables used within the different studies are not the same. After confidence intervals are calculated for each study for a given comparison, the results are pooled and weighted by sample size to obtain a single value. This value, with an associated confidence interval, represents the aggregate effect across the reviewed studies.

For most purposes, the null hypothesis is represented by the value zero (0) because the null hypothesis proposes that there will be "no difference" between groups. If the confidence interval contains 0, there is no statistically significant difference between groups. If the confidence interval does not contain 0, there is a statistically significant difference between groups. When using confidence intervals to determine the significance of odds ratios and relative risk ratios, a significant difference is identified when the interval does not contain the number one (1). This is because a ratio of 1 means that the risks for the groups being compared are equal.

The mathematical complexities of meta-analysis are often elegantly summarized in a "forest plot." In fact, the central part of the logo for the Cochrane Collaboration is a stylized forest plot for a meta-analysis, reproduced as Figure 26-2. The vertical line represents "no difference" between comparison groups, and we will assume that values to the left of the line favor treatment (perhaps this is a meta-analysis of seven studies of a popular weight-loss program and values to the left represent weight loss) and values to the right of the line favor the control condition. The seven horizontal lines represent the seven different studies. The first and sixth studies in the meta-analysis demonstrate significant weight loss because their confidence intervals do not encompass the "no difference" point. The second, third, and fifth studies tend toward the weight-loss side of the plot, but do not represent significant differences because they encompass the "no difference" point. The fourth and seventh studies do not show significant differences and tend toward the "no difference" point. The diamond at the bottom of the plot represents the pooled effect across all of the studies. The vertical axis of the diamond gives the mean pooled effect, and the horizontal axis gives the confidence interval for the pooled effect. The conclusion from the Cochrane Collaboration forest plot is that the program results in modest weight losses when considered across these seven studies.

In an actual meta-analysis, many separate analyses may be done. For example, in our hypothetical review of CPM after TKA (assuming more than the

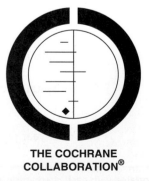

**THE COCHRANE
COLLABORATION®**

Figure 26-2 Logo of the Cochrane Collaboration, depicting a stylized forest plot of meta-analysis results.

seven studies that are presented in tables throughout this chapter), we might calculate pooled effects for the comparison between usual care and CPM for each of five different dependent variables and then do an additional five analyses for the comparison between long- and short-duration CPM. For example, Figure 26-3 illustrates a forest plot from de Goede and colleagues'[14] meta-analysis of therapy effects in Parkinson's disease, showing the results of one of the four analyses that were done for different dependent variables (activities of daily living, walking speed, stride length, and neurological signs).

One of the major statistical concerns about meta-analysis revolves around the concept of whether the different study results are homogeneous or heterogeneous. Homogeneity is desirable and "means that the results of each individual trial are mathematically compatible with the results of any of the others."[37] When the individual confidence intervals that are plotted on a forest plot overlap, the trials are said to be homogeneous. Conversely, when some lines do not overlap with any other lines, the trials are said to be heterogeneous, and they are often thought to represent different clinical populations of interest. More formal testing for heterogeneity is often done with a chi-square test

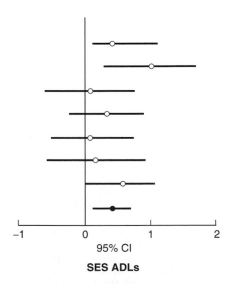

Figure 26-3 Forest plot showing significant impact of therapy on activities of daily living (ADLs) for individuals with Parkinson's disease. Visual analysis shows that the trials are homogeneous and the summary effect size (SES) is significant. (From de Goede CJT, Keus SHJ, Kwakkel G, Wagenaar RC: The effects of physical therapy in Parkinson's disease: A research synthesis, *Arch Phys Med Rehabil* 82:509–515, 2001.)

(see Chapter 21). Heterogeneity can be managed by "correcting" for covariates such as age, by doing separate meta-analyses for different clinical subgroups, or with a variety of other statistical maneuvers that require the assistance of a skilled meta-analyst.

Specify Problems That Need Further Study

Just as original research studies lead to recommendations for further study, the results of systematic reviews with or without meta-analysis generally suggest areas for further study. For some variables, the review may demonstrate consistent, rigorous results that can be considered definitive. For other variables, the review may reveal inconsistencies in the literature that need further study, may identify gaps in the literature that require more study, or may reveal methodological limitations of the literature that need to be rectified with more rigorous studies. As a result of their review, English and associates reported a paucity of information on the amount and patterns of time spent in sedentary and physical activity, as well as time spent in different intensity levels of activity. They further noted that studying the time spent in, and patterns of, sedentary and physical activity is complicated by the varied definitions of sedentary and physical activity time.[26]

For the actual meta-analysis on CPM after TKA, Milne and colleagues[27] found improvements in active knee flexion and analgesic use, as well as reduced length of stay and need for manipulation under anesthesia, with CPM and physical therapy compared with physical therapy alone. They concluded that CPM combined with physical therapy "may" be beneficial but noted that the potential benefits need to be weighed against the inconvenience and cost of CPM. Furthermore, they concluded that more research is needed to determine whether there are differences in effectiveness with different durations and intensities of CPM intervention. Note that these actual meta-analysis results are different from what might be concluded from the incomplete, hypothetical review presented in Tables 26-1 to 26-3, supporting the need to use complete, systematic methods to synthesize the literature.

REPORTING ON SYSTEMATIC REVIEWS

Reports of systematic reviews follow the format typical of a research article, with introduction, methods, results, and discussion sections. Reporting issues unique to systematic reviews are highlighted, including those specific to meta-analyses.[39]

Describing Review Methods

The methods section of a systematic review needs to be explicit and reproducible. This means that it is important to provide detailed information on search strategies, on how studies were selected for inclusion, and on how data were extracted from the studies. The PRISMA statement[17] includes a flowchart to help authors organize information about how they chose the literature ultimately appearing in the systematic review. The possibility of publication bias should be addressed in the narrative or with analytic techniques if a meta-analysis was performed. If, as is good practice, more than one reviewer independently selected studies and extracted data, information about the interrater reliability of the raters needs to be provided. In addition, the method for resolving any inconsistencies between raters needs to be specified. If a meta-analysis was done, a data analysis section with statistical information needs to be included, especially information about the homogeneity of the trials.

Any systematic review needs to include a listing of studies that were included in the review. Sometimes this is done in a separate table or appendix; other times the study citations are simply included in the reference list of the paper. Sometimes authors will also include a table or appendix of excluded studies so that readers can evaluate the results of the selection process used in the review.

Presenting Review Results

A typical systematic review tabulates basic information from each step of the synthesis. Tables 26-1, 26-2, and 26-3 are typical of the tables that would be included in a published report of a systematic review. Results of meta-analyses can be presented in tables, but they are often also presented in forest plots similar to those in Figures 26-2 and 26-3.

SUMMARY

Synthesis of the literature is needed for evidence-based practice, developing research proposals, and identifying research methods, experts, and funding sources in a given area. There are three general approaches to synthesizing research results across several different studies: (1) narrative review, (2) systematic review without meta-analysis, and (3) systematic review with meta-analysis.

Narrative reviews, although the norm in the past, are being replaced by systematic reviews, which are designed to be systematic, explicit, and reproducible.

When enough studies in a review meet certain mathematical requirements, a systematic review with meta-analysis may be done to pool results across many studies. Systematic reviews require a clearly stated purpose, a comprehensive search strategy, and clearly stated inclusion and exclusion criteria. Synthesis steps in a systematic review include identifying important characteristics of each study, determining the quality of each study, identifying important constructs across studies, making descriptive or statistical comparisons across studies, and specifying problems that need further study. Reports of systematic reviews follow the format of a traditional research article, with explicit methods, tabulations of information from each step of the synthesis, and, when appropriate, tables or forest plots of meta-analytic results.

REFERENCES

1. Ilott I: Challenging the rhetoric and reality: Only an individual and systemic approach will work for evidence-based occupational therapy, *Am J Occup Ther* 57:351–354, 2003.
2. Lieberman D, Scheer J: AOTA's evidence-based literature review project: An overview, *Am J Occup Ther* 56:344–349, 2002.
3. Fink A: *Conducting Research Literature Reviews: From the Internet to Paper*, 4th ed, Thousand Oaks, Calif, 2014, Sage.
4. Victor N: The challenge of meta-analysis: Discussion. Indications and contraindications for meta-analysis, *J Clin Epidemiol* 48:5–8, 1995.
5. Finney DJ: A statistician looks at meta-analysis, *J Clin Epidemiol* 48:87–103, 1995.
6. Pogue J, Yusurf S: Overcoming the limitations of current meta-analysis of randomised controlled trials, *Lancet* 351:47–52, 1998.
7. Glass GV: Primary, secondary and meta-analysis of research, *Educ Res* 5:3–9, 1976.
8. Findley TW: Research in physical medicine and rehabilitation. II. The conceptual review of the literature or how to read more articles than you ever want to see in your entire life, *Am J Phys Med Rehabil* 68:97–102, 1989.
9. Hesse S, Werner C, von Frankenberg S, Bardeleben A: Treadmill training with partial body weight support after stroke, *Phys Med Rehabil Clin North Am* 14:S111–S123, 2003.
10. Geertzen JHB, Martina JD, Rietman HS: Lower limb amputation. Part 2: Rehabilitation—a 10 year literature review, *Prosthet Orthot Int* 25:14–20, 2001.
11. Sommers RK, Logsdon BS, Wright JM: A review and critical analysis of treatment research related to articulation and phonological disorders, *J Commun Disord* 25:3–22, 1992.
12. Bilney B, Morris ME, Perry A: Effectiveness of physiotherapy, occupational therapy, and speech pathology for people with Huntington's disease: A systematic review, *Neurorehabil Neural Repair* 17:12–24, 2003.
13. Peurala SH, Kantanen MP, Sjögren T, et al: Effectiveness of constraint-induced movement therapy on activity

and participation after stroke: A systematic review and meta-analysis of randomized controlled trials, *Clin Rehabil* 26:209–223, 2011.

14. de Goede CJT, Keus SHJ, Kwakkel G, Wagenaar RC: The effects of physical therapy in Parkinson's disease: A research synthesis, *Arch Phys Med Rehabil* 82:509–515, 2001.

15. Flippin M, Reszka S, Watson LR: Effectiveness of the Picture Exchange Communication System (PECS) on communication and speech for children with autism spectrum disorders: A meta-analysis, *Am J Speech-Language Pathol* 19:178–195, 2010.

16. McCallum CA, Mosher PD, Jacobson PJ, et al: Quality in physical therapist clinical education: A systematic review, *Phys Ther* 93:1298–1311, 2012.

17. PRISMA Statement. Available at: http://www.prisma-statement.org/. Accessed December 16, 2014.

18. Law M, Philip I: Systematically reviewing the evidence. In Law M, editor: *Evidence-Based Rehabilitation: A Guide to Practice*, Thorofare, NJ, 2002, Slack.

19. MacDonald SJ, Bourne RB, Rorabeck CH, et al: Prospective randomized clinical trial of continuous passive motion after total knee arthroplasty, *Clin Orthop* 380:30–35, 2000.

20. Chen B, Zimmerman JR, Soulen L, DeLisa JA: Continuous passive motion after total knee arthroplasty: A prospective study, *Am J Phys Med Rehabil* 79:421–426, 2000.

21. Chiarello CM, Gundersen L, O'Halloran T: The effect of continuous passive motion duration and increment on range of motion in total knee arthroplasty patients, *J Orthop Sports Phys Ther* 25:119–127, 1997.

22. Gose JC: Continuous passive motion in the postoperative treatment of patients with total knee replacement: A retrospective study, *Phys Ther* 67:39–42, 1987.

23. Basso DM, Knapp L: Comparison of two continuous passive motion protocols for patients with total knee implants, *Phys Ther* 67:360–363, 1987.

24. Yashar AA, Venn-Watson E, Welsh T, et al: Continuous passive motion with accelerated flexion after total knee arthroplasty, *Clin Orthop* 345:38–43, 1997.

25. Pope RO, Corcoran S, McCaul K, Howie DW: Continuous passive motion after primary total knee arthroplasty: Does it offer any benefits? *J Bone Joint Surg B* 79:914–917, 1997.

26. English C, Manns PJ, Tucak C, Bernhardt J: Physical activity and sedentary behaviors in people with stroke living in the community: A systematic review, *Phys Ther* 94:185–196, 2014.

27. Milne S, Brosseau L, Robinson V, et al: Continuous passive motion following total knee arthroplasty, *Cochrane Database Syst Rev* 3:CD004260, 2003.

28. Garrard J: *Health Sciences Literature Review Made Easy: The Matrix Method*, 4th ed, Burlington, Mass, 2014, Jones & Bartlett.

29. Darrah J, Hickman R, O'Donnell M, et al. AACPDM Methodology to Develop Systematic Reviews of Treatment Interventions, rev 1.2. 2008. Available at https://www.aacpdm.org/resources/outcomes/systematicReviewsMethodology.pdf. Accessed May 14, 2014.

30. Lipsey MW, Wilson DB: *Practical Meta-Analysis*, Thousand Oaks, Calif, 2000, Sage.

31. Hunter JE, Schmidt FL: *Methods of Meta-Analysis: Correction Error and Bias in Research Findings*, 3rd ed, Thousand Oaks, Calif, 2014, Sage.

32. Rosenthal R: *Meta-Analytic Procedures for Social Research*, Newbury Park, Calif, 1991, Sage.

33. Petiti DM: *Meta-analysis, Decision-Analysis, and Cost-Effectiveness Analysis*, Oxford, UK, 1994, Oxford University Press.

34. Geller NL, Proschan M: Meta-analysis of clinical trials: A consumer's guide, *J Biopharm Stat* 6:377–394, 1996.

35. Basu A. How to Conduct a Meta-Analysis. Available at: http://www.pitt.edu/~super1/lecture/lec1171/001.htm. Accessed December 16, 2014.

36. Comprehensive Meta-Analysis. Available at: www.meta-analysis.com. Accessed December 16, 2014.

37. Greenhalgh T: How to read a paper: Papers that summarize other papers: Systematic reviews and meta-analyses, *BMJ* 315:672–675, 1997.

38. Sutton AJ, Abrams KR, Jones DR: An illustrated guide to the methods of meta-analysis, *J Eval Clin Pract* 7:135–148, 2001.

39. Stroup DF, Thacker SB, Olson CM, et al: Characteristics of meta-analyses related to acceptance for publication in a medical journal, *J Clin Epidemiol* 54:655–660, 2001.

CHAPTER 27

Implementing a Research Project

CHAPTER OUTLINE

The Research "Backstory"
Proposal Preparation
General Proposal Guidelines
Elements of the Research
Proposal
Title
Investigators
Problem Statement
Purposes
Methods
Dissemination
Budget
Work Plan
Appendices
Approvals

Human Participants Protection
Institutional Review Boards
Levels of Review
Informed Consent
Funding
Budget
Institution Funding
Corporation Funding
Foundation Funding
Types of Foundations
Identifying Foundations
Applying for Foundation Funds
Government Funding
Obtaining Participants
Inpatient Recruitment

Outpatient Recruitment
Recruitment of the Lay Public
Data Collection
Data Collection Procedures
Safeguarding Data
Protecting Participant Identity
Data Recording Forms
Pilot Study
Scheduling Participants and Personnel
Data Collection
Data Analysis
Data Coding
Data Entry
Statistical Analysis
Summary

Although the primary purpose of this text is to provide readers with the knowledge they need to use research evidence in practice, some readers will want to extend that knowledge by implementing projects of their own. Students, in fact, may *have* to extend their knowledge because research projects may be required for classes and as requirements for master's or first professional (e.g., DPT) degrees; implementation of research certainly will be required for research degrees (e.g., Ph.D.).

We should acknowledge, particularly for the first two student categories mentioned above, a certain artificiality. That is, students are put in a position in which they must—all of a sudden—become "interested" enough in a topic to develop and implement a research project. Furthermore, especially as a class assignment, the time constraint of a semester is not typical in the world of research. With that acknowledgment, it is our

experience that students forced to complete a research project almost always find it beneficial, if not entirely enjoyable. Because they do not have extensive experience, beginning students in particular typically are interested in enough topics to appreciate the learning they glean from carrying out research.

The final two chapters of this text, then, are designed to provide practitioners and students with some "nuts and bolts" guidance about implementing research and disseminating the results of that research (see Chapter 28). However, research is rarely an individual venture; most studies are undertaken by multiple authors who contribute different types of expertise to the project. Individuals beginning a research program are encouraged to identify mentors and colleagues who can provide the diverse array of skills needed to mount a successful project, as suggested in Whyte's "scientific autobiography,"[1] which sheds light on the complex way in which research agendas in rehabilitation grow and develop. Students completing research for a course will typically have neither the "team" relationship of research nor a designated mentor. However, students should be willing to use their course professor as a resource and perhaps even other instructors in (and potentially outside) the department. Students completing a thesis for a master's or first professional degree or a doctoral dissertation will have a designated faculty mentor as well as a thesis or dissertation committee. Guidelines for establishing the mentor relationship and developing a committee can be found in several sources dedicated to theses and dissertations.[2-4]

A look at any research journal will reveal that the vast majority of research is completed by more than one person—a team. Houser and Bokovoy[5] summarize some of the benefits of a team approach to research. They cite (1) the possible reduction in workload for any one person, (2) the diversity of viewpoints in defining and refining questions, and (3) moral support.

This chapter first identifies three preliminary steps that must be completed before any data are collected: (1) a research plan, or proposal, must be prepared and submitted for approval through appropriate academic or administrative channels; (2) the researchers must seek the approval of human or animal subject protection committees, if appropriate; and (3) the researchers must secure the funds needed to implement the study. Next, the chapter presents guidelines for implementing all phases of a research project, from participant selection to data analysis. Methods of obtaining participants are discussed first, followed by the development and use of research instrumentation. Tips for managing data collection and recording are then presented, and the chapter ends with suggestions for data analysis, including guidelines for using computer statistical programs and statistical consultants.

THE RESEARCH "BACKSTORY"

Before proceeding, we wish to inform the reader—particularly the research novice—of some realities of implementing research because the following sections may seem quite straightforward and even idealized. Hegde[6] suggests that we view research in its "formal" aspects and in its "formative" aspects. The *formal aspects* are those features we see in a research article. The *formative aspects*, on the other hand, are all the planning, missteps, serendipitous findings, reworkings of research questions, errors, debates, and more that go on both before and during a research project. The formal aspects are the *results* of all those formative ones. The reader—especially the beginning researcher—should realize and, in fact, embrace the fact that research, as a human act, will include much more than the research report or article would have us believe occurred. That said, we present guidelines for at least the formal aspects.

PROPOSAL PREPARATION

The research proposal is a blueprint for the conduct of a research study. The proposal is also the mechanism by which the researcher sells the study idea to those individuals who are in a position to approve and perhaps fund it. Thus, the proposal must be written in a fashion that makes the purpose and methods of the study intelligible to those outside the researcher's sphere of interest. In this section of the chapter, general guidelines for proposal preparation are given, followed by specific suggestions related to each basic element of a research proposal. Detailed suggestions for proposal preparation have been provided by others.[7-9]

General Proposal Guidelines

Ideas with merit may never get to the implementation stage if the proposal does not meet the technical standards of the agency to which it is submitted, if the language is confusing, or if the appearance of the document makes it difficult to read. Thus, researchers need to prepare their proposal in the format, style, and appearance preferred by the agency to which they are submitting it. Whether one is submitting the proposal to a doctoral dissertation committee, to an institutional review board for assessment of whether the proposal contains adequate safeguards for the human participants involved in the research, or to a foundation for funding, there will be guidelines to follow for preparation of the proposal. If there is a page limit, do not exceed it. If required to submit one original and three copies, do not submit an original and two copies. If the proposal must be in someone's office by a certain date, do not simply mail the proposal on that date, and pay attention to deadlines for electronic submissions, including time of day and time zone. In short, follow the directions of the group to whom the proposal will be submitted. The proposal may need to be modified to meet different needs at different times. The format that students must use for the proposal they submit to their research advisors will likely differ from the format required for submission of the proposal to the human participants review committee, and the format required for foundation funding will probably differ from the other two formats.

The proposal must be well organized and contain clear, concise language appropriate for the individuals who will be reviewing it. The *Publication Manual of the American Psychological Association*[10] is an excellent source for language use in the rehabilitation professions. A proposal submitted to one's academic advisors can be written with the assumption that the audience has basic knowledge of the area of study; a proposal submitted to a family-run philanthropic foundation must be written so that lay individuals can grasp the essential elements and importance of the proposal. The appearance of the document must both invite the reader and convey the investigator's competence. Misspellings convey the message that the proposal writer does not pay attention to details and may make the reviewer wonder whether adequate attention would be paid to the

details of the research. Cramped type, narrow margins, draft-quality print, and poor photocopying all make the document difficult to read. Attractive documents have a good balance between text and white space, achieved through adequate margins, lots of headings for skimming, and numbered or bulleted lists. Some sources for thesis and dissertation preparation were cited previously.[2,3] In addition, entering "preparing theses and dissertations" in any major search engine will yield many Web sites devoted to the topic.

Elements of the Research Proposal

In many ways, the elements of a research proposal are similar to those of a research article. In fact, a good proposal can serve as the outline for the first draft of a research article. Box 27-1 outlines the typical sections of a proposal.

Box 27-1

Components of a Research Proposal

Title
  Key words
  Variables of interest
Investigators
  Names and credentials
  Affiliation
  Curricula vitae in appendix
Abstract
Problem
  Based in the work of the profession
  Backed up with literature
Purposes
  Specific objectives of the study
  Researchers' hypotheses about results
Methods
  Subject selection and assignment
    Procedures
    Provisions for confidentiality
  Procedures
    Justified by literature
    Detailed enough to assess benefits and risks
    Qualifications of investigators or others to
      perform procedures
    Provisions for protection of participants during
      testing or treatment
    Reference to informed consent form in
      appendix, if appropriate

Data analysis
  Based on best-case scenario
  May include contingency plans
References
Dissemination
  Conferences at which presentations may be given
  Journal to which results will be submitted first
  Other means by which results may be
    disseminated to the communities of interest
Budget
  Personnel, salaries, and benefits
  Supplies
  Equipment
  Mailing, printing, etc.
  Participant stipends
  Data analysis
  Presentation and publication preparation
  Presentation travel
Work plan
  All phases, from implementation to dissemination
Appendices
  Curricula vitae of investigators
  Informed consent form
  Very detailed procedures

Title

The proposal title should be concise yet precise and should identify the general problem area, the variables (for experiments and quasi-experiments), and the target populations. Some good examples from recent research are "Relative and Absolute Reliability [dependent variables] of a Vertical Numerical Pain Rating Scale Supplemented with a Faces Pain Scale [problem area and independent variable] After Stroke [target population]"[11]—an experimental study—or "Early Predictors of Language and Social Communication Impairments [general problem area and outcome measures] at Ages 9-11 Years: A Follow-Up Study of Early-Referred Children [target population]"[12]—a nonexperimental study. When seeking funding for a study, researchers may include in the title of their study words similar to those listed as priorities by the funding agency. For example, if an agency lists the funding of research related to Down syndrome as one of its priorities, researchers studying children with hypotonia (including some with Down syndrome) might do well to title their proposal "Assessment of Children with Down Syndrome and Other Hypotonic Conditions" rather than "Assessment of Children with Hypotonia."

Investigators

The names, credentials, and institutional affiliations of the investigators should be given. If cooperating institutions with whom the researchers are not formally affiliated will be involved in the research, they should be specified here. A curriculum vitae, or scholar's résumé, of each investigator is often included in an appendix to the proposal.

Problem Statement

The problem statement in a research proposal is generated and placed in the context of related literature. A persuasive paragraph or two are needed to convince the prospective sponsors of the study's importance, perhaps using the "given, however, therefore" framework presented in Chapter 4. That is, the literature review should provide both a background and rationale for the statement of the problem or the questions to be investigated. The problems need to be consistent with the goals and mission of the institution at which the research will be performed and with the purposes for which an agency is making funds available.

Problem statements can be brief and separate but most often are embedded within the literature review. After all, the purpose of a literature review is to develop a rationale for the study, and there must be some sort of problem or the study would have no purpose.

Purposes

The purposes section of a proposal enumerates how the problem will be approached in the study. All statements of purpose (or, alternatively, research questions) should (1) be clear, (2) be derived from problems noted in the literature review, (3) specify research variables, and (4) capture the nature of the study in one or two paragraphs. If there are several purposes, they should be listed in a logical sequence according to factors such as importance, underlying concepts, or timing. The format of the purposes varies depending on the type of research being proposed. Using the examples cited previously, we can look at those authors' statements of purpose/research questions. Li-Ling and colleagues noted, "no scale has yet been developed specifically for pain after stroke,"[11](p. 130) and, further, "Therefore, a vertical scale incorporating the NPRS [Numerical Pain Rating Scale] and FPS [Faces Pain Scale] could be used by all people with stroke."(p. 130) They then went on to describe their purpose as follows:

> The aim of the present study was to determine the relative and absolute reliabilities of the vertical NPRS incorporated with the 6-face FPS for assessing pain in the affected arm in people with stroke.(p. 130)

From this, without having read the whole article, we know that the investigators will (1) be assessing two outcomes (absolute and relative reliability) of a possible method (NPRS+FPS) for measuring pain in one limb of affected stroke patients. We have a good preview of the measures, methods, and population to be used.

In a hypothetical example, if the research is exploratory in nature, the purposes may take the form of broad questions, as in the following statement:

The purpose of this study is to answer four questions:

1. To what extent do health professions students feel isolated from the clinical environment during their first year of study?

2. What difficulties do newly licensed clinicians experience in making the transition from student to professional?

3. Does participation in a program in which students are matched with clinician advisors decrease feelings of isolation from the clinic?

4. Does participation in the clinician advisor program ease the transition from student to professional?

If the research is in a more developed area, more formalized research hypotheses may be appropriate.

Proposals for qualitative research, especially those using grounded theory (see Chapter 14), may pose unique issues because the exact method might not be predictable. Sandelowski and Barroso[13] offer helpful suggestions, as do Holloway and Wheeler[14] and Knafl and Deatrick.[15]

The last-named authors offer their "Top 10 Tips" for a successful qualitative research proposal, and we find several that are unique to qualitative research. Some are (1) make the case for the idea, not the method; (2) identify your qualitative method (see Chapter 14) without giving readers a tutorial on that method; (3) give examples that can provide the reviewer a clear understanding of how the study is likely to unfold; (4) emphasize quality controls such as training research assistants in the methodology.

Methods

The methods section of a research proposal should include information on participant selection, material or apparatus, procedures, and data analysis. Description of the sample must include the source of participants for the study; the sample size anticipated; the methods of assigning participants to groups, if appropriate; and the means by which the informed consent of the participants will be obtained and their safety ensured, if appropriate. A copy of the informed consent document should be included as an appendix to the proposal (guidelines for writing informed consent statements are presented later in this chapter).

Procedures should be discussed in detail (though see the comments above regarding qualitative research), with reference to the literature that provides justification for the choice of procedures. Any independent and dependent variables should be defined clearly. The means by which extraneous variables are controlled should be noted, and the reasons for leaving any extraneous variables uncontrolled should be given.

The data analysis procedures in the proposal are usually based on a best-case scenario but may include contingency plans for nonnormal data or if the number of anticipated participants does not materialize. There should be a data analysis element for every research hypothesis or question. If statistical consultants have been used to develop the data analysis section of the proposal or will be available to assist with data analysis, this should be indicated here.

Dissemination

Readers of the proposal may want to know how the researchers will disseminate the study findings. Conference presentation and journal article publications are the most common means of dissemination (see Chapter 28).

Budget

There are costs associated with any research project. If a project is self-funded by the researcher or internally funded by an organization, these costs are frequently hidden because the individuals doing the research are donating their time or the institution in which the research is being conducted simply does not actually calculate the loss of revenue from the decreased clinical productivity of the individuals involved. Externally funded projects require detailed budgets that account for both the direct and indirect costs of the research. Direct costs include equipment, supplies, computers, salaries and benefits of individuals working on the project, and the like. Indirect costs include administrative costs, overhead, and salaries and benefits of individuals peripherally involved with the study. See the "Funding" section of this chapter for more detailed information on developing a budget for the research project.

Work Plan

The work plan specifies when tasks will be accomplished and who will accomplish them. All phases from planning through implementation and dissemination need to be included in the work plan. Researchers need to be realistic in estimating the amount of time needed to accomplish the project, making sure that adequate slack is included to manage unforeseen complications. Time constraints on students or considerations of the clinic may dictate that certain events happen at certain times. When this is the case, the researchers should develop the work plan by proceeding backward from a set date to ensure that all necessary preliminary tasks are accomplished. Table 27-1 shows a work plan developed for a study required for completion of an academic degree. In this example, data collection will occur at a burn clinic held only once a month. The work plan therefore revolves around the set dates on which the clinic is held.

Appendices

In the appendices, the researcher provides detailed information that may be required by reviewers of the proposal but is not required for a basic understanding of what the proposal entails. Common items include the curricula vitae of the investigators, informed consent forms, calibration logs, and very detailed procedures such as diagrams of equipment, specific maneuvers, and materials presented to research participants in writing or orally.

Approvals

After the proposal is prepared, it requires approval, sometimes from individuals at several different levels. Student proposals require the approval of research advisors and committees. Clinical research proposals require administrative approval at one or more levels in an organization. Proposals for studies using human

Table 27-1

Work Plan for a Research Project

Submit first draft to advisor	Start
Finish revisions to first draft	30 days later
Advisor approves proposal for degree requirements	1 week later
Submit approved proposal to burn clinic director at hospital	3 days later
Burn clinic director reviews proposal and makes suggestions or approves	1 month later
Make protocol revisions if necessary	10 days later
Submit institutional review board (IRB) materials for university approval	1 week later
University IRB holds meeting	10 days later
Build measuring device and test with researchers	Same day
Submit IRB materials for hospital approval	3 days later
Hospital IRB holds meeting	2 weeks later
Reserve video equipment for pilot and test days	3 days later
Develop data collection forms	Same day
Pilot test with one or two patients	10 days later
Revise forms and photocopy for data collection	3 days later
Collect data at burn clinic	3 days later
Arrange for photography for presentation and publication	10 days later
Collect data at burn clinic	2 weeks later
Enter data into computer program	10 days later
Analyze data	2 weeks later
Submit first draft of academic paper to advisor	5 weeks later
Submit second draft of paper to advisor	9 weeks later
Develop presentation script and submit to advisor	30 days later
Advisor approves presentation script	30 days later
Generate presentation visuals	3 weeks later
Submit abstract for presentation at conference	2 weeks later
Oral presentation to faculty	10 days later
Submit third draft of paper to advisor	3 weeks later
Submit final draft of paper to advisor	1 week later
File approved copies of paper with university	1 week later
Revise academic paper for journal publication	30 days later
Submit for publication	2 weeks later

or animal subjects require approval by human or animal subject protection committees. The procedures for obtaining academic and administrative approval vary widely from institution to institution and are not discussed further. In contrast, the procedure for obtaining approval from human participants protection committees tends to be similar at most institutions.

HUMAN PARTICIPANTS PROTECTION

Researchers in the rehabilitation professions must undertake many procedures to ensure the protection of the human participants they use in their studies. Researchers who use animal subjects must submit their proposals for approval from comparable animal subjects protection committees.

To protect their participants from harm, researchers must design sound studies in which dangers to participants are minimized, secure the informed consent of participants, and implement the research with care and consideration for the participants' safety (see also Chapter 5). Review committees are the mechanisms by which these elements of participant safety are ensured. The generic term for these committees is institutional review board (IRB). Since 1971, federal regulations in the United States have specified that research conducted with government funds be subject to review by a committee concerned with the rights and welfare of participants.[16] In addition, most scientific journals today require evidence that research with animal or human subjects has undergone a review, irrespective of the funding source of the research.

Although specific committee procedures vary from institution to institution, many IRBs base their work on federal guidelines. Consequently, most of the guidelines presented here are based on the guidelines of the federal government. These guidelines, along with thoughtful discussion of ethical issues posed within the clinical research process, have been well summarized by several authors.[17-21]

Institutional Review Boards

Federal regulations[22] specify that an IRB be composed of at least five members with varying backgrounds representative of the type of research conducted at the institution: Individuals of different genders and races should be represented, at least one member must have a nonscientific background, and one member should be unaffiliated with the institution. This composition is designed to ensure that a closely knit group of scientists does not make the decisions about their own or their colleagues' projects.

The purpose of the IRB is to review research conducted under the auspices of the institution to ensure that the rights of human participants are protected. This includes protected information defined by the Health Insurance Portability and Accountability Act (HIPAA). These rights are protected when research designs minimize risks to participants, when participant selection and assignment are equitable, when researchers have made provisions for the confidentiality of information, and when participants are provided with the information they need to make an informed decision about whether to participate in the research. The IRB accomplishes its purpose through regular meetings during which it reviews written proposals submitted in a format specified by the IRB and by monitoring the progress of research that it has approved.

Levels of Review

IRBs typically have three levels of review of research projects: exempt, expedited, and full. Research that is exempt from review includes the following:

- Research that involves normal educational practices
- Survey or interview procedures that do not involve sensitive areas of behavior and in which responses are recorded in such a way that they cannot be attributed to a particular individual
- Observations of public behavior
- Study of existing data that are not protected health information

Although such research is often exempt from review by the IRB, institutions usually require researchers to submit materials (such as a proposal and questionnaires) to the IRB so that the members can confirm whether the research fits the exempt category. An exempt study in rehabilitation might involve a mailed survey of clinicians to determine their opinions about contemporary practice issues.

Expedited reviews are permitted for studies that involve minimal risks to participants. Such procedures include the following:

- Collection of hair, nails, or external secretions
- Recording of noninvasive data
- Study of small amounts of blood through venipuncture
- Study of the effects of moderate exercise in healthy volunteers

Expedited reviews are typically done by just a few members of the IRB and do not require a meeting of the full committee. An expedited study in rehabilitation might involve measuring range of motion in a patient group, having patients complete self-reported quality-of-life tools, or assessing mobility gains of normal participants following an exercise program.

The IRB conducts a full review of the following:

- Research projects that involve more risks than those identified for exempt or expedited review
- Studies of lower-risk procedures in children or others who are unable to provide meaningful consent

Examples of rehabilitation studies that would require full review include assessment of the fitness level of patients with cardiovascular disease or a trial of an oral-motor program in children with cerebral palsy.

Informed Consent

In the context of research, informed consent refers to an interaction between the researcher and the potential participant.[23] The researcher provides the potential participant with the information he or she needs to make an informed decision about whether to participate in the research. The potential participant then makes his or her decision and communicates it to the researcher, usually by either signing or declining to sign a written consent form. Special consideration in the informed consent process needs to be taken with individuals, such as minors and those with dementia, who are unable to provide their own consent and rely on others to protect their interests.[24-26] A fuller discussion of the principles of informed consent was provided in Chapter 5.

Consent forms must be written in language that is understandable to the individuals who will be giving consent. The typical reading level of participants should be considered, as should visual acuity and native language. A copy of the consent form itself should be provided to the participant. Box 27-2 lists the elements

---

Box 27-2

Elements of a Consent Form

Statement that the study constitutes research
Explanation of study's purposes
Explanation of basis of participant selection and
   duration of participant involvement
Explanation of provisions for subject confidentiality
Description of procedures, with experimental
   procedures identified
Description of risks and discomforts
Description of potential benefits to participants and
   others
Description of alternative treatments, if available
Statement of whether compensation is available for
   injuries
Name of person to contact if questions or injuries arise
Statement emphasizing that participation is
   voluntary
Statement that the participant has the right to
   withdraw from the study at any time
Statement of disclosure of information gained
   in the study that might influence participant's
   willingness to continue participation
Explanation of payment arrangements, if applicable
Consent statement
Date line
Participant's signature line
Investigator's signature line
Investigator's institutional affiliation and telephone
   number

---

of an informed consent statement, and Figure 27-1 presents a sample consent form document. Consent forms may not contain exculpatory language—that is, language that asks participants to waive any of their legal rights or releases the investigator or institution from liability for negligent acts associated with the research project. Ideally, the form is contained on a single sheet of paper, with front and back sides used as needed. If more pages are needed, they should be numbered "1 of 3," "2 of 3," and the like so that participants are assured that all the needed information has been received.

The researcher should keep the signed consent forms in a secure location, and contemporary IRBs will want to know how the researcher will securely maintain informed consent and other documents associated with the study. The length of time the forms are retained depends on the nature and length of the research and on the latency and duration of foreseeable complications related to the research procedures. Researchers should recognize that the signed consent form is usually the only point at which each participant's name is linked to the study. Therefore, secure storage of signed consent forms is an important part of maintaining participants' confidentiality.

There are two general situations in which consent forms may not be needed or appropriate. The first is the collection of data through a mailed survey. In this case, the elements of informed consent should be contained within the cover letter written by the researcher to the potential respondent, and return of the questionnaire by the respondent is taken as evidence of consent. The second situation is a study that is of a sensitive nature, and signed consent forms would be a means by which the study participants could be identified. In this situation, informed consent may be obtained verbally if approved by the IRB.

FUNDING

Conducting research is costly. A challenge for researchers is to find funding to support their research interests. Funds generally come from one of four sources: institutions (especially a researcher's own), corporations, foundations (including those of professional associations and societies), or the government. This section of the chapter presents a typical budget for a research study and then discusses the peculiarities of the four funding sources.

Budget

Table 27-2 presents a budget for a descriptive study that would require data collection by two clinicians and support services from one aide and one secretary. Personnel costs are determined by estimating the proportion of time each individual would be involved in the study, multiplying the salary by that proportion, and adding a reasonable percentage for benefits. Equipment costs should be estimated, including service and repair costs if appropriate. Consultants are individuals who are engaged on a daily or hourly basis to fulfill a special need of the research project. Statistical, computer, engineering, and artistic consultants are common examples. The cost of disseminating the results of the research includes manuscript preparation, creation of photographs and graphs, use of copyrighted materials, platform or poster presentations, and traveling to conferences to present the research. Overhead costs for the institution sponsoring the research is often figured as a percentage of the direct costs. This percentage may be specified by the funding agency or calculated by the institution in which the research is conducted.

University of Anytown
1256 Holt Road
Department of Rehabilitation

Anytown, Indiana 46234
(317) 555-4300

CONSENT TO PARTICIPATE IN A RESEARCH STUDY

TITLE OF STUDY: Comparison of Integrated Electromyographic Activity and Strength Measures in the Supraspinatus Muscle in Two Positions.

You are invited to participate in a research study that measures the electrical activity and strength of the supraspinatus muscle, which is located in the back of the shoulder. You have been invited to participate based on the assumption that you have a shoulder which is free of injury or disability. Your participation would require attendance at a single measurement session lasting approximately one hour.

Prior to your participation, an investigator will take a brief medical history to determine whether you have had previous shoulder problems which would make you ineligible to participate. Weight, height, age, and sex will also be recorded. You will be assigned a participant number so that your name will not be associated with any of the findings of this study.

The research procedure consists of measurement of muscle electrical activity and strength in two positions. The electrical activity of your supraspinatus muscle will be measured by an experienced electromyographer. He will insert a 27-gauge sterile needle containing two fine-wire electrodes into your muscle. After positioning the wires, the needle will be removed and the wires will remain in place for testing in both positions. The wires will be removed on completion of data collection in both positions.

Strength will be measured with a handheld dynamometer, which is a stationary device held by the researcher and placed at the back of your wrist. You will be asked to use your shoulder muscles to push against the device as hard as you can. This will be repeated three times in each of the two positions.

In the first position you will be seated, with your arm straight in front of you with your thumb pointing down. In the second position you will lie on your stomach with your arm out straight in front of you and with your thumb pointing up.

PAGE 1 of 2

_____ (Participant's Initials)

Figure 27-1 Example of a consent form.

CONSENT TO PARTICIPATE IN A RESEARCH STUDY (Continued)

TITLE OF STUDY: Comparison of Integrated Electromyographic Activity and Strength Measures in the Supraspinatus Muscle in Two Positions.

The risks of participation in this study include muscle fatigue or soreness from exercise, temporary discomfort from needle insertion, infection from the needle electrode, bleeding from needle insertion, and a small risk of puncture of the chest cavity which could lead to pain, difficulty breathing, and would require medical attention. To protect from infection, sterile needles and electrodes will be used and will be disposed of after each use. To protect from the risk of chest cavity puncture, the electromyographer will use needle placement designed to minimize this risk. If muscle soreness occurs, you will be instructed in procedures to minimize discomfort. No compensation is available for injuries resulting from participation in this research.

By determining the position in which the supraspinatus muscle is most effective, the results of this research may benefit patients and athletes who wish to strengthen their shoulder muscles.

If you have questions about this research or need to report an injury related to your participation in this research, contact xxxxx at (xxx) xxx-xxxx. Your participation in this research is voluntary, and your decision whether or not to participate will not affect your standing at this institution. If you elect to participate in the study, you have the right to withdraw from the study at any time without affecting your standing at the institution. You will receive a copy of this form.

CONSENT

I, _____, voluntarily consent to participate in this research study as described above. I have had a chance to ask questions of the researcher, and have had any questions answered to my satisfaction.

_____
Participant Signature

_____
Researcher Signature

_____
Date

PAGE 2 of 2

Figure 27-1—cont'd

Institution Funding

Much of rehabilitation research is funded by the institution in which it is conducted. Department managers who believe in research as an essential element of professionalism may allow staff to conduct limited amounts of research on work time. However, because research time does not produce revenue like patient care does, even the most research-oriented managers have difficulty releasing clinicians from patient care to perform research. This is particularly true in the contemporary cost-cutting, high-productivity environment that is prevalent in rehabilitation settings in the United

Table **27-2**

Research Project Budget

Item	Explanation	Cost
Personnel		
Joyce McWain	10% time for 1 year	$10,400
Principal investigator	Benefits 30% of salary	
	Annual salary $80,000	
Randall Myers	5% time for 1 year	$4550
Co-investigator	Benefits 30% of salary	
	Annual salary $70,000	
Ben Riley	5% time for 6 months	$650
Rehabilitation aide	Benefits 30% of salary	
	Annual salary $20,000	
Sally Knapp	5% time for 6 months	$813
Administrative assistant	Benefits 30% of salary	
	Annual salary $25,000	
Equipment		
Handheld dynamometers	Two at $1200 each	$2400
Consultants		
Statistician	30 hours at $150/hour	$4500
Dissemination		
Photocopying	1000 pages at $.10/page	$100
Visuals	Black and white diagrams $250	$650
	Poster 4×8 feet $400	
Travel	Principal investigator and co-investigator to annual conference, $2000 each	$4000
Subtotal		$28,063
Overhead	30% of $28,063	$8419
Total		**$36,482**

States. For that reason, most institutional sources of research funding are universities, where research is considered a normal part of faculty activity.

Corporation Funding

A corporation may fund a research project directly through its operating funds or indirectly through a grant from a foundation associated with the company. When a corporation provides research funds through direct giving, it is usually to support activities directly related to the corporation's function. For example, equipment manufacturers may be willing to provide equipment for and pay the salaries of researchers who are conducting studies that showcase their products. Some manufacturers are willing to loan equipment for the duration of a project; many students, who typically conduct research on a shoestring budget, have obtained loaner equipment simply by contacting the manufacturer or a local sales representative.

Researchers who accept funds directly from corporations need to be sure they understand who has control of the data and their dissemination. A corporation may wish to retain ownership of the data so that it has the prerogative of not releasing any data that are not favorable toward its product. Researchers who contact companies for support must decide whether they are willing to accept such terms, should the company request them. The reader should review the material on conflict of interest in the chapter on ethics (see Chapter 5).

Foundation Funding

Foundations are private entities that distribute funds according to the priorities set by their donors or their boards of trustees. There are different types of foundations with unique requirements for individuals seeking funding.

Types of Foundations

Foundations that provide research grants can be broadly divided into independent, company-sponsored, and community foundations. The funds of an independent foundation usually come from a single source, such as a family, an individual, or a group of individuals. Independent foundations give grants in fields specified by the few individuals who administer the fund; giving is often limited to the local geographical region in which the fund is located. Independent foundations that support rehabilitation research in the United States include the American Occupational Therapy Foundation, the Foundation for Physical Therapy, and the American Speech-Language-Hearing Foundation. Note that these foundations are financially and functionally independent of the corresponding professional associations. Comparable foundations, such as the United Kingdom's Physiotherapy Research Foundation, exist in other countries.[27]

A company-sponsored foundation is an independent entity that is funded by contributions from a company. Although the foundation is independent from the corporation, it tends to give grants in fields related to the company's products or customers. Giving is often limited to the geographical region or regions in which the company is located.

Community foundations are publicly supported by funds derived from many donors. The mission of a community foundation is to meet the needs of its locale; thus the projects it funds must be directly related to the welfare of the community.

Identifying Foundations

Large institutions supported by several grant agencies have grants administration officers who can help researchers identify appropriate funding sources. The Foundation Center, a nonprofit organization, publishes comprehensive references that can also help researchers identify foundations that fund studies in their area

of interest. Readers should note that the very important "Foundation Directory" is available online and is updated annually.[28,29] These references are available in hard copy and electronic formats in many university or public libraries. Readers should note that the "Corporate Foundation Profiles" appears not to have been updated since 2002. The information provided for each foundation includes the size of the fund, the amount given annually, the names of agencies to whom funds were given, and the types of projects funded (e.g., scholarships, construction of new facilities, education, or research). Several specialized indexes and journals focus on funding projects in health or health-related areas, such as disabled populations.[30,31]

Applying for Foundation Funds

The procedure for applying for foundation funds varies greatly from foundation to foundation. Funding decisions in independent foundations may rest with a very few individuals. Consequently, applying for funds is relatively informal. A letter of inquiry describing the research in general terms should be sent to the foundation. Ways in which the research meets the goals of the foundation should be emphasized. The reply from the foundation will indicate whether the idea is appealing to them and will ask for additional information if it is. The additional information required is likely to be fairly brief and can be assembled in a format determined by the researcher.

Corporate-sponsored foundations often have more formalized grant application procedures. However, the letter of inquiry is still the first means by which the researcher contacts the foundations. If the general area of the research is within the scope of the foundation's activities, the foundation will respond with directions for formal application for funds.

Government Funding

The federal government is a major provider of research grants in the United States. Box 27-3 provides a partial listing of the government agencies that provide funding for health sciences research. Probably the best two sources for finding government funding (at least at the federal level) are the Catalog of Federal Domestic Assistance[32] and the Web site of the Department of Health and Human Services' section on grants.[33] Other references provide detailed information about strategies for applying for government grant funds.[34]

The procedure for obtaining federal grant funding is far more formal than that for obtaining foundation funding. First, the grant funds must be made available. To do this, Congress must both authorize the grant-funding

Box 27-3

Partial Listing of U.S. Federal Government Funding Sources for Health Research

Department of Health and Human Services
Administration for Children and Families
Centers for Disease Control and Prevention
National Institute for Occupational Safety and Health
National Institutes of Health
National Cancer Institute
National Heart, Lung, and Blood Institute
National Institute of Arthritis and Musculoskeletal and Skin Diseases
National Institute of Child Health and Human Development
National Institute of Neurological Disorders and Stroke
National Institute on Aging
National Institute for Dental Research
National Center for Medical Rehabilitation Research
National Institute of Deafness and Other Communication Disorders
National Institute of Mental Health
Office of Alternative Medicine
National Science Foundation
Department of Education
National Institute for Disability and Rehabilitation Research
Veterans Health Administration

program and then, in a separate legislative step, appropriate funds for the program. Administration of appropriated funds is delegated to a large grants administration bureaucracy in Washington, D.C. When funds are appropriated for a grant program, notice is placed in the *Federal Register,* the daily federal government news publication. After notice is placed in the register, application materials can be released to potential grant recipients. Applications are highly formalized, and grant applicants must certify that they are in compliance with a variety of federal regulations related to nondiscrimination and protection of human participants. Although the process is formalized, the individuals who direct the various grant programs are available to discuss the application process with grant writers.

The awarding of federal grants is usually accomplished by a peer review committee. Experienced researchers are assembled to review the submitted proposals and make recommendations about their disposition. Often only one or two reviewers read the entire proposal; the rest of the committee members read only the abstract of the study and hear the primary reviewers' descriptions and evaluations of the project. It is therefore imperative that the abstract of the grant proposal accurately reflect the scope of the project for which funding is sought.

Federal grant proposals will have one of three outcomes: approval with funding, approval without funding, or disapproval. A proposal is disapproved if the study does not meet the purpose of the grant or its design is not acceptable. Proposals that meet the technical requirements are approved and given a certain priority level. Only those with the highest priority level are funded.

After writing the research proposal, obtaining administrative and IRB approval, and securing the funds needed to implement a project, the researcher must contend with the substantial logistical details of implementing a project.[35,36] The second half of this chapter addresses a number of these concerns, including recruitment of participants, data collection, and data analysis.

OBTAINING PARTICIPANTS

The time and effort required to obtain research participants are often far greater than the researcher anticipates. For example, assume that we wish to implement a study of older adults who have undergone total knee arthroplasty. We plan to study two groups who undergo different inpatient and outpatient postoperative rehabilitation. Measurement of certain outcomes will be taken at discharge, 3 months postoperatively, and 6 months postoperatively. If we know that 100 such surgeries are performed in a 6-month period at our facility, we may assume that there will be no difficulty obtaining two study groups of 40 participants each for our study. Table 27-3 shows, however, several ways in which the number of available participants will be far fewer than the 100 patients who undergo the surgery. If the scenario in Table 27-3 were realized, we would be faced with a situation in which fewer than 20 participants were available per group during the 6 months in which participants were to be recruited.

Researchers need to plan their participant recruitment strategy carefully to ensure an adequate number of participants. Different strategies are appropriate when recruiting inpatients, outpatients, or the general public. In all cases, recruitment of participants should take place after an IRB has approved both the conduct of the study and the procedures to be used for ensuring the informed consent of participants.

Table 27-3

Eventual Sample from a Potential 100 Patients

Reason for Participation or Nonparticipation	N	N Remaining
Total knee arthroplasties performed in 6 months	100	100
Young patient with hemophilia	3	97
Patient with perioperative complications	5	92
Patient lives more than 60 miles away or has received outpatient care at another clinic	10	82
Patient's surgeon does not wish to participate	12	70
Patient does not consent to be in study	10	60
Patient does not complete outpatient care	12	48
Patient dies before 6-month visit	2	46
Patient moves or cannot be located to schedule 6-month appointment	4	42
Patient does not come to the scheduled 6-month follow-up appointment	6	36

Inpatient Recruitment

In the inpatient setting, the admitting physician is clearly in control of the care that the patient receives while in the hospital. Thus, securing inpatients for study requires careful work with the medical staff of the institution. In fact, the best way to secure participants for study is to invite key physicians to collaborate in the entire research endeavor. In addition, the administrative chain of command within the facility will need to be followed to secure permission to implement the project.

After securing the permission of the admitting physician, the researcher contacts participants directly to secure their informed consent. As with all participant recruitment methods, patients must be approached in a manner that conveys that, regardless of whether

they choose to participate, their care will not be compromised. Researchers and physicians should determine together the best procedure for securing patient consent: The physician may mention the study to the patients first and indicate that the researcher will visit with details; the researcher may accompany the physician on rounds so that they can jointly present the study to patients, assuring them that the different professionals are working together on the research endeavor; or the researcher may present the study first, giving patients the opportunity to discuss the study later with the physician before consenting.

Outpatient Recruitment

Outpatient recruitment is somewhat easier than inpatient recruitment because the physician is not necessarily the point of control for the research. If a descriptive, correlational, or methodological study is being conducted that does not involve any procedures contraindicated by the current condition of the patient, the researcher can feel free to proceed without obtaining referring physician consent. As is the case with inpatients, it is wise to inform the referring physicians of the ongoing project so that they will not be alarmed if patients tell them that they have participated in a research study.

After the study, it is courteous to send the referring physicians of participants a summary of the study results, along with your assessment of how the results will allow for serving their patients better in the future. Alternatively, collaboration with physicians may prove rewarding for both parties as well as having the added benefit of providing researchers with easier access to some participants.

If the research protocol requires a departure from a physician's orders, permission must be sought and gained from both the physician and the patient, as described under the "Inpatient Recruitment" section. Again, collaboration or communication with the physicians about the study results may make them more willing to have their patients participate in future studies.

Recruitment of patients who have completed their course of treatment requires careful consideration of the confidentiality of their medical records, particularly since the implementation of HIPAA in the United States (and similar acts in other countries). Consider a case in which a university-based researcher contacts a clinic to request access to patient records to identify participants who meet certain inclusion criteria. The clinic, being interested in the project, agrees to participate in the study and provides the researcher with the names and addresses of patients with the particular diagnosis. Patients would have good reason to be concerned about breaches of confidentiality if they received a letter from an unknown researcher requesting their participation in a study based on the fact that they had had a certain surgery and were seen for treatment at a certain clinic. In today's environment, such a recruitment procedure would probably not be approved by an IRB. Alternate procedures would involve having a clinic employee—who already has access to the clinic records—write a letter to eligible patients explaining the study and asking for their permission to release their name and address to the researcher.

Recruitment of the Lay Public

When a study requires the participation of the lay public rather than patients, researchers are challenged by the need to balance their desire for convenient access to a particular group of participants with the hope that results will be generalizable beyond the particular sample studied. In the past, this balance has often been lacking: Use of health professions students as a convenient source of participants has limited the generalizability of many studies to young, healthy individuals, who make up the majority of health professions students.

Groups that consist of individuals with a wide range of educational, racial, ethnic, and socioeconomic (among other) characteristics are desirable for many studies. If one works in a large organization, recruiting participants from employees at all levels—from upper administration to maintenance staff—often provides the sort of variety that is desired.

Researchers who require specific types of participants need to be creative in identifying existing groups from which to recruit. Examples of groups that may yield good participant pools for certain populations include religious institutions, senior citizen or retirement centers, apartment complexes, health clubs, day care centers, and youth or adult sport leagues. For example, if one wished to study balance in well elderly people, participants might be found in groups in religious institutions, senior bowling leagues, residential retirement centers, or senior citizen centers with daytime programs. The choice of which group to use would depend on the contact the researcher has with members of the groups and how seriously biased the group membership is in light of the particular research question. For instance, if a researcher's great aunt bowls 3 days a week in a senior league, she might be able to recruit plenty of participants for a balance study. However, if the researcher believes that the senior bowlers would be biased in the direction of better balance than most of

the well elderly, the bowling league may not be a good choice, no matter how easy it would be to obtain participants from the group.

After a researcher has determined that a particular group is suitable for study, the appropriate administrative approval is needed, whether from the director of personnel, the manager of the bowling alley, the leader of the religious institution, or the administrator of the retirement center. When seeking such approval, the researcher needs to prepare a brief version of the study proposal, written in terms understandable to the person whose approval is sought. A blank consent form should be included along with documentation of the IRB approval. To gain administrative approval, the researcher will need to convince the official that the study has value; that participation in the study will not greatly disrupt the facility's routine; that participants are at minimal risk of harm and will be treated with dignity and respect; and, if appropriate, that participants may enjoy the participation and interaction with others that it affords.

After administrative approval has been given to recruit participants from a particular facility, the researcher needs to make initial contact with potential participants. This may be done by discussing the study at a group meeting, writing letters to particular potential participants, or posting flyers in areas frequented by the members of the desired group. Whatever the format, this initial information should include the purpose of the study, the actual activities in which the participant would be participating, the time commitment required to participate, and the means by which interested parties can contact the researcher.

DATA COLLECTION

Although there are many types of data collection tasks, the number is not large. Three major types of data collection tools used by rehabilitation researchers are biophysiological instruments, interviews, and questionnaires. Also common are responses to oral or written verbal materials, stimuli, or instructions, verbal responses (oral, written, or signed) to manipulated environments (including language environments), responses to standardized tests, and reported responses to perceptual tasks. Details regarding the development and administration of interviews and questionnaires are presented in Chapters 14 and 17 and are not repeated here. This section of the chapter focuses on general principles of data collection or specific data collection issues related to the use of biophysiological instruments.

Data Collection Procedures

When using existing instrumentation, the researcher must be familiar with both the manufacturer's instructions for use of the equipment and the protocols that other researchers have followed with the equipment. From this information, decisions can be made about the procedures for data collection. Although a general procedure for data collection will have been developed for the research proposal, very detailed procedural guidelines should be established and written down so that they can be implemented uniformly within the study. For example, a procedure such as height measurement seems simple and would not require detailed description in a proposal. However, before data collection is begun, the specific procedure for taking the height measurement should be developed: Will the measurement be taken with participants barefoot, stocking footed, or in shoes? Will participants be instructed to stand comfortably or stand tall? Should the head be comfortably erect or in military axial extension? Written standardization procedures are particularly important if more than one researcher will be measuring participants.

Accuracy checks of the equipment should be conducted when applicable. Goniometers can be checked against known angles, scales can be checked against known weights, and calibration of equipment can be accomplished according to manufacturer's instructions or published standards. In some instances, the researcher may wish to have an engineer or manufacturer's technician give the equipment a mechanical or electrical checkout to determine that it is operating properly before data are collected. Calibration should be periodic and informal checks of equipment carried out daily.

Safeguarding Data

When collecting data, the researcher needs to take steps to ensure quality and completeness. Although specific suggestions for data collection are provided in the following sections, all researchers must consider the overriding concern for the safety of data that have been collected. Briefcases get lost, cars get stolen, hard drives crash, dogs chew, and buildings can be destroyed by fires or floods. Given the many possible disasters that can threaten one's data, it makes sense to maintain backup copies of the information one has collected. If the data are collected and stored on computer disk, make a backup copy of the disk. If the data are collected on handwritten forms, either make copies of the completed forms or transfer the information to a data file soon after collecting it.

The two copies of the data should be stored in two different locations; it does no good to have two copies of the data if both are in the same file that was stored directly under the pipe that burst. If several researchers collaborate with one another, different researchers should probably keep the data in different locations. The IRB will want to know how data storage and backup procedures protect the confidentiality of the participants, particularly if the data set includes information that could identify participants.

Protecting Participant Identity

When each participant enters the trial, he or she should be assigned a number or alias and, if appropriate, a study group according to one of the plans developed in Chapter 9. A master list specifying each participant's name, contact information if appropriate, study identification number, and group membership should be maintained. If data recorders and participants are blind to group membership, generally only one researcher has access to the master list. This researcher should keep the master list in a secure location where other researchers will not accidentally come across the information; a second copy should be kept separately from the original copy, but still in a secured location.

Data Recording Forms

Researchers must design forms for data collection if not already supplied, such as for standardized tests. The form may be a pen-and-paper form or, more likely nowadays, one that is filled out directly on a computer or even an electronic handheld device (there's probably an app for that). The form should contain space for each participant's identification number but not name. The order of items on the form should be carefully considered to coincide with the order in which the information will be collected. Adequate space should be left for a readable response to the information. Data collection forms for interviews and other processes for qualitative research may need more flexibility, but actually may result in simpler forms.

In general, the information should be collected at the highest measurement level possible. For example, adult ages should be recorded as age at last birthday. Even if the researcher plans to categorize participants into age groups, such as those younger than 60 and those 60 and older, it is wise to collect the information as actual age and then code it into groups. In this way, if a later research question requires actual age, that information is available. If just the group membership (younger than 60 or 60 and older) is recorded originally, there is no way to later determine participants' actual ages.

If data require coding (e.g., conversion of letters into numbers and collapse of actual ages into age groups)

for analysis, the form should be designed to facilitate the coding process. Figure 27-2 shows a completed data collection form with space for data coding for the hypothetical total knee arthroplasty study described in Section 7 of this text (see Tables 20-1 and 20-2).

TOTAL KNEE ARTHROPLASTY REHABILITATION STUDY

BACKGROUND INFORMATION

Case Number (CN)   *1* *5*

Clinic Attended (CL)
1 = Community Hospital
2 = Memorial Hospital
3 = Religious Hospital   *2*

Patient Sex (SEX)
0 = Male
1 = Female   *1*

Patient Age in years at last birthday (AGE)   *6* *8*

Type of Prosthesis (PRO)
1 = Total condylar
2 = Posterior stabilizer
3 = Flat tibial plateau   *2*

Miscellaneous Information
Surgeon   *Bennett*
Side of Surgery   *(R)*
Date of Surgery   *2-12-2014*
Diagnosis   *OA*

THREE-WEEK POSTOPERATIVE DATA

Date   *3-5-2014*

Three-week ROM, degrees (W3R)
Clinician   *80*   *0* *7* *6*

SIX-WEEK POSTOPERATIVE DATA

Date   *3-25-2014*

Clinician   *80*

Six-week ROM, degrees (W6R)   *0* *7* *0*

SIX-MONTH POSTOPERATIVE DATA

Date   *8-15-2014*

Six-month ROM, degrees (M6R)   *0* *9* *5*

Six-month Extension Torque, N•m (E)   *1* *7* *0*

Figure 27-2 Data collection form, with coding column.

Six-Month Flexion Torque, N•m (F) $\underline{1}$ $\underline{0}$ $\underline{2}$

Gait Velocity, cm/s (V) $\underline{1}$ $\underline{6}$ $\underline{5}$

Flexion Contracture at Six Months (DFC)

Value $\underline{8°}$

1 = >15 degrees
②= 6 to 15 degrees
3 = 0 to 5 degrees $\underline{2}$

Varus/Valgus Angulation in Stance (DVV)

Value $\underline{4° varus}$

1 = >10 degrees valgus
2 = >5 degrees varus or 6 to 10 degrees valgus
③= 5 degrees varus to 5 degrees valgus $\underline{3}$

Mediolateral Stability (DML)
1 = Marked instability
②= Moderate instability
3 = Stable $\underline{2}$

Anteroposterior Stability with Knee at 90° Flexion (DAP)
1 = Marked instability
②= Moderate instability
3 = Stable $\underline{2}$

Distance Walked (ADW)
5 = Unlimited
④= 4 to 6 blocks
3 = 2 to 3 blocks
2 = Indoors only
1 = Transfers only $\underline{4}$

Assistive Device (AAD)
5 = None
4 = Cane outside
③= Cane full time
2 = Two canes, crutches
1 = Walker or unable $\underline{3}$

Stair Climbing (ASC)
⑤= Reciprocal, no rail
4 = Reciprocal, with rail
3 = One at a time, with or without rail
2 = One at a time, with rail and assistive device
1 = Unable to climb stairs $\underline{5}$

Rising from Chair (ARC)
⑤= No arm assistance
4 = Single arm assistance
3 = Difficult with two arm assistance
2 = Needs assistance of another
1 = Unable to rise $\underline{5}$

Figure 27-2—cont'd

The blank spaces on the right-hand side of the form are for the pieces of information that will be entered in the computer data file. Some information such as the date and the name of the researcher collecting the data may not be relevant to the final data set, but may be useful to have if there is a question about a piece of information. For two of the deformity variables, actual angular value is reduced to a category; however, there is room on the form for both the actual value and the code that corresponds to the category in which the angular value belongs.

Pilot Study

A pilot study is crucial to the smooth running of a research trial. In a pilot study, the researchers go through a "dress rehearsal" of the research protocol, using a few volunteers similar to those who will participate in the study. The pilot study allows the researchers to take care of small possible mishaps in the procedure and reveals the little details that need attending to: How long does it actually take to collect the data? Is the planned sequence cumbersome? Is another assistant needed for one part of the study? How much paper is used for the computer printout, and is there enough available to complete the study? Is an extension cord or extra batteries needed to power the equipment? Should office supplies be handy?

Scheduling Participants and Personnel

The pilot study allows the researcher to make educated guesses about how the data collection will proceed. Participants in the actual study should expect the researcher to provide a realistic estimate of the time it will take to complete their participation. Participants may not mind participating in a study that requires 5 hours of data collection as long as they know up front that this is the time that will be involved. Participants will understandably be upset and may withdraw from participation if they are initially led to believe that data collection will require 1 hour and are still waiting to finish after 3 hours.

Adequate personnel need to be available for data collection. The types of tasks that need to be accomplished are greeting participants as they arrive, explaining the study and securing informed consent (if not done in advance), telephoning participants who have not arrived as expected, gathering background information and screening participants to ensure that they meet inclusion criteria, preparing participants for data collection, collecting the actual data, spotting participants for safety, and thanking participants for their assistance. In some studies, one researcher could handle all these tasks; in others, five or six researchers might be required.

Data Collection

All of the preparations mentioned thus far allow the researcher to collect data. There are several considerations and choices to make. For the most part, researchers collect data from one participant at a time, but there may be times when it is advantageous to work with participants in a group (e.g., to discuss ramifications of a type of treatment). Researchers need to decide how long data collection sessions will be and will want to consider participants' health or other relevant status,

without taxing participants physically or mentally. Researchers, in considering session length, will want to consider whether to include a rest period.

Regardless of the data collection methodology, researchers must be prepared for sessions and should practice before actually collecting data. Response or other data collection forms should have been developed and should be ready. Researchers must be absolutely familiar with materials or equipment used to elicit responses.

DATA ANALYSIS

The ease with which the data analysis is accomplished depends greatly on whether the researcher has (1) written a well-developed proposal with a sound plan for data analysis and (2) collected data carefully with an eye to the analysis stage. In discussing data analysis, this section presumes that a computer statistical package and a statistical consultant are available for studies with any quantitative data. For all but the smallest data sets, both are necessary. After a discussion of the roles of computers and consultants, suggestions are provided for the three steps of data analysis: data coding, data entry, and statistical analysis.

Many computer statistical packages are available for use on personal or mainframe computers. Three widely used statistical packages are SPSS, Statistical Analysis System (SAS), and Biomedical Data Processing (BMDP); all three are available in mainframe or personal computer versions. Many other programs are also available. For example, the *British Journal of Mathematical and Statistical Psychology* has regular reviews of new statistical software. The basic procedure for all of the computer statistical packages is that the variables of interest are defined, the data are coded and entered into a data file, and then the analyses are run.

Statistical consultants can be used in several different ways. First, they can be consulted during the planning stages of a project to help determine whether the planned design can be analyzed in a way that will answer the research question. Second, they can help the researcher determine the sample size needed to obtain statistically significant results given certain assumptions about the size of differences between groups and the extent of variability within groups. Third, they can provide access to and are knowledgeable about statistical software. Fourth, they can check any analysis the researcher might have done on his or her own. Finally, they can review the written report of a research project to ensure that what the researcher has written about the statistical analysis is in fact what was done.

Before working with statistical consultants, the researcher must have a clear idea of the purposes of his or her research. A list of proposed variables and the values they may take is essential because statistical decisions will be based in part on the measurement characteristics of the data. Consultants may also wish to review published reports of studies similar to the one being planned so that they can see the type of analysis that is the norm in the discipline or for a particular journal.

The researcher and consultant must be clear about who will do which tasks associated with the analysis. Will the consultant enter data, run the analysis, prepare summary tables, and summarize the results for the researcher? Or will the researcher enter the data, receive a stack of printouts, and contact the consultant only if there are any questions? Because the consultant will likely work for an hourly fee, the researcher should ask the consultant for an estimate of the number of hours that will be required for the level of involvement desired.

Data Coding

The first step of data analysis is to develop a coding scheme for the data. The coding scheme for our hypothetical total knee arthroplasty data was initially presented in Table 20-1. Figure 27-2 shows how the coding scheme is translated into a form that encourages simultaneous data collection and coding.

Responses that are letters or descriptors (A, B, C, and D on multiple-choice items; "strongly agree," "agree," "neutral," "disagree," and "strongly disagree" for Likert-type items) are generally converted into numbers for data analysis. Some statistical programs permit the researcher to enter the letter and convert it to a number; others require that numbers be entered.

The researcher needs to decide how to handle missing data points. One option is to simply leave them as blanks in the data set. In other instances, the researcher may want frequency counts of missing data or may wish to analyze a subgroup of individuals who did not respond to a certain question. In these cases, missing data need to be given their own code. The number 9 or 99 is often used as the code for missing data. For some analyses, researchers "impute" values by, for example, entering the mean value for any missing data.

Some questionnaire items may permit multiple responses. For example, a multiple-choice item may ask respondents to indicate all the choices that apply to their situation. Coding of multiple responses is often best accomplished by converting the single item into several yes/no items. Assume that in our coding system, a "yes" response is coded 1, and a "no" response is coded 0. The response for a respondent who checked A, C, and E out of A through F responses for a multiple-answer item would be coded as follows: A=1, B=0, C=1, D=0, E=1, and F=0.

After the coding scheme is accomplished, the researcher should go through the data and convert them to codes as necessary. Although some researchers may be able to sit in front of the computer with raw data and simultaneously code and enter them, most will have a more accurate data set, and will save time in the long run, if they perform coding and entering separately. After the data have been coded initially, the codes need to be rechecked and corrected by either the original coder or another member of the research team.

Data Entry

After the data are coded, they need to be entered into the computer for analysis. In many instances, the data file can be created through a standard spreadsheet program and then transferred into a format that can be used by the statistical software. Although the actual procedures for data entry vary from package to package, the basic structure of a data file is that the variables are represented by columns and the participants by rows, as shown initially in Table 20-2 for the hypothetical study of patients with total knee arthroplasty.

When data have already been coded before they are entered, the researcher can enter data quickly without needing to think about what the numbers actually mean. Some researchers find that data entry goes more quickly if one person reads the numbers aloud and another enters them.

After data entry, the data set needs to be edited against the data-coding sheets. For some variables, it is possible to do "logical" tests of the data; if a variable can take values of 1 through 5, then the presence of a few 6s in the database must be errors. Only after the data set is edited, or "cleaned," is the researcher ready to run the statistical analyses that will answer the research questions.[37,38]

Statistical Analysis

Too often, investigators test their research hypotheses without first gaining a sense of the character of the data set. The first statistical procedure done should be running frequencies and descriptive data for each variable within the data set as a whole. In doing so, the researcher can get a sense of the distribution, means and standard deviations, and frequencies of the variables overall. If there are very extreme values for some variables, the researcher should recheck them against the original data sheets for accuracy. If the person collecting the data thought there might be an irregularity, it may be noted on the original data collection sheet. Extreme values are known as outliers and may sometimes be deleted from a data set with justification. A statistical consultant can help the researcher decide when it is reasonable to delete outliers.

Next, the researcher should divide the total sample into groups, if appropriate to the study purposes. For example, after the descriptive information about the total knee arthroplasty sample has been examined, frequencies, means, and standard deviations for each of the clinics under study should be run. This tells the researcher whether data are normally distributed and whether there is homogeneity of variance within the subgroups of interest. This information is essential to determining whether the assumptions for parametric testing are met. If they are not, then the researcher adopts the nonparametric contingency plan for the variables that have not met parametric assumptions.

Only after the data have been examined as noted previously can the statistical tests of interest be conducted. Many of the programs have a dizzying array of options from which to choose for a given statistical test. If uncertain about which options are appropriate, the researcher should use the services of a statistical consultant.

SUMMARY

A research proposal is a blueprint for a study, specifying the investigators, research problem, purposes, methods, references, methods of dissemination of results, budget, and work plan. Research proposals must be approved by facility administrators, an academic committee, an IRB, or some combination of these entities. The role of the IRB is to ensure that the investigators have put into place procedures needed to safeguard the rights of their participants, including their privacy rights. Research proposals are also used to secure funding for the study. Major sources of funding include institutions, corporations, foundations, and the government. Increasing levels of formalization of the grant application and award process are exerted as the research moves from institutional funding to government funding. Many private foundations and government agencies sponsor research that is of interest to rehabilitation professionals.

Implementation of a research project requires attention to detail at every step of the process. Recruitment of participants involves consideration of physician consent, participant consent, administrative approval, and generalizability of research findings. Researchers must attend to many details related to data collection, including specific procedures, ensuring the safety of the data,

protecting the identity of participants, developing data collection forms, conducting pilot studies, and scheduling participants and personnel. Data analysis for all but the smallest data sets requires the use of a computer statistical package and a statistical consultant.

REFERENCES

1. Whyte J: Building a program of outcomes research: Personal reflections, *Am J Phys Med Rehabil* 80:865–874, 2001.
2. Thomas RM, Brubaker DL: *Theses and Dissertations: A Guide to Planning, Research, and Writing*, 2nd ed, Thousand Oaks, Calif, 2008, Corwin Press.
3. Cone JD, Foster SL: *Dissertations and Theses from Start to Finish: Psychology and Related Fields*, 2nd ed, Washington, DC, 2006, American Psychological Association.
4. Wisker G: *The Good Supervisor: Supervising Postgraduate and Undergraduate Research for Doctoral Theses and Dissertations*, 2nd ed, Bastingstoke, UK, 2012, Palgrave Macmillan.
5. Houser J, Bokovoy J: *Clinical Research in Practice: A Guide for the Bedside Scientist*, Sudbury, Mass, 2006, Jones & Bartlett.
6. Hegde MN: *Clinical Research in Communicative Disorders*, 3rd ed, Austin, Tex, 2003, Pro-Ed.
7. Denicolo P, Becker LM: *Developing Research Proposals*, Los Angeles, Calif, 2012, Sage.
8. Punch K: *Developing Effective Research Proposals*, 2nd ed, London, UK, 2006, Sage.
9. Krathwohl DR, Smith NL: *How to Prepare a Dissertation Proposal: Suggestions for Students in Education and the Social and Behavioral Sciences*, Syracuse, NY, 2005, Syracuse University Press.
10. American Psychological Association: *Publication Manual of the American Psychological Association*, 6th ed, Washington, DC, 2010, Author.
11. Li-ling C, Ching-yi W, Keh-chung L, Ching-ju H: Relative and absolute reliability of a vertical numerical pain rating scale supplemented with a faces pain scale after stroke, *Phys Ther* 94:129–138, 2014.
12. Chiat S, Roy P: Early predictors of language and social communication impairments at ages 9-11 years: A follow-up study of early-referred children, *J Speech Lang Hear Res* 56:1824–1836, 2013.
13. Sandelowski M, Barroso J: Writing the proposal for a qualitative research methodology project, *Qual Health Res* 13:781–820, 2003.
14. Holloway I, Wheeler S: *Qualitative Research in Nursing and Healthcare*, 3rd ed, Chichester, UK, 2010, Wiley-Blackwell.
15. Knafl KA, Deatrick JA: Top 10 tips for successful qualitative grantsmanship, *Res Nurs Health* 28:441–443, 2005.
16. U.S. Department of Health and Human Services. Title 45 CFR Part 46 Protection of Human Subjects. Available at: http://www.hhs.gov/ohrp/policy/ohrpregulations.pdf. Accessed December 17, 2014.
17. Coleman CH, editor: *The Ethics and Regulation of Research with Human Subjects*, Newark, NJ, 2005, LexisNexis Matthew Bender.
18. Emanuel EJ, editor: *The Oxford Textbook of Clinical Research Ethics*, Oxford, UK, 2008, Oxford University Press.
19. Oliver P: *The Student's Guide to Research Ethics*, 2nd ed, Maidenhead, UK, 2010, Open University Press.

20. Beauchamp TL, Frey RG, editors: *The Oxford Handbook of Animal Ethics*, Oxford, UK, 2011, Oxford University Press.

21. Hammersley M, Traianou A: *Ethics in Qualitative Research: Controversies and Contexts*, Thousand Oaks, Calif, 2012, Sage.

22. U.S. Dept. of Health and Human Services. Institutional Review Boards (IRBs). Available at: http://www.hhs.gov/ohrp/assurances/irb/index.html. Accessed December 17, 2014.

23. Federman DD, Hanna KE, Rodriguez LL, for the Institute of Medicine (US) Committee on Assessing the System for Protecting Human Research Participants: *Responsible Research: A Systems Approach to Protecting Research Participants*, Washington, DC, 2003, National Academies Press.

24. Lambert V, Glacken M: Engaging with children in research: Theoretical and practical implications of negotiating informed consent/assent, *Nurs Ethics* 18:781–801, 2011.

25. Mayo AM, Wallhagen MI: Considerations of informed consent and decision-making competence in older adults with cognitive impairment, *Res Gerontol Nurs* 2:103–111, 2009.

26. Karlawish J, Cary M, Moelter ST, et al: Cognitive impairment and PD patients' capacity to consent to research, *Neurology* 81:801–807, 2013.

27. Wiles R: Physiotherapy Research Foundation: Review of activity 1995–2001, *Physiotherapy* 89:138–139, 2003.

28. Foundation Center. The Foundation Directory. Available at: foundationcenter.org/. Accessed December 17, 2014.

29. Foundation Center: *Corporate Foundation Profiles*, 12th ed, New York, NY, 2002, Author.

30. Foundation Center: *Grant$ for the Physically and Mentally Disabled*, New York, NY, no date, Foundation Center.

31. Foundation Center: *Grants for People with Disabilities*, New York, NY, 2006, Author.

32. Catalog of Federal Domestic Assistance. Available at: www.cfda.gov. Accessed December 17, 2014.

33. U.S. Dept. of Health and Human Services. Find Grants. Available at: http://www.grants.gov/web/grants/home.html. Accessed December 17, 2014.

34. Reif-Lehrer L: *Grant Application Writer's Handbook*, 4th ed, Boston, Mass, 2005, Jones & Bartlett.

35. Ward D: *Effective Grants Management*, Sudbury, Mass, 2010, Jones & Bartlett.

36. Council on Foundations: *Best Practices in Grants Management*, Washington, DC, 2001, Author.

37. Polit DF: *Statistics and Data Analysis for Nursing Research*, 2nd ed, Upper Saddle River, NJ, 2010, Pearson Education.

38. Roberts BL, Anthony MK, Madigan EA, Chen Y: Data management: Cleaning and checking, *Nurs Res* 46:350–352, 1997.

28

Publishing and Presenting Research

CONTENTS

Publication of Research
  Types of Publications
  Peer Review Process
  Authorship and Acknowledgment

  Multiple Publication
  Style Issues
  Components of a Research Article
Presentation of Research

  Platform Presentations
  Poster Presentations
Summary

Research can never influence practice if it remains in a file drawer. Therefore, the culmination of the research endeavor is the dissemination of results. When made public, research can fulfill its goal of adding to the body of evidence clinicians draw on when working with patients or clients. This is not to say, however, that all research that is conducted should be disseminated. Some research is so flawed that valid conclusions cannot be drawn from the results. Given this caveat, after an investigator has obtained results that have something to add to the body of knowledge, he or she needs to find the appropriate way to disseminate the results. There are two main mechanisms for doing so: publication and presentation.

This chapter describes the publication and presentation process and presents guidelines for developing effective publications and presentations. Guidelines for manuscript preparation, a complete manuscript in two different formats, and a presentation script and visuals are provided in Appendices D through G, respectively.

PUBLICATION OF RESEARCH

The main vehicle for publication of research results is the journal article. This section differentiates between types of publications and journals; discusses the peer review process, authorship, and acknowledgment issues in publication; and presents a variety of language and usage issues that arise when writing about research.

Types of Publications

Professional publications usually fall into one of three categories: journals, magazines, and newsletters. Newsletters present news of interest to subscribers or members. They may occasionally highlight important research findings but generally do not report original research. Many state chapters of professional associations publish newsletters regularly.

Magazines are publications with full-length articles about general topics of interest to professionals. Some magazine articles may refer to original research, but they do not ordinarily report original research. Articles on practice management, overviews of patient care for certain groups, and discussions of professional issues are appropriate topics for professional magazines.

In general, journals have as their primary purpose the reporting of original research findings in a defined area, although some journals have as their mission the publication of review articles. When publication of original research is the primary focus of a journal, this does not preclude publication of review articles, editorials, or other features such as book reviews or the news of a professional association. There are two types of journals: peer reviewed or non–peer reviewed. In considering a manuscript submitted for publication, editors of peer reviewed, or "refereed," journals contact professionals who are knowledgeable about the content area of a manuscript to determine whether the manuscript has scientific rigor and significantly adds to knowledge in the discipline. The final decision about whether a paper is published is made by an editor who is a scholar within the discipline. Publication decisions for non–peer reviewed, or non-refereed, journals may be made by individuals who are professional editors rather than scholars within the discipline. A journal's peer review status may be mentioned in its instructions to authors and can be found in directories of serials that are in the reference section of the library.[1,2]

Peer Review Process

The personnel involved in the peer review process typically include the journal editor, an editorial board chaired by the editor, and manuscript reviewers. All of these individuals are scholars or practitioners in the discipline or related areas. The journal editor is appointed by the managing body that publishes the journal; the editorial board is usually appointed by the editor, with the consent of the managing body that publishes the journal; and the editorial board establishes qualifications for being a manuscript reviewer and accepts applications from interested professionals. For many journals, all these positions are voluntary; however, the editors of larger journals may receive a stipend or honorarium.

When a manuscript is submitted to a peer reviewed journal for consideration for publication, a chain of events is triggered. The editor or staff reviews the manuscript to determine whether it meets technical requirements (e.g., length, reference style) and whether it fits the general mission of the journal. If either of these conditions is not met, the manuscript is returned to the authors without further review. If the manuscript meets the technical and mission criteria, it is retained for further review.

The manuscript is usually assigned for review to one editorial board member and one or more manuscript reviewers. The board and manuscript reviewers are selected on the basis of their area of expertise in the profession or their knowledge of the research methods used by the authors. The board member and reviewers critique the manuscript to determine the soundness of the research design, the importance and usefulness of the research in light of other literature and the needs of practitioners, and the clarity and readability of the manuscript.

The manuscript reviewers summarize their opinions of the manuscript to the editorial board member and indicate whether they believe it merits publication. The editorial board member synthesizes his or her opinion with the input from the various reviewers and renders an opinion about the paper to the editor.

Based on the information from the editorial board member and reviewers, the editor makes a decision about publication of the manuscript. A manuscript generally has one of four fates: acceptance, provisional acceptance pending revision, rejection with suggestion to rewrite, or rejection without suggestion to rewrite. Very few manuscripts are accepted for publication without revisions. A manuscript may be accepted provisionally pending revisions when the content and structure of the study seem sound and useful but the article format needs to be polished. A rejection with a suggestion to rewrite usually means that the topic is important to the profession, but the article as written is too incomplete or disorganized to permit judgment about the credibility of the research. A rejection without a suggestion to rewrite usually means that the topic is simply not a high priority for the journal or that the research methods are too flawed to permit valid conclusions.

As might be inferred by the process just described, peer review is time consuming. Several months may elapse between submission and a first decision about the manuscript. Author revisions may take several more months, as will final editing of the manuscript by the journal staff. Moreover, because many journals have a backlog of articles waiting to be published, publication of an accepted paper may be delayed several more months. It is not uncommon for more than a year to elapse between submission of a manuscript and its eventual publication. A recent approach to ameliorate this delay is to publish articles electronically as soon as they are accepted, for example as in the *Journal of Speech, Language, and Hearing Research*.[3]

Authorship and Acknowledgment

Today, most journal articles are coauthored by multiple researchers. In addition to the authors, there are often individuals who have contributed to the study and deserve acknowledgment at the conclusion of the article. Because authorship and acknowledgment involve prestige and recognition, there are often controversies about who should be an author, in what order the authors should be presented, and who should be acknowledged.

Various groups provide guidelines to help researchers make authorship and acknowledgment decisions.[4-6] The International Committee of Medical Journal Editors (ICMJE) encourages editors of all journals to develop "a contributorship policy, as well as a policy on identifying who is responsible for the integrity of the work as a whole."[4(p. 2)] ICMJE is typical in its definition of "author" and requires that anyone listed as an author "be someone who has made substantive intellectual contributions to a published study."[4(p. 2)] Further, the designation of author "should be based on 1) substantial contributions to conception and design, acquisition of data, or analysis and interpretation of data; 2) drafting the article or revising it critically for important intellectual content; and 3) final approval of the version to be published."[4(p. 2)] ICJME provides further guidance for authorship by large, multicenter groups, common in scientific studies. These criteria are essentially echoed by the American Psychological Association (APA).[6] The order in which the authors' names are listed should reflect the relative strength of the contributions they have made to the project, with the first author contributing the most and the last author contributing the least. This order should be discussed when tasks are being divided among the researchers in the early stages of a project. The order may change somewhat as the project progresses; before submission of the paper for publication, the authors should negotiate among themselves what the final order will be.

Authors should acknowledge individuals who have made contributions to the project that do not qualify them as authors. Such contributors may include those who collected or analyzed some of the data, colleagues who loaned facilities or fabricated equipment, or peers who provided critical review of early drafts of the manuscript. All acknowledged individuals should receive a copy of the manuscript and give their permission to be named.

Multiple Publication

Journals hold the copyright to materials they publish, requiring that authors transfer the copyright of a work to them in the event it is published. Therefore, journals require authors to disclose prior publication and do not typically accept for consideration papers that have been published in full elsewhere. In addition, journals do not typically permit multiple submission of articles. That is, authors cannot submit the same article for consideration by more than one journal at a time. Therefore, authors identify the journal they think is a best fit for their work, submit the article to that journal for consideration, and wait for a decision from that journal. If the first journal to which an article is submitted rejects the article, the authors are then free to submit it to another journal.

Style Issues

The research article is a specialized form of writing. Its hallmarks are precision, conciseness, and consistency. The novelist uses words to paint pictures and uses different words to convey similar meanings in different contexts. Whereas creative use of language makes novels enjoyable, it makes research articles infuriating if different terms are used to represent the same construct.

Each journal publishes its own instructions for authors. These instructions typically specify the types of articles accepted for review, the editorial process, the format that the manuscript should take, the reference style to use, procedures for manuscript submission, and the style manual that should be used to prepare the paper. These instructions can be found in selected issues of the journal or on the journal's Web site.

A style manual is a document of technical information for authors. Most journals that publish rehabilitation research have adopted the style, or a variant of the style, described in the *American Medical Association Manual of Style*[7] or the *Publication Manual of the American Psychological Association*.[6] The major difference between the two styles is the way that references are cited in the text and the format of the reference list. Box 28-1 shows the two different styles for in-text citations and reference lists. Style manuals specify such things as when numbers are presented as numerals (e.g., 227) and when they are written out (e.g., two hundred twenty-seven), what levels of headings and subheadings to use, how to present mathematical symbols, how to set up tables, how to cite literature in the text of an article, and what format to follow for the reference list at the end of the article. They also present useful writing style and grammar suggestions, including how to differentiate among confusing terms (e.g., affect and effect), when to use certain punctuation marks, and how to avoid exclusionary language. Table 28-1 presents several style problems that commonly appear in the papers of novice authors. This table can help writers eliminate these mistakes from their papers, but it is no substitute for frequent reference to a style manual. In addition to style manuals, a search for "scientific writing style" or "medical writing style" on any search engine will result in several excellent references providing general guidelines for scientific and medical writing.[8,9] In addition, these days writers are greatly assisted by available software at least for putting citations in the proper format for a number of styles. A search using terms like "citation format" in a good search engine will yield several possibilities.

A set of style guidelines that should be of particular importance to rehabilitation professionals relates to references about people with disabilities. Authors (and clinicians) should pay close attention to the implications of the words they use to refer to this population. Table 28-2 presents a set of guidelines for writing about people with disabilities.[10]

Box 28-1

Comparison of American Medical Association and American Psychological Association Styles for In-Text Citation and Reference Lists

American Medical Association Manual of Style[7]

Like Basso and Knapp[1] in the 1980s, Chen and colleagues[2] concluded that use of continuous passive motion after total knee arthroplasty did not have an effect on postoperative edema.

REFERENCES

1. Basso DM, Knapp L. Comparison of two continuous passive motion protocols for patients with total knee implants. *Phys Ther.* 1987; 67: 360-363.
2. Chen B, Zimmerman JR, Soulen L, DeLisa JA. Continuous passive motion after total knee arthroplasty: a prospective study. *Am J Phys Med Rehabil.* 2000; 79: 421-426.

Publication Manual of the American Psychological Association[6]

Like Basso and Knapp (1987), Chen, Zimmerman, Soulen, and DeLisa (2000) concluded that use of continuous passive motion after total knee arthroplasty did not have an effect on postoperative edema.

REFERENCES

Basso, D. M., & Knapp, L. (1987). Comparison of two continuous passive motion protocols for patients with total knee implants. *Physical Therapy, 67,* 360-363.

Chen, B., Zimmerman, J. R., Soulen, L., & DeLisa, J. A. (2000). Continuous passive motion after total knee arthroplasty: A prospective study. *American Journal of Physical Medicine and Rehabilitation, 79,* 421-426.

Components of a Research Article

The components of a research article are as follows:
1. Title and title page
2. Abstract
3. Introduction
4. Methods
5. Results
6. Discussion
7. Conclusions
8. Acknowledgments
9. References
10. Tables
11. Figures

Appendix D provides a numbered list of guidelines for the preparation of each section; Appendix E and Appendix F present the same hypothetical manuscript in American Medical Association (AMA) and APA style, respectively. Each hypothetical manuscript is annotated with numbers that correspond to the items in Appendix D. Writers should consult the appropriate style manual for additional guidance. In addition, those who expect to present a great deal of graphical data may benefit from consulting detailed texts for guidance.[11,12]

PRESENTATION OF RESEARCH

Presentation is the second major format by which research results are disseminated. Most, if not all, professional associations in the rehabilitation professions hold meetings at which research presentations are made. The process of selecting a paper for presentation usually involves submission of an abstract of the study, generally many months in advance of the conference. Some associations use peer review to select abstracts for presentation; others accept any abstracts that meet the technical guidelines and can be accommodated within the conference schedule. Some associations specify that abstracts must be of studies that have not been presented previously. However, because conference presentations are less permanent and less accessible than publications, some conference organizers permit presentation of studies that have been presented elsewhere, particularly if they target a different audience. Thus, as long as it is permitted by the conference organizer, researchers may feel comfortable presenting the results of a study at both a local and national meeting or at meetings for different professional groups. For example, a study related to the roles of physical therapists and athletic trainers in the clinical setting might be appropriate for presentation at a conference of physical therapists and at a conference for athletic trainers, as long as the conference organizer for the later conference is willing to accept previously presented work.

There are two major formats for conference presentations: platform presentations and poster presentations. Guidelines are available to help individuals plan effective research presentations.[9,12-14] Each presentation format is described and illustrated in the following sections.

Platform Presentations

A platform presentation is made by a researcher to an audience of peers attending the conference. The presentation time is usually short; anywhere from 10 to 20 minutes is common. High-quality visuals are expected to accompany the presentation, and most

Table 28-1

Common Style Problems in Manuscripts of Novice Authors

Problem	Example of Problem	Corrected Text
Abbreviation is used without being identified at the first use.	Many children with CP experience communication difficulties. The type of CP has an impact on …	Many children with cerebral palsy (CP) experience communication difficulties. The type of CP has an impact on …
Sentence begins with a numeral.	224 responses were received.	Two hundred twenty-four responses were received. OR We received 224 responses.
Abbreviation of units of measurement is inconsistent or nonstandard (standard units do not have to be spelled out the first time they are used).	Velocity was measured in centimeters per second, with the younger group walking at a rate of 180 cm/sec.	Velocity was measured in cm/s, with the younger group walking at a rate of 180 cm/s.
Language includes jargon or informal terms understood by a small group of professionals.	The participants completed 20 reps of quad sets.	The participants completed 20 repetitions of isometric quadriceps femoris muscle contractions.
Punctuation after quotation marks is incorrect.	Boswell stated that "complacency rules in many professions".	Boswell stated that "complacency rules in many professions."
Author refers to himself or herself in the third person. First person language is preferred today, even in scientific writing.	This author believes that Mayberry overstated his findings.	I believe that Mayberry overstated his findings.
Comparative terms are used, but no comparison is made.	Johnson found an increase in strength of the middle deltoid muscle.	Johnson found an increase in strength of the middle deltoid muscle after completion of the exercise program.
Exclusionary terms are used, or awkward constructions are made.	The therapist should not let his emotions cloud his judgment. OR The therapist should not let his/her emotions cloud his/her judgment.	Therapists should not let their emotions cloud their judgment. OR Emotions should not cloud the therapist's judgment.
Male or female is used as a noun rather than an adjective.	We studied 50 females.	We studied 50 women.
Author unnecessarily hyphenates prefixed words.	The post-test scores for the non-injured hand were …	The posttest scores for the noninjured hand were …

major conferences today use digital projection systems, enabling researchers to incorporate text, tables and graphs, clip art, still photography, and digital video as appropriate to the presentation. A suggested sequence for development of a research presentation is presented here. Appendix G provides a script and visuals for a presentation of the manuscript presented in Appendices E and F.

1. Complete a draft of the manuscript. A manuscript provides the complete picture of the study to be described in the presentation. However, because most presentations precede submission of the work

Table 28-2

Guidelines for Writing About People with Disabilities

Sensational or Negative Portrayal	Straightforward, Positive Portrayal
Traumatic brain injury patient [focuses on the injury rather than the person]	Individual with a traumatic brain injury [focuses on the person rather than the injury; use patient only if the person is, in fact, undergoing health care]
Physically challenged [euphemisms imply that disabilities cannot be dealt with in a straightforward manner]	Person with a disability [puts the person first, then the disability; acknowledges the disability directly]
Special children [attempts to glorify differences]	Children with disabilities [straightforward portrayal]
Wheelchair-bound [evokes a confined image contrary to the active role of many people who use wheelchairs]	Uses a wheelchair [describes the wheelchair as the tool that it is]
Suffers from multiple sclerosis [sensationalizes the disease]	Has multiple sclerosis [states the disease matter-of-factly]

Modified from The Life Span Institute, Research and Training Center on Independent Living, University of Kansas. Guidelines for Reporting and Writing About People with Disabilities. Available at: http://www.rtcil.org/products/RTCIL%20publications/Media/Guidelines%20for%20Reporting%20and%20Writing%20about%20People%20with%20Disabilities.pdf. Accessed December 18, 2014.

for publication, the author does not often have a final version of the manuscript available to guide the development of the presentation. However, a draft of the manuscript can help the presenter decide which elements are essential and which can be deleted for the presentation. In addition, because most research presentations follow the same sequence as a journal article, a draft manuscript provides a ready-made outline for the presentation.

2. Determine which manuscript content is essential for the presentation. Because conference research presentations are brief, presenters need to be selective about the information they include in the presentation. Examine each paragraph of the draft manuscript to determine whether it is essential to an understanding of the project. A guideline for developing the presentation is to spend approximately:
   • 10% of the allotted time establishing the problem and context of the study
   • 20% of the time describing the methods
   • 30% of the time presenting the results
   • 30% of the time discussing the results
   • 10% of the time summarizing the conclusions and/or responding to audience questions

The introduction section of the paper can be shortened by deleting many specific references to the related literature and developing the problem conceptually. The methods section can be shortened by eliminating detail about measurement procedures and minimizing technical information about

the instruments used. Remember that a presentation audience just needs to understand the methods and does not need enough detail to replicate them in a future study.

Whereas research papers often include separate instrumentation and procedures sections, a presentation may flow more smoothly if the two are combined. Similarly, some repetition may be eliminated if the data analysis, results, and some parts of the discussion sections of the presentation are integrated. Conclusions should be clear and concise, providing the audience with a few memorable "take-home" points.

3. Divide the manuscript into segments. A general guideline for preparation of a conference presentation is to have each visual displayed for between 10 and 20 seconds, for an average of 4 visuals per minute. A 10-minute presentation might therefore have 40 visuals. This requires that the researcher divide the essential content into small "sound bites" in which each can be illustrated with a visual. Varying the length of the segments helps maintain audience interest.

4. Design the visuals. For each text segment, decide whether it is best illustrated with text, a table, a photograph, a drawing, a video, or a graph. Most conferences are set up for horizontal projection, so the presenter should design visuals in a horizontal format. Presentation software is widely available within standard integrated office software packages.

Slides of text should generally contain no more than 10 lines of text and no more than six words per line. The style should be telegraphic, using phrases rather than complete sentences. Text should not exactly repeat the script of the presentation; audiences do not like to have visuals read to them. Use of uppercase and lowercase letters is thought to be more readable than using all capital letters; simple sans serif typefaces are preferred.

Tables of information should contain no more than three columns and no more than seven rows. Use of data tables as they appear in the manuscript is rarely suitable because they contain far more information than can be absorbed in 10 to 20 seconds. Graphs are often more effective than tables in a presentation.

Photographs should be clear enough that the audience can locate the item of interest quickly. Photographers should strive for an uncluttered background that contrasts well with the subject. Sometimes photographs are simply not the best way to get a visual message across. For example, a line diagram of a particular piece of equipment may be able to focus attention on the relevant portion of the instrument; an illustration of an anatomical part may be more effective than a photograph.

Graphs should be used to illustrate the relationships between different numbers within the data set. Pie charts show proportions well, bar graphs effectively illustrate differences in quantities between groups, and line graphs are ideal for illustrating change across time. Because the visual will be displayed for a limited time, the graph should be as simple and clear as possible. Labels should be large enough to read; words should be kept to a minimum.

5. Draft the visuals. Most large conferences use electronic data projection systems to display presentation graphics directly from the presenter's laptop computer. Presentation software, such as PowerPoint, is a common component of integrated software packages that include word processing, spreadsheet, and presentation capabilities, enabling researchers or their support staff to create their own presentations. Occasionally, smaller conferences may still rely on slide projection; in this case, researchers can use hospital or university media services departments to assist in producing slides from their graphics program or commercial slide production services, which are available in most large cities.

6. Integrate text and visuals. After the visuals have been produced, practice delivering the text and visuals together. Manuscript text is often too sterile for presentation purposes and needs to be redrafted into

a more conversational tone. In addition, the text that goes with each visual should help integrate the visuals with the text without repeating exactly the same information. Integrating the text and visuals is an iterative process that may require a few rounds of revision of visuals and text until they match well and tell the research story effectively. Figure 28-1 shows a sample graph with presentation text that highlights its important points. Session moderators will cut off presenters who run beyond their allotted time, so it is important to time the practice run-throughs and make adjustments as needed to meet the time limits of the conference.

Presenters need to decide whether they want to use a script, notes, or just their visuals to guide the presentation. Although some experienced presenters do not use any prompts other than their visuals, most novice presenters benefit from written materials to guide their talk. Even in a high-tech environment, some presenters like to use 3-×5-inch cards on which a script or notes for each visual is written. Others like to use standard-sized paper on which the script or notes for each visual are written in paragraph form, with marks inserted to indicate when to change the visual. Still others like to use the "notes" feature of their graphics program to print out hard copies of the visuals with accompanying text. Appendix G shows the text and visuals for a presentation of the hypothetical paper provided in Appendices E and F.

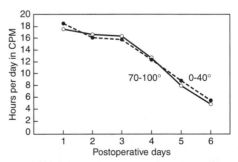

The two CPM groups received nearly identical hours per day in CPM, as shown by the two lines on this graph. Observe the gradual reduction in hours of CPM per day, starting at about 18 hours per day and ending up at less than 6 hours per day by the sixth postoperative day.

Figure 28-1 Example of visual and text for a platform presentation. Text highlights important features of the graph shown in the visual. CPM = continuous passive motion.

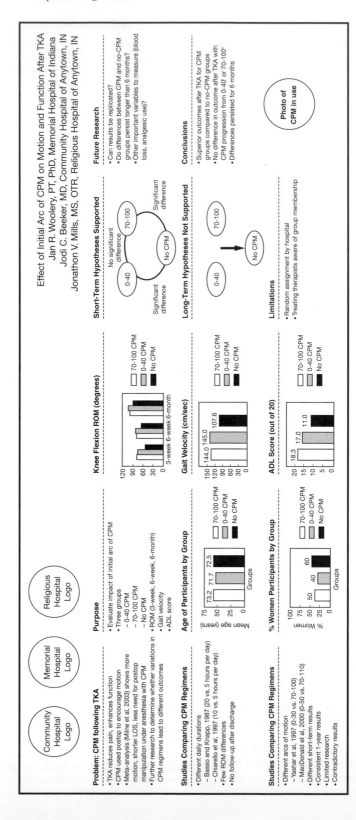

Figure 28-2 Schematic diagram for a poster presentation. ADL = activities of daily living; CPM = continuous passive motion; ROM = range of motion. (From Woolery JR, Beeker JC, Mills JV: Effect of initial arc of CPM on motion and function after TKA [hypothetical article presented in Appendices E to G].)

Poster Presentations

Poster presentations are a common feature at conferences and are becoming increasingly accepted as a means of disseminating scientific information. A poster session consists of a collection of large posters describing research studies. The posters are generally displayed for a relatively long time (e.g., one and a half hours), and presenters are required to be with their posters for at least a certain portion of the display time, if not all of it. The advantages of a poster session over a platform presentation are (1) conference attendees can view the posters when they have time, and (2) the researcher has more opportunity to interact with interested colleagues.

The space available for the posters is generally about 4×8 feet. At most large conferences, the norm is now an attractive single-panel poster that is unrolled from a tube and tacked up onto the board. Although these posters are often designed by professional graphic artists working with the researcher through the media services department of a hospital or university, it is possible for researchers without access to these resources to design attractive posters in standard graphics packages and send them to a commercial printer for production. It is, however, still acceptable to create a multiple-panel poster by designing a series of mini-posters that are easily printed on a standard color printer and mounted and laminated at a local copy shop. Researchers who prepare posters should ensure that the type is readable from a distance of 2 to 3 feet and that the sequence in which the poster should be examined is clear. Figure 28-2 shows a schematic diagram of a poster.

SUMMARY

Research results are disseminated through either publication or presentation. Publication of research results in journals is a formal process guided by peer review. Journal articles usually follow a standard sequence: introduction, methods, results, discussion, and conclusions. Presentation of research usually occurs at conferences through a platform talk with accompanying visuals or through a poster session in which the researcher can interact with conference attendees less formally than in the platform format. Presentations usually follow the same sequence as journal articles.

REFERENCES

1. EBSCO. The Serials Directory. Available at: http://www.ebscohost.com/public/the-serials-directory. Accessed December 18, 2014.
2. ProQuest. Ulrichsweb.com. Available at: http://www.ulrichsweb.com/UlrichsWeb/faqs.asp#About_Ulrichs. Accessed December 18, 2014.
3. American Speech-Language-Hearing Association. Journal of Speech, Language, and Hearing Research. Available at: http://jslhr.pubs.asha.org/justaccepted.aspx. Accessed December 18, 2014.
4. International Committee of Medical Journal Editors. Uniform Requirements for Manuscripts Submitted to Biomedical Journals: Writing and Editing for Biomedical Publication. Available at: http://www.icmje.org/recommendations/archives/2008_urm.pdf. Accessed December 18, 2014.
5. Council of Science Editors. CSE's White Paper on Promoting Integrity in Scientific Journal Publications, 2012 Update. Available at: http://www.councilscienceeditors.org/i4a/pages/index.cfm?pageid=3331. Accessed December 18, 2014.
6. American Psychological Association: *Publication Manual of the American Psychological Association*, 6th ed, Washington, DC, 2010, Author.
7. Flanagin A, Christiansen S, editors: *AMA Manual of Style: A Guide for Authors and Editors*, 10th ed, New York, NY, 2007, Oxford University Press.
8. Day RA, Gastel B: *How to Write and Publish a Scientific Paper*, 6th ed, Westport, CT, 2006, Greenwood Press.
9. Browner WS: *Publishing and Presenting Clinical Research*, 2nd ed, Philadelphia, Pa, 2006, Lippincott, Williams & Wilkins.
10. Life Span Institute, Research and Training Center on Independent Living, University of Kansas. Guidelines for Reporting and Writing About People with Disabilities. Available at: http://www.rtcil.org/products/RTCIL%20publications/Media/Guidelines%20for%20Reporting%20and%20Writing%20about%20People%20with%20Disabilities.pdf. Accessed December 18, 2014.
11. Cleveland WS: *The Elements of Graphing Data*, revised ed, Murray Hill, NJ, 1994, AT&T Bell Laboratories.
12. Nicol AA, Pexman PM: *Displaying Your Findings: A Practical Guide for Creating Figures, Posters, and Presentations*, 6th ed, Washington, DC, 2010, American Psychological Association.
13. Anholt RRH: *Dazzle 'em with Style: The Art of Oral Scientific Presentation*, 2nd ed, Philadelphia, Pa, 2006, Elsevier Academic.
14. Alley M: *The Craft of Scientific Presentations: Critical Steps to Succeed and Critical Errors to Avoid*, 2nd ed, New York, NY, 2013, Springer.

A

Random Numbers Table

Table of 14,000 Random Units

Line/Col.	(1)	(2)	(3)	(4)	(5)	(6)	(7)	(8)	(9)	(10)	(11)	(12)	(13)	(14)
1	10480	15011	01536	02011	81647	91646	69179	14194	62590	36207	20969	99570	91291	90700
2	22368	46573	25595	85393	30995	89198	27982	53402	93965	34095	52666	19174	39615	99505
3	24130	48360	22527	97265	76393	64809	15179	24830	49340	32081	30680	19655	63348	58629
4	42167	93093	06243	61680	07856	16376	39440	53537	71341	57004	00849	74917	97758	16379
5	37570	39975	81837	16656	06121	91782	60468	81305	49684	60672	14110	06927	01263	54613
6	77921	06907	11008	42751	27756	53498	18602	70659	90655	15053	21916	81825	44394	42880
7	99562	72905	56420	69994	98872	31016	71194	18738	44013	48840	63213	21069	10634	12952
8	96301	91977	05463	07972	18876	20922	94595	56869	69014	60045	18425	84903	42508	32307
9	89579	14342	63661	10281	17453	18103	57740	84378	25331	12566	58678	44947	05585	56941
10	85475	36857	43342	53988	53060	59533	38867	62300	08158	17983	16439	11458	18593	64952
11	28918	69578	88231	33276	70997	79936	56865	05859	90106	31595	01547	85590	91610	78188
12	63553	40961	48235	03427	49626	69445	18663	72695	52180	20847	12234	90511	33703	90322
13	09429	93969	52636	92737	88974	33488	36320	17617	30015	08272	84115	27156	30613	74952
14	10365	61129	87529	85689	48237	52267	67689	93394	01511	26358	85104	20285	29975	89868
15	07119	97336	71048	08178	77233	13916	47564	81056	97735	85977	29372	74461	28551	90707
16	51085	12765	51821	51259	77452	16308	60756	92144	49442	53900	70960	63990	75601	40719
17	02368	21382	53404	60268	89368	19885	55322	44819	01188	65255	64835	44919	05944	55157
18	01011	54092	33362	94904	31273	04146	18594	29852	71585	85030	51132	01915	92747	64951
19	52162	53916	46369	58586	23216	14513	83149	98736	23495	64350	94738	17752	35156	35749
20	07056	97628	33787	09998	42698	06691	76988	13602	51851	46104	88916	19509	25625	58104
21	48663	91245	85828	14346	09172	30168	90229	04734	59193	22178	30421	61666	99904	32812
22	54164	58492	22421	74103	47070	25306	76468	26384	58151	06646	21524	15227	96909	44592
23	32639	32363	05597	24200	13363	38005	94342	28728	35806	06912	17012	64161	18296	22851
24	29334	27001	87637	87308	58731	00256	45834	15398	46557	41135	10367	07684	36188	18510
25	02488	33062	28834	07351	19731	92420	60952	61280	50001	67658	32586	86679	50720	94953
26	81525	72295	04839	96423	24878	82651	66566	14778	76797	14780	13300	87074	79666	95725
27	29676	20591	68086	26432	46901	20849	89768	81536	86645	12659	92259	57102	80428	25280
28	00742	57392	39064	66432	84673	40027	32832	61362	98947	96067	64760	64584	96096	98253
29	05366	04213	25669	26422	44407	44048	37937	63904	45766	66134	75470	66520	34693	90449
30	91921	26418	64117	94305	26766	25940	39972	22209	71500	64568	91402	42416	07844	69618
31	00582	04711	87917	77341	42206	35126	74087	99547	81817	42607	43808	76655	62028	76690
32	00725	69884	62797	56170	86324	88072	76222	36086	84637	93161	76038	65855	77919	88006
33	69011	65797	95876	55293	18988	27354	26575	08625	40801	59920	29841	80150	12777	48501
34	25976	57948	29888	88604	67917	48708	18912	82271	65424	69774	33611	54262	85963	03547
35	09763	83473	73577	12908	30883	18317	28290	35797	05998	41688	34952	37888	38917	88050
36	91567	42595	27958	30134	04024	86385	29880	99730	55536	84855	29080	09250	79656	73211
37	17955	56349	90999	49127	20044	59931	06115	20542	18059	02008	73708	83517	36103	42791
38	46503	18584	18845	49618	02304	51038	20655	58727	28168	15475	56942	53389	20562	87338
39	92157	89634	94824	78171	84610	82834	09922	25417	44137	48413	25555	21246	35509	20468
40	14577	62765	35605	81263	39667	47358	56873	56307	61607	49518	89656	20103	77490	18062
41	98427	07523	33362	64270	01638	92477	66969	98420	04880	45585	46565	04102	46880	45709
42	34914	63976	88720	82765	34476	17032	87589	40836	32427	70002	70663	88863	77775	69348
43	70060	28277	39475	46473	23219	53416	94970	25832	69975	94884	19661	72828	00102	66794
44	53976	54914	06990	67245	68350	82948	11398	42878	80287	88267	47363	46634	06541	97809
45	76072	29515	40980	07391	58745	25774	22987	80059	39911	96189	41151	14222	60697	59583
46	90725	52210	83974	29992	65831	38857	50490	83765	55657	14361	31720	57375	56228	41546
47	64364	67412	33339	31926	14883	24413	59744	92351	97473	89286	35931	04110	23726	51900
48	08962	00358	31662	25388	61642	34072	81249	35648	56891	69352	48373	45578	78547	81788
49	95012	68379	93526	70765	10593	04542	76463	54328	02349	17247	28865	14777	62730	92277
50	15664	10493	20492	38391	91132	21999	59516	81652	27195	48223	46751	22923	32261	85653
51	16408	81899	04153	53381	79401	21438	83035	92350	36693	31238	59649	91754	72772	02338
52	18629	81953	05520	91962	04739	13092	97662	24822	94730	06496	35090	04822	86772	98289
53	73115	35101	47498	87637	99016	71060	88824	71013	18735	20286	23153	72924	35165	43040
54	57491	16703	23167	49323	45021	33132	12544	41035	80780	45393	44812	12515	98931	91202
55	30405	83946	23792	14422	15059	45799	22716	19792	09983	74353	68668	30429	70735	25499
56	16631	35006	85900	98275	32388	52390	16815	69298	82732	38480	73817	32523	41961	44437
57	96773	20206	42559	78985	05300	22164	24369	54224	35083	19687	11052	91491	60383	19746
58	38935	64202	14349	82674	66523	44133	00697	35552	35970	19124	63318	29686	03387	59846
59	31624	76384	17403	53363	44167	64486	64758	75366	76554	31601	12614	33072	60332	92325

Table of 14,000 Random Units—cont'd

Line/Col.	(1)	(2)	(3)	(4)	(5)	(6)	(7)	(8)	(9)	(10)	(11)	(12)	(13)	(14)
60	78919	19474	23632	27889	47914	02584	37680	20801	72152	39339	34806	08930	85001	87820
61	03931	33309	57047	74211	63445	17361	62825	39908	05607	91284	68833	25570	38818	46920
62	74426	33278	43972	10119	89917	15665	52872	73823	73144	88662	88970	74492	51805	99378
63	09066	00903	20795	95452	92648	45454	09552	88815	16553	51125	79375	97596	16296	66092
64	42238	12426	87025	14267	20979	04508	64535	31355	88064	29472	47689	05974	52468	16834
65	16153	08002	26504	41744	81959	65642	74240	56302	00033	67107	77510	70625	28725	34191
66	21457	40742	29820	96783	29400	21840	15035	34537	33310	06116	95240	15957	16572	06004
67	21581	57802	02050	89728	17937	37621	47075	42080	97403	48626	68995	43805	33386	21597
68	55612	78095	83197	33732	05810	24813	86902	60397	16489	03264	88525	42786	05269	92532
69	44657	66999	99324	51281	84463	60563	79312	93454	68876	25471	93911	25650	12682	73572
70	91340	84979	46949	81973	37949	61023	43997	15263	80644	43942	89203	71795	99533	50501
71	91227	21199	31935	27022	84067	05462	35216	14486	29891	68607	41867	14951	91696	85065
72	50001	38140	66321	19924	72163	09538	12151	06878	91903	18749	34405	56087	82790	70925
73	65390	05224	72958	28609	81406	39147	25549	48542	42627	45233	57202	94617	23772	07896
74	27504	96131	83944	41575	10573	08619	64482	73923	36152	05184	94142	25299	84387	34925
75	37169	94851	39117	89632	00959	16487	65536	49071	39782	17095	02330	74301	00275	48280
76	11508	70225	51111	38351	19444	66499	71945	05422	13442	78675	84081	66938	93654	59894
77	37449	30362	06694	54690	04052	53115	62757	95348	78662	11163	81651	50245	34971	52924
78	46515	70331	85922	38329	57015	15765	97161	17869	45349	61796	66345	81073	46106	79860
79	30986	81223	42416	58353	21532	30502	32305	86482	05174	07901	54339	58861	74818	46942
80	63798	64995	46583	09765	44160	78128	83991	42865	92520	83531	80377	35909	81250	54238
81	82486	84846	99254	67632	43218	50076	21361	64816	51202	88124	41870	52689	51275	83556
82	21885	32906	92431	09060	64297	51674	64126	62570	26123	05155	59194	52799	28225	85762
83	60336	98782	07408	53458	13564	59089	26445	29789	85205	41001	12535	12133	14645	23541
84	43937	46891	24010	25560	86355	33941	25786	54990	71899	15475	95434	98227	21824	19585
85	97656	63175	89303	16275	07100	92063	21942	18611	47348	20203	18534	03862	78095	50136
86	03299	01221	05418	38982	55758	92237	26759	86367	21216	98442	08303	56613	91511	75928
87	79626	06486	03574	17668	07785	76020	79924	25651	83325	88428	85076	72811	22717	50585
88	85636	68335	47539	03129	65651	11977	02510	26113	99447	68645	34327	15152	55230	93448
89	18039	14367	61337	06177	12143	46609	32989	74014	64708	00533	35398	58408	13261	47908
90	08362	15656	60627	36478	65648	16764	53412	09013	07832	41574	17639	82163	60859	75567
91	79556	29068	04142	16268	15387	12856	66227	38358	22478	73373	88732	09443	82558	05250
92	92608	82674	27072	32534	17075	27698	98204	63863	11951	34648	88022	56148	34925	57031
93	23982	25835	40055	67006	12293	02753	14827	22235	35071	99704	37543	11601	35503	85171
94	09915	96306	05908	97901	28395	14186	00821	80703	70426	75647	76310	88717	37890	40129
95	50937	33300	26695	62247	69927	76123	50842	43834	86654	70959	79725	93872	28117	19233
96	42488	78077	69882	61657	34136	79180	97526	43092	04098	73571	80799	76536	71255	64239
97	46764	86273	63003	93017	31204	36692	40202	35275	57306	55543	53203	18098	47625	88684
98	03237	45430	55417	63282	90816	17349	88298	90183	36600	78406	06216	95787	42579	90730
99	86591	81482	52667	61583	14972	90053	89534	76036	49199	43716	97548	04379	46370	28672
100	38534	01715	94964	87288	65680	43772	39560	12918	86537	62738	19636	51132	25739	56947
101	13284	16834	74151	92027	24670	36665	00770	22878	02179	51602	07270	76517	97275	45960
102	21224	00370	30420	03883	96648	89428	41583	17564	27395	63904	41548	49197	82277	24120
103	99052	47887	81085	64933	66279	80432	65793	83287	34142	13241	30590	97760	35848	91983
104	00199	50993	98603	38452	87890	94624	69721	57484	67501	77638	44331	11257	71131	11059
105	60578	06483	28733	37867	07936	98710	98539	27186	31237	80612	44488	97819	70401	95419
106	91240	18312	17441	01929	18163	69201	31211	54288	39296	37318	65724	90401	79017	62077
107	97458	14229	12063	59611	32249	90466	33216	19358	02591	54263	88449	01912	07436	50813
108	35249	38646	34475	72417	60514	69257	12489	51924	86871	92446	36607	11458	30440	52639
109	38980	46600	11759	11900	46743	27860	77940	39298	97838	95145	32378	68038	89351	37005
110	10750	52745	38749	87365	58959	53731	89295	59062	39404	13198	59960	70408	29812	83126
111	36247	27850	73958	20673	37800	63835	71051	84724	52492	22342	78071	17456	96104	18327
112	70994	66986	99744	72438	01174	42159	11392	20724	54322	36923	70009	23233	65438	59685
113	99638	94702	11463	18148	81386	80431	90628	52506	02016	85151	88598	47821	00265	82525
114	72055	15774	43857	99805	10419	76939	25993	03544	21560	83471	43989	90770	22965	44247
115	24038	65541	85788	55835	38835	59399	13790	35112	01324	39520	76210	22467	83275	32286
116	74976	14631	35908	28221	39470	91548	12854	30166	09073	75887	36782	00268	97121	57676
117	35553	71628	70189	26436	63407	91178	90348	55359	80392	41012	36270	77786	89578	21059
118	35676	12797	51434	82976	42010	26344	92920	92155	58807	54644	58581	95331	78629	73344

Continued

Table of 14,000 Random Units—cont'd

Line/Col.	(1)	(2)	(3)	(4)	(5)	(6)	(7)	(8)	(9)	(10)	(11)	(12)	(13)	(14)
119	74815	67523	72985	23183	02446	63594	98924	20633	58842	85961	07648	70164	34994	67662
120	45246	88048	65173	50989	91060	89894	36063	32819	68559	99221	49475	50558	34698	71800
121	76509	47069	86378	41797	11910	49672	88575	97966	32466	10083	54728	81972	58975	30761
122	19689	90332	04315	21358	97428	11188	39062	63312	52496	07349	79178	33692	57352	72862
123	42751	35318	97513	61537	54955	08159	00337	80778	27507	95478	21252	12746	37554	97775
124	11946	22681	45045	13964	57517	59419	58045	44067	58716	58840	45557	96345	33271	53464
125	96518	48688	20996	11090	48396	57177	83867	86464	14342	21545	46717	72364	86954	55580
126	35726	58643	76869	84622	39098	36083	72505	92265	23107	60278	05822	46760	44294	07672
127	39737	42750	48968	70536	84864	64952	38404	94317	65402	13589	01055	79044	19308	83623
128	97025	66492	56177	04049	80312	48028	26408	43591	75528	65341	49044	95495	81256	53214
129	62814	08075	09788	56350	76787	51591	54509	49295	85830	59860	30883	89660	96142	18354
130	25578	22950	15227	83291	41737	79599	96191	71845	86899	70694	24290	01551	80092	82118
131	68763	69576	88991	49662	46704	63362	56625	00481	73323	91427	15264	06969	57048	54149
132	17900	00813	64361	60725	88974	61005	99709	30666	26451	11528	44323	34778	60342	60388
133	71944	60227	63551	71109	05624	43836	58254	26160	32116	63403	35404	57146	10909	07346
134	54684	93691	85132	64399	29182	44324	14491	55226	78793	34107	30374	48429	51376	09559
135	25946	27623	11258	65204	52832	50880	22273	05554	99521	73791	85744	29276	70326	60251
136	01353	39318	44961	44972	91766	90262	56073	06606	51826	18893	83448	31915	97764	75091
137	99083	88191	27662	99113	57174	35571	99884	13951	71057	53961	61448	74909	07322	80960
138	52021	45406	37945	75234	24327	86978	22644	87779	23753	99926	63898	54886	18051	96314
139	78755	47744	43776	83098	03225	14281	83637	55984	13300	52212	58781	14905	46502	04472
140	25282	69106	59180	16257	22810	43609	12224	25643	89884	31149	85423	32581	34374	70873
141	11959	94202	02743	86847	79725	51811	12998	76844	05320	54236	53891	70226	38632	84776
142	11644	13792	98190	01424	30078	28197	55583	05197	47714	68440	22016	79204	06862	94451
143	06307	97912	68110	59812	95448	43244	31262	88880	13040	16458	43813	89416	42482	33939
144	76285	75714	89585	99296	52640	46518	55486	90754	88932	19937	57119	23251	55619	23679
145	55322	07589	39600	60866	63007	20007	66819	84164	61131	81429	60676	42807	78286	29015
146	78017	90928	90220	92503	83375	26986	74399	30885	88567	29169	72816	53357	15428	86932
147	44768	43342	20696	26331	43140	69744	82928	24988	94237	46138	77426	39039	55596	12655
148	25100	19336	14605	86603	51680	97678	24261	02464	86563	74812	60069	71674	15478	47642
149	83612	46623	62876	85197	07824	91392	58317	37726	84628	42221	10268	20692	15699	29167
150	41347	81666	82961	60413	71020	83658	02415	33322	66036	98712	46795	16308	28413	05417
151	38128	51178	75096	13609	16110	73533	42564	59870	29399	67834	91055	89917	51096	89011
152	60950	00455	73254	96067	50717	13878	03216	78274	65863	37011	91283	33914	91303	49326
153	90524	17320	29832	96118	75792	25326	22940	24904	80523	38928	91374	55597	97567	38914
154	49897	18278	67160	39408	97056	43517	84426	59650	20247	19293	02019	14790	02852	05819
155	18494	99209	81060	19488	65596	59787	47939	91225	98768	43688	00438	05548	09443	82897
156	65373	72984	30171	37741	70203	94094	87261	30056	58124	70133	18936	02138	59372	09075
157	40653	12843	04213	70925	95360	55774	76439	61768	52817	81151	52188	31940	54273	49032
158	51638	22238	56344	44587	83231	50317	74541	07719	25472	41602	77318	15145	57515	07633
159	69742	99303	62578	83575	30337	07488	51941	84316	42067	49692	28616	29101	03013	73449
160	58012	74072	67488	74580	47992	69482	58624	17106	47538	13452	22620	24260	40155	74716
161	18348	19855	42887	08279	43206	47077	42637	45606	00011	20662	14642	49984	94509	56380
162	59614	09193	58064	29086	44385	45740	70752	05663	49081	26960	57454	99264	24142	74648
163	75688	28630	39210	52897	62748	72658	98059	67202	72789	01869	13496	14663	87645	89713
164	13941	77802	69101	70061	35460	34576	15412	81304	58757	35498	94830	75521	00603	97701
165	96656	86420	96475	86458	54463	96419	55417	41375	76886	19008	66877	35934	59801	00497
166	03363	82042	15942	14549	38324	87094	19069	67590	11087	68570	22591	65232	85915	91499
167	70366	08390	69155	25496	13240	57407	91407	49160	07379	34444	94567	66035	38918	65708
168	47870	36605	12927	16043	53257	93796	52721	73120	48025	76074	95605	67422	41646	14557
169	76504	77606	22761	30518	28373	73898	30550	76684	77366	32276	04990	61667	64798	66276
170	46967	74841	50923	15339	37755	98995	40162	89561	69199	42257	11647	47603	48779	97907
171	14558	50769	35444	59030	87516	48193	02945	00922	48189	04724	21263	20892	92955	90251
172	12440	25057	01132	38611	28135	68089	10954	10097	54243	06460	50856	65435	79377	53890
173	32293	29938	68653	10497	98919	46587	77701	99119	93165	67788	17638	23097	21468	36992
174	10640	21875	72462	77981	56550	55999	87310	69643	45124	00349	25748	00844	96831	30651
175	47615	23169	39571	56972	20628	21788	51736	33133	72696	32605	41569	76148	91544	21121
176	16948	11128	71624	72754	49084	96303	27830	45817	67867	18062	87453	17226	72904	71474
177	21258	61092	66634	70335	92448	17354	83432	49608	66520	06442	59664	20420	39201	69549
178	15072	48853	15178	30730	47481	48490	41436	25015	49932	20474	53821	51015	79841	32405

Table of 14,000 Random Units—cont'd

Line/Col.	(1)	(2)	(3)	(4)	(5)	(6)	(7)	(8)	(9)	(10)	(11)	(12)	(13)	(14)
179	99154	57412	09858	65671	70655	71479	63520	31357	56968	06729	34465	70685	04184	25250
180	08759	61089	23706	32994	35426	36666	63988	98844	37533	08269	27021	45886	22835	78451
181	67323	57839	61114	62192	47547	58023	64630	34886	98777	75442	95592	06141	45096	73117
182	09255	13986	84834	20764	72206	89393	34548	93438	88730	61805	78955	18952	46436	58740
183	36304	74712	00374	10107	85061	69228	81969	92216	03568	39630	81869	52824	50937	27954
184	15884	67429	86612	47367	10242	44880	12060	44309	46629	55105	66793	93173	00480	13311
185	18745	32031	35303	08134	33925	03044	59929	95418	04917	57596	24878	61733	92834	64454
186	72934	40086	88292	65728	38300	42323	64068	98373	48971	09049	59943	36538	05976	82118
187	17626	02944	20910	57662	80181	38579	24580	90529	52303	50436	29401	57824	86039	81062
188	27117	61399	50967	41399	81636	16663	15634	79717	94696	59240	25543	97989	63306	90946
189	93995	18678	90012	63645	85701	85269	62263	68331	00389	72571	15210	20769	44686	96176
190	67392	89421	09623	80725	62620	84162	87368	29560	00519	84545	08004	24526	41252	14521
191	04910	12261	37566	80016	21245	69377	50420	85658	55263	68667	78770	04533	14513	18099
192	81453	20283	79929	59839	23875	13245	46808	74124	74703	35769	95588	21014	37078	39170
193	19480	75790	48539	23703	15537	48885	02861	86587	74539	65227	90799	58789	96257	02708
194	21456	13162	74608	81011	55512	07481	93551	72189	76261	91206	89941	15132	37738	59284
195	89406	20912	46189	76376	25538	87212	20748	12831	57166	35026	16817	79121	18929	40628
196	09866	07414	55977	16419	01101	69343	13305	94302	80703	57910	36933	57771	42546	03003
197	86541	24681	23421	13521	28000	94917	07423	57523	97234	63951	42876	46829	09781	58160
198	10414	96941	06205	72222	57167	83902	07460	69507	10600	08858	07685	44472	64220	27040
199	49942	06683	41479	58982	56288	42853	92196	20632	62045	78812	35895	51851	83534	10689
200	23995	68882	42291	23374	24299	27024	67460	94783	40937	16961	26053	78749	46704	21983

From Beyer WH, editor: *Standard Mathematical Tables,* Boca Raton, Fla, 1984, CRC Press, pp 555–558.

B

Areas in One Tail of the Standard Normal Curve

This table shows the shaded area

z	.00	.01	.02	.03	.04	.05	.06	.07	.08	.09
0.0	.500	.496	.492	.488	.484	.480	.476	.472	.468	.464
0.1	.460	.456	.452	.448	.444	.440	.436	.433	.429	.425
0.2	.421	.417	.413	.409	.405	.401	.397	.394	.390	.386
0.3	.382	.378	.374	.371	.367	.363	.359	.356	.352	.348
0.4	.345	.341	.337	.334	.330	.326	.323	.319	.316	.312
0.5	.309	.305	.302	.298	.295	.291	.288	.284	.281	.278
0.6	.274	.271	.268	.264	.261	.258	.255	.251	.248	.245
0.7	.242	.239	.236	.233	.230	.227	.224	.221	.218	.215
0.8	.212	.209	.206	.203	.200	.198	.195	.192	.189	.187
0.9	.184	.181	.179	.176	.174	.171	.169	.166	.164	.161
1.0	.159	.156	.154	.152	.149	.147	.145	.142	.140	.138
1.1	.136	.133	.131	.129	.127	.125	.123	.121	.119	.117
1.2	.115	.113	.111	.109	.107	.106	.104	.102	.100	.099
1.3	.097	.095	.093	.092	.090	.089	.087	.085	.084	.082
1.4	.081	.079	.078	.076	.075	.074	.072	.071	.069	.068
1.5	.067	.066	.064	.063	.062	.061	.059	.058	.057	.056
1.6	.055	.054	.053	.052	.051	.049	.048	.048	.046	.046
1.7	.045	.044	.043	.042	.041	.040	.039	.038	.038	.037
1.8	.036	.035	.034	.034	.033	.032	.031	.031	.030	.029
1.9	.029	.028	.027	.027	.026	.026	.025	.024	.024	.023
2.0	.023	.022	.022	.021	.021	.020	.020	.019	.019	.018
2.1	.018	.017	.017	.017	.016	.016	.015	.015	.015	.014
2.2	.014	.014	.013	.013	.013	.012	.012	.012	.011	.011
2.3	.011	.010	.010	.010	.010	.009	.009	.009	.009	.008
2.4	.008	.008	.008	.008	.007	.007	.007	.007	.007	.006
2.5	.006	.006	.006	.006	.006	.005	.005	.005	.005	.005
2.6	.005	.005	.004	.004	.004	.004	.004	.004	.004	.004
2.7	.003	.003	.003	.003	.003	.003	.003	.003	.003	.003
2.8	.003	.002	.002	.002	.002	.002	.002	.002	.002	.002
2.9	.002	.002	.002	.002	.002	.002	.002	.001	.001	.001
3.0	.001									

Reprinted with permission from Colton T: *Statistics in Medicine,* Boston, Mass, 1974, Little, Brown.

Questions for Narrative Evaluation of a Research Article

STEP ONE

Classification of Research and Variables

- Was data collection prospective or retrospective? (Chapters 6, 7, and 12)
- Was the purpose of the research description, relationship analysis, difference analysis, or some combination? (Chapters 6, 7, and 12)
- Was the study experimental or nonexperimental? (Chapters 6 and 12)
- Was the study conducted according to the assumptions and methods of the quantitative, qualitative, or single-system paradigms? (Chapter 6)
- What were the independent variables? (Chapter 7)
- What were the dependent variables? (Chapter 7)

STEP TWO

Analysis of Purposes and Conclusions

- Is there a conclusion for every purpose?
- Is there a purpose for every conclusion?
- Are there significant results that should be evaluated for possible alternative explanations and clinical importance? (Chapter 20)
- Are there nonsignificant results that should be evaluated for power and clinical importance? (Chapter 20)

STEP THREE

Analysis of Design and Control Elements

- What was the design of the study? (Chapters 10 through 15)
- Was the independent variable implemented in a laboratory-like or clinic-like setting? (Chapters 6 and 7)
- Was selection of subjects done randomly, by cluster, by convenience, or purposively? (Chapter 9)

- Were subjects assigned to groups through individual random assignment, block assignment, systematic assignment, matched assignment, or consecutive assignment? (Chapter 9)
- Were extraneous experimental-setting variables under tight laboratory-like control or loose, clinic-like control? (Chapter 7)
- Were extraneous subject variables under laboratory-like or clinic-like control? (Chapter 7)
- What was the level of control over measurement techniques? (Chapters 6, 18, and 19)
- Was information controlled through incomplete information, participant masking, or researcher masking? (Chapters 6 and 8)

STEP FOUR

Validity Questions

- Construct validity (Chapter 8)
  - Were the variables in the study defined and implemented in meaningful ways?
- Construct underrepresentation
  - Were variables well developed and defined?
  - Were there enough levels of the independent variable? Was treatment administered as an all-or-none phenomenon or in varying levels?
  - Do the dependent variables provide information in all areas important to the phenomenon under study?
  - Was the independent variable administered at a lower intensity or in a different manner than would be typical in a clinical setting?
- Experimenter expectancies
  - Were the experimenter's expectations transparently obvious to participants?
  - Were there differences between the construct as labeled and the construct as implemented, based on the influence of the experimenter?

- Interaction of different treatments
  - What uncontrolled treatments might have interacted with the independent variable?
- Interaction of testing and treatment
  - Could any of the measurements used in the study have contributed to a treatment effect?
- Internal validity (Chapter 8)
  - Was the independent variable the probable cause of differences in the dependent variables?
- History and interaction of history and assignment
  - What events other than implementation of the independent variable occurred during the study that might have plausibly caused changes in the dependent variable?
  - If any historical events took place, did the events have an equal impact on treatment and control groups?
- Maturation and interaction of maturation and assignment
  - Could changes in the dependent variable have been the result of the passage of time, rather than the implementation of the independent variable?
  - If a control group was present, were the same maturational influences at work for them as for the treatment group?
- Testing
  - Is familiarity with testing procedures a likely explanation for differences in the dependent variable?
  - Were tests conducted with equal frequency for treatment and control groups so that any testing effects were consistent for all groups within the study?
- Instrumentation and interaction of instrumentation and assignment
  - Were instruments calibrated appropriately?
  - Were measurements taken under controlled environmental conditions such as temperature or humidity?
  - If the instrument was a human observer, what measures were taken to ensure consistency of observations?
  - Were instruments expected to be equally sensitive across the values expected for both the treatment and control groups?
- Statistical regression to the mean
  - Were participants selected for the study based on an extreme score on a single administration of a test?
  - Can improvements or declines in performance be attributed to statistical regression rather than true change?

- Assignment
  - Were participants assigned to groups randomly?
  - If not assigned randomly, what factors other than the one of interest might have influenced their assignment?
- Mortality
  - What proportions of participants were lost from the treatment and control groups?
  - Were the proportions of participants lost equal for the treatment and control groups?
  - What are possible explanations for differential loss of participants from the groups?
- Diffusion or imitation of treatments
  - Were treatment and control group members able to share information about their respective routines?
  - Was either the treatment or control regimen likely to have been perceived as more desirable by participants in the other group?
- Compensatory equalization of treatments
  - Were researchers aware of which participants were in which group?
  - Were those implementing the treatments likely to have paid extra attention to control group members because of the presumed inferiority of care they received?
- Compensatory rivalry or resentful demoralization
  - Did participants know whether they were in the treatment or control group?
  - Were control group members likely to have either tried harder or withdrawn their efforts because they knew they were in the control group and perceived it to be a less desirable alternative than being in the treatment group?
- Statistical conclusion validity (Chapters 8 and 20)
  - Were statistical tools used appropriately?
- Low power
  - Are statistically insignificant results related to small sample size, high within-group variability, or small between-groups differences?
  - Do statistically insignificant differences seem clinically important?
- Lack of clinical importance
  - Are statistically significant results clinically important?
- Error rate problems
  - If multiple statistical tests were performed, did the researcher set a conservative alpha level to compensate for alpha-level inflation?
  - Are identified significant differences isolated and difficult to explain, or is there a pattern of significant differences that suggests true differences rather than type I errors?

- Violated assumptions
  - Were tests used appropriately for independent and dependent samples?
  - Were assumptions about normal distribution of data and homogeneity of variance satisfied?
- Failure to use intention-to-treat analysis
  - Was everyone who was entered into the study included in the final data analysis according to the treatment they were intended to have, whether or not they completed the study?
  - If not, did the authors present a sound rationale for using a completer analysis instead of an intention-to-treat analysis?
- External validity (Chapters 7 and 8)
  - To whom and under what conditions can the research results be generalized?
- Selection
  - Were volunteers used for study? In what ways do these volunteers differ from clinical populations?
  - Are results from normal participants generalized to patient populations?
  - Do the authors limit their conclusions to participants similar to those studied?
- Setting
  - To what extent did the experimental setting differ from the setting to which the researchers wish to generalize the results?
  - Were control elements implemented fastidiously, as in a laboratory, or pragmatically, as in a clinic?
- Time
  - How much time elapsed between the collection of the data in the study and the present time?

- Do differences in overall clinical management of patients make the studied procedures less appropriate today than when the study was implemented?

STEP FIVE

Place Study into Literature Context

- Do results confirm or contradict the findings of others?
- Does this study correct some of the deficiencies identified in other studies?
- Does the study examine constructs or variables unstudied by others?
- How do the sample size and composition compare with those of other studies?
- How does the validity of this study compare with that of related studies?

STEP SIX

Personal Utility Questions

- Are your setting and the research setting similar enough to warrant application of the results of the research to your clinical practice?
- Does the study cause you to question some of the assumptions under which you have managed patients?
- Do the methods of this study suggest ways in which you can improve on the design of a study that you are planning?

APPENDIX D

Basic Guidelines for Preparing a Journal Article Manuscript

This appendix contains basic guidelines for preparing a journal article manuscript in either American Medical Association (AMA)[1] or American Psychological Association (APA)[2] style. Additional suggestions about general scientific writing have been included as well, based on the work of Day and Gastel[3] and Browner.[4] These guidelines can help jump-start the writing process or answer some questions when other resources are not available. They are not, however, a substitute for regular consultation of more detailed and authoritative references: the style manual specified by a journal, the instructions for authors for specific journals, and general books and articles about scientific writing.

1. General Guidelines
   1.1. Double-space everything, including block quotes, tables, and references.
   1.2. Margins should be a minimum of 1 inch; some journals request more generous margins.
   1.3. Do not right-justify the text or hyphenate words at the ends of lines. These adjustments may make an attractive document but hinder the editing process.
   1.4. Generally plan for about 15 pages of text, plus title page, abstract page, tables, references, and figures. Consult journal instructions to authors for more specific length guidelines. Note that articles describing qualitative research may be longer than typical and follow a somewhat different outline; refer to examples in the literature for guidance.
   1.5. Manuscript pagination is as follows: Title page is page 1 but may or may not include the page number; abstract page is page 2; text begins on page 3. Tables follow the references. Each table begins on a new page, and table pages are numbered consecutively with the manuscript. The final numbered manuscript page is the one on which the figure legends are written; it starts on a separate page following the tables. APA style does not specify the location of the page numbers, but because each page must also have the running head, it makes sense to have both at the top in a header, beginning with the title page. AMA style does not specify; refer to specific journal guidelines.
   1.6. Determine formats for headings and subheadings and use them consistently. APA style requires the following for papers with three heading levels:

Method
Participants
Facility A

AMA style does not specify but indicates that the format for headings needs to be consistent throughout the paper and follow any guidelines set by the specific journal.

2. Title and Title Page
   2.1. Title should be concise, yet specific. Include important variables under study (see also Chapter 27). "Knee Function After Total Knee Arthroplasty" is too concise if the study is really one of "Effect of Two Continuous Passive Motion Regimens on Knee Function Six Months After Total Knee Arthroplasty."
   2.2. Titles are generally descriptive (such as "Effect of Continuous Passive Motion on Knee Range of Motion After Total Knee Arthroplasty") but may be assertive (such as "Continuous Passive Motion Does Not Improve Knee Range of Motion After Total Knee Arthroplasty"). Some believe that assertive titles place too much emphasis on the conclusion without considering the context that the full article provides.
   2.3. Consider using terms that are indexed in the databases interested readers are likely to search; for example, use "total knee arthroplasty" rather than "total knee replacement" because "arthroplasty" is indexed and "replacement" is not.

2.4. Title in APA style is in uppercase and lowercase letters, centered on the page. AMA style does not specify and refers authors to specific journal guidelines.

2.5. APA style specifies a two-part byline including the author's name without titles and degrees and the institutional affiliation of the author, centered on separate lines beneath the title. More detailed information about authors goes in an author note at the end of the paper or on the title page if the manuscript is undergoing a masked review. AMA style includes highest degrees and refers authors to specific journal guidelines for additional details.

3. Abstract

3.1. In AMA style, limit the abstract to 250 words. APA refers authors to the abstract guidelines of each journal.

3.2. Summarize the study's purpose, procedures, results, and major conclusions. For reports of original research, AMA style requires use of a structured abstract with headings: "Context," "Objective," "Design," "Setting," "Participants," "Intervention," "Outcome Measures," "Results," "Conclusions."

3.3. Use major indexing terms within the abstract because users of electronic bibliographic databases often search abstracts as well as titles.

3.4. Do not cite references or provide p values because these are meaningful only in the context of the study.

4. Introduction

4.1. No heading is used for the introduction. Repeat the title and then begin the first paragraph (APA) or just begin the first paragraph (AMA).

4.2. In a paper of 15 pages, the introduction section is typically 2 to 3 pages.

4.3. Cite only the most relevant citations about the topic area. A journal article does not contain an exhaustive review of the literature; rather, it places the problem into the context of the literature.

4.4. In-text citation of references is very different in AMA and APA styles (see Box 28-1 for a comparison of the two citation styles).

4.4.1. AMA style uses numerical citations with superscripts, numbered in the order in which they are cited. If superscripts are unavailable, then the number should be enclosed in parentheses.

4.4.1.1. If the text refers to an author's name, the numeral follows the name directly. If the author's name is not mentioned and the entire sentence is related to the citation, the numeral goes at the end of the sentence. If the citation refers to only part of the sentence, the numeral is placed at the conclusion of that part of the sentence.

4.4.1.2. If there are two authors, always include both surnames when citing names in the text. For citations with three or more authors, use the first author's surname with "et al," "and colleagues," "and coworkers," or "and associates." When using a numbered reference style like the AMA, writers often cite references with the author name and publication date in parentheses in early drafts of the paper. This prevents repeated renumbering of references as the paper is edited. For the final draft, the names and parentheses are removed and the correct numbers inserted. Alternately, many authors use bibliographic management software to manage references and prevent the need for repeated renumbering of citations as a paper evolves. Note that in AMA style, "et al" is used without punctuation, consistent with other AMA conventions that minimize punctuation for abbreviations and initials.

4.4.2. APA style uses author-date citation style in which author surnames and publication dates are entered at the appropriate point in the manuscript. If the text refers to the author's name, then only the publication date needs to be included in parentheses following the use of the author's name. If the author's name is not mentioned in the text, then the author surname and date are included in parentheses at the appropriate point in the text. When there are two authors, include both surnames in the parenthetical citation (Brown & Preston, 2003). When there are three to five authors, include all names at first reference (Brown, Preston, & Glass, 2003) and shorten with et al. in subsequent citations (Brown et al., 2003). With six or more authors, use "et al." at first reference. Note that in APA style, "et al." is used with punctuation, consistent with other APA conventions for abbreviations and punctuation.

4.5. Suggested first paragraph: Broadly state the problem, with documentation as needed.

4.6. Suggested second through fourth paragraphs, as needed: Summarize what is known about the problem, that is, what others have found out about the problem in their own research.

4.7. Suggested last paragraph: Identify the gap in the literature that needs to be filled, and then state the purpose of your research. State research hypotheses if appropriate. Identify major variables, using the names that you will use throughout the rest of the paper. If you have several purposes, place them in order of importance or in the order that they will be discussed in the rest of the paper.

5. Methods

5.1. The methods section is usually subdivided into "Participants," "Instruments," "Procedures," and "Data Analysis" or similar subheadings.

5.2. In a paper of 15 pages, the methods section is typically 3 to 5 pages long.

5.3. Cite literature needed to justify the methods you used, or cite others' procedures if they are too lengthy to be repeated in your article.

5.4. The participants subsection should describe inclusion and exclusion criteria, sampling and assignment methods, and source of the participants. This section must also include the methods of assuring participants' protection and a statement (when appropriate) about Institutional Review Board (IRB) clearance.

5.5. The instruments subsection should describe each instrument used in data collection.

5.5.1. Present instruments in the order that you will eventually present the rest of your methods and results. For example, if you have taken range of motion, strength, and functional measures and plan to discuss them in that order, describe the goniometers first, the dynamometers second, and the functional scale last.

5.5.2. If you developed the instrument, provide details about the instrument development process.

5.5.3. If you performed reliability or validity testing with the instruments but this was not the primary purpose of the research, present reliability or validity information here. If the research is methodological, then reliability or validity information belongs in the results section.

5.5.4. Figures of instrument arrays should be detailed enough to allow other researchers to replicate the instrumentation.

5.6. The procedures subsection should describe what you did in enough detail that others can replicate the study. Refer to other authors if necessary to justify your procedures.

5.7. Consider combining the instrument subsection with the procedures subsection if the equipment used is nontechnical and familiar to most professionals to whom the article would be of interest.

5.8. The data analysis subsection should include data reduction procedures and statistical testing for each variable.

5.8.1. If possible, present information about the data analysis in the order of variables presented earlier in the paper.

5.8.2. State the statistical package used and alpha level if appropriate.

5.8.3. If necessary, justify or clarify your use of statistical procedures with references.

6. Results

6.1. Sometimes the results section is subdivided by variables or classes of variables.

6.2. Text is often short, with much of the information presented in tables and figures. Tables and figures should substitute for information in the text, not repeat it. Tables and figures are numbered separately in order of their appearance in the text (see Sections 11 and 12 below).

6.3. Present variables in previously established order.

6.4. Do not discuss the implications of the results here; just present the appropriate descriptive and statistical information.

6.5. In a paper of 15 pages, the results section is typically only 1 to 2 pages long, supplemented by figures and tables.

7. Discussion

7.1. The discussion is the heart of the paper, the place for interpretation of the results.

7.2. In a paper of 15 pages, the discussion is typically 3 to 4 pages long.

7.3. Additional references are often cited to place the results into a broader context.

7.4. Suggested first section: Interpret the major results in terms of your original hypotheses.

7.5. Suggested second section: Examine the results that were as predicted by your hypothesis, reinforcing the theory that led you to the hypothesis.

7.6. Suggested third section: Examine the results that were not as predicted, speculating about the meaning of the inconsistent results.

7.7. Suggested fourth section: Discuss the limitations of the study.

7.8. Suggested fifth section: Discuss the clinical implications of the findings.

7.9. Suggested sixth section: Discuss directions for future research.

8. Conclusions

8.1. Not all articles have a conclusions section. APA style manuscripts do not typically have a separate conclusions section. If the conclusions are not a separate section, they are integrated into the discussion.

8.2. In a paper of 15 pages, the conclusions are typically less than a page long. The conclusions are stated concisely, in the order in which the questions were posed in the purpose section of the study.

8.3. Avoid making sweeping conclusions that are not grounded in your results.

9. Author Note and Acknowledgments

9.1. In AMA style, author information is on the title page and acknowledgments are placed on a separate page between the end of the text and the references. In APA style, author notes, including acknowledgments, are placed between the references and the tables, unless the paper will be undergoing masked review, in which case they are placed on the title page.

9.2. Each person acknowledged should have given permission to be acknowledged.

9.3. Be specific about the contribution of each person, for example: "critical review," "manuscript preparation," or "data collection."

10. References

10.1. Begin references on a separate page.

10.2. Double-space references.

10.3. List only references cited in the study.

10.4. AMA style numbers references in the reference list in the order they are cited in text. APA style puts references in order alphabetically by the surname of the first author and does not number the references.

10.5. Place references into proper format. Pay attention to punctuation, capitalization, and italicization in the various elements of the reference (see Table 28-1 for a comparison of the two styles).

10.6. Consult the appropriate style manual for detailed directions on specific formats for other types of references (e.g., book, chapter in a book, dissertation).

11. Tables

11.1. Tables consist of rows and columns of numbers or text.

11.2. Vertical lines are not used in tables; use horizontal lines only.

11.3. Tables should not repeat information in the text. If a table can be summarized in a sentence or two, then it should probably not be a table.

11.4. Number tables (e.g., Table 1, Table 2, Table 3) according to their order in the paper. Refer to each table in the text, highlighting the most important information. If there is only one table, it is not numbered.

11.5. Table titles should describe the specific information contained within the table—for example, "Data" is too general a title; "Mean Knee Function Variables by Clinic" is more specific.

11.6. Each table begins on a separate page placed after the references. Tables may be continued onto additional pages.

12. Figures

12.1. Figures are illustrative materials such as graphs, diagrams, or photographs.

12.2. Figures should not repeat information in text or tables. They should be used only when visual information is more effective than tabular or text information.

12.3. Figures are numbered (e.g., Figure 1, Figure 2, Figure 3) in order of their appearance in the paper. If there is only one figure, it is not numbered.

12.4. Figure legends are listed on a separate sheet following the tables. The legend should make the figure meaningful on its own by explaining any abbreviations and describing concisely the important points being illustrated. The figure legend page is the last numbered page of the manuscript.

12.5. The figure itself is not labeled or numbered on its face. Figures are identified outside the figure area or on the back of the figure; be careful not to damage the figure by labeling it.

12.6. Identification of figures in theses or dissertations will deviate from this format. Because they are used in the format prepared by the author, rather than being typeset in a journal, figure numbers and legends must accompany the figures themselves, and figure pages are numbered.

REFERENCES

1. *American Medical Association Manual of Style*, 10th ed, Oxford, UK, 2009, Oxford University Press.
2. *Publication Manual of the American Psychological Association*, 6th ed, Washington, DC, 2010, American Psychological Association.
3. Day RA, Gastel B: *How to Write and Publish a Scientific Paper*, 6th ed, Westport, Conn, 2006, Greenwood Press.
4. Browner WS: *Publishing and Presenting Clinical Research*, 3rd ed, Philadelphia, 2012, Lippincott Williams & Wilkins.

American Medical Association Style: Sample Manuscript for a Hypothetical Study

The following short, hypothetical manuscript on continuous passive motion following total knee arthroplasty is based, with a few changes in the demographic variables, on the hypothetical data set presented in Chapter 20 in Tables 20-1 and 20-2. The circled numbers in the manuscript correspond to guidelines listed in Appendix D.

Effect of Initial Arc of Continuous Passive Motion on Motion
and Function Following Total Knee Arthroplasty   ←(2.1)

Jan R. Woolery, PhD;

Jodi C. Beeker, MD;   ←(2.5)

Jonathon V. Mills, MS

JR Woolery is Research Therapist, Department of Physical Therapy,
Memorial Hospital of Indiana, 555 Main Street, Anytown, IN 46234
(USA). Address all correspondence to Dr. Woolery. E-mail:
jrwoolery@memorialindiana.org   ←(9.1)

JC Beeker is Orthopedic Surgeon, Department of Orthopedic
Surgery, Community Hospital of Anytown, Anytown, IN.

JV Mills is Staff Therapist, Occupational Therapy Department,
Religious Hospital of Anytown, Anytown, IN.

Presented at the 2004 Annual Conference of the Association of
Hip and Knee Surgeons, New Orleans, La, February 20-24, 2004.

This study was approved by the institutional review boards of
Memorial Hospital of Indiana, Community Hospital of Anytown,
and Religious Hospital of Anytown.

2

ABSTRACT

(3.2) **Context:** Optimal progression of range of motion (ROM) in continuous passive motion (CPM) devices following total knee arthroplasty (TKA) is not well established, despite their use for over 20 years. **Objective:** To compare the effects of two CPM regimens with different initial arcs of motion to no CPM on knee motion and function up to 6 months after TKA. One CPM regimen began with motion set at 70° to 100° of knee flexion and progressed toward full extension; the other began with motion set at 0° to 40° of knee flexion and progressed toward full flexion. **Design:** Controlled trial with 6-month follow-up. **Setting:** Three community hospitals in the Midwestern region of the United States. **Participants:** Ten consecutive patients over the age of 50 years following unilateral TKA at each of three different hospitals. **Interventions:** Patients were assigned by hospital to receive 6 days of CPM starting at 70° to 100° of flexion, CPM starting at 0° to 40° of flexion, or no CPM. **Outcome Measures:** Knee flexion ROM 3 and 6 weeks postoperatively and knee flexion ROM, gait velocity, and activities of daily living (ADL) score 6 months postoperatively. **Results:** Significant differences among groups were identified for all dependent variables, with higher scores for CPM groups. There were no significant differences between the CPM groups. **Conclusions:** CPM groups had better outcomes than the no-CPM group, regardless of the initial arc of motion.

(4.1)→   Total knee arthroplasty is a common surgical procedure used to reduce pain and enhance function for individuals with knee impairment secondary to osteoarthritis. Continuous passive motion (CPM) is used to encourage early motion of the knee joint after total knee arthroplasty (TKA). Milne and colleagues[1] ←(4.4.1) conducted a meta-analysis of 14 randomized controlled trials of CPM following TKA, showing that CPM combined with PT resulted in more active knee flexion at discharge, a shorter length of stay, and less need for postoperative manipulation than PT alone. They recommended further research to determine whether there are differences in CPM effectiveness with different CPM protocols or with different patient or diagnostic groups.   ←(4.5)

Studies comparing different CPM regimens have identified few short-term differences among groups and no long-term differences. Groups receiving different daily durations of CPM were compared by Basso and Knapp[2] and Chiarello and colleagues[3]; in both cases no ROM differences between groups were identified at discharge. (4.6)→ Pope and colleagues[4] found no ROM differences between groups receiving CPM with different initial arcs of motion (0° to 40° versus 0° to 70° of knee flexion). Finally, Yashar and associates[5] and MacDonald and colleagues[6] compared groups receiving CPM with an initial flexion arc of motion from 0° to up to 50° to those receiving CPM with an accelerated initial flexion arc of motion from 70° to up to 110°. Yashar and colleagues[5] identified a short-term advantage for the accelerated group on knee flexion ROM, but no long-term differences. MacDonald and colleagues[6] found no short-term or long-term differences between CPM groups or a control group receiving usual care without CPM. Thus, on one potentially important CPM variable, initial arc of motion, the research is limited and the results are contradictory.

Therefore, we designed a study to further evaluate the impact of the initial arc of motion of CPM on short-term and long-terms outcomes after TKA. Specifically, the purpose of this study was to determine whether there were differences between two CPM protocols (initial arc of motion of 0° to 40° versus 70° to 100°) ←(4.7) and no CPM on knee flexion ROM at 3 and 6 weeks postoperatively and on knee flexion ROM, gait velocity, and ADL score at 6 months postoperatively. We hypothesized that there would be no differences between CPM groups at any time, that there would be differences between the no-CPM group and both CPM groups at 3 and 6 weeks postoperatively, and that there would be no differences among groups at 6 months postoperatively.

METHODS

Participants   ←(5.1)

Participants were patients who were at least 50 years old, had a diagnosis of osteoarthritis, and underwent TKA in 2003 at one of three hospitals in Anytown, Indiana: Community Hospital, Memorial Hospital, and Religious Hospital. Before beginning this study, the characteristics of patients undergoing TKA was compared across the three participating hospitals and found to be similar for age, sex, diagnosis, and type of prosthesis   ←(5.4) implanted. Because of the similarity of patients at the three hospitals, we assigned the CPM protocol randomly to hospitals rather than individually to patients. Patients at Community Hospital received an initial arc of 70° to 100° of CPM, patients at Religious Hospital received an initial arc of 0° to 40°, and patients at Memorial Hospital received no CPM. The first 10 patients in 2003 who met the inclusion criteria and consented to participate were entered into the trial at each hospital. Twelve eligible patients (three at Community, five at Religious, and four at Memorial) did not consent to participate in the study.

For the 30 patients who entered the trial, half were women and the mean (SD) age was 72.5 (4.7) years. The sex distribution and mean age across groups was similar: 50% women, 73.2 (5.6) years for the 70° to 100° CPM group; 40% women, 71.7 (6.5) years for the 0° to 40° CPM group; and 60% women, 72.5 (4.7) years for the no-CPM group. All 30 patients completed the trial.

Instruments ←(1.6)

CPM Units. ACME CPM (ACME Orthopedics, Roadrunner, Ariz) units were used to deliver the CPM treatment at all three facilities.

(5.5)→ **Goniometers.** ROM measurements were taken with the 12-inch, full-circle, plastic universal goniometers available at each facility.

(11.4)→ **ADL Scale.** We modified the Brigham and Women's Knee Rating Scale[7] to assess ADL (Table 1). The values for each of the four subscales (distance walked, assistive device, stair climbing, and rising from a chair) were added for each person to give a single ADL score that could range from a low of 4 to a high of 20.

Procedure

Patients underwent the assigned postoperative rehabilitation protocol. For the two CPM groups the units were applied in the recovery room and used for 20 hours on the first postoperative day. On subsequent days the ROM was advanced 10° (toward more   ←(5.6) flexion for the 0° to 40° group and toward extension for the

70° to 100° group) per day and the time in the unit was reduced by about 2 hours per day. Each day the time spent in CPM was recorded for each patient. Knee flexion ROM measurements were taken with patients supine according to the procedures described by Norkin and White,[8] with values recorded to the nearest degree. ←(5.3) The 3-week and 6-week measures were taken by the treating therapists at each hospital when patients came for their routine outpatient physical therapy visits. The 6-month measures were all taken in the physical therapy department at Community Hospital by an independent investigator (JVM) who was unaware of group assignment. Velocity was measured by having the participant walk at a comfortable pace across a 20-m measured distance. Each participant was timed with a stopwatch during the center 10 m of the walk and time was converted to cm/s for analysis. Within the modified Brigham and Women's Knee Rating Scale, use of an assistive device, rising from a chair, and stair climbing were actually observed and rated; distance walked was a self-reported measure.

Data Analysis

Analysis of variance (ANOVA) was used to test for differences between groups for each of the following dependent variables: 3-week ROM, 6-week ROM, and 6-month ROM; gait velocity; and ADL score. The Newman-Keuls procedure was used for

(5.8)→ post hoc analysis. Alpha was set at .05 for each analysis. SPSS for Windows 10.02 was used for the data analysis (SPSS Inc,

(5.8.2)→ Chicago, Ill).

RESULTS

Average time spent in CPM per day was similar for the two CPM

(6.2)→ groups (Figure). There were significant differences between groups for all variables (Table 2). For all variables, post hoc analysis showed that the CPM groups were not statistically different from one another, but that both were significantly different from the no-CPM group.

DISCUSSION

Of our three hypotheses, two were supported: (1) that there would be no differences between the CPM groups at any time and (2) that there would be 3- and 6-week differences between the   ←(7.4) no-CPM group and both the CPM groups. The significant differences between the no-CPM and CPM groups is consistent with the meta-analysis findings of Milne and colleagues,[1] strengthening the case for using CPM to improve short-term postoperative ROM after TKA. In addition, our findings suggest that the benefits extend beyond ROM to include gait and other functional outcomes.

The lack of differences between the CPM groups is consistent with the work of Yashar and colleagues[5] and MacDonald and associates[6] who also found no difference in ROM outcomes between groups receiving different initial arcs of motion. Further, the ←(7.5) addition of gait velocity and ADL measures in our study provides evidence that both impairment and disability level outcomes are similar regardless of the direction in which ROM is progressed with CPM.

Our final hypothesis, that differences between the no-CPM group and the CPM groups would not be present at 6 months, was not supported. We plan to continue the study to determine ←(7.6) if differences in all variables disappear by 1 year postoperatively, as has been found by others.[4-6]   ←(7.3)

The functional importance of our gait and ADL findings is apparent if one looks at the mean values for the different groups. The no-CPM group had an average gait velocity of only 107.6 cm/s, well below the averages of the two CPM groups (144.0 and 145.6 cm/s). The ADL scores of the CPM groups were approximately 18 and 17 of 20, respectively. This indicates minor impairment on two of the components or moderate impairment on one. In contrast, the average ADL score for the no-CPM group was 11, indicating moderate to severe impairment in one or more of the ADL components.

In interpreting these results, several limitations or alternative explanations must be considered. First, because the treatments were assigned by hospital and not by patient, systematic differences between the hospitals could explain the ← 7.7 difference in results. Second, because the treating therapists could not be masked to the group membership of the participants, their expectations may have influenced subject performance. Despite these limitations, the results have clinical implications for facilities using CPM for patients after TKA. Our results seem to indicate that patients who receive CPM—regardless of the initial arc of motion—do better on important outcome measures until at least 6 months after surgery compared with patients who do not receive CPM.

7.9 → Further research must be done to see if these results can be replicated, to see whether differences between CPM and no-CPM groups persist longer than 6 months, and to determine whether there are other important differences among CPM groups (e.g., blood loss or analgesic use) that would suggest an optimal direction for increasing motion after surgery.

CONCLUSIONS

Patients who underwent TKA and received CPM with different initial arcs of motion (starting at 70° to 100° of flexion or starting at 8.2→ 0° to 40° of flexion) had significantly better knee flexion ROM at 3 weeks and 6 weeks and significantly better knee flexion ROM, gait velocity, and ADL scores at 6 months postoperatively than did those who did not receive CPM.

ACKNOWLEDGMENTS ←(9.1)

We thank Ben Counter, PhD, for assistance with the statistical analysis of the study and Ellen Redline, PT, PhD, for her critical review of an earlier draft of the manuscript. ←(9.3)

REFERENCES ←(10.1)

(10.4)→ 1. Milne S, Brosseau L, Robinson V, Noel MJ, Davis J, Drouin H, et al. Continuous passive motion following total knee arthro-

(10.2)→ plasty (Cochrane Review). In: *The Cochrane Library*. Chichester, UK: John Wiley & Sons; 2003: Issue 4.

2. Basso DM, Knapp L. Comparison of two continuous passive motion protocols for patients with total knee implants. *Phys Ther*. 1987;67:360-363.

3. Chiarello CM, Gundersen L, O'Halloran T. The effect of continuous passive motion duration and increment on range of motion in total knee arthroplasty patients. *J Orthop Sports Phys Ther*. 1997;25:119-127.

4. Pope RO, Corcoran S, McCaul K, Howie DW. Continuous passive motion after primary total knee arthroplasty: does it offer any benefits? *J Bone Joint Surg Br*. 1997;79:914-917.

5. Yashar AA, Venn-Watson E, Welsh T, Colwell CW, Lotke P. Continuous passive motion with accelerated flexion after total knee arthroplasty. *Clin Orthop*. 1997;345:38-43.

6. MacDonald SJ, Bourne RB, Rorabeck CH, McCalden RW, Kramer J, Vaz M. Prospective randomized clinical trial of continuous passive motion after total knee arthroplasty. *Clin Orthop*. 2000;380:30-35.

7. Ewald FC, Jacobs MA, Miegel RE, Walker PS, Poss R, Sledge CB. Kinematic total knee replacement. *J Bone Joint Surg Am.* 1984;66:1032-1040.

8. Norkin CC, White DJ. *Measurement of Joint Motion: A Guide to Goniometry.* Philadelphia, Pa: FA Davis Co; 1995:142-143.

Table 1. Modified Brigham and Women's Knee Rating Scale[7]   ←(11.5)

Variable ←(11.1)	Scoring Criteria ←(11.2)
Distance walked	5 = Unlimited
	4 = 4 to 6 blocks
	3 = 2 to 3 blocks
	2 = Indoors only
	1 = Transfers only
Assistive device	5 = None
	4 = Cane outside
	3 = Cane full time
	2 = Two canes or crutches
	1 = Walker or unable
Stair climbing	5 = Reciprocal, no rail
	4 = Reciprocal, rail
	3 = One at a time, with or without rail
	2 = One at a time, with rail and assistive device
	1 = Unable

16

(11.6)→ Table 1 (continued). Modified Brigham and Women's Knee

Rating Scale[7]

Variable	Scoring Criteria
Rising from a chair	5 = No arm assistance
	4 = Single arm assistance
	3 = Difficult with two arm assistance
	2 = Needs assistance of another
	1 = Unable

17

Table 2. Outcomes for 70° to 100° CPM, 0° to 40° CPM,

and No-CPM Groups

Outcomes	Group Means (SD)			ANOVA	
	70°-100° CPM	0°-40° CPM	No CPM		
	(n=10)	(n=10)	(n=10)	F	P
3-week flex-ion ROM (°)	77.6 (19.8)	72.6 (18.9)	49.1 (14.6)	7.21	.003
6-week flex-ion ROM (°)	78.9 (17.1)	82.8 (12.3)	58.6 (12.3)	8.53	.003
6-month flex-ion ROM (°)	100.0 (7.1)	103.3 (4.1)	85.8 (10.0)	15.63	<.001
Gait velocity (cm/s)	144.0 (19.6)	145.6 (20.7)	107.6 (29.4)	8.25	.002
ADL score	18.3 (2.2)	17.0 (2.4)	11.0 (4.1)	16.24	<.001

CPM = continuous passive motion; ROM = range of motion;

ADL= activities of daily living.

(12.4)→ **FIGURE LEGEND**

Figure. Mean daily time in continuous passive motion (CPM) for patients in each CPM group.   ←(12.5)

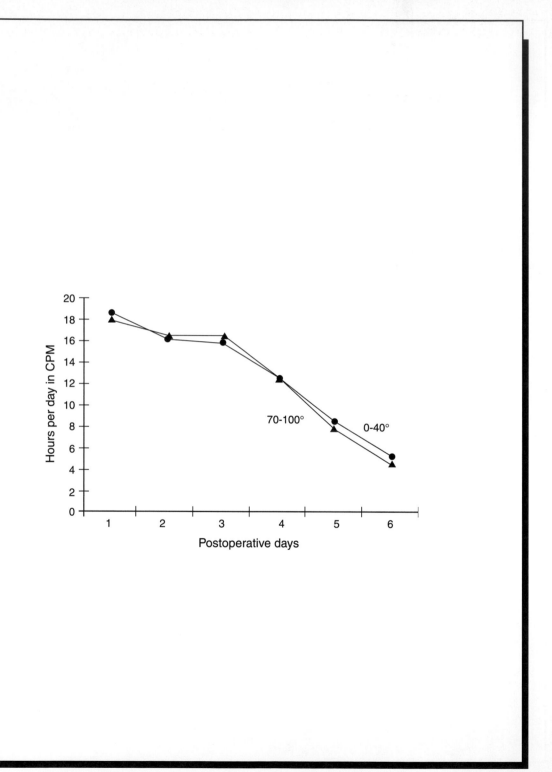

F

American Psychological Association Style: Sample Manuscript for a Hypothetical Study

The following short, hypothetical manuscript on continuous passive motion following total knee arthroplasty is based, with a few changes in the demographic variables, on the hypothetical data set presented in Chapter 20 in Tables 20-1 and 20-2. The circled numbers in the manuscript correspond to guidelines listed in Appendix D.

Running head: INITIAL ARC OF MOTION FOR CPM

Effect of Initial Arc of Continuous Passive Motion on Motion   ←(2.1)

and Function Following Total Knee Arthroplasty

Jan R. Woolery

Memorial Hospital of Indiana, Anytown, IN   ←(2.5)

Jodi C. Beeker

Community Hospital of Anytown (IN)

Jonathon V. Mills

Religious Hospital of Anytown (IN)

2   Initial Arc of Motion

Abstract

(3.1)→ Two continuous passive motion (CPM) regimens with different initial arcs of motion (70° to 100° and 0° to 40° of knee flexion) were compared to no CPM on knee motion and function up to 6 months after total knee arthroplasty (TKA). Ten consecutive patients over the age of 50 years following unilateral TKA were studied at each of three different community hospitals. Group assignments were made randomly by hospital. CPM groups scored higher on all measures, including knee range of motion, gait velocity, and function. There were no significant differences between the CPM groups. The findings are consistent with past research supporting the use of CPM following TKA, with little differentiation between groups receiving different CPM regimens.

Effect of Initial Arc of Continuous Passive Motion on
4.1→   Motion and Function Following Total
Knee Arthroplasty

Total knee arthroplasty is a common surgical procedure used
to reduce pain and enhance function for individuals with knee
impairment secondary to osteoarthritis. Continuous passive
motion (CPM) is used to encourage early motion of the knee
joint after total knee arthroplasty (TKA). Milne et al. (2003) ←4.4.2
conducted a meta-analysis of 14 randomized controlled trials of
CPM following TKA, showing that CPM combined with PT resulted
in more active knee flexion at discharge, a shorter length of
stay, and less need for postoperative manipulation than PT
alone. They recommended further research to determine whether
there are differences in CPM effectiveness with different CPM
protocols or with different patient or diagnostic groups.

Studies comparing different CPM regimens have identified few
short-term differences among groups and no long-term
4.6→ differences. Groups receiving different daily durations of CPM
were compared by Basso and Knapp (1987) and Chiarello,
Gundersen, and O'Halloran (2000); in both cases no ROM
differences between groups were identified at discharge. Pope,
Corcoran, McCaul, and Howie (1997) found no ROM differences
between groups receiving CPM with different initial arcs of

4   Initial Arc of Motion

motion (0° to 40° versus 0° to 70° of knee flexion). Finally, Yashar, Venn-Watson, Welsh, Colwell, and Lotke (1997) and MacDonald et al. (2000) compared groups receiving CPM with an initial flexion arc of motion from 0° to up to 50° to those receiving CPM with an accelerated initial flexion arc of motion from 70° to up to 110°. Yashar et al. (1997) identified a short-term advantage for the accelerated group on knee flexion ROM, but no long-term differences. MacDonald et al. (2000) found no short-term or long-term differences between CPM groups or a control group receiving usual care without CPM. Thus, on one potentially important CPM variable, initial arc of motion, the research is limited and the results are contradictory.

Therefore, we designed a study to further evaluate the
(4.7)→ impact of the initial arc of motion of CPM on short-term and long-terms outcomes after TKA. Specifically, the purpose of this study was to determine whether there were differences between two CPM protocols (initial arc of motion of 0° to 40° versus 70° to 100°) and no CPM on knee flexion ROM at 3 and 6 weeks postoperatively and on knee flexion ROM, gait velocity, and ADL score at 6 months postoperatively. We hypothesized that there would be no differences between CPM groups at any time, that there would be differences between the no-CPM group and both CPM groups at 3 and 6 weeks postoperatively, and that

there would be no differences among groups at 6 months postoperatively.

Methods

Participants   ←(5.1)

Participants were patients who were at least 50 years old, had a diagnosis of osteoarthritis, and underwent TKA in 2003 at one of three hospitals in Anytown, Indiana: Community Hospital, Memorial Hospital, and Religious Hospital. Before beginning this study, the characteristics of patients undergoing TKA was

(5.4)→ compared across the three participating hospitals and found to be similar for age, sex, diagnosis, and type of prosthesis implanted. Because of the similarity of patients at the three hospitals, we assigned the CPM protocol randomly to hospitals rather than individually to patients. Patients at Community Hospital received an initial arc of 70° to 100° of CPM, patients at Religious Hospital received an initial arc of 0° to 40°, and patients at Memorial Hospital received no CPM. The first 10 patients in 2003 who met the inclusion criteria and consented to participate were entered into the trial at each hospital. Twelve eligible patients (three at Community, five at Religious, and four at Memorial) did not consent to participate in the study.

6   Initial Arc of Motion

For the 30 patients who entered the trial, half were women and the mean (SD) age was 72.5 (4.7) years. The sex distribution and mean age across groups was similar: 50% women, 73.2 (5.6) years for the 70° to 100° CPM group; 40% women, 71.7 (6.5) years for the 0° to 40° CPM group; and 60% women, 72.5 (4.7) years for the no-CPM group. All 30 patients completed the trial.

Instruments

(1.6)→   **CPM units.** ACME CPM (ACME Orthopedics, Roadrunner, Ariz) units were used to deliver the CPM treatment at all three facilities.

Goniometers. ROM measurements were taken with the 12-inch, (5.5)→ full-circle, plastic universal goniometers available at each facility.

ADL scale. We modified the Brigham and Women's Knee Rating (11.4)→ Scale (Ewald, et al., 1984) to assess ADL (Table 1). The values for each of the four subscales (distance walked, assistive device, stair climbing, and rising from a chair) were added for each person to give a single ADL score that could range from a low of 4 to a high of 20.

Procedure

Patients underwent the assigned postoperative rehabilitation protocol. For the two CPM groups the units were applied in the

recovery room and used for 20 hours on the first postoperative   ←(5.6)
day. On subsequent days the ROM was advanced 10° (toward more
flexion for the 0° to 40° group and toward extension for the 70°
to 100° group) per day and the time in the unit was reduced by
about 2 hours per day. Each day the time spent in CPM was
recorded for each patient. Knee flexion ROM measurements were
taken with patients supine according to the procedures
described by Norkin and White (1995) with values recorded to   ←(5.3)
the nearest degree. The 3-week and 6-week measures were taken
by the treating therapists at each hospital when patients came
for their routine outpatient physical therapy visits. The
6-month measures were all taken in the physical therapy
department at Community Hospital by an independent investigator
(JVM) who was unaware of group assignment. Velocity was
measured by having the participant walk at a comfortable pace
across a 20-m measured distance. Each participant was timed
with a stopwatch during the center 10 m of the walk and time
was converted to cm/s for analysis. Within the modified
Brigham and Women's Knee Rating Scale (1984), use of an assistive device, rising from a chair, and stair climbing were actually observed and rated; distance walked was a self-reported
measure.

8   Initial Arc of Motion

Data Analysis

(5.8)→ Analysis of variance (ANOVA) was used to test for differences between groups for each of the following dependent variables: 3-week ROM, 6-week ROM, and 6-month ROM; gait velocity; and ADL score. The Newman-Keuls procedure was used for post hoc analysis. Alpha was set at .05 for each analysis. SPSS for Windows 10.02 was used for the data analysis (SPSS Inc, Chicago, Ill).   ←(5.8.2)

Results

Average time spent in CPM per day was similar for the two CPM groups (Figure 1). There were significant differences between groups for all variables (Table 2). For all variables,   ←(6.2) post hoc analysis showed that the CPM groups were not statistically different from one another, but that both were significantly different from the no-CPM group.

Discussion

Of our three hypotheses, two were supported: (1) that there would be no differences between the CPM groups at any time and (7.4)→ (2) that there would be 3- and 6-week differences between the no-CPM group and both the CPM groups. The significant differences between the no-CPM and CPM groups is consistent with the meta-analysis findings of Milne et al. (2003) strengthening the case for using CPM to improve short-term postoperative ROM after TKA. In addition, our findings suggest that the benefits extend beyond ROM to include gait and other functional outcomes.

The lack of differences between the CPM groups is consistent (7.5)→ with the work of others (Yashar et al., 1997; MacDonald et al., 2000) who also found no difference in ROM outcomes between groups receiving different initial arcs of motion. Further, the addition of gait velocity and ADL measures in our study provides evidence that both impairment and disability level outcomes are similar regardless of the direction in which ROM is progressed with CPM.

Our final hypothesis, that differences between the no-CPM (7.6)→ group and the CPM groups would not be present at 6 months, was not supported. We plan to continue the study to determine if differences in all variables disappear by 1 year postopera- tively, as has been found by others (Yashar et al., 1997; Pope (7.3)→ et al., 1997; MacDonald et al., 2000).

The functional importance of our gait and ADL findings is apparent if one looks at the mean values for the different groups. The no-CPM group had an average gait velocity of only 107.6 cm/s, well below the averages of the two CPM groups (144.0 and 145.6 cm/s). The ADL scores of the CPM groups were approximately 18 and 17 of 20, respectively. This indicates

10   Initial Arc of Motion

minor impairment on two of the components or moderate impair-

ment on one. In contrast, the average ADL score for the no-CPM

group was 11, indicating moderate to severe impairment in one

or more of the ADL components.

In interpreting these results, several limitations or

alternative explanations must be considered. First, because the

treatments were assigned by hospital and not by patient,   ←(7.7)

systematic differences between the hospitals could explain the

difference in results. Second, because the treating therapists

could not be masked to the group membership of the partici-

pants, their expectations may have influenced subject perform-

ance. Despite these limitations, the results have clinical

implications for facilities using CPM for patients after TKA.

Our results seem to indicate that patients who receive CPM—

regardless of the initial arc of motion—do better on important

outcome measures until at least 6 months after surgery compared

with patients who do not receive CPM.

Further research must be done to see if these results can be

replicated, to see whether differences between CPM and no-CPM

(7.9)→ groups persist longer than 6 months, and to determine whether

there are other important differences among CPM groups (e.g.,

blood loss or analgesic use) that would suggest an optimal

direction for increasing motion after surgery.

(8.1)→   In summary, patients who underwent unilateral TKA and

received CPM with different initial arcs of motion (starting at

70° to 100° of flexion or starting at 0° to 40° of flexion) had significantly better knee flexion ROM at 3 weeks and 6 weeks and significantly better knee flexion ROM, gait velocity, and ADL scores at 6 months postoperatively than did those who did not receive CPM.

12   Initial Arc of Motion

References   ←(10.1)

Basso, D. M., Knapp, L. (1987). Comparison of two continuous
(10.4)→ passive motion protocols for patients with total knee
    implants. *Physical Therapy, 67,* 360-363.   ←(10.2)

Chiarello, C. M., Gundersen, L., & O'Halloran, T. (1997). The
    effect of continuous passive motion duration and increment on
    range of motion in total knee arthroplasty patients. *Journal
    of Orthopaedic and Sports Physical Therapy, 25,* 119-127.

Ewald, F. C., Jacobs, M. A., Miegel, R. E., Walker, P. S.,
    Poss, R., & Sledge, C. B. (1984). Kinematic total knee
    replacement. *Journal of Bone and Joint Surgery American,
    66,* 1032-1040.

MacDonald, S. J., Bourne, R. B., Rorabeck, C. H., McCalden,
    R.W., Kramer, J., & Vaz, M. (2000). Prospective randomized
    clinical trial of continuous passive motion after total knee
    arthroplasty. *Clinical Orthopedics and Related Research,
    380,* 30-35.

Milne, S., Brosseau, L., Robinson, V., Noel, M. J., Davis, J.,
    Drouin, H., et al. (2003). Continuous passive motion following
    total knee arthroplasty (Cochrane Review). In: *The Cochrane
    Library* (Issue 4). Chichester, UK: John Wiley & Sons.

Norkin, C. C., & White, D.J. (1995). *Measurement of joint
    motion: A guide to goniometry* (pp. 142-143). Philadelphia,
    PA: FA Davis.

Pope, R. O., Corcoran, S., McCaul, K., & Howie, D.W. (1997)
    Continuous passive motion after primary total knee arthro-
    plasty: does it offer any benefits? *Journal of Bone and
    Joint Surgery British, 79,* 914-917.

Yashar, A.A., Venn-Watson, E., Welsh, T., Colwell, C. W., &
    Lotke, P. (1997) Continuous passive motion with accelerated
    flexion after total knee arthroplasty. *Clinical Orthopedics
    and Related Research, 345,* 38-43.

14   Initial Arc of Motion

(9.1)→ **Author Note**

Jan Woolery, Department of Physical Therapy, Memorial Hospital

of Indiana; Jodi Beeker, Department of Orthopedic Surgery,

Community Hospital of Anytown, Anytown, IN; Jonathon Mills,

Occupational Therapy Department, Religious Hospital of Anytown,

Anytown, IN.

We thank Ben Counter, PhD, for assistance with the statistical

analysis of the study, and Ellen Redline, PT, PhD, for her

(9.3)→ critical review of an earlier draft of the manuscript.

Correspondence concerning this article should be addressed to

Jan Woolery, Department of Physical Therapy, Memorial Hospital

of Indiana, 555 Main Street, Anytown, Indiana 46234 (USA).

E-mail: *jrwoolery@memorialindiana.org*

(11.6)→ Table 1
Modified Brigham and Women's Knee Rating Scale[a]   ←(11.5)

_____

(11.1)→ Variable   Scoring Criteria   ←(11.2)

_____

Distance walked   5 = Unlimited

                         4 = 4 to 6 blocks

                         3 = 2 to 3 blocks

                         2 = Indoors only

                         1 = Transfers only

Assistive device   5 = None

                         4 = Cane outside

                         3 = Cane full time

                         2 = Two canes or crutches

                         1 = Walker or unable

Stair climbing   5 = Reciprocal, no rail

                         4 = Reciprocal, rail

                         3 = One at a time, with or without

                             rail

                         2 = One at a time, with rail and

                             assistive device

                         1 = Unable

_____

16   Initial Arc of Motion

Table 1(continued)

Modified Brigham and Women's Knee Rating Scale[a]

Variable	Scoring Criteria
Rising from a chair	5 = No arm assistance
	4 = Single arm assistance
	3 = Difficult with two arm assistance
	2 = Needs assistance of another
	1 = Unable

[a]See Ewald, et al. (1984).

Table 2

Outcomes for 70° to 100° CPM, 0° to 40° CPM, and No-CPM Groups

Outcomes	Group Means (SD)			ANOVA	
	70°-100° CPM (n=10)	0°-40° CPM (n=10)	No CPM (n=10)	*F*	*P*
3-week flexion ROM (°)	77.6 (19.8)	72.6 (18.9)	49.1 (14.6)	7.21	.003
6-week flexion ROM (°)	78.9 (17.1)	82.8 (12.3)	58.6 (12.3)	8.53	.003
6-month flexion ROM (°)	100.0 (7.1)	103.3 (4.1)	85.8 (10.0)	15.63	<.001
Gait velocity (cm/s)	144.0 (19.6)	145.6 (20.7)	107.6 (29.4)	8.25	.002
ADL score	18.3 (2.2)	17.0 (2.4)	11.0 (4.1)	16.24	<.001

CPM = continuous passive motion; ROM = range of motion;

ADL = activities of daily living.

18   Initial Arc of Motion

(12.4)→   Figure Caption

Figure 1. Mean daily time in continuous passive motion (CPM) for

patients in each CPM group.

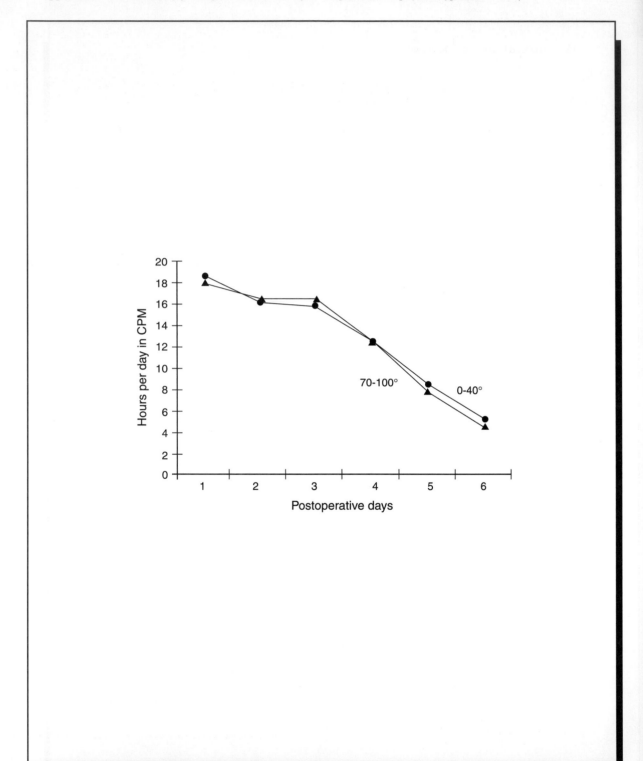

G

Sample Platform Presentation Script with Slides

1. Good afternoon. I'm pleased to be here in New Orleans to present the results of our study of the effect of the initial arc of continuous passive motion on knee motion and function following total knee arthroplasty. No author has any financial interest bearing on this study.

Effect of Initial Arc of CPM on Motion and Function Following TKA

Jan R. Woolery, PT, PhD
Jodi C. Becker, MD
Jonathon V. Mills, MS, OTR

Memorial Hospital of Indiana, Anytown, IN
Community Hospital of Anytown, IN
Religious Hospital of Anytown, IN

---

2. As we all know, total knee arthroplasty, or TKA, is a common surgical procedure used to reduce pain and enhance function for individuals with knee impairment secondary to osteoarthritis. Continuous passive motion, or CPM, is used to encourage early motion of the knee joint after total knee arthroplasty. Recently, Milne and colleagues published a Cochrane Review of 14 randomized controlled trials of CPM following TKA. They found small but significant benefits of CPM combined with PT—it resulted in more active knee flexion at discharge, a shorter length of stay, and less need for postoperative manipulation than PT alone. However, they recommended further research to determine whether there are differences in CPM effectiveness with different CPM protocols or with different patient or diagnostic groups.

Problem: CPM Following TKA

- TKA reduces pain, enhances function
- CPM used postop to encourage motion
- Meta-analysis (Milne et al, 2003) shows more motion, shorter LOS, less need for postop manipulation under anesthesia with CPM
- Further research to determine whether variations in CPM regimens lead to different outcomes

---

3. There are only a few studies out there that examine differences between CPM regimens. Groups receiving different daily durations of CPM were compared by Basso and Knapp and Chiarello and colleagues; in both cases, few ROM differences between groups were identified at discharge, and there was no follow-up to see what happened after discharge.

Studies Comparing CPM Regimens

- Different daily durations
  - Basso and Knapp, 1987 (20 vs 5 hours per day)
  - Chiarello et al, 1997 (10 vs 5 hours per day)
- Few ROM differences
- No follow-up after discharge

---

4. Two studies compared CPM using different arcs of motion. Yashar and associates and MacDonald and colleagues both compared groups receiving CPM with an initial flexion arc of motion from 0° to up to 50° to those receiving CPM with an accelerated initial flexion arc of motion from 70° to up to 110°. Yashar identified a short-term advantage for the accelerated group on knee flexion ROM, but MacDonald did not. Neither study found differences at 1 year postop. Thus, on this potentially important CPM variable, initial arc of motion, the research is limited and the results are contradictory.

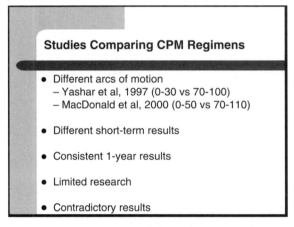

5. Another aspect of the CPM literature is that authors have often reported on impairment and cost outcomes such as range of motion and length of hospital stay. Disability level outcomes such as gait velocity or activities of daily living have rarely been reported.

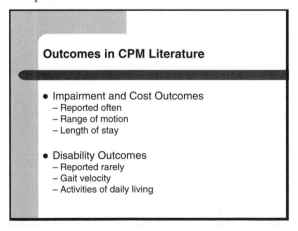

6. Therefore, we designed a study to evaluate the impact of the initial arc of motion of CPM on short-term and long-term outcomes in CPM protocol. Specifically, the purpose of this study was to determine whether there were differences between a CPM protocol starting at 0 to 40 degrees, a CPM protocol starting at 70 to 100 degrees, and no CPM. The dependent variables we looked at were ROM at 3 weeks, 6 weeks, and 6 months; gait velocity; and ADL score.

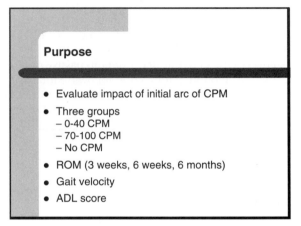

7. We hypothesized that in the short term there would be differences between the no-CPM group and both CPM groups at 3 and 6 weeks postoperatively, but no difference between the two CPM groups.

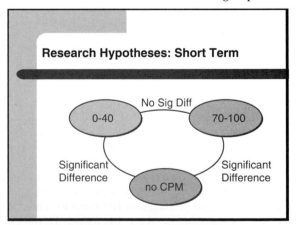

8. For the long term, we hypothesized that there would be no differences among groups at 6 months postoperatively.

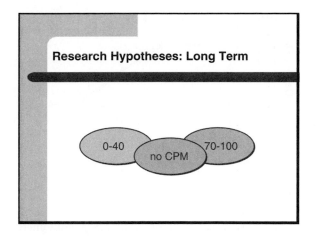

9. Participants were patients who were at least 50 years old, had a diagnosis of osteoarthritis, and underwent a unilateral TKA in 2003 at one of three hospitals in Anytown, Indiana: Community Hospital, Memorial Hospital, and Religious Hospital. The study was approved by the IRBs of the hospitals.

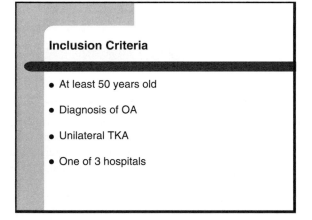

10. Before beginning this study, the characteristics of patients undergoing TKA were compared across the three participating hospitals and found to be similar for age, sex, diagnosis, type of prosthesis implanted, and so forth. Because of the similarity of patients at the three hospitals, we assigned the CPM protocol randomly to hospitals rather than individually to patients. Patients at Community Hospital received an initial arc of 70 to 100 degrees of CPM, patients at Religious Hospital received an initial arc of 0 to 40 degrees, and patients at Memorial Hospital received no CPM.

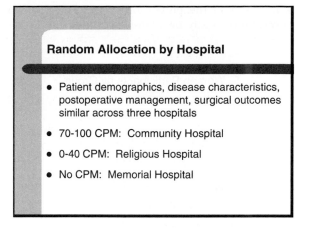

11. The first 10 patients in 2003 who met the inclusion criteria and consented to participate were entered into the trial at each hospital. Twelve eligible patients did not consent to participate in the study. Our patients really came through for us, and all 30 who were entered into the study completed all the measurement sessions.

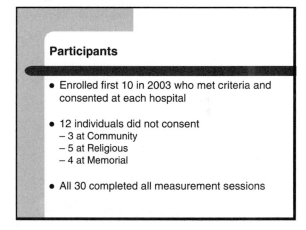

12. The average age of participants in the three groups was very similar, as shown in the graph.

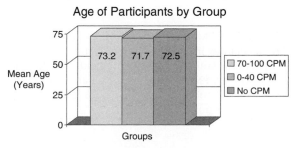

13. In addition, the proportion of men and women was fairly evenly distributed across the groups, as shown.

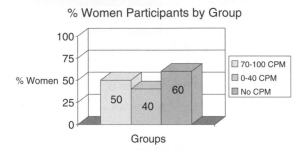

% Women Participants by Group

14. For the two CPM groups, the units were applied in the recovery room and used for 20 hours on the first postoperative day. On subsequent days, the ROM was advanced 10 degrees (toward more flexion for the 0- to 40-degree group and toward extension for the 70- to 100-degree group) per day, and the time in the unit was reduced by about 2 hours per day. Each day, the time spent in CPM was recorded for each patient.

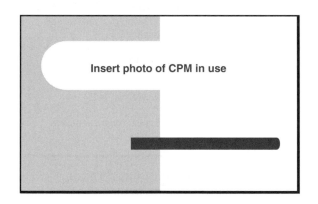

15. The two CPM groups received nearly identical hours per day in CPM, as shown by the two lines on this graph. You can observe the gradual reduction in hours of CPM per day, starting at about 18 hours per day and ending up at less than 6 hours per day by the sixth postoperative day.

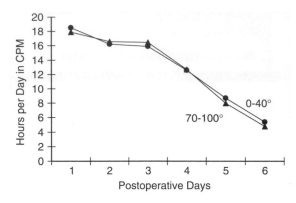

16. We took knee flexion measures as shown in the slide. We used a 12-inch, full-circle goniometer according to the procedures outlined by Norkin and White.

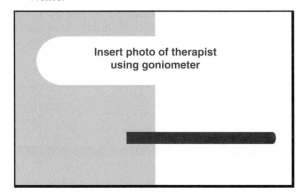

17. Gait velocity measures were taken 6 months after surgery as shown, by timing the participant with a stopwatch during the middle 10 meters of a 20-meter walkway. The data were converted to centimeters per second.

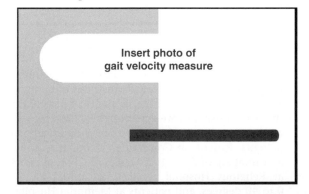

18. The Modified Brigham and Women's Knee Function Scale was administered 6 months after surgery. The distance each participant was able to walk was a self-reported measure, but we directly observed assistive device use, stair climbing, and rising from a chair. The four activity scores are summed to create a single ADL score, with the highest level of function scored as 20.

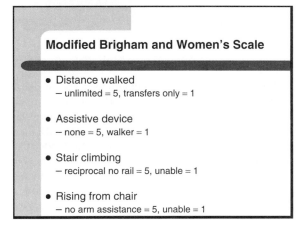

Modified Brigham and Women's Scale

- Distance walked
  – unlimited = 5, transfers only = 1

- Assistive device
  – none = 5, walker = 1

- Stair climbing
  – reciprocal no rail = 5, unable = 1

- Rising from chair
  – no arm assistance = 5, unable = 1

19. We used an analysis of variance to test for differences between groups for each of the dependent variables. The Newman-Keuls procedure was used for post hoc analysis. Alpha was set at .05 for each analysis. Data were analyzed using SPSS.

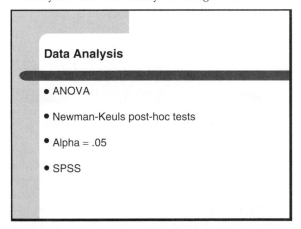

Data Analysis

- ANOVA

- Newman-Keuls post-hoc tests

- Alpha = .05

- SPSS

20. Mean knee flexion range of motion at 3 weeks, 6 weeks, and 6 months after surgery can be seen to increase across time for all groups. The CPM groups both achieved better than an average of 90 degrees of flexion by 6 months, but the group that did not receive CPM had an average of slightly less than 90 degrees of flexion by then.

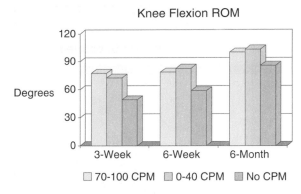

21. Mean gait velocity for both CPM groups was more than 140 centimeters per second; for the no-CPM group, it was less than 110 centimeters per second.

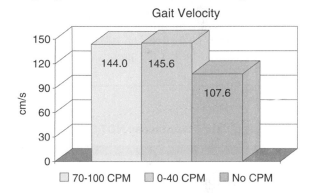

22. The mean ADL scores for the two CPM groups were 18 and 17 out of 20; the mean score for the no-CPM group was 11.

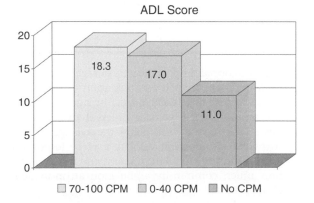

23. Our short-term hypotheses were supported, as the two CPM groups were better than the no-CPM group on all variables, but there were no differences between the two CPM groups.

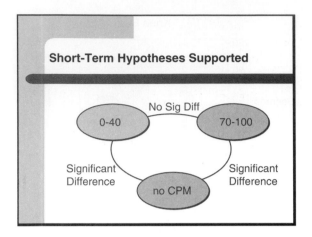

24. Our long-term hypotheses were not supported. We had thought that all three groups would have similar outcomes by 6 months postoperatively. We were surprised to find that the no-CPM group was still lagging behind both CPM groups on all variables after 6 months.

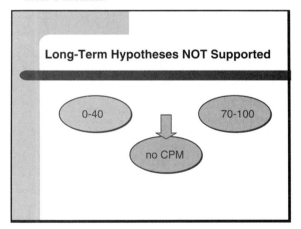

25. The functional importance of our gait and ADL findings is apparent if we look again at the mean values for the different groups. The no-CPM group had an average gait velocity of less than 110 centimeters per second, well below the averages of the two CPM groups. Gait velocity may be important for community ambulation safety, and it may affect how much community ambulation an individual chooses to do.

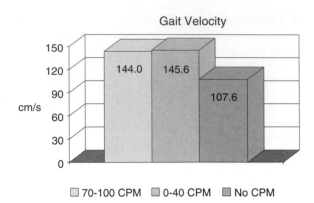

26. The ADL scores of the CPM groups were approximately 18 and 17 of 20, respectively. This indicates minor impairment on two of the components or moderate impairment on one. In contrast, the average ADL score for the no-CPM group was 11, indicating moderate to severe impairment in one or more of the ADL components. If, for example, stair climbing and distance walked are limited, this can reduce community ambulation, important life activities such as grocery shopping, and recreational activities such as travel.

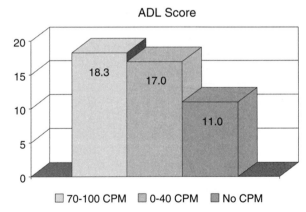

27. There are two main limitations of our research design. First, because the treatments were assigned by hospital and not by patient, there may have been systematic differences between care at the hospitals that could explain the differences in results. Second, because the treating therapists were aware of group membership of the participants, their expectations may have influenced patient performance.

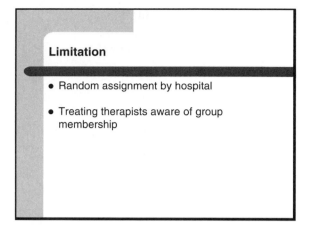

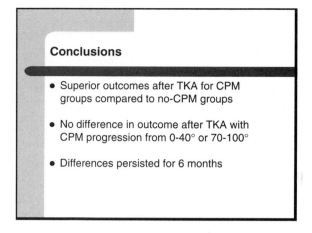

28. Future research in the area should focus on replicating these results, studying whether differences between the CPM and no-CPM groups persist longer than 6 months, and determining whether other important variables—such as postoperative blood loss or analgesic use—are affected by differences in CPM regimens.

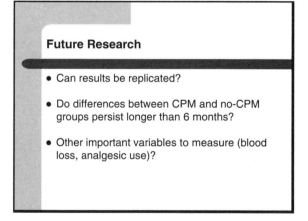

29. There are really three messages that I hope you take home from this presentation today. First, there were superior outcomes after total knee arthroplasty for both CPM groups compared with no-CPM. Second, there was no difference in outcome after total knee arthroplasty based on the arc of motion at which the CPM was started. And third, these differences persisted for 6 months after surgery. Based on this work, we plan to continue to use CPM on a routine basis at our facilities, but will leave the initial arc of motion to the discretion of the physician and therapist.

30. I'd like to publicly thank the study participants, who all showed up for all the measurement sessions; the treating therapists at all three hospitals, who do such a great job day in and day out; Dr. Ben Counter, our statistics whiz; and Dr. Ellen Redline, who helped us design this presentation.

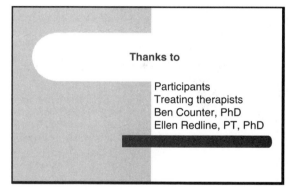

31. I'd be happy to take any questions at this time.

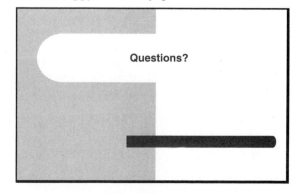

Index

Note: Page numbers followed by *b* indicate boxes, *f* indicate figures and *t* indicate tables.

A

A-B-A designs, 124
A-B designs, 123–124
AACPDM. *See* American Academy of Cerebral Palsy and Developmental Medicine (AACPDM)
Abscissa, 72
Absolute reliability, 244, 329–330
Abstract, review of, 367
Acceptance region, 276
Accessible population, 92–93, 93*t*
  characteristics defining, 93
Accreditation Council for Graduate Medical Education, 7
Acoustic condition, independent variable of, 68
Action
  codes of ethics for, 47–51
  moral principles of, 43–46
    conflict of interest, 45
    nondiscrimination, 45–46
    principle of autonomy, 45
    principle of beneficence, 44
    principle of nonmaleficence, 44
    principle of utility, 44–45
Active control group, 111
Active-controlled research design, 48–49
Active variables, 69–70
Adjusted rate, 180–181, 182*t*
Advanced analysis of variance, techniques of, 298–307
Alpha factoring, 341
Alpha level, 272–273
  statistical power and, 276
Alpha level inflation, 272
  error rate problem and, 278
Alternating-treatment designs, 129–132, 131*t*, 132*f*
  combined with multiple-baseline designs, 131
  graphing data for, 137–138, 137*t*, 138*t*, 139*f*
American Academy of Cerebral Palsy and Developmental Medicine (AACPDM), 31
  evidence hierarchy for, 23
American Council on Occupational Therapy Education, 7–8
American Medical Association
  citation and reference lists for, 402*b*
  style manual of, 401
American Occupational Therapy Association (AOTA)
  code of ethics for, 50–51
  goal of, 7

American Physical Therapy Association (APTA)
  code of ethics for, 50
  goal of, 7
American Psychological Association
  citation and reference lists for, 402*b*
  style manual of, 401
American Speech-Language-Hearing Association
  code of ethics for, 50
  educational standards for, 7–8
  evidence-based practice and, 155
  goal of, 7
Analysis of covariance (ANCOVA), 305, 305*f*, 306*f*, 306*t*
Analysis of differences, 149–151
  prospective, 151
  retrospective, 150–151
Analysis of relationships, 148–149
  among variables, 148
  prospective, 149
  retrospective, 149
  statistical, basics of, 318–328
Analysis of variance (ANOVA)
  advanced, 298–307
  between-subjects two-way, 299–302, 299*t*, 300*f*, 300*t*, 301*f*, 301*t*
  differences across several dependent variables in, 304–305
  differences between more than one independent variable in, 298–304
  Friedman's, 296–297
  mixed-design, 298–299
  mixed-design two-way, 302–304, 302*t*, 303*f*
  multivariate, 304, 305*t*
  one-way, 289–291, 295, 304
  repeated measures of, 295–296, 296*t*
  two-factor between-subjects, 299*t*
  two-factor mixed-design, 302*t*
  two-way, 299
  univariate, 304
Analysis phase, of power, 316
ANCOVA. *See* Analysis of covariance (ANCOVA)
Animal subjects, ethical concerns about, 5
ANOVA. *See* Analysis of variance (ANOVA)
AOTA. *See* American Occupational Therapy Association (AOTA)
Appendices, for research proposal, 381
Approvals, for research proposal, 381–382

APTA. *See* American Physical Therapy Association (APTA)
Archival data, 144–145
    decision rules and, 146
Article. *See also* Research article; Review articles
    about therapy, questions for, 356*b*
    questions for
        about diagnosis, screening, prognosis, and harm, 357*b*
        about therapy, 356*b*
    review, generic evaluation of, 353–354
        article identification and selection strategies in, 354
        assessment of clarity of review question in, 353–354
        assessment of validity in, 354
        personal utility of review in, 354
        results against strength of evidence in, 354
Artifacts, 170–171
    in environment, 171
ASHA. *See* American Speech-Language-Hearing Association
    (ASHA)
Assigned variables, 69–70
Assignment
    to groups, 100–103, 100*t*
        as threat to internal validity, 83
    of participants, 92–105
    significance of, 92
Asymmetrical distribution, 265
Attribute, 69
Attrition, as threat to internal validity, 83–84
Autism, nonexperimental research and, 144
Autism spectrum disorder, 190
Autonomy, principle of, 45

B
"Backstory," of research, 378
Backward regression strategy, 335–336
Bar graph, 72–73, 74*f*
Basement effect, 84
Basic science research, 154
Behavioral research, single-subject paradigm and, 63
Behavioral view, of treatment diffusion, 85
Bench research, 154, 154*f*
Beneficence
    principle of, 44
    research and, 23
Between-groups design, 110–111, 117–118
Between-groups difference, statistical probability
    and, 273
Between-groups sum of squares (SSB), 289
    calculation of, 290*t*
Between-groups variability, 289
Between-subjects design, 110–111, 117–118
Between-subjects factors, 298–299
Between-subjects two-way analysis of variance, 299–302,
    299*t*, 300*f*, 300*t*, 301*f*, 301*t*
Bias, 331*f*, 332*f*
Bibliographic search. *See* Reference lists
Bibliographies, 39
Bimodal distribution, 265
Biophysiological measurement, 241

Block, random assignment by, 101*t*, 102
Body-weight-supported treadmill training (BWSTT),
    review on, 364
Bonferroni test, 291
Boolean operations, 35–36, 39*f*
Bruininks-Oseretsky Test of Motor Proficiency (BOTMP), 246
Budget
    for research project, 384–385, 387*t*
    for research proposal, 381

C
Calibration, 81
Canadian Occupational Performance Measure (COPM),
    202
Canonical correlation, 321
    characteristics of, 321*t*
Carryover effects, 113
Case-control design, 145*t*, 150
Case-control studies, 188*f*, 189–191
    documentation of, 191
    positive and negative features of, 190–191
Case report, 145*t*, 146
    contributions of, to theory and practice, 154–155, 154*f*
    format of, 157
    prospective, 153
    purposes of, 155–157
        clinical experience, sharing of, 155
        evidence-based practice, illustration of, 155
        persuading and motivating, 156–157
        practice guidelines and pathways, development of, 157
        problem-solving skill, 156
        research hypothesis, 156
        testing theory, 156
    retrospective, 153
Case study, 146, 153, 160–161, 161*t*
"Case-to-case generalizability", 121
CAT. *See* Computer Adaptive Testing (CAT)
CATs. *See* Critically Appraised Topics (CATs)
Causal-comparative research, 149
Cause-and-effect relationship, 68
CCAM. *See* Continuing Care Activity Measure (CCAM)
Ceiling effect, 84
Celeration line analysis, of single-subject designs, 308,
    308*f*, 310*f*, 310*t*
Census, retrospective data and, 146
Central tendency, 265
    as descriptive measure, 267
    measures of, 265
        mean, 265
        median, 265
        mode, 265
Cerebrovascular accident (CVA), interventions for, 74
Changing-criterion designs, 133–134, 133*f*
Chi-square distribution
    example of, 282*f*
    as squared *z* scores, 282
    for statistical tests, 282
Chi-square test of association, 288, 292–293, 292*t*

CINAHL. *See* Cumulative Index of Nursing and Allied Health Literature (CINAHL)
Citation. *See* Reference lists
Classical measurement theory, 240–241
"Clever Hans", 57
Clinical case reports, 153–158. *See also* Case report
Clinical research, 154, 154*f*
   issues in, structured evaluation by, 355–356
Clinical trials, 154, 154*f*
Clinician-researcher dichotomy, 5–6
   solution to barrier of, 6
Closed-format survey items, types of
   Likert type, 217
   multiple choice, 217
   Q-sort, 217–218
   semantic differential, 217
Cluster sampling, 97–98
   example of, 98*f*
   simple random sampling *versus*, 97
Cochrane Collaboration, 372
   logo for, 372*f*
Cochrane Library, 38
Coding system, 171
Coefficient. *See also* Correlation coefficients
   of determination, 323–324
   statistical significance of, 324–325
   strength of, 322–323
Cohort, definition of, 113
Cohort design, 145*t*, 150, 188–189, 188*f*
   characteristics of, 191
   variants of, 191
Cohort studies, 25, 191–192
Commission on Accreditation in Physical Therapy Education, 7–8
Communication Profile for the Hearing Impaired (CPHI), 203*t*
Community foundations, 388
Company-sponsored foundation, 388
Compensatory equalization of treatments, as threat to internal validity, 85
Complete observer model, 169
Completely randomized design, 116–117
Completer analysis, 278
Computer Adaptive Testing (CAT), 201
Concurrent cohort studies, 188–189, 188*f*, 191
Condition-specific tools, for rehabilitation, 201–202, 203*t*
Confidence intervals
   around coefficient, 325
   foundations for testing of, 314
   hypothesis testing with, 313–315, 372
   interpretation and examples of, 314–315
   of sampling distribution, 270–271
Confidentiality, HIPAA and, 45
Conflict of interest, 45
Confounding variables, 70
Consecutive assignment, 102–103
Consecutive sampling, 99

Consent form, 384. *See also* Informed consent
   elements of, 384*b*
   example of, 385*f*
Constant, 68
   prevalence and, 178
Construct underrepresentation, as threat to construct validity, 86
Construct validity, 76, 85–88, 244–245
   concerns with, 351
   evaluation of, 27*t*, 29
   external validity *versus*, 88
   for methodological research, 253–254
   threats to, 86
      construct underrepresentation as, 86
      experimenter expectancies as, 86–87
      interaction between different treatments as, 87
      interaction between testing and treatment as, 87–88
Content analysis, 144–145
Content validity, 245
   for methodological research, 254
Continuing Care Activity Measure (CCAM), 277–278
Continuous variable, 234
Continuum, 72–73
Contrast, 291
Control group
   active, 111
   for controlling maturation effects, 79
Controlled manipulation, 121
Convenience, samples of, 98–99, 99*f*
COPM. *See* Canadian Occupational Performance Measure (COPM)
Corporation funding, of research project, 387–388
Correlation, 318–326
   measurement theory and, 320–321
   point-biserial, 321
Correlation coefficients, 237, 239*t*
   alternative, 320–321
   assumptions of, 321–322
      homoscedasticity, 321–322, 323*f*
      relationships between variables in, 321, 322*f*
      variability of variables, 322, 324*f*
   characteristics of, 321*t*
   interpretation of, 322–325
      coefficient of determination in, 323–324
      coefficient strength in, 322–323
      confidence intervals in, 325
      limits of, 325, 325*f*
      statistical significance in, 324–325
   literature examples of, 325–326
Correlation matrix, 320, 320*t*
   for factor analysis, 340–341, 340*t*
Correlational research, 145*t*, 148
Cover letter, for questionnaire, 224*f*, 225*f*
Cox regression model, 313
CPHI. *See* Communication Profile for the Hearing Impaired (CPHI)
Cramer's V, 321, 326
   characteristics of, 321*t*

Criterion-referenced change, history threat and, 79
Criterion-referenced measurement, 240
Criterion validity, 245–246
  for methodological research, 254–255
Critical incident report, for observations, 170
Critically Appraised Topics (CATs), 29–30
Cross-products, 319
Cross-sectional case-control design, 151
Cross-sectional studies, 188*f*, 189
Crude rate, 180–181, 181*f*
C statistic, 311–312
Culture, 161
Cumulative Index of Nursing and Allied Health Literature
  (CINAHL), 36–37
Cumulative relationships, among types of validity, 90
Curvilinear relationships, analysis of, 321
Cutoff score, 185, 185*f*
CVA. *See* Cerebrovascular accident (CVA)

D
DASH. *See* Disabilities of the Arm, Shoulder, and Hand
  (DASH)
Data
  forms for recording of, 392–394, 393*f*
  generating meaning of, 172, 173*f*
  missing, techniques for dealing with, 207
  organization of, 171
  recording of
    categorically, 170
    narrative, 170
  safeguarding, 392
  statistical, across studies, 372–373
  survival analysis of, 207–208, 208*f*
Data analysis
  in qualitative research, 171–174
  for research project, 395–397
    data coding in, 396
    entry in, 396
    statistical analysis and, 396–397
    statistical consultants for, 395
    statistical packages for, 395
  in research proposal, 381
  verification of, 172–174
Data coding, in research project, 396
Data collection
  nonexperimental, retrospective nature of, 350
  for qualitative research, 165–171
  for research project, 391–395
    procedures for, 392
    protecting participant identity in, 392
    recording forms in, 392–394, 393*f*
    safeguarding, 392
Data entry, for research project, 396
Data management, 171–172
Data set
  central tendency and, 265
  examples of, 260*t*, 262*t*
  mean of, 265

Data set (*Continued*)
  statistical reasoning and, 260
  variability of, 265–267
Database, for systematic review, 368
Declaration of Helsinki, 47, 51
Degrees of freedom, 266
Delphi method, 148
Delphi study, 226
Delphi technique, 226
Demoralization, as threat to internal
  validity, 85
Denominator
  for incidence, 179
  prevalence and, 178
Dependent sample, 284
  differences between two, 293–295, 293*t*
Dependent variables, 69–70
  operationally defined, 70
Descriptive measures, central tendency and variability
  as, 267
Descriptive research
  purpose of, 144
  variables in, 144
Descriptive statistics, 265
Descriptive theory, 12–13
Determination, coefficient of, 323–324
Developmental research, 145*t*
DHHS. *See* U.S. Department of Health and Human Services
  (DHHS)
Diagnosis, epidemiological research and, 184–188
"Direct" replication, 90
Directional hypothesis, 287
Disabilities of the Arm, Shoulder, and Hand (DASH), 203*t*,
  255
Discrete variable, 234
Discriminant analysis, 339
Dissemination, for research proposal, 381
Dissertation Abstracts International, 38
Distributions. *See also* Frequency distribution; Normal
  distribution
  for analysis of differences, 281–282, 282*f*
  for statistical tests, 281–282
Document, definition of, 170
Dummy coding, 335

E
EBM. *See* Evidence-based medicine (EBM)
EBPT. *See* Evidence-based physical therapy (EBPT)
Economic risks, of research, 52
Editorial board, 400
Educational Resource Information Center (ERIC), 37
Effect size, statistical probability and, 274
Effectiveness, 195–196
Efficacy, 195
Electronic database. *See also* Web-based database
  library catalogs as, 38
EMBASE, 36
Empiricism, 56–57

Epidemiological research, 145*t*, 146
  proportions for test usefulness in, 184
    sensitivity and specificity in, 184–187, 184*f*, 185*f*
Epidemiology, 146, 176–193
  definition of, 176
Equalization of treatments, compensatory, as threat to
  internal validity, 85
ERIC. *See* Educational Resource Information Center (ERIC)
Error, 274–276. *See also* Statistical error
  standard error of mean, 313–314
  type I, 275
  type II, 275, 316
Error rate problems, 278
Ethical dilemmas, single-subject designs and, 140
Ethics. *See* Research, codes of ethics for
Ethnographic interview, 168
Ethnography
  nature of, 162
  as qualitative design, 161–163, 161*t*
Evaluation research, 145*t*, 146
  outcomes of a program and, 146
Evidence
  evaluation of, 363
    one article at a time, 345–362
  levels of, 355*t*
    for different domains of medical practice and medical
      research, 24*t*
    evaluation of, 356–358
  synthesizing bodies of, 363–375
  use of, in health care practice, 23
Evidence-based medicine (EBM)
  definition of, 345
  model
    definition of, 23
    domains of, 23–25, 24*t*
    evidence hierarchy for, 23
Evidence-based physical therapy (EBPT), 26
Evidence-based practice, 23–32
  ASHA and, 155
  illustration of, case reports and, 155
  implementation of, 26, 26*b*
  institution of, 30–31
  limitations of, 31
  PICO and, 26
  process for, 26
Evidence-Based Review Databases, 38
  Cochrane Library as, 38
  Hooked on Evidence as, 38
  Physiotherapy Evidence Database as, 38
Evidence hierarchy
  levels of, 23–25, 24*t*
  randomized control trial and, 23
Examination, in prospective descriptive research, 147
Experiment, 68
  goals of, 70
  requirements of, 107
Experimental attrition, controlling, 84
Experimental manipulation, in single-subject research, 65

Experimental research, definition of, 107
Experimenter expectancies, as threat to construct validity,
  86–87
Explanatory theory, 13, 14*f*
External validity, 76, 88–90
  concerns with, 352
  evaluation of, 27*t*, 29
  group designs and, 121
  internal/construct validity *versus*, 88
  in qualitative research, 90
  in single-subject research, 89–90
  threats to
    selection as, 88–89
    setting as, 89
    time as, 89
Extraction techniques, 341
Extraneous factors, control of, 59, 65
Extraneous variables, 70
  controlling, 70
  related to participants, 70

F
F distribution, 282, 289
  example of, 282*f*
  for statistical tests, 282
F ratio, 289
F statistic, generation of, 289
Factor analysis, 339–343
  correlation matrix for, 340*t*
  literature examples for, 342–343
  steps in, 340–342
  uses of, 339–340
Factor loadings, 341, 341*t*, 342*t*
Factorial design
  line graph and, 73
  nested design *versus*, 115–116, 115*f*, 116*f*, 117*f*, 118*f*
Factorial experiment, 71–72, 72*f*, 72*t*
Familiarization sessions, testing threat and, 81
Fatigue Questionnaire, 203*t*
FCMs. *See* Functional Communication Measures (FCMs)
Field study, 154, 154*f*
FIM. *See* Functional Independence Measure (FIM)
Floor effect, 84
Focus-group interviews, 147
Focus on Therapeutic Outcomes, Inc. (FOTO), 206
Formal aspects, of research, 378
Forward regression strategy, 335–336
FOTO. *See* Focus on Therapeutic Outcomes, Inc. (FOTO)
Foundation funding, of research project, 388
  applying for, 388
  identifying, 388
  types of, 388
Framingham study, 149
Frequency distribution, 235, 235*t*
  definition of, 261–264
  grouped, with percentages, 263–264
  histogram of, 235*f*, 264, 264*f*
  median of, 265

Frequency distribution *(Continued)*
   mode of, 265
   with percentages, 261–264, 263t
   stem-and-leaf plot, 264, 264t
Friedman's analysis of variance, 296–297
   calculation of, 296–297
   hypotheses for, 296
Functional Communication Measures (FCMs), 202
Functional Independence Measure (FIM), 206
Functional relationships, 70–72, 71f
   types of, 71
Funding
   availability and sources of, 8
   lack of, as research barrier, 4
   of research project, 384–389
      budget in, 384–385, 387t
      corporation, 387–388
      foundation, 388
      government, 388–389, 389b
      institution, 386–387

G

Gait, theory of, 13, 14f
GAS. *See* Goal Attainment Scaling (GAS)
Gate control theory, of pain, 17
Generality by replication, 89–90
Generalizability
   of research, 58
   of results, 57
      single-subject designs and, 140
Generalizability theory, 241
General theory. *See* Middle-range theory
Geocentric theory, 14
GMFM. *See* Gross Motor Function Measure (GMFM)
Goal Attainment Scaling (GAS), 202
Google Scholar, 37
Government funding, of research project, 388–389
   grant proposals for, 389
   institutional review boards for, 389
   procedure for, 388–389
   sources of, 389b
Grand mean, 289
Grand theory, 15–17
Graphs/graphing, 72–74
   for alternating-treatments designs, 137–138, 137t, 138t, 139f
   in research manuscript, 405, 405f
   for single-subject data, 134–138, 135f, 135t, 136f, 136t
"Gray" literature, 367–368
Gross Motor Function Measure (GMFM), 251–252
Grounded theory, 161t, 163–164
   goal of, 164
Group designs, 107–119
   assumptions of, 108
   external validity and, 121
   problems with, 120–121

Grouped frequency distribution
   histogram presenting, 264, 264f
   with percentages, 263–264, 264t
Groups, assignment to, 100–103, 100t

H

Health Information Portability and Accountability Act (HIPAA), 45
   provisions of, 47
Health-related quality of life, 199–201
Heterogeneity, in meta-analysis, 373
Highwire Press, 37–38
HIPAA. *See* Health Information Portability and Accountability Act (HIPAA)
Hislop's pathokinesiological framework for physical therapy, 16, 16f
Histogram, grouped frequency distribution with, 264, 264f
Historical cohort studies, 188–189
Historical research, 145t, 146
History, as threat to internal validity, 77–79
Homogeneity, in meta-analysis, 373
Homoscedasticity, 321–322, 323f
Hooked on Evidence, 38
Horizontal axis, 72
Human instrument, 81
Human occupation, model of, 16–17
Human participants, ethical concerns about, 5
Hypothesis
   definition of, 13
   development for research, 156
   testing
      with confidence intervals, 313–315, 372
      review of, 313–314
      traditional, 372

I

IADL. *See* Lawton Instrumental Activities of Daily Living (IADL)
ICF. *See* International Classification of Functioning, Disability, and Health (ICF)
ICIDH. *See* International Classification of Impairments, Disabilities, and Handicaps (ICIDH)
Image factoring, 341
In-house databases, 205
Incidence, 179–180
   denominator of, 179
   numerator of, 179
   prevalence and, 180
Independent foundations, 388
Independent groups, differences between two or more, 289–293, 289t
Independent sample, 284
Independent *t* test, 287–288
   formula for, 286t, 287
   use of, 287–288
Independent variables, 68
   levels of, 68
   linear relationship and, 71, 71f, 71t

Independent variables *(Continued)*
  nonlinear relationship and, 71, 71*t*, 72*f*
  parameter and, 73, 73*f*
  treatment and, 68
Inferential statistics, 271
Informed consent
  components of, 46
  elements of, 384*b*
  example of, 385*f*
  information needed for, 46
  of research project participants, 383–384
Inpatient recruitment, for research project, 390
Institution funding, for research project,
    386–387
Institutional review boards (IRBs), 47
  federal regulations for, 383
  levels of review of, 383
  purpose of, 383
Instrument reliability, 241–242
Instrumentation, as threat to internal validity, 81
Insurance claims database, 205
Intention-to-treat analysis, 278–279
Interaction designs, 132–133
Internal validity, 76–85
  concerns with, 351
  evaluation of, 27*t*, 29
  external/construct validity *versus*, 88
  increasing, 77
  threats to, 77
    assignment as, 83
    compensatory equalization of treatments as, 85
    history as, 77–79
    instrumentation as, 81
    interactions between, 84–85
    maturation as, 79–81
    rivalry and demoralization as, 85
    statistical regression to mean as, 81–83, 82*f*
    subject attrition as, 83–84
    testing as, 81
    treatment diffusion as, 85
  threats to, single-subject designs and, 140
  within-subjects/repeated measures designs
      for, 77
International Classification of Functioning, Disability, and
    Health (ICF), 196–198, 197*f*
  diagram of, 15*f*
  parts of, 15
International Classification of Impairments, Disabilities,
    and Handicaps (ICIDH), 196, 197*f*
Internet surveys
  advantages and limitations of, 226
  feasibility of, 226
  process for, 226
  software for, 226
Interrater reliability, 242–243
Interval scales, 233
Intervening variables, 70
  effect of removal of, 305–307, 305*f*

Interventions
  duration and frequency of, 139
  presentation pattern and, 129
  randomized controlled trial and, 108
Interview(s)
  advantages and disadvantages of, 219*t*
  as data collection method, for qualitative research, 165–168
  ethnographic, 168
  how to, 167
  implementation details for, 227–228
  open-format items for, 216
  participants for
    access to, 227
    motivating, 227
    number of, 166
  in prospective descriptive research, 147–148
  purpose of
    establishing relationship in, 168
    getting information in, 167–168
    giving information in, 168
  schedule for, 227
  semistructured, 166
  setting for, 167
  structured, 165–166
  style of, 166
  unstructured, 166
Intraclass correlation, characteristics of, 321, 321*t*
Intraclass correlation coefficients, 332–334
  calculations of, 333*t*
  repeated measures and, 332–333
Intrarater reliability, 242
Intrasubject reliability, 243
Introduction section, of research manuscript, 404
Investigators, for research proposal, 380
IRBs. *See* Institutional review boards (IRBs)
IRT. *See* Item response therapy (IRT)
Item response therapy (IRT), 201

J
Jadad scales
  criteria and scoring for, 358
  randomized control trial, in scoring quality of, 359*t*
Journal editor, 400
Journals
  authorship and acknowledgement in, 400–401
  for observations, 170
  peer review process for, 400
  purpose of, 399–400
  style issues in, 401, 403*t*

K
Kappa, 321, 334–335
  calculation of, 334*t*
  characteristics of, 321*t*
Kendall's tau, 321
  characteristics of, 321*t*
Knee flexion, measurements of, frequency distribution
    of, 235*t*

Known-groups approach, 254
Kruskal-Wallis test, 289, 291–292
  conduction of, 292
  multiple-comparison procedure for, 292

L

Latin square technique, in selecting treatment, 114, 114*f*
Lawton Instrumental Activities of Daily Living (IADL), 245
Lay public, recruitment of, for research project, 391
Level analysis, of single-subject designs, 308–311, 309*f*
Levels-of-evidence approach
  criticism for, 356
  evaluation of, 358
  Medical Research Council and, 356–358
  to systematic review, 368–370
Library catalogs, advantages of, 38
Likelihood ratio, 186–187
  negative test, 187
  positive test, 187
Likert type survey items, 217
Line graph, 72–73
  factorial design and, 73
  single-subject designs and, 73, 73*f*
Linear functional relationship, independent variable and,
    71, 71*f*, 71*t*
Linear regression, 326–328, 326*f*, 327*f*
Literature. *See* Research literature
Log-rank test, 313
Logical positivism, 56
Logistic regression, 338–339
  literature examples for, 339
  rationale for, 338, 338*f*
Lysholm Knee Rating Scale, 208–209

M

MACTAR scale. *See* McMaster Toronto Arthritis (MACTAR)
    scale
Magazines, 399
Mailed survey, 220–226. *See also* Questionnaire
  access to sampling frame in, 220
  advantages and disadvantages of, 220
  follow-up for, 223
  implementation details for, 223–226
  motivating prospects to respond to, 223
  participants for, 220
  questionnaire development in, 220–223
  researcher-developed *versus* existing instruments
    in, 220
Mann-Whitney test, 288, 288*t*
  with Bonferroni adjustment of alpha, 292
  hypothesis for, 288
  performance of, 288
  z score and, 288
MANOVA. *See* Multivariate analysis of variance (MANOVA)
Mantel-Haenszel test, 313
Manuscript reviewers, 400
Matched assignment, 101*t*, 102
Material traces, 170

Maturation, as threat to internal validity, 79–81, 80*f*
MCID. *See* Minimal clinically important difference (MCID)
McMaster Toronto Arthritis (MACTAR) scale, 202
McNemar test, 294–295, 295*t*
  performance of, 294–295
Mean, 235
  of data set, 265
Mean designs, 252–253
Mean square between groups (MSB), 291
Mean square within each group (MSW), 291
Measurement
  definition of, 231–232
  determining scale of, 234
  frameworks of, 239–240
  of properties, 232
  reliability of, 240–244
    range of scores in, 252
    sources of variability in, 249–250
    standardization levels in, 250–251
  responsiveness to change, 246–247
  scales of, 232–234
    interval, 233
    nominal, 232
    ordinal, 232–233
    ratio, 233–234
  standard error of, 237–239, 252
  validity of, 148, 149, 244–246
    construct validity, 244–245
    content validity, 245
    criterion validity, 245–246
  variable classification for, 234
Measurement theory, 59, 231–248
  correlation and, 320–321
  statistical foundations of, 235–239
    correlation coefficient, 237, 239*t*
    frequency distribution, 235, 235*t*
    mean, 235
    normal curve, 236–237, 237*f*, 238*f*
    standard deviation, 236
    variance, 235–236
Median, 265, 265*t*
  calculation of, 265
Medical Outcomes Study (MOS), 200
Medical randomized controlled trials, 109
Medical records
  abstracts of, 204–205
  review of, 204
Medical Research Council, levels-of-evidence approach
    and, 356–358
Medline (PubMed), 36
Member checking, 172
Mentors, lack of, as research barrier, 4–5
Meta-analysis, 145*t*, 150
  basic concept behind, 364–365
  central concepts of, 372
  concept behind, 151
  definition of, 364–365
  mathematical complexities of, 372

Meta-analysis *(Continued)*
  presenting results of, 372*f*, 373*f*, 374
  of randomized control trial, 23–25
  statistical concerns about, 373
  systematic review with, 364–365
  systematic review without, 364
Metatheory, 15
Methodological research, 145*t*, 249–257
  goals of, 249
  optimization designs for, 252–253
    mean designs, 252–253
    standardization designs, 252
  reliability designs for, 249–253
    participant selection for, 251–252
    range of scores in, 252
    sources of variability in, 249–250
    standardization levels in, 250–251
  responsiveness designs for, 255–256
  validity designs for, 253–255
Methods section
  of research paper, 404
  of research proposal, 381
    data analysis in, 381
    information in, 381
    procedures in, 381
  of systematic review, 374
Middle-range theory, 17
  gate control theory of pain as, 17
  physical stress theory as, 17
  sensory integration model as, 17
Minimal clinically important difference (MCID), 277–278
Minimal detectable difference (MDD), 277–278
Mixed design, 117–118
Mixed-design analysis of variance, 298–299
Mixed-design two-way analysis of variance, 302–304, 302*t*, 303*f*
Mode, 265*t*
  of frequency distribution, 265
Model of human occupation (MOHO), 16–17
MOHO. *See* Model of human occupation (MOHO)
MOS. *See* Medical Outcomes Study (MOS)
MSB. *See* Mean square between groups (MSB)
MSW. *See* Mean square within each group (MSW)
Multiple-baseline designs, 127–129, 128*f*, 130*f*
Multiple baseline measures, for controlling maturation effects, 79, 80*f*
Multiple choice survey items, 217
Multiple-comparison procedure
  common, 291
  for Kruskal-Wallis test, 292
  as post hoc test, 291
  twists to, 291
Multiple correlation, 321
  characteristics of, 321*t*
Multiple-factor experimental designs, 114–118
  between-groups, within-group, and mixed, 117–118
  completely randomized *versus* randomized-block designs, 116–117

Multiple-factor experimental designs *(Continued)*
  factorial *versus* nested designs in, 115–116, 115*f*, 116*f*, 117*f*, 118*f*
  questions leading to, 114–115
Multiple regression, 335–338
  equation
    interpretation of, 336–338, 337*f*
    predictability of, enhancing, 337
  literature examples of, 338
  variable entry in, 335–336
Multivariate analysis of variance (MANOVA), 304, 305*t*
  discriminant analysis and, 339

N
Nagi model, 196, 197*f*
Narrative reviews, 363–364
Narrative validity analysis, 368–370
National Institute on Disability and Rehabilitation Research (NIDRR), 206
National Institutes for Health (NIH), 8
National outcomes databases, 205–207
National Spinal Cord Injuries Database, 206
Naturalistic paradigm. *See* Qualitative paradigm
Negative predictive value, 184*f*, 185*f*, 187, 187*f*
Nested design, factorial design *versus*, 115–116, 115*f*, 116*f*, 117*f*, 118*f*
Newman-Keuls procedure, 291
Newsletters, 399
NIDRR. *See* National Institute on Disability and Rehabilitation Research (NIDRR)
NIH. *See* National Institutes for Health (NIH)
Nominal scales, 232
Nonconcurrent cohort studies, 188–189, 188*f*, 191, 192
Nondiscrimination, 45–46
Nonequal intervals between points, 232–233, 233*f*
Nonequivalent control-group design, 112–113, 112*t*
Nonexperimental analysis of differences, 149, 151
Nonexperimental epidemiological designs, 188–192, 188*f*
Nonexperimental research
  analysis of relationships in, 148–149
  definition of, 143
  determining effectiveness of, 195–196
  format for, 148
  overview of, 143–152
  relationship analysis studies as, 318
  types of, 145*t*
Nonlinear functional relationship, independent variable and, 71, 71*t*, 72*f*
Nonmaleficence
  principle of, 44
  research and, 23
Nonmethodological studies, reliability in, 253
Nonparametric statistical tests, 283
  Kruskal-Wallis test as, 291–292
  Mann-Whitney or Wilcoxon rank sum tests, 288
  requirements for, 283
Nonprobabilistic sampling method, 93

Nonprobability sampling, 98–100
  forms of
    purposive sampling, 99–100
    samples of convenience, 98–99, 99*f*
    snowball sampling, 99
Nonproportional stratified sampling, 95–96
Norm-referenced measures, 239
Normal curve, 236–237, 237*f*, 238*f*
  definition of, 267
Normal distribution, 267–269
  percentages of, 268–269, 268*f*
  sampling distribution and, 269–271
Normative research, 145*t*, 149
Null hypothesis, 271–272
  acceptance region for, 276
  alpha level and, 272–273
  representation of, 372
Numeral, definition of, 231–232
Numerator
  for incidence, 179
  prevalence and, 178
Nuremberg Code, 47

O
Observation
  categories in, 170
  of conversation, factors to account for, 170*b*
  as data collection method, for qualitative research,
    168–170
  ethical issues in, 169
  in prospective descriptive research, 147
  techniques and processes of, 169–170
Observational measurements, 241
Observer-as-participant model, 169
Obtained probability level, 272
Odds ratio, 181–184
Omnibus *F* test, 291
One-tailed probability, 287
One-way analysis of variance, 289–291, 295, 304
  calculation of, 290*t*
Open-format survey items
  difficulty with, 217
  for interviews, 216
  questionnaires, 217
Opportunistic research, 168
Optimization research
  mean designs for, 252–253
  standardization designs for, 252
Order effects, 113
Ordinal measurement, 283
Ordinal scales, 232–233
  nonequal intervals on, 232–233, 233*f*
Ordinate, 72
Oswestry Disability Index, 203*t*
Outcomes research, 194–214
  analysis issues for, 207–209
    comparisons across scales, 208–209, 209*f*
    multivariate statistics, 209

Outcomes research *(Continued)*
  case mix adjustments and, 207
  condition-specific tools for, 201–202, 203*t*
  data for
    missing, techniques for dealing with, 207
    survival analysis of, 207–208, 208*f*
  database research for, 204–207
    administrative databases, 205
    in-house databases, 205
    insurance claims database as, 205
    medical records as, 204
    national outcomes databases as,
      205–207
  design issues for, 204–209
  effectiveness and, 195–196
  efficacy and, 195
  frameworks for, 196–198, 197*f*
    ICF as, 196–198, 197*f*
    ICIDH as, 196, 197*f*
    Nagi model as, 196, 197*f*
  measurement tools for, 198–204
    PROMIS, 200–201
    quality of life, 199
    self-assessment and rating scales as, 198–199
    Short Form-36, of MOS, 200
  patient-specific instruments for, 202
  purpose of, 195–196
  satisfaction and, 202–204
Outpatient recruitment, for research project,
  390–391

P
Pain, gate control theory of, 17
Paired-*t* test, 293
Parameters, 73, 73*f*
  central tendency and variability as, 267
Parametric statistical tests, 283
  assumptions about
    homogeneity of variance, 283
    level of measurement, 283–284
    participants for, 283
Partial correlation, 321
  characteristics of, 321*t*
Participants
  exclusion of, 93
  selection and assignment of, 92–105, 350
  subject *versus*, 42
Participant-as-observer model, 169
Participant observation, 161–162
Pathokinesiological framework for physical therapy, 16, 16*f*
Patient Reported Outcome Measurement Information
  System (PROMIS), 200–201
  CAT and, 201
  instruments, current and under development, 201
  IRT and, 201
  validation of, 201
Patient-specific instruments, 202
Pattern, of variable performance, 122

Pearson product moment correlation
    calculation of, 319–320, 319t, 320f
    characteristics of, 321t
    with extensions, 329–332, 330t
    strategies for, 330
    usefulness of, 330
PEDro scale
    criteria and scoring for, 358
    randomized control trial, in scoring quality of, 359t, 360t
Peer-reviewed journal, case reports in, 157
Peer review process, 400
Percentages, 177
    frequency distribution with, 261–264, 263t
    grouped frequency distribution with, 263–264, 264t
    of normal distribution, 268–269, 268f
Period prevalence, 178–179
Phenomenology, as qualitative design, 161t, 163
Phi, 321
    characteristics of, 321t
Photographs, in research manuscript, 405
Physical risks, of research, 51–52
Physical stress theory (PST), 17
Physical therapy
    evidence-based, 26
    pathokinesiological framework for, 16, 16f
Physiotherapy Evidence Database (PEDro), 38
PICO, 26
PICS. See Picture Exchange Communication System (PECS)
Picture Exchange Communication System (PECS), 364–365
Pilot study, for research project, 395
    participants and personnel for, 395
Placebo-controlled research design, 48–49
Planned orthogonal contrasts, 291
Platform presentations, of research, 402–405
POEC-S. See Proficiency in Oral English Communication Screening (POEC-S)
Point-biserial correlation, 321
    characteristics of, 321t
Point in time, 178–179
Point prevalence, 178–179
Policy research, 145t
Population
    characteristics defining, 93
    samples versus, 92–93
    types of, 92–93
Population standard deviation
    computation of, 267t
    definition of, 266–267
Population variance
    computation of, 267t
    definition of, 266–267
    use of, 266
Positive predictive value, 184f, 185f, 187, 187f
Positivism, 56
Poster presentations, of research, 406f, 407
Postpositivism, 65

Posttest-only control-group design, 111–112, 112t
Posttest-only design, testing threat and, 81
Power, 316
    alpha level and, 276
    low, as statistical conclusion validity threat, 277
    in research, 276
    sample size and, 276
    of test, 276–277
    within-group variability and, 276
Power analysis, 315–316
    analysis phase, 316
    design phase, 315–316
    type II error and, 316
Power tables or programs, 276
Practice, research and, boundaries between, 42–43
Practice theory, 17
Predictive theory, 13
Predictive validity, 255
Predictive value, 187–188
    characteristic of, 188
    positive and negative, 187
    prevalence and, 187f
Presentation pattern, interventions and, 129
Pretest-posttest control-group design, 110–111, 110t, 111t
Pretreatment baseline, history threat and, 78
Prevalence, 178–179
    constant and, 178
    denominator for, 178
    incidence and, 180
    numerator for, 178
    point in time, 178–179
Principal components extraction, 341
Priori theory, 58
Probabilistic sampling method, 93
Probability
    computation of, 267t
    of errors, 274–276
Probability sampling, 94–98
    types of
        cluster sampling, 97–98, 98f
        simple random sampling, 94–95, 94t
        stratified sampling, 95–97, 96t
        systematic sampling, 95, 96t
Problem-solving skills, building, 156
Problem statement, for research proposal, 380
Profession, characteristics of, 3b
Professional associations
    code of ethics for, 50
    goals of, 7
Professional publications, 399
    journals as, 399–400
    magazines as, 399
    newsletters as, 399
Proficiency in Oral English Communication Screening (POEC-S), 149
Project home, 146
PROMIS. See Patient Reported Outcome Measurement Information System (PROMIS)

Proportional stratified sampling, 95–96
Proportions, 177
    hypothetical data for, 177*t*
Proposal, for research project, 378–382
    elements of, 379–382, 379*b*
        appendices, 381
        approvals, 381–382
        budget, 381
        dissemination, 381
        investigators, 380
        methods section of, 381
        problem statement, 380
        purposes section, 380–381
        title, 380
        work plan, 381, 382*t*
    guidelines for, 378–379
Prospective analysis of differences, 151
Prospective case report, 153
Prospective descriptive research, 147–148
    examination in, 147
    interview in, 147–148
    observation in, 147
    questionnaire in, 148
Prospective study, 68, 189
"Proxy" consent, 46–47
PST. *See* Physical stress theory (PST)
Psychological risks, of research, 52
Psychophysics
    concepts from, 184
    receiver-operating characteristic curve in,
        185–186, 186*f*
PsycINFO, 37
Published research. *See also* Research article; Review
    articles
    appropriate wording in, 348*t*
    guidelines for
        discussing, 347
        writing about, 348*t*
    inappropriate wording in, 348*t*
PubMed (Medline), 36
Purposes section, of research proposal, 380–381
Purposive sampling, 99–100
    logic and power of, 100
Pygmalion effect, 87

Q

Q-sort, 217–218
Qualitative designs, 160–164
    case study, 160–161
    ethnography, 161–163, 161*t*
    grounded theory, 161*t*, 163–164
    hypothetical research problems matching, 161*t*
    phenomenology, 161*t*, 163
Qualitative paradigm, 60–63
    alternate names for, 56, 56*b*
    assumptions of, 57*t*, 60–62, 160
        interdependence of investigator and subjects, 60
        multiple constructed realities, 60, 60*b*

Qualitative paradigm *(Continued)*
        no causation, 61
        results specific to time and context, 61
        value laden, 61–62
    methodological issues relating to
        manipulation and control as, 62–63
        measurement tool, 62
        subject selection, 62
        theory within, 62
    methods of, 58*t*
Qualitative research, 145*t*, 159–175
    data analysis in, 171–174
    data collection methods for, 165–171
        interview, 165–168
        observation in, 168–170
    external validity in, 90
    goal of, 61
    idiographic, 61
    methods of, 164–174
        sampling, 164–165
    natural setting for, 62–63
Quality of life
    elements of, 199
    health-related, 199–201
Quantitative paradigm, 56–59
    alternate names for, 56, 56*b*
    assumptions of, 56–58, 57*t*
        determining causation, 57
        generalizability of results, 57
        independence of investigator and subjects, 57
        research as value free, 58
        single objective reality, 56–57
    methodological issues relating to
        control of extraneous factors, 59
        manipulation, 59
        measurement, 59
        subject selection, 58–59
        theory within, 58
    methods of, 58*t*
Quantitative research
    goal of, 56–57
    as nomothetic, 57
Questionnaire
    advantages and disadvantages of, 219*t*
    cover letter for, 224*f*, 225*f*
    Delphi technique for, 148, 226
    development of, 220–223
        drafting items for, 220–221
        expert review of, 221
        final revision of, 223
        first revision of, 221–222
        pilot testing of, 222–223
    example of, 222*f*
    for mailed surveys, 220–223
    as open-format survey item, 217
    prospect for, 223
    in prospective descriptive research, 148
Questionnaire generation tool, 226

Questions
  for articles
    about diagnosis, screening, prognosis, and harm, 357b
    about therapy, 356b
  research, developing answerable, 18

R

Random assignment, 100
  methods of
    by block, 101t, 102
    consecutive assignment as, 102–103
    deciding on, 103
    by individual, 101t, 102
    matched assignment as, 101t, 102
    systematic assignment as, 101t, 102
Random order with rotation, in selecting treatment, 114, 114f
Random sampling, 99–100
Randomized-block design, 116–117
Randomized controlled trial (RCT), 23, 108–110
  AACPDM and, 31
  cautions about, 109–110
  evaluation of, 358
  intervention effect and, 108–109
  meta-analyses of, 23–25
  practical considerations in, 109
  as prospective and experimental, 108
  scales for scoring quality of, 359t
    PEDro scale, 359t, 360t
  systematic review of, 23–25
Range, as variability measure, 266
Rates, 177–178
  as crude, specific, and adjusted, 180–181, 181f, 181t, 182t
  hypothetical data for, 177t
Rating scale
  comparisons across, 208–209, 209f
  construction and use of, 198
  for dependent variable, 69–70
  development of, 199
  purpose of, 199
  in speech-language pathology, 202
  validity and, 199
Ratio, 177
  hypothetical data for, 177t
  scales, 233–234
RCT. See Randomized controlled trial (RCT)
Reactive measures, 81
Receiver-operating characteristic curve, 185–186, 186f
  cutoff score and, 186, 186f
  sensitivity and specificity and, 186
Reciprocal relationship, validity and, 90
Reciprocal threats, validity and, 90
Records, definition of, 171
Reference lists, 39
  review of, 367–368
Regression. See Logistic regression; Multiple regression
Regression equation, 327
  multiple, interpretation of, 336–338, 337f
  reliability analysis and, 330, 331f

Rehabilitation database, common, 36–38
  CINAHL, 36–37
  Dissertation Abstracts International, 38
  EMBASE, 36
  Evidence-Based Review Databases, 38
  Google Scholar, 37
  Highwire Press, 37–38
  PsycINFO, 37
  PubMed (Medline), 36
  SPORTDiscus, 37
  Web of Science, 38
Rehabilitation literature. See Research literature
Rehabilitation practitioner
  educational standards for, 7–8
  professional associations for, 7
Rehabilitation research, 1–10
  barriers to, 4–7
    clinician-researcher dichotomy, 5–6
    ethical concerns, 5
    familiarity with research process, 5
    funds, lack of, 4
    mentors, 4–5
    overcoming, 6
    statistical support, 5
    time, 5
  measures reported in, 277–278
  multiple-factor experimental designs in, 114
  publications for, 7
  reason for developing, 3–4
    body of knowledge, 3
    intervention effectiveness, 3–4
    for patient and client care improvement, 4
  status of, 7–8
    educational standards, 7–8
    funding, 8
    professional association goals, 7
    publication vehicles, 7
  theory in, 11–22
Rejection region, 275
Relationship analysis. See Analysis of relationships
Relative reliability, 243–244, 329–330
Relative risk, 181–184
  calculation of, 183f
  standard table for determining, 182f
Reliability
  components of, 241–243
    instrument, 241–242
    interrater, 242–243
    intrarater, 242
    intrasubject, 243
  definition of, 148, 240
  forms of, 329–330
  of measurement
    range of scores in, 252
    sources of variability in, 249–250
    standardization levels in, 250–251
  in nonmethodological studies, 253
  paired measurements and, 329–330

Reliability *(Continued)*
    quantification of, 243–244
        absolute, 244
        relative, 243–244
    theories of, 240–241
Reliability analysis, 329–335
    regression equation and, 330, 331*f*
Reliability coefficients, 329
Reliability study
    participant selection for, 251–252
    standardization levels for, 250–251
Repeated measures, intraclass correlation coefficients and, 332–333
Repeated measures analysis of variance, 295–296
    summary of, 296*t*
Repeated measures designs, 77, 113–114
Repeated treatment designs, 113–114
    maturation effects in, 79
Replication
    direct *versus* systematic, 90
    history threat and, 79
Research
    analysis of relationships in, 148–149
    artifacts of, 170–171
    backstory of, 378
    Belmont definition of, 43
        innovative therapies, 43
        intent, 43
        plan, 43
    characteristics of, 2
        challenging status quo, 2
        as creative, 2
        as systematic, 2–3
    codes of ethics for, 47–51
        design justifies study, 48–49
        independent review, 50
        privacy and confidentiality, 49
        publication integrity, 50
        risk and benefit, 49–50
        suffering and injury, avoidance of, 49
    definitions of, 2–3
    evaluation of, 26–30, 347–353
        classification of research and variables in, 349
        comparison of purposes and conclusions in, 349–350
        databases of, 31
        description of design and control elements in, 350–351
        identification of threats to validity in, 351–352
        personal utility in, 353
        placement of study in context of other research in, 352–353
        quality score in, assignment of, 358
        steps in, 348
        validity of, 26–29, 27*t*
        written, 29–30
    existing, in development of new problems, 19, 20*t*
    hypothesis for, development of, 156
    informed consent for, 46–47

Research *(Continued)*
        competence, 46–47
        components of, 46
        disclosure and, 46
        information needed for, 46
        patient comprehension and, 46
        voluntariness, 46
    practice and, boundaries between, 42–43
    presentation of, 402–407
        platform presentations, 402–405
        poster presentations, 406*f*, 407
        selection of, 402
    publication of, 399–402
        authorship and acknowledgment of, 400–401
        multiple, 401
        peer review process for, 400
        types of, 399–400
    publishing and presenting of, 399–407
    quantitative, goal of, 56–57
    risks in, 51–52
        economic, 52
        physical, 51–52
        psychological, 52
        social, 52
    theory and practice, relationships among, 11–12, 12*f*
    trustworthiness of, 347
    types of, matrix of, 144*f*
    utility of, 347
    value free, 58
Research article. *See also* Published research; Review articles
    components of, 402
    elements of, 345–347, 346*t*
    style issues in, 401, 403*t*, 404*t*
Research design, 350
    evidence, levels of, 355*t*
    maximizing power within, 315
Research ethics, 42–54
    explicit attention to, 50
Research evidence. *See* Evidence
Research literature
    evaluation of, 348
        EBP model of, 29
    finding, 33–41
        electronic (Web-based) not site specific, 35
    information in, 34
    organizing search for, 39–40
    reference lists and bibliographies for, 39
    searching for, reasons for, 33–34
    single-journal indexes or databases for, 39
    synthesizing
        approaches to, 363
        characteristics of individual studies in, 368, 369*t*
        comparisons across studies in, 370–372
        constructs across studies in, 370, 371*t*
        included studies for, 369*t*
        pool statistical data across studies in, 372–373
        problems that need further study, 373

Research literature *(Continued)*
  quality of individual studies, 368–370, 370*t*
  reasons for, 363
  steps in, 368
  systematic review of, 366*f*
  types of, 34–35
Research manuscript
  draft of, 403–404
  graphs in, 405, 405*f*
  instrumentation and procedures sections of, 404
  introduction section of, 404
  methods section of, 404
  peer review process for, 400
  photographs in, 405
  presentation of, time allotment for, 404
  slides for, 404–405
  tables for, 405
Research methods, identification and selection of, 20
Research paradigms, 55–67
  alternate names for, 56, 56*b*
  assumptions about, 57*t*
  importance of, 55
  methods of, 58*t*
  qualitative, 60–63
  quantitative, 56–59
  relationships among, 65–66
  single-subject, 63–65
  terminology for, 56
Research participant, subject *versus*, 42
Research problems, evaluation of, 20–21
  feasible, 20–21
  interesting, 21
  novel, 21
  relevant, 21
  studied ethically, 21
Research process, lack of familiarity with, as research barrier, 5
Research project
  data analysis for, 395–397
    data coding in, 396
    data entry in, 396
    statistical analysis and, 396–397
    statistical consultants for, 395
    statistical packages for, 395
  data collection for, 391–395
    procedures for, 392
    protecting participant identity in, 392
    recording forms in, 392–394, 393*f*
    safeguarding, 392
  funding of, 384–389
    budget in, 384–385, 387*t*
    corporation, 387–388
    foundation, 388
    government, 388–389, 389*b*
    institution, 386–387
  implementing, 377–398
  institutional review boards for, 383
  participants for

Research project *(Continued)*
    informed consent of, 383–384, 384*b*, 385*f*
    inpatient recruitment for, 390
    lay public, 391
    obtaining, 389–391
    outpatient recruitment for, 390–391
    protection of, 382–384
    sample of, 390*t*
  pilot study for, 395
    participants and personnel for, 395
  preliminary steps for, 378
  proposal for, 378–382
    elements of, 379–382, 379*b*
    guidelines for, 378–379
  team for, benefits of, 378
Research proposal. *See* Proposal
Research questions, answerable, developing, 18
Research validity, 76–91
  areas of, evaluation of, 29
  evaluation of, 26–29, 27*t*, 355
    construct validity, 27*t*, 29
    external validity, 27*t*, 29
    internal validity, 27*t*, 29
    statistical validity, 27*t*, 29
    written, 29–30
  sources for determining, 29–30, 30*b*
  types of, 76
    construct validity, 76, 85–88
    external validity, 76, 88–90
    internal validity, 76–85
    relationships among, 90
    statistical conclusion validity, 76
Researcher
  complete observer model, 169
  as complete participant, 168
  as observer, 162
  observer-as-participant model, 169
  as participant, 162
  participant-as-observer model, 169
Residual, 326–327
Responsiveness designs, 255–256
Retrospective analysis of differences, 150–151
Retrospective analysis of relationships, 149
Retrospective case report, 153
Retrospective descriptive research, purpose of, 144–147
Retrospective design
  case-control design and, 150
  cohort design and, 150
  meta-analysis and, 150
Retrospective study, 189
"Reversal" design, 126
Review articles. *See also* Published research; Research article
  generic evaluation of, 353–354
    article identification and selection strategies in, 354
    assessment of clarity of review question in, 353–354
    assessment of validity in, 354
    personal utility of review in, 354
    results against strength of evidence in, 354

Risk ratio, 181–184
    calculation of, 183*f*
Rivalry, as threat to internal validity, 85
Rosenthal effect, 87
Rotated factor loadings, 341*t*, 342*t*
Rotation techniques, 341
Running record, for observations, 170

S
Safety, in research, 49
Sample size, 103–104, 103*t*, 104*f*
    power analysis of, 315
    sampling distribution and, 274*f*
    statistical power and, 276
    statistical probability and, 274
    variables needed for, 276
Sample standard deviation
    computation of, 267*t*
    definition of, 266–267
Sample variance
    computation of, 267*t*
    definition of, 266–267
    symbol for, 266
Samples
    independence or dependence of, 284
    population *versus*, 92–93
Samples of convenience, 98–99, 99*f*
Sampling distribution, 269–271
    confidence intervals of, 270–271
    mean, sample variance, and standard deviation for, 269*t*
    sample size and, 274*f*
Sampling error, 93
Sampling frame, 93, 220
Sampling method
    probabilistic, *versus* nonprobabilistic, 92
    for qualitative research, 164–165
    significance of, 92
Scheffé test, 291
Science training, 6
Scientist-practitioner
    development of, 6–7
    in EBP process, 26
    PICO and, 26
    roles of, 6–7
Scoring approach, to systematic review, 368–370
Scree method, 341
Screening, epidemiological research and, 184–188
Search fields, 35
Secondary analysis, 145*t*, 216
SEE. *See* Standard error of estimate (SEE)
Selection
    of participants, 92–105
    as threat to external validity, 88–89
Self-assessment scale, 198–199
    in audiology, 202
Self-report measurements, 241
Semantic differential survey items, 217
Semistructured interviews, 166

Sensitivity, 184–187, 184*f*
    calculation of, 184–187
    likelihood ratio and, 187
Sensory integration model, 17
Setting, as threat to external validity, 89
Short Form-36, of Medical Outcomes Study, 200
Shoulder Pain and Disability Index (SPADI), 255–256
Sickness Impact Profile (SIP), 203*t*
Significant difference, 271–274
    alpha level and, 272–273
    null hypothesis and, 271–272
Simple random sampling, 94–95, 94*t*
    cluster sampling *versus*, 97
    comprehending *versus* implementing of, 95
    preferred method for, 94–95
Simultaneous treatments designs, 129
Single-case experimental design, 63
Single data point, 123
Single-factor experimental designs, 110–114
    types of
        nonequivalent control-group design, 112–113, 112*t*
        posttest-only control-group design, 111–112, 112*t*
        pretest-posttest control-group design, 110–111, 110*t*, 111*t*
        repeated measures/repeated treatment designs, 113–114
        single-group pretest-posttest design, 112, 112*t*
        time series design, 113, 113*t*
Single-group pretest-posttest design, 112, 112*t*
Single-journal indexes or databases, 39
Single-subject data, graphing, 134–138, 135*f*, 135*t*, 136*f*, 136*t*
Single-subject design(s), 120–141
    analysis of, 307–312, 307*f*
        celeration line, 308, 308*f*
        level, trend, slope and variability, 308–311, 309*f*
        two standard deviation band, 311, 312*f*
    characteristics of, 121–122
    considerations for, 139–140
    development of, 120
    experimental nature of, 122
    external validity in, 89–90
    features of, 140
    limitations of, 140
        ethical dilemmas as, 140
        generalizability of results as, 140
        internal validity threat as, 140
        statistical analysis as, 140
    line graphs for, 73, 73*f*
    prospective nature of, 122
    testing threat and, 81
    threats to
        history as, 78
        maturation as, 79–81
    use of, 120
    variations of, 122
        A-B designs as, 123–124
        alternating-treatment designs as, 129–132, 131*t*, 132*f*
        changing-criterion designs as, 133–134, 133*f*

Single-subject design(s) *(Continued)*
  interaction designs as, 132–133
    multiple-baseline designs as, 127–129, 128*f*, 130*f*
    withdrawal designs as, 124–126, 125*f*, 127*f*
Single-subject paradigm, 63–65
  alternate names for, 56, 56*b*
  assumptions about, 57*t*, 63
  methodological issues relating to
    manipulation and control as, 65
    measurement, 64
    subject selection, 64
    theory within, 64
  methods of, 58*t*
Single-subject data, 307*f*
SIP. *See* Sickness Impact Profile (SIP)
Skin cancer screening, case report and, 157
Slides, in research manuscript, 404–405
Slope analysis, of single-subject designs, 308–311, 309*f*
Snowball sampling, 99, 165
Social risks, of research, 52
Social Science Citation Index, 38
SPADI. *See* Shoulder Pain and Disability Index (SPADI)
Spearman's rho, 321
  characteristics of, 321*t*
Specific rate, 180–181, 181*f*, 181*t*
Specific theory, 17
Specificity, 184–187, 184*f*
  calculation of, 185*f*
  likelihood ratio and, 187
SPORTDiscus, 37
Squared *z* scores, 282
SSB. *See* Between-groups sum of squares (SSB)
S-shaped curve, 338, 338*f*
SSW. *See* Within-group sum of squares (SSW)
Standard deviation, 236
  computation of, 267*t*
  definition of, 266–267
  as variability measure, 266–267
Standard error of estimate (SEE), 326–327
  for multiple regression equation, 336
Standard error of mean (SEM), 269–270, 313–314
Standard error of measurement (SEM), 237–239, 252, 269–270
Standard normal distribution, 268
Standardization designs, 252
Standardization levels, in measurement protocol, 250–251
  highly standardized approach, 250–251
  nonstandardized approach, 250
  partially standardized approach, 251
Statistical analysis
  for research project, 396–397
  of single-subject designs, 140
Statistical analysis of differences, 285–297
  advanced, 298–317
  basics of, 281–297
Statistical analysis of relationships
  advanced, 329–343
  basics, 318–328

Statistical conclusion validity, 76
  clinical importance of, lack of, 277–278
  concerns with, 352
  threats to, 277
    error rate problems, 278
    intention-to-treat analysis, failure to use, 278–279
    low power, 277
    violated assumptions, 278
Statistical error, type I and type II, 275, 275*f*
Statistical Package for the Social Sciences, 285
Statistical power
  alpha level and, 276
  sample size and, 276
  within-group variability and, 276
Statistical probabilities, 273
  between-groups difference and, 273
  effect size and, 274
  sample size and, 274
  within-group variability and, 273–274
Statistical reasoning, 259–280
Statistical regression to mean, as threat to internal validity, 81–83, 82*f*
Statistical support, lack of, as research barrier, 5
Statistical test of differences
  basic, 286*t*
  as nonparametric, 283
  as parametric, 283
  steps in, 284–285, 285*t*
Statistical validity, evaluation of, 27*t*, 29
Statistics, definition of, 267
Status quo, research challenging, 2
Stem-and-leaf displays, for ROM scores, 295*t*
Stem-and-leaf plot, 264, 264*t*
Stepwise regression strategy, 335–336
Stratified sampling, 95–97, 96*t*
Stroke-adapted Sickness Impact Profile, 203*t*
Structured interview, 165–166
Style issues, in research article, 401, 403*t*, 404*t*
Subject, participant *versus*, 42
Subject attrition, as threat to internal validity, 83–84
Subject selection, as threat to internal validity, 83
Survey
  definition of, 215
  format for, 216
    closed-format items, 217–218
    open-format items, 216–217
  implementation methods for, 219*t*
  information obtained through, 216
  retrospective data and, 146
Survey research, 145*t*, 215–229
  definition of, 215
  Internet surveys for, 226
  interview surveys for, 226–228
    access to prospective participants for, 227
    implementation details for, 227–228
    motivating prospects to participate in, 227
    schedule for, 227

Survey research *(Continued)*
  mailed surveys for, 220–226
    access to sampling frame in, 220
    advantages and disadvantages of, 220
    follow-up for, 223
    implementation details for, 223–226
    motivating prospects to respond to, 223
    participants for, 220
    questionnaire development in, 220–223
    researcher-developed versus existing instruments
      in, 220
  need for rigor in, 218
  sample size for, 218–220
  sampling for, 218–220
  scope of, 215–216
Survey software products, 226
Survival analysis, of data, 207–208, 208f, 312–313
  elements needed for, 312
Survival curves, 312
  differences between, 313
Symmetrical distribution, 265
Systematic assignment, 101t, 102
"Systematic" replication, 90
Systematic review, 150
  criticism of, 368
  format for, 373
  listing of studies for, 374
  with meta-analysis, 364–365, 366f
  methods section of, 365, 374
  preparation for, 365–368
    identify literature, 367
    rationale and purpose of, 365–367
    studies for inclusion, 367–368
  presenting results of, 372f, 373f, 374
  of randomized control trial, 23–25
  reporting on, 373–374
  reproducibility of, 368
  without meta-analysis, 364
Systematic sampling, 95
  bias in, 96t

T
Tables, in research manuscript, 405
Target population, 92–93
  characteristics defining, 93
t distribution
  compared to z distribution, 282
  example of, 282f
  for statistical tests, 282
Tendon transfers, for quadriplegia, case reports on,
    156–157
Test of Infant Motor Performance (TIMP), 245, 255
Test-retest reliability, 241
Test/testing
  power of, 276
  as threat to internal validity, 81
  treatment and, interaction as threat to construct
    validity, 87–88

Theory
  definitions of, 12–15
    levels of restrictiveness in, 12–13, 12t
    tentativeness of, 14–15
  descriptive, 12–13
  evaluation of, 17–18
  explanatory, 13, 14f
  geocentric, 14
  measurement, 59
  modification of, 11–12
  predictive, 13
  priori, 58
  purpose of, 18
  putting into practice, 18–21
    answerable research questions, 18
    problem, 19
    question identification and selection, 19–20
    research methods, 20
    theoretical framework identification and selection, 19
    topic, 18
  in qualitative paradigm, 62
  in quantitative paradigm, 58
  research and practice, relationships among, 11–12, 12f
  scope of, 15–17
    grand theory, 15–17
    metatheory, 15
    middle-range theory, 17
    practice theory, 17
    specific theory, 17
  in single-subject paradigm, 64
  testability of, 15
Tier 2 intervention, 70
Time
  lack of, as research barrier, 5
  as threat to external validity, 89
Time series design, 113, 113t
Title, of research proposal, 380
Total sum of squares (TSS), 289
  calculation of, 290t
Treatment
  compensatory equalization of, as threat to internal
    validity, 85
  outcome satisfaction of, 202–204
  selection strategy for, 114, 114f
    Latin square technique, 114
    random order with selection in, 114
  testing and, interaction between, as threat to construct
    validity, 87–88
  type, independent variable of, 68
Treatment diffusion, as threat to internal validity, 85
Treatment reversal, 78
Trend analysis, of single-subject designs, 308–311, 309f
Triangulation, 243
TSS. *See* Total sum of squares (TSS)
t test, independent, 286t, 287–288
Tukey HSD test, 291
Tuskegee Syphilis Study, 47, 48b
Two-factor between-groups design, 118

Two-factor between-subjects analysis of variance, 299*t*
Two-factor mixed-design analysis of variance, 302*t*
Two standard deviation band analysis, 311, 312*f*
Two-tailed probability, 287
Two-way analysis of variance, 299
Type I error, 275
Type II error, 275
    power analysis and, 316

U

U statistic, 288
UDSMR. *See* Uniform Data System for Medical
    Rehabilitation (UDSMR)
Uniform Data System for Medical Rehabilitation
    (UDSMR), 206
Univariate analysis of variance, 304
Unstructured interviews, 166
U.S. Department of Health and Human Services (DHHS), 47
Utility, principle of, 44–45

V

Validity. *See also* Construct validity; External validity;
    Internal validity
    of measurement, 244–246
        construct validity, 244–245
        content validity, 245
        criterion validity, 245–246
    research, 76–91
        threats to, 351–352
        types of, 76
            construct validity, 76, 85–88
            external validity, 76, 88–90
            internal validity, 76–85
            relationships among, 90
            statistical conclusion validity, 76
    self-assessment and rating scales and, 199
    of statistical conclusion, 277–279
Validity designs, 253–255
    construct validity, 253–254
    content validity, 254
    criterion validity, 254–255
Variability
    analysis, of single-subject designs, 308–311, 309*f*
    of data set, 265–267
    as descriptive measure, 267
    measures of
        range, 266
        standard deviation, 266–267
        variance, 266
    sources of, 249–250, 250*b*
Variable(s), 68–75
    active, 69–70
    assigned, 69–70
    classification of, 349
    correlation of, 318–326
    functional relationships and, 70–72
    graphs and, 72–74
    independent, 68
        levels of, 68

Variable(s) *(Continued)*
    intervening, effect of removal of,
        305–307, 305*f*
    measuring changes in, 232
    properties of, 232
    relationships among, 148
    for sample size, 276
    types of, 234, 234*t*
        continuous or discrete, 234
Variance, 235–236
    computation of, 236*t*, 267*t*
    symbol for, 266
    as variability measure, 266
Vertical axis, 72
Vignette, 217
Voluntary consent, 47

W

Web-based database, features of, 35
    Boolean operations, 35–36, 39*f*
    languages in, 36
    search fields, 35
    search limits, 36
Web of Science, 38
Western Ontario and McMaster University Osteoarthritis
    Index (WOMAC), 203*t*
Wilcoxon rank sum test, 288, 288*t*, 294*t*, 313
    conduction of, 294
    paired-*t* test and, 294
Wilks' lambda test, 304
Withdrawal designs, 124–126, 125*f*, 127*f*
    changing-criterion design *versus*, 133
    phase change for, 139
    phase length of, 126
Within-group design, 117–118
Within-group sum of squares (SSW), 289
    calculation of, 290*t*
Within-group variability
    statistical power and, 276
    statistical probability and, 273–274, 273*f*
Within-subjects design, 77, 117–118
WOMAC. *See* Western Ontario and McMaster University
    Osteoarthritis Index (WOMAC)
Work plan, for research proposal, 381, 382*t*
World Health Organization (WHO)
    ICF and, 196–198, 197*f*
    ICIDH and, 196, 197*f*
    International Classification of Functioning, Disability,
        and Health
        diagram of, 15*f*
        parts of, 15
World Medical Association, Declaration of Helsinki, 47

Z

z distribution, *t* distribution compared to, 282
z score, 267–268
    computation of, 267*t*
    Mann-Whitney test and, 288